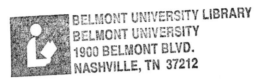

Vascular Nursing

Vascular Nursing

Third Edition

Victora A. Fahey, RN, MSN, CVN

Advanced Practice Nurse/Clinical Nurse Specialist
Vascular Surgery
Northwestern Memorial Hospital
Chicago, Illinois

W.B. SAUNDERS COMPANY
A *Harcourt Health Sciences Company*
St. Louis Philadelphia London Sydney Toronto

W.B. SAUNDERS COMPANY
A *Harcourt Health Sciences Company*

The Curtis Center
Independence Square West
Philadelphia, Pennsylvania 19106

Library of Congress Cataloging-in-Publication Data

Vascular nursing / [edited by] Victora A. Fahey.—3rd ed.

p.   cm.

Includes bibliographical references and index.

ISBN 0–7216–7657–X

1. Blood vessels—Diseases—Nursing.   I. Fahey, Victora A.   [DNLM:
   1. Vascular Diseases—nursing.   WY 152.5 V331 1999]

RC674.V37   1999   616.1′3—dc21

DNLM/DLC   98–37280

VASCULAR NURSING   ISBN 0–7216–7657–X

Printed in the United States of America.

Last digit is the print number: 9   8   7   6   5   4   3

CONTRIBUTORS

Shahab Abdessalam, M.D.

General Surgery Resident, University of Nebraska Medical Center, Omaha, Nebraska
Mesenteric Ischemia

B. Timothy Baxter, M.D.

Professor of Surgery, University of Nebraska Medical Center, Omaha, Nebraska
Mesenteric Ischemia

John J. Bergan, M.D.

Clinical Professor of Surgery, University of California, San Diego, and Uniformed
University of the Health Sciences, Bethesda, Maryland; Attending, Scripps Memorial
Hospital, La Jolla, California
Lymphedema

Donna R. Blackburn, R.N., M.S., R.V.T.

Technical Director, Vascular Laboratory, Northwestern Memorial Hospital,
Chicago, Illinois
Noninvasive Vascular Testing

Lynn M. Borgini, R.N.

Staff Nurse, Vascular/Thoracic Surgery, Northwestern Memorial Hospital,
Chicago, Illinois
Intraoperative Nursing Care of the Vascular Patient

Mimi Bradley, R.N., B.S.N.

Clinical Research Coordinator, Northwestern Memorial Hospital, Chicago, Illinois
Extracranial Cerebrovascular Disease

Alyson J. Breisch, R.N., M.S., A.N.P.

Nurse Practitioner, Division of Cardiology, Department of Medicine, Duke University
Medical Center, Durham, North Carolina
Renovascular Hypertension

Carol Cox, R.N.

Vascular/Thoracic Operating Room Nurse Specialist, Northwestern Memorial Hospital, Chicago, Illinois
Intraoperative Nursing Care of the Vascular Patient

Michael C. Dalsing, M.D.

Professor of Surgery, Indiana University School of Medicine, Indianapolis, Indiana
Chronic Venous Disease

Jennie P. Daugherty, R.N., M.S.N., C.S.

Clinical Nurse Specialist, Edwards-Eve Clinic Association, Nashville, Tennessee
Vascular Trauma

Mitzi A. Ekers, R.N., M.S., A.R.N.P.

Vascular Nurse Practitioner and Consultant, Clearwater, Florida
Vascular Medicine and Vascular Rehabilitation

Victora A. Fahey, R.N., M.S.N., C.V.N.

Advanced Practice Nurse/Clinical Nurse Specialist, Vascular Surgery, Northwestern Memorial Hospital, Chicago, Illinois
Clinical Assessment of the Vascular System; Arterial Reconstruction of the Lower Extremity

Marsha B. Ford, R.N., B.S.N.

Peripheral Vascular Nurse Clinician, Ann Arbor Veterans Affairs Medical Center, affiliated with University of Michigan Medical Center, Ann Arbor, Michigan
Arterial Disease

Linda M. Graham, M.D.

Professor of Surgery, University of Michigan Medical School; Staff Surgeon, Ann Arbor Veterans Affairs Medical Center, affiliated with University of Michigan Medical Center, Ann Arbor, Michigan
Arterial Disease

David Green, M.D., Ph.D.

Professor of Surgery, Northwestern University Medical School; Attending Physician, Northwestern Memorial Hospital, Chicago, Illinois
Thrombotic Disorders in Vascular Patients

Tara L. Hahn, M.D.

General Surgery Resident, Indiana University School of Medicine, Indianapolis, Indiana
Chronic Venous Disease

Jacqueline Helt, R.N., B.S.N., C.V.N.

Clinical Assistant Liaison Nurse, Division of Vascular Surgery, St. Luke's–Roosevelt Hospital Center, New York, New York
Amputation in the Vascular Patient

Alan T. Hirsch, M.D.

Director, Vascular Medicine Program, University of Minnesota Health Center, Minneapolis, Minnesota

Joan Jacobsen, R.N., M.S.N., C.V.N

Clinical Nurse Specialist/Case Manager, Meriter Hospital, Madison, Wisconsin
Vascular Access Surgery; Amputation in the Vascular Patient

Judith M. Jenkins, R.N., M.S.N.

Research Coordinator, Clinical Nurse Specialist, Trauma Patient Care Center, Vanderbilt University Medical Center, Nashville, Tennessee
Vascular Trauma

Linda Kennedy, R.N., R.V.T.

Vascular Nurse Technologist, Northwestern Memorial Hospital, Chicago, Illinois
Noninvasive Vascular Testing

John F. Lee, M.D., F.A.C.S.

Clinical Assistant Professor, Division of Vascular Surgery, University of South Florida; Attending, St. Anthony's Hospital, St. Petersburg, Florida
Upper-Extremity Problems

Jon S. Matsumura, M.D.

Assistant Professor of Surgery, Northwestern University Medical School; Attending Surgeon, Northwestern Memorial Hospital, and Chicago VA Medical Center, Lakeside Division, Chicago, Illinois
Surgery of the Aorta

Walter J. McCarthy, M.D.

Associate Professor of Surgery, Department of Cardiovascular-Thoracic Surgery, Rush Medical School; Chief of Vascular Surgery, Rush-Presbyterian-St. Luke's Medical Center, Chicago, Illinois
Arterial Reconstruction of the Lower Extremity

Cynthia J. McNeave, R.N.

Clinical Practice, St. Anthony's Hospital, St. Petersburg, Florida
Upper-Extremity Problems

Janice D. Nunnelee, Ph.D.(C), R.N., C.V.N., A.N.P.

Assistant Professor, University of Missouri-St. Louis; Adult Nurse Practitioner, Unity Health System, St. Louis, Missouri
Medications Used in Vascular Patients

William H. Pearce, M.D.

Professor of Surgery, Northwestern University Medical School, Attending Surgeon and Chief, Division of Vascular Surgery, Northwestern Memorial Hospital, Chicago, Illinois
Extracranial Cerebrovascular Disease

Karen L. Rice, R.N., M.S.N., C.C.R.N.

Clinical Instructor, Graduate School of Nursing, Louisiana State Medical Center; Adult Nurse Practitioner/Geriatric Clinical Specialist, Alton Ochsner Medical Foundation Hospital, New Orleans, Louisiana
Venous Thrombosis and Pulmonary Embolism

Michael J. Rohrer, M.D.

Associate Professor of Surgery, University of Massachusetts Medical School; Director, Venous Clinic, University of Massachusetts Hospital, Worcester, Massachusetts
The Systemic Venous System: Basic Considerations

Przemyslaw Twardowski, M.D.

Staff Physician, Department of Oncology and Therapeutics Research, City of Hope National Medical Center, Duarte, California
Thrombotic Disorders in Vascular Patients

Robert L. Vogelzang, M.D.

Professor of Radiology, Northwestern University Medical School; Chief of Vascular and Interventional Radiology, Northwestern Memorial Hospital, Chicago, Illinois
Percutaneous Vascular Intervention and Imaging Techniques

M. Eileen Walsh, R.N., M.S.N., C.V.N.

Vascular Clinical Nurse Specialist/Case Manager, Jobst Vascular Center, The Toledo Hospital, Toledo, Ohio
Venous Thrombosis and Pulmonary Embolism

Larry R. Williams, M.D.

Clinical Assistant Professor, Division of Vascular Surgery, University of South Florida; Attending, St. Anthony's Hospital, St. Petersburg, Florida
Upper-Extremity Problems

FOREWORD

At present, vascular surgery has emerged as a distinct specialty in the field of surgery. A wide variety of revascularization procedures, including radiologic interventions and endovascular grafts, are now available to help prevent stroke, extend life, and preserve limbs. Additionally, new diagnostic and imaging techniques are being introduced to provide noninvasive assessment of vascular problems. Because of these immense strides in the diagnosis and treatment of vascular disease as well as the increased responsibility of nurses caring for vascular patients, the nurse must be thoroughly conversant with the multifaceted problems of vascular disease.

Vascular Nursing is now in its third edition. As can be seen from the table of contents, the text provides a comprehensive overview of vascular disease and its most current treatment. The volume is divided into five parts. The first part discusses basic considerations of pathophysiology of arteries, veins, and lymphatics. The second part reviews current perioperative evaluation and management, including newer imaging and interventional techniques. The chapter on intraoperative care emphasizes the essentials of perioperative nursing of the vascular patient. The chapter on thrombotic disorders explains newer findings in coagulation problems in vascular patients. The third through fifth parts are composed of several chapters addressing specific problems related to arterial and venous disease, vascular access surgery, amputation, and vascular trauma. A comprehensive chapter focusing on a medical approach to peripheral arterial disease has been incorporated.

A unique feature of this book is the joint effort of vascular surgeons and nurses as contributing authors. Each author specializing in the vascular field has been selected for his or her clinical expertise. Most important, the chapters provide essential information on which nursing practice is based.

This book is a valuable resource to a variety of audiences, including medical/surgical, intensive care, and operating room nurses; vascular technologists; clinical nurse specialists; and nurse practitioners and educators. Although primarily directed toward nurses, this text will be useful to other members of the health care team caring for vascular patients, including physical and occupational therapists, dietitians, medical students, residents, and primary care physicians.

JAMES S.T. YAO, M.D., Ph.D.
Magerstadt Professor of Surgery
Acting Chair, Department of Surgery
Northwestern University Medical School
Chicago, Illinois

PREFACE

Vascular diseases encompass a wide array of arterial, venous, and lymphatic problems. A significant portion of the population is afflicted with the effects of stroke, myocardial infarction, or peripheral arterial disease, as well as acute or chronic venous disease. Most patients with vascular disease present with complex nursing problems because of advanced age, associated medical conditions such as hypertension or diabetes, and the multiple systems affected by atherosclerosis.

Since the second edition of this book, significant advancements have occurred in the treatment of vascular disease. Progress continues through improved technology in vascular imaging and endovascular intervention. We see a renewed interest in venous disease, a better understanding of hematologic and biochemical factors, and the expanded role of vascular medicine in the treatment of arterial disease. The focus on prevention of vascular disease provides nurses with a new opportunity to have an impact on patient care.

Vascular nursing was established as a specialty with the founding of the Society for Vascular Nursing in 1982. The growth of this organization reflects the recognition by nurses of the unique needs of vascular patients as well as the need for nursing education in this field.

In the current era of cost containment comes increased responsibility for nurses caring for vascular patients. As hospital stays have become abbreviated, nurses are challenged to provide quality care during a shortened inpatient period. Greater emphasis is placed on the outpatient coordination prior to intervention as well as assessment of home care needs after discharge. Clinical pathways have been incorporated in this text to serve as guidelines to patient care as well as to assist in the delivery of cost effective care without compromising clinical outcomes.

Delivery of optimal care requires a thorough understanding of vascular disease as well as current methods of diagnosis and treatment. This third edition maintains the tradition of the first and second editions with one primary objective: to provide a comprehensive review of vascular disease and its nursing management. It is hoped that the contents of this text will encourage excellence in vascular nursing by establishing standards of vascular nursing practice, ultimately resulting in quality patient care.

VICTORA A. FAHEY

ACKNOWLEDGMENTS

This book would not be possible without the contributions of the following people. I would like to express my gratitude and sincere appreciation to the dedicated contributing authors for their time and expertise; John J. Bergan, MD, William Flinn, MD, Jon Matsumura, MD, Walter J. McCarthy, MD, William H. Pearce, MD, and James S.T. Yao, MD, for their contributions to my knowledge of vascular disease and mentorship; my family and friends for their encouragement; my nursing colleagues for their advice and support; Northwestern Memorial Hospital Department of Nursing and the Division of Vascular Surgery, Northwestern University Medical School, for their support; staff at W.B. Saunders, and Lynette Dangerfield and Janeen Fitzpatrick, for their diligent assistance in preparation of the manuscript, and last but not least my patients, for teaching me the most important lessons of life.

CONTENTS

PART THREE
ARTERIAL DISEASES

PART FOUR
VENOUS DISEASES

PART FIVE
SPECIFIC PROBLEMS

PART ONE

BASIC CONSIDERATIONS

1

Arterial Disease

Linda M. Graham, MD, and Marsha B. Ford, RN, BSN

❧ · ❧

Atherosclerosis is the most common disease in the United States, with atherosclerotic coronary disease the number one cause of death. Cerebrovascular disease manifested as strokes afflicts more than 500,000 patients each year.[1] The incidence of atherosclerotic occlusive disease involving the extremities is difficult to estimate because many patients tolerate the effects of disease by modifying their lifestyle, and do not seek medical attention. More than 583,000 peripheral vascular surgical procedures (not including coronary artery bypass procedures or amputations) were performed in 1992, a 31 percent increase over the number performed 11 years earlier.[2] In addition, the number of patients seen with less severe arterial disease that does not require surgery seems to be increasing. This may be a reflection of increasing life expectancy.

To better evaluate and appropriately care for patients with arterial disease, it is important to have a basic understanding of its etiology and pathophysiology. This contributes to accurate assessment, planning, and implementation of comprehensive nursing care and patient education.

ANATOMY/PHYSIOLOGY

Arteries consist of three distinct layers: the intima (formally, the tunica intima), media (tunica media), and adventitia (tunica adventitia) (Figs. 1–1 and 1–2). The innermost layer, the intima, consists of a monolayer of endothelial cells on the luminal surface of the vessel resting on a layer of connective tissue. The internal elastic membrane separates the intima from the media. The media is a relatively thick layer containing smooth muscle cells, collagen, and elastic fibers. The external elastic membrane separates the media from the adventitia. The adventitia is the outer layer of the artery and is composed of connective tissue with collagen and some elastic fibers. It provides a major portion of the total strength of the arterial wall. The intima and the inner portion of the media receive nutrients by diffusion from the arterial lumen, but the outer portion of the media and the adventitia are provided with nutrients by vasa vasorum, small blood vessels that penetrate the outer wall of the artery.

Arteries may be classified by their size, the constituents of the vessel wall, or their function (conductive or distributive). Conductive arteries follow relatively straight courses and have comparatively few branches. For the lower extremity, these include the common and external iliac arteries, the common and superficial femoral arteries, and the popliteal arteries. The anterior and posterior tibial arteries and the peroneal artery have features of both conductive and distributive vessels. The distributive vessels arise from the conductive

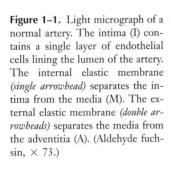

Figure 1–1. Light micrograph of a normal artery. The intima (I) contains a single layer of endothelial cells lining the lumen of the artery. The internal elastic membrane *(single arrowhead)* separates the intima from the media (M). The external elastic membrane *(double arrowheads)* separates the media from the adventitia (A). (Aldehyde fuchsin, × 73.)

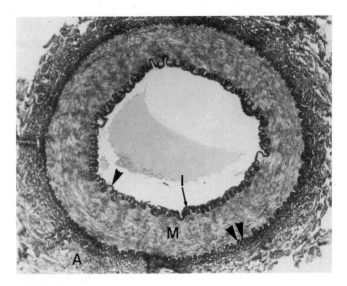

arteries and divide into multiple branches. These include the arteries to the abdominal viscera, the internal iliac arteries, and the profunda femoris arteries. Conductive arteries tend to be most severely affected by atherosclerosis, particularly at branch points. Anatomy of the cerebral vasculature, upper and lower extremities, abdomen, and viscera (Fig. 1–3) is discussed in their respective chapters.

Changes occur in the intima and media with aging; they generally affect larger and medium-sized vessels while sparing small arteries and arterioles. Most pronounced are changes in the intima, with the thickness and collagen content increasing and the elasticity decreasing.[3] Degeneration of the internal elastic membrane, disruption and calcification of elastic tissue, and degeneration of smooth muscle in the media are seen when diffuse intimal thickening inhibits the diffusion of nutrients from the lumen.

The maintenance and regulation of regional blood flow depend on resistance in the muscular arteries and arterioles, which is altered by a number of local factors including intrinsic myogenic tone and metabolic parameters, such as tissue oxygen tension, carbon dioxide tension, and potassium and lactic acid levels.[4]

Physical factors, such as heat and cold, also affect the circulation. Effects of circulating agents, such as epinephrine and angiotensin, are generalized in the cardiovascular system, whereas effects of other substances, such as prostaglandins and endothelial cell–derived relaxing and constricting factors, may be confined to local region(s).

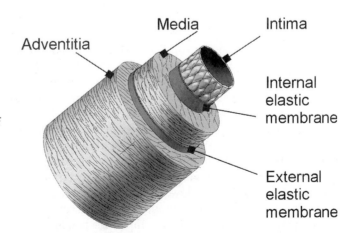

Figure 1–2. Schematic drawing of artery wall layers.

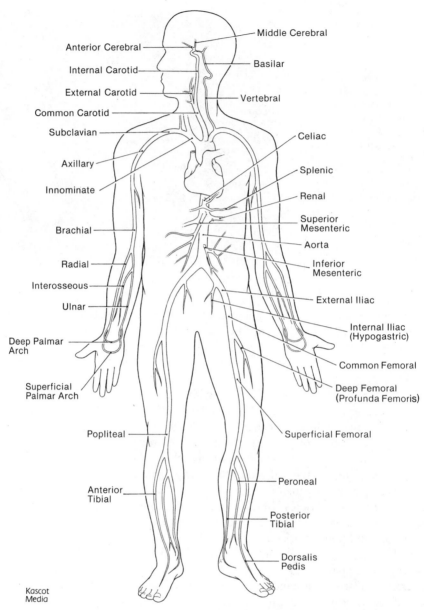

Figure 1–3. Arterial anatomy.

In addition to local control, neural control of limb blood flow is important. Resistance blood vessels in skin and skeletal muscle are innervated through the sympathetic adrenergic system, but skeletal muscle also receives some cholinergic vasodilator fibers. Sympathetic denervation increases limb blood flow, particularly to the skin and through nonnutritive arteriovenous anastomoses.

Resistance in the peripheral vascular bed is variable. The normal resting resistance is relatively high but decreases with exercise by vasodilation at the arteriolar level, allowing increased blood flow to exercising muscles. The amount of increase is limited, however, by intrinsic arterial narrowing in patients with arterial occlusive disease. Changes in blood pressure and flow in the lower limbs with exercise provide the basis for noninvasive diagnostic testing. The magnitude of the pressure drop and the time for recovery to resting pressures after exercise are important parameters.

ETIOLOGY

Causes of arterial disease are extremely varied. Atherosclerosis is the most common arteriopathy in this country. A variety of nonatherosclerotic arterial diseases exist, however. These are less common and often less well defined than is atherosclerotic disease. An introduction to some of these diseases is essential for the evaluation and care of patients with all varieties of arterial disease.

Atherosclerosis

Atherosclerosis is responsible for the majority of arterial disease, both occlusive and aneurysmal. Although the exact cause of atherosclerosis is not defined, several hypotheses have been proposed, including reaction to serum lipids, response to vessel wall injury, and cellular transformation. These hypotheses are not necessarily mutually exclusive. The predominance of lesions at branch points and vessel origins suggests the role of hemodynamic factors in determining the location of atherosclerotic lesions. Alterations in shear stress, both increased and decreased, may play a role in the development of arterial disease.[5-7]

The lipid oxidation theory (Fig. 1–4) of atherosclerosis suggests that high serum levels promote infiltration of lipids into the arterial wall, where these lipids are oxidized. The

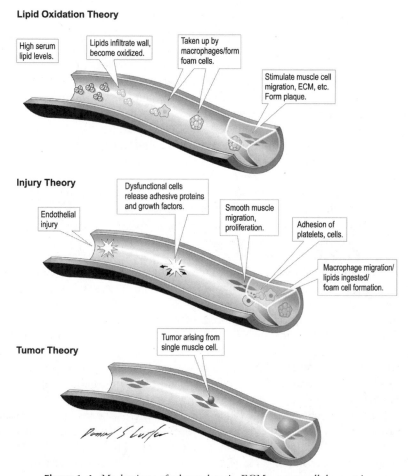

Figure 1–4. Mechanisms of atherosclerosis. ECM = extracellular matrix.

oxidized lipids are taken up by macrophages to form foam cells, and stimulate migration and proliferation of smooth muscle cells and extracellular matrix production, resulting in formation of atherosclerotic plaque. In addition, these lipids alter normal cell function, resulting in impaired vasodilation, increased thrombogenicity, and decreased ability of endothelial cells to migrate into an area of injury. The hypothesis of a causative role of oxidized lipids in atherogenesis is supported by experimental studies showing that atherosclerosis is induced by a high-fat diet and antioxidants have a protective effect.[8]

The injury hypothesis (see Fig. 1–4) suggests that atherosclerosis begins with an endothelial injury that causes cellular dysfunction with release of growth factors and increased expression of adhesive proteins on the endothelial cell surface.[9] The growth factors induce smooth muscle cell migration and proliferation. Platelets, monocytes, and lymphocytes attach to the endothelial cells. Macrophages migrate beneath the endothelium and ingest lipids to become foam cells. Hypercholesterolemia may cause subtle endothelial injury with alteration in permeability, stimulation of monocyte migration, and release of growth factors from platelets or other cells to initiate the process. The continued release of growth factors and cytokines leads to progression of the lesion.

A final hypothesis is that each arterial plaque begins as a benign tumor arising from a single smooth muscle cell (see Fig. 1–4). Experimental evidence has suggested that 80 percent of human fibrous plaques are monoclonal in character.[10]

A number of risk factors have been identified as contributing to the atherosclerotic process, the three major ones being hypercholesterolemia, cigarette smoking, and hypertension.[11] Other factors that contribute to atherosclerosis include diabetes mellitus, obesity, hypertriglyceridemia, hyperuricemia, sedentary living, stress, and a family history of cardiovascular disease. A number of clinical studies have demonstrated the association between elevated serum cholesterol—particularly low-density lipoprotein (LDL) cholesterol—and atherosclerosis.[12] On the other hand, there is an inverse relationship between high-density lipoprotein (HDL) cholesterol levels and clinical manifestations of atherosclerosis because HDL is involved in the transport of cholesterol from extrahepatic tissues to the liver, where it can be removed. The harmful effects of smoking are numerous and include vasoconstriction, increased blood pressure, decreased cardiac index, increased myocardial oxygen demand, endothelial cell injury, alteration of platelet–vessel wall interactions, increased platelet aggregation and blood viscosity, and increased cholesterol.[13] Even chronic exposure to secondhand smoke has these harmful effects and increases the risk of atherosclerosis.[14] Finally, hypertension not only is an independent risk factor for atherosclerosis but also acts synergistically with other risk factors, particularly elevated cholesterol, to enhance the development of atherosclerotic lesions.

Recognition of these risk factors provides the basis for conservative therapy of lower-extremity atherosclerotic occlusive disease. This includes the cessation of cigarette smoking, institution of an exercise program, control of hypertension, proper management of diabetes mellitus, and reduction of hyperlipidemia. Dietary management should be aimed at attaining ideal weight, reducing the amount of total fat intake, shifting to polyunsaturated fats, and restricting cholesterol intake.[15] Recent clinical trials demonstrate that reducing cholesterol levels decreases the risk of recurrent events in patients with heart disease and decreases total mortality by 30 percent in the 5.4-year median follow-up period.[16, 17] The beneficial effects of cholesterol-lowering therapy extend to all groups studied including men, women, diabetics, and patients over the age of 60.[16] Cholesterol lowering appears to help in the restoration of normal endothelial cell function and anticoagulant activity.

The histopathologic changes that occur in atherosclerosis consist of migration and replication of smooth muscle cells, deposition of connective tissue matrix with increased collagen and proteoglycans, lymphocyte and macrophage infiltration, and accumulation of lipids in the cells and surrounding matrix.[9] The fatty streak is considered by some to be the earliest lesion of atherosclerosis. It is commonly found in children and consists of lipid-laden macrophages, lymphocytes, and smooth muscle cells surrounded by lipid deposits. Some fatty streaks may regress, but others appear to progress to become fibrous plaques, the next lesion in the spectrum of atherosclerosis. Fibrous plaques consist of a cap of dense connective tissue and smooth muscle cells and macrophages with intracellular and extracellular lipid. Beneath the cellular layer may be areas of degeneration with necrotic debris, cholesterol crystals, and calcification. Some fibrous plaques progress to become complex lesions with an accumulation of atheromatous debris, intramural hemorrhage, and intimal calcification. Calcification of the vessel wall causes loss of elastic properties, thereby affecting hemodynamics of blood flow. Hemorrhage into a plaque may produce a sudden narrowing, or it may be a precursor of intimal disruption with the formation of an ulcerated lesion. Microemboli of platelet aggregates, thrombus, or atheromatous debris from an area of ulceration may occlude small vessels downstream from the atherosclerotic lesion. Although this commonly produces symptoms in the cerebrovascular circulation, symptomatic atheroemboli are less frequent in the lower-extremity circulation.

The atherosclerotic process may affect primarily the intima and inner media, with development of stenosis or occlusion, or it may cause degeneration of the media, with weakening of the vessel wall and aneurysmal dilation. The exact reason that some patients with atherosclerosis develop occlusive disease while others develop aneurysmal degeneration is not known. In certain conditions such as Marfan's syndrome, defects in the structural integrity of the vessel wall or abnormalities in collagen and elastic content are found. However, most adults who develop aneurysms do not have an obvious inherited disorder. The elastin and collagen content of an atherosclerotic aneurysm is altered by increased activity of elastase and/or collagenase or by decreased activity of their inhibitors. The paucity of vasa vasorum in the abdominal aorta may also promote aneurysm formation because of inadequate nutrition, with resultant weakening of the vessel wall. In addition, certain hemodynamic factors may contribute to aneurysm formation and determine their frequent location at major bifurcations. Finally, an inflammatory cell infiltrate may affect aneurysm formation and progression because of proteolytic enzymes released from leukocytes.

Although atherosclerotic occlusive disease is a diffuse process, certain segments of the arterial tree are more commonly involved, including the coronary arteries, the common carotid artery bifurcation and proximal portion of the internal carotid artery, the aortic bifurcation, and the iliac and common femoral arteries. The lesion of the common femoral artery often extends for a short distance into the profunda femoris artery. The superficial femoral artery is usually diffusely diseased, with the most severe involvement in the region of the adductor hiatus. The distal popliteal artery is commonly diseased, particularly in diabetics.

Atherosclerotic disease of the lower extremity tends to occur in a symmetric fashion and may be divided into aortoiliac disease, femoropopliteal disease, and tibial-peroneal disease. On examining volunteers, Widmer and colleagues[18] found the superficial femoral artery to be the peripheral artery most commonly diseased, being occluded in 50 percent of people with vascular disease. On the basis of angiographic or surgical findings, Haimovici[19] found combined femoral-popliteal-tibial disease in approximately 50 percent of cases. In patients with single-segment involvement, however, the tibial vessels were most commonly affected, being diseased in 29.2 and 23.9 percent of patients with atherosclerotic occlusive disease, with or without diabetes, respectively.[19]

Diabetics have not been found to have a unique form of vascular disease, although diabetes seems to alter the progression and distribution of atherosclerotic disease. Atherosclerosis is more common in diabetics than nondiabetics, and it occurs at a younger age. More than 80 percent of diabetics surviving 20 years after diagnosis have some form of vascular disease.[20] Vascular disease, particularly coronary artery disease and cerebral vascular disease, accounts for approximately 75 percent of deaths of diabetic patients.[20] Diabetics tend to have a lower incidence of aortoiliac occlusive disease of the distal popliteal artery and tibial vessels, and more frequent and diffuse involvement of the profunda femoris artery, than nondiabetics. Medial calcification develops in lower-extremity arteries of diabetics, but this is not necessarily associated with atherosclerotic narrowing of the vessels. The artery becomes incompressible, however, making noninvasive blood pressure measurement inaccurate.

The distal distribution of occlusive disease, diminished sensation due to diabetic neuropathy, and decreased resistance to infection in poorly controlled diabetes account for the high incidence of gangrenous changes of the feet in diabetic patients. The amputation rate is much higher in diabetics than in nondiabetics, with more than 50 percent of patients requiring amputation for gangrene being diabetic.[21, 22] An increased use of arterial reconstructive procedures has resulted in a decrease in amputation rate.[23] However, long-term survival is still compromised; approximately 50 percent of diabetic patients survive 4 years after emergency operation for foot infection or gangrene.[24]

The peripheral neuropathy of diabetics may produce deficits in the sensory, motor, and sympathetic nerve supply of the lower extremity. Poor sensation as a result of the neuropathy leads to an increased likelihood of trauma. Deficits in motor innervation to intrinsic muscles of the foot produce weakness, resulting in deformities of the foot and toes with abnormal weight distribution predisposing to callus formation and ulceration, particularly in the area of the metatarsal heads. In addition, the autonomic neuropathy produces an autosympathectomy, causing arteriovenous shunts to open, increasing nonnutrient blood flow.

Arteritis

Arteritis is an inflammatory process that involves the arterial wall (Fig. 1–5). A variety of arteritides have been identified. Porter and associates have classified immune arteritides into four groups: Buerger's disease, granulomatous or giant-cell arteritides, polyarteritis nodosa group, and hypersensitivity arteritides.[25]

Buerger's Disease

Buerger's disease, also known as thromboangiitis obliterans, appears to be a unique clinical and pathologic disease entity associated with heavy cigarette smoking. It occurs primarily in men less than 40 years of age, but approximately 20 percent of the patients with Buerger's disease are women.[26] Patients present with occlusions of the distal arteries of the upper and lower extremities. Rest pain and ischemic ulceration occur early in the course of the disease, and patients have a higher incidence of subsequent limb loss than do patients with atherosclerosis. The survival rate of patients with thromboangiitis obliterans, however, is distinctly better than that of patients with atherosclerosis.[25, 27]

Histologic studies demonstrate preservation of the general architecture of the vessel wall with a segmental transmural inflammatory process involving small and medium-sized arteries as well as adjacent veins and nerves.[25] The infiltration of lymphocytes and, occasionally, giant cells is accompanied by fibroblast proliferation. This inflammatory process is often followed by thrombosis, with fibrotic obliteration of the vessels and fibrotic encasement of the adjacent nerve. An arteriogram will show segmental occlusion of the smaller arteries. Treatment consists of abstinence from tobacco in any form. The distal vessel involvement in this disease process usually precludes bypass surgery, but regional sympathectomy is sometimes of benefit in healing superficial ulcerations.

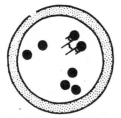

1) Circulating soluble immune complexes in antigen excess

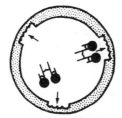

2) Increased vascular permeability via platelet derived vasoactive amines and IgE mediated reactions

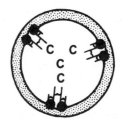

3) Trapping of immune complexes along basement membrane of vessel wall and activation of complement components (C)

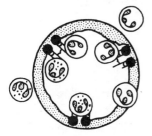

4) Complement derived chemotactic factors (C3 a, C5a, C567) cause accumulation of PMNs

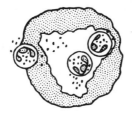

5) PMNs release lysosomal enzymes (collagenase, elastase)

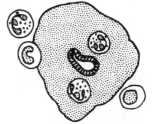

6) Damage and necrosis of vessel wall, thrombosis, occlusion, hemorrhage

Figure 1–5. Mechanism of arterial damage due to immune arteritis. PMN = polymorphonuclear leukocyte. (From Faci AS, Hayes BF, Katz P: The spectrum of vasculitis. Ann Intern Med 1978; 89:660–676.)

Giant-Cell Arteritis

Giant-cell arteritis includes Takayasu's arteritis and temporal arteritis.[25] Takayasu's disease most commonly affects young women between the ages of 10 to 30.[28] The majority of cases occur in Asia, but many cases have also been reported in the United States, Mexico, and Europe. The typical patient has malaise, fever, night sweats, anorexia, and weight loss. The transmural inflammatory process involves the aortic arch and the vessels arising from the arch (type I—8 percent), the abdominal aorta and visceral vessels (type II—11 percent), both the arch and the abdominal aorta (type III—65 percent), or the pulmonary arteries (type IV—15 percent).[29] Cardiovascular symptoms may develop, and hypertension occurs in up to 70 percent of the cases, with resulting heart failure not unusual.[28] Neurologic symptoms frequently accompany involvement of the aortic arch vessels, but cerebrovascular accidents are unusual. Arterial biopsy reveals diffuse sclerosis, with extensive destruction of elastic fibers of the media, and a transmural inflammatory process with lymphocytes and giant cells. Angiography reveals irregularity of the artery, with areas of stenosis, poststenotic dilatation, occlusion of proximal portions of branches of the aorta, and saccular aneurysms of the aorta and its branches in 10–15 percent of the cases.[29, 30] Active arteritis may continue for years after the onset of the disease. Often steroids are effective in decreasing the activity of the disease process, but bypass surgery is frequently necessary to control hypertension and improve cerebral or visceral perfusion.

Temporal arteritis is a second disease in the giant-cell arteritides. The typical patient is over the age of 50, and the ratio of affected females to males ranges from 2:1 to 4:1.[30] Symptoms frequently include a flu-like illness with malaise, fever, polymyalgias, stiffness of the neck and shoulder girdle, and headache with tenderness along the course of the temporal artery. Diagnosis is based on an elevated erythrocyte sedimentation rate and a positive temporal artery biopsy that shows inflammatory changes with thickening of the intima, patchy areas of necrosis in the media, and infiltration of the media and adventitia by monocytes and eosinophils as well as giant cells.[31] In most cases, the inflammatory process subsides in less than 1 year, but in others it lasts several years.[30]

The major complication of this disease is visual changes or permanent visual loss secondary to ischemic optic neuritis or central retinal artery occlusion, which occurs approximately 3 months after onset.[30] Other complications, including stenosis or aneurysms of the aorta or its main branches, occur about 8 months after onset. Prompt steroid therapy may control the inflammatory response, thereby improving blood flow through the affected vessels. Furthermore, surgical therapy often fails unless high-dose steroids are administered concomitantly. Death is rare but may occur after aortic dissection, rupture of the aorta, myocardial infarction, or cerebral infarction.[30]

Polyarteritis Nodosa

The polyarteritis nodosa group of vasculitides includes classic polyarteritis nodosa, Kawasaki disease, Cogan's syndrome, Behçet's disease, and drug abuse arteritis.[25] Polyarteritis nodosa is a systemic disease that causes fibrinoid necrosis of small and medium-sized arteries; it afflicts males twice as frequently as females, with a peak incidence in the fifth decade of life.[25] Renal involvement occurs in more than 80 percent of the cases.[32] Visceral ischemia as well as aneurysmal disease may occur as a result of polyarteritis nodosa. Histologic examination reveals a transmural inflammatory process, with destruction of the media causing aneurysm formation.

Kawasaki disease is an acute, febrile, mucocutaneous condition with an associated arteritis similar to polyarteritis nodosa, except that it occurs in young children.[33] Coronary artery involvement leads to cardiac arrhythmias or infarcts, which are the usual cause of death.

Cogan's syndrome is a rare condition manifested as interstitial keratitis, bilateral deafness, and systemic vasculitis similar to polyarteritis nodosa, with focal degeneration, fibrosis, and inflammatory infiltration of large veins and muscular arteries.[34, 35] Systemic manifestations include congestive heart failure, gastrointestinal hemorrhage, adenopathy, splenomegaly, hypertension, musculoskeletal involvement, and eosinophilia.

Behçet's disease, originally described as relapsing iridocyclitis with ulcers of the mouth and genitalia, is a systemic vasculitis that affects both arteries and veins.[36] Superficial or deep venous thrombosis is common. Although aneurysms of large arteries have been reported, thrombosis of small arteries causing involvement of multiple organ systems is more common.

Drug abusers may develop a necrotizing arteritis similar to polyarteritis nodosa, or they may sustain arterial damage secondary to inadvertent intra-arterial injection of drugs.[37] The necrotizing angiitis can lead to aneurysm formation or to stenosis and occlusion secondary to intimal proliferation and medial fibrosis. Patients present with renal failure, hypersensitivity, pulmonary edema, or pancreatitis.

Hypersensitivity Arteritis

Hypersensitivity angiitis is the name applied to a variety of vasculitides involving small arteries. These include classic hypersensitivity angiitis, arteritis of collagen vascular diseases, mixed cryoglobulinemia arteritis, and arteritis associated with malignancy.[25] These conditions appear to result from arterial damage secondary to the formation of antigen-antibody complexes within small arteries, although the cause is never identified in some patients. The typical patient develops a skin rash, fever, and evidence of organ dysfunction.

Vasospastic Phenomenon

Raynaud's syndrome is the classic vasospastic disorder in which the vast majority of patients affected are women. The term *Raynaud's disease* has been used to imply a benign syndrome without demonstrable cause, whereas *Raynaud's phenomenon* is used when there is an underlying immunologic basis for Raynaud's syndrome. The distinction is not always clear, however. Raynaud's syndrome is characterized by episodic digital vasospasm precipitated by cold or emotional stress.[38] The classic Raynaud's attack consists of profound blanching of the digits accompanied by numbness but little pain, followed by cyanosis after prolonged warming, and finally by reactive hyperemia with intense erythema and burning pain. Patients may have normal vessels but an exaggerated vasoconstrictive response to stimuli; however, approximately 60 percent have a normal vasoconstrictive response with underlying digital artery occlusion.[39] Of these latter patients, more than half have an immunologic or connective tissue disorder, most commonly scleroderma. Approximately 10 percent of patients with occlusive disease eventually develop digital gangrene. Treatment is primarily palliative, with blocking agents (most recently calcium channel blockers) being of some benefit.

Vasospasm may also be drug-induced through excessive use of ergotamine tartrate for the treatment of migraine headaches. Ergot-induced vasospasm usually involves the lower extremities, beginning in the superficial femoral arteries and becoming more severe distally.[40] Isolated upper-extremity vasospasm secondary to ergotism is rare.[41] Angiography demonstrates bilateral symmetric arterial spasm, sometimes accompanied by thrombus formation. Treatment consists of withdrawal of ergotamine preparations, hydration, heparinization, and administration of vasodilators. Oral nifedipine has been used with excellent results, and intravenous nitroprusside is effective.

Fibromuscular Dysplasia

Fibromuscular dysplasia is a heterogeneous group of arterial occlusive diseases characterized by abnormalities in the mesenchymal cells and fibrous connective tissue of the arterial wall. Most patients with fibromuscular dysplasia are women under the age of 40. The renal arteries are affected more commonly than any other artery in the body. Fibromuscular dysplasia is the second most common type of renal artery disease causing renovascular hypertension. Arterial fibrodysplasia less commonly affects the internal carotid arteries, vertebral arteries, and external iliac arteries. Fewer than 1 percent of patients undergoing carotid arteriography have fibromuscular dysplasia of the internal carotid or vertebral artery,[42] but this can cause neurologic symptoms identical to those of atherosclerotic disease.[43] When the disease causes symptoms, surgical treatment with gradual dilation is recommended. Renal and iliac lesions are amenable to treatment by percutaneous transluminal angioplasty or surgery.

Four types of renal fibromuscular dysplasia are recognized: intimal fibroplasia, medial hyperplasia, medial fibroplasia, and perimedial dysplasia.[44] *Intimal fibroplasia*, accounting for 5 percent of fibromuscular disease, is most frequently encountered in infants and young adults. Angiographically, it appears as long, tubular stenoses and is characterized by subendothelial accumulations of mesenchymal cells in fibrous connective tissue. *Medial hyperplasia* is seen in 1 percent of cases and is characterized by an excess of medial smooth muscle cells without fibrosis. *Medial fibroplasia* accounts for 85 percent of dysplastic lesions and appears angiographically as a "string of beads." Disorganization of smooth muscle cells, appearance of myofibroblasts, and accumulations of excessive ground substance in the media characterize these stenotic lesions. Adjacent to such narrowings are often areas of marked medial thinning that can progress to macroaneurysms. *Perimedial dysplasia* makes up 10 percent of dysplastic lesions and appears as a series of stenoses without intervening aneurysms. Excessive accumulation of elastic tissue in the inner adventitia is characteristic of this lesion.

Trauma

Arterial injuries can result from penetrating or blunt trauma. Penetrating trauma includes stab wounds, gunshot wounds, or iatrogenic injuries from vessel catheterization. Blunt trauma may result in direct injury of vessels, but it commonly results in fractures or dislocations of long bones, which secondarily injure vessels. The vessels of the extremities are the most commonly injured because they are long and superficially located. When trauma occurs adjacent to a joint, vascular damage is particularly common because vessels are in a relatively fixed position and thus vulnerable to injury (see Chapter 21).

Compartment Syndrome

Compartment syndromes are due to swelling within the osteofascial compartments of the leg or arm, which causes increased intracompartmental pressure and results in decreased vascular perfusion. This most commonly occurs with revascularization after prolonged ischemia, particularly that subsequent to arterial trauma or emboli. However, compartment syndromes may develop spontaneously or as a result of external compression or bleeding within the compartment. When the pressure of the compartment exceeds capillary perfusion pressure, nutritive blood flow to the tissues is compromised. This usually occurs with intracompartmental pressures over 30–40 mmHg, but it may occur at lower intracompartmental pressures in the face of hypotension. Nerves appear to be most susceptible to ischemia-induced injury, with muscle necrosis occurring later. Clinical findings include paresthesias, pain (especially with passive movement of the muscle), weakness of the involved muscle, and tenseness of the compartment. Loss of pulses is a very late sign. The diagnosis is made on clinical grounds, but it may be confirmed by measuring compartment pressures. Fasciotomy is the appropriate treatment.

Arterial Infection

Arterial infection may result from a variety of processes.[45] Bacterial endocarditis may produce septic emboli that can lodge in normal arteries, resulting in infection followed by weakening of the arterial wall and aneurysm formation. A local abscess may spread to an adjacent arterial wall, causing its destruction and pseudoaneurysm formation. Trauma to the artery with concomitant contamination may also result in an infected pseudoaneurysm. Finally, during an episode of bacteremia, microorganisms may lodge in an atherosclerotic plaque or aneurysm, where they begin to multiply.

The bacteriology of arterial infections varies with the type of process. Cultures of arterial lesions secondary to bacterial endocarditis most often grow pneumococci or *Streptococcus*, *Enterococcus*, *Staphylococcus*, *Escherichia coli*, or *Proteus* organisms.[45, 46] *Staphylococcus* and members of the family Enterobacteriaceae are the bacteria encountered most commonly in peripheral mycotic aneurysms that are not associated with bacterial endocarditis.[45] Infected aortic aneurysms most frequently grow staphylococci or salmonella.[47, 48] *Salmonella* appears to have a predilection for atherosclerotic arterial walls, particularly in the abdominal aorta. Syphilitic aneurysms and tuberculous aneurysms were common before antibiotic therapy but are rarely seen today.

Compression Syndrome

Several arterial compression syndromes in which the artery is compressed by an abnormal muscle or fibrous band have been described. The most common is the thoracic outlet syndrome, in which the brachial plexus, subclavian artery, or subclavian vein is compressed or irritated as it passes between the first rib and the clavicle. Patients who develop this syndrome often have congenital anomalies, such as a cervical rib or an abnormal fibrous band resulting in a narrow thoracic outlet. Callus formation after clavicular fracture may also result in narrowing of the thoracic outlet with resultant compression syndrome. Symptoms most commonly result from irritation of the brachial plexus (90–95 percent of cases), and less often from compression of the artery or vein (less than 5 percent of cases).[49] Physical therapy and other conservative treatments should be tried before operative intervention in patients with neurogenic symptoms only.

A second compression syndrome is popliteal artery entrapment, in which the artery is compressed by the medial head of the gastrocnemius muscle or by fibrous bands. The popliteal artery may have an abnormal location, deviating medially around a normal medial head of the gastrocnemius muscle (50 percent); the attachment of the medial head of the gastrocnemius muscle may be lateral to its normal location (25 percent); or muscle slips of the medial head of the gastrocnemius muscle may compress the artery.[50] Popliteal entrapment syndrome is most commonly encountered in young men, but it has been diagnosed in older patients and is bilateral in approximately one-third of the cases. Repeated trauma to the popliteal artery may result in the development of atherosclerosis, aneurysms, or thrombus and embolization.

Patients with popliteal entrapment present with symptomatic arterial occlusion or intermittent claudication. Active plantar flexion of the foot while the knee is extended, or passive dorsiflexion of the foot, may diminish pulses or alter waveforms. The diagnosis is confirmed on angiography by medial deviation of the popliteal artery or at the time of surgical intervention. In any patient in whom the diagnosis is made, operative therapy should be undertaken to divide the offending muscle band if the artery is patent and free of disease or to bypass the artery if stenosis, occlusion, or aneurysm is present.

Another arterial compression syndrome has been called the adductor canal compression syndrome. The distal superficial femoral artery is compressed by the tendinous insertion of the adductor magnus onto the femur or by an abnormal musculotendinous band arising from the adductor magnus.[51] Treatment involves division of the tendon, with arterial reconstruction if necessary.

Radiation Arteritis

Irradiation of vascular tissue in the treatment of malignant disease causes endothelial damage, with altered permeability, inflammatory changes, and thrombosis of small vessels.[52] Larger vessels develop intimal thickening, proliferation of smooth muscle cells, degenerative changes in the media, and inflammatory infiltration of the adventitia. Segmental or diffuse narrowing, fibrotic occlusion, and atherosclerotic changes are common consequences of radiation therapy and may develop years after irradiation. Surgical therapy is complicated by the dense periarterial fibrous tissue.

Cystic Adventitial Disease

Cystic adventitial disease is an unusual condition in which a cyst filled with mucinous material forms in the adventitia or subadventitial layer of the vessel wall. The condition most commonly affects males and most frequently involves the popliteal artery, but it may occur in other arteries and even in veins.[53] The cause of adventitial cystic disease is not known, but the condition may represent a true ganglion or result from mucin-secreting cells retained within the arterial wall. Treatment by evacuation or enucleation of the cyst is effective.

Congenital Conditions

Congenital anomalies of the arterial system are many and varied and include duplication anomalies, agenesis, hypoplasia, and anomalous courses. An abnormal origin of the right subclavian artery is the most common congenital anomaly of the aortic arch, and such anomalous arteries seem to have an increased incidence of aneurysm formation.[54] Aortic coarctation, a congenital narrowing or stricture of the aorta, most commonly affects a short segment of the thoracic aorta in the region of the isthmus but may involve the abdominal aorta. Patients with aortic coarctation may have hypertension or manifestations of lower-extremity ischemia.

Hypoplasia of the aortoiliac system, characterized by an unusually small caliber of these arteries, is occasionally encountered in patients with lower-extremity ischemic symptoms and seems to have a particular predilection for women.[55] These women are frequently heavy smokers and present at a relatively early age, usually in their early 40s.

Arteriomegaly, an unusual form of arterial disease characterized by excessively large arteries, is identified in 5 percent of arteriograms.[56] The cause and natural history are poorly understood, but arteriomegaly seems to represent a variant of atherosclerosis that appears at an earlier age. Histologic examination of the arterial wall shows fragmentation of the internal elastic membrane and loss of elastic tissue in the media. Arteriography demonstrates large, tortuous arteries, with associated aneurysm formation in 30–66 percent of the patients.[56, 57] The high incidence of thrombotic and embolic complications justifies surgical treatment of these aneurysms, although reconstructive procedures are often complex.

Fetal arteries may persist into adulthood. For example, the sciatic artery, which is present in the embryo but is normally replaced by the femoral artery, may persist into adulthood, traveling through the sciatic foramen and connecting distally to the popliteal artery. The superficial femoral artery may be normal or hypoplastic in such patients, whereas the persistent sciatic artery seems to have a propensity for aneurysmal degeneration.[58]

Congenital arteriovenous fistulae and malformations range from capillary hemangiomas, which usually regress in early childhood, to large arteriovenous connections, causing bony and soft-tissue hypertrophy, distal ischemic changes, and varicosities and ulceration secondary to chronic venous insufficiency. Congenital arteriovenous fistulae are equally distributed between men and women and affect the lower extremity more frequently than the upper extremity.[59] Treatment of simple cutaneous hemangiomas consists of observation because most will regress. Conservative therapy is advocated for large congenital arteriovenous fistulae because of the low incidence of cardiac problems and because of their refractoriness to surgical therapy, which is due to the multitude of arteriovenous connections.

Other congenital arterial disorders include isolated aneurysms caused by a localized defect in the elastic tissue and aneurysms associated with disorders of connective tissue metabolism. Cystic medial necrosis, a condition characterized by hyaline degeneration of the media and manifested by aortic dissection and spontaneous arterial rupture, may result from a variety of metabolic conditions that alter the composition and structure of collagen, elastin, or mucopolysaccharide ground substance, causing a generalized weakening of the arterial wall.[25] Patients with Marfan's syndrome have premature degeneration of vascular elastic tissue, manifested by mitral valvular insufficiency, aortic dissection, and aortic aneurysms. These complications lead to death by the age of 32 in 50 percent of the patients.[60] Another group of disorders affecting vessel wall strength is Ehlers-Danlos syndrome, which is characterized by defects in collagen production. The type IV variety is known as the "arterial" type because defective synthesis of one type of collagen causes decreased strength of major vessels, resulting in the formation of true and false aneurysms and arteriovenous fistulae, spontaneous arterial ruptures, and dissections.[61] Neurofibromatosis has been associated with a variety of vascular disorders, including renal artery stenosis, abdominal aortic coarctation, and aneurysm formation.[25]

Homocystinemia is an inborn error of metabolism with a deficiency of the enzyme cystathionine synthetase, which results in elevated blood levels of homocystine.[62] These patients have rapidly progressive atherosclerosis.

Inherited deficiencies of certain circulating inhibitors of clotting factors may result in repeated episodes of arterial and, particularly, venous thromboses. A deficiency of anti-thrombin III has been related to recurrent episodes of venous thromboembolism and arterial thromboses. A deficiency of protein C, an enzyme that, when activated, functions as an anticoagulant by inactivating factors V and VIII, is also associated with recurrent thromboses.[63] A deficiency in protein S, another antithrombotic plasma protein that serves as a cofactor for protein C, predisposes to recurrent venous thromboses.

Hyperviscosity Syndromes

A variety of conditions can cause increased blood viscosity, which may lead to venous thrombosis or occlusion of digital vessels. These include polycythemia vera with an increased hematocrit value, elevated fibrinogen levels, myeloma, cryoglobulinemia, myeloid metaplasia, macroglobulinemia, and leukemia.[25]

PATHOPHYSIOLOGY

Basic principles of fluid dynamics help to describe the consequences of arterial occlusive or aneurysmal disease, as well as the changes that occur with arteriovenous fistulae. Energy losses from fluid flowing through a stenosis account for the clinical manifestations of occlusive disease. Aneurysmal rupture results when tension on the arterial wall exceeds its strength.

Poiseuille's law describes the relationship between pressure and flow of fluid through cylindrical tubes:

$$\Delta P = \bar{V}\, 8l\eta/\, r^2 = Q\, 8l\eta/\, \pi r^4$$

where ΔP is the pressure drop along the tube, $\bar{V}$ is the mean flow velocity, l is tube length, η is the viscosity coefficient, r is the inside radius of the tube, and Q is the volume flow.[64] Thus, with laminar flow in a cylindrical tube, the pressure drop is inversely proportional to the fourth power of the radius. A small decrease in radius causes a significant change in pressure.

Occlusive Disease

The degree of arterial narrowing required to produce a measurable decrease in blood pressure or flow is called a critical stenosis. The decrease in pressure or energy losses associated with a narrowing are inversely proportional to the fourth power of the radius according to Poiseuille's law. In general, significant changes in pressure occur when the arterial lumen has been reduced by 50 percent of its diameter or 75 percent of its cross-sectional area ($A = \pi r^2$). Blood viscosity, blood flow velocity, and the length of the stenosis are also factors in determining the hemodynamic significance of the stenosis. The pressure drop across a given stenosis increases with rising flow velocity. Thus, a stenosis that is not significant at rest may become critical when flow rates are increased by exercise. It is often difficult to predict the hemodynamic significance of a lesion strictly on the basis of the apparent reduction in diameter seen on an angiogram. Therefore, blood pressure measurement made before and after an increase of flow with exercise, reactive hyperemia, or the injection of a vasodilator allows detection of a significant stenosis.

Although the length of a stenosis will affect energy loss, such losses are due primarily to entrance and exit effects. Therefore, two separate stenoses will have a more significant effect than a single stenosis of the same diameter and a length equal to the sum of the two stenoses. Multiple subcritical stenoses can cause energy losses with a pressure drop similar to that of a single critical stenosis.[65]

Single-level atherosclerotic occlusive disease of the peripheral circulation is usually well tolerated. However, multiple stenoses at several levels increase energy losses, causing symptomatic ischemia, the severity of which depends on the extent of disease. The majority of patients with a superficial femoral occlusion will not have symptoms. If the same lesion is combined with a significant aortoiliac stenosis, however, symptoms will result. Correction of the proximal lesion will generally suffice to relieve symptoms.

As a critical stenosis is formed, collateral circulation develops. Collateral vessels are pre-existing pathways that enlarge when flow through a parallel major artery is reduced (Fig. 1–6). The stimulus for collateral development appears to be the presence of an abnormal pressure gradient across the system and also distal ischemia.[66, 67] Collateral vessels are smaller, longer, and more numerous than the major arteries they replace. The

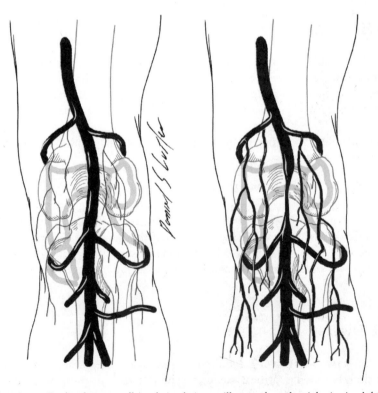

Figure 1–6. Popliteal artery collateral circulation as illustrated on the right (patient's left).

number, size, and functional capacity of collateral vessels are related to the level and severity of occlusive lesions, as well as the duration of obstruction. Resistance through collateral vessels, however, is always greater than through the normal artery, limiting the increase in flow that can occur with exercise. A regular exercise program will stimulate collateral development, gradually increasing the capacity of the collateral bed, and will improve symptoms of intermittent claudication. In addition, muscles may adapt at a subcellular level to use available oxygen more efficiently during exercise.

An acute arterial occlusion, such as that resulting from an embolus, causes ischemia to a peripheral bed without allowing time for collateral development. This results in more severe hemodynamic and metabolic consequences than does occlusion of a vessel with chronic stenosis. In addition, emboli tend to lodge at major bifurcations, eliminating sources of collateral flow.

Aneurysmal Disease

Aneurysms result from the degeneration of structural components and weakening of the arterial wall. Rupture occurs if tension on the arterial wall exceeds the tensile strength of the wall. Laplace's law defines tension (T) as:

$$T = P \times r$$

where P is the pressure exerted by the fluid (dyne/cm^2), and r is the radius (cm). It can be seen from the above formula that as the radius of an aneurysm increases, the tension on the arterial wall becomes greater. Thus, the aneurysm rupture rate rises with increased aneurysmal size and with elevated blood pressure. Therefore, blood pressure control is essential when a patient with a small aneurysm is being monitored.

Arteriovenous Fistulae

Arteriovenous fistulae, whether congenital or traumatic, provide a "short circuit" between the high-pressure arterial system and the low-pressure venous system, which may lead to marked hemodynamic and anatomic changes.[68] The magnitude of the pathophysiologic changes depends on the size and location of the arteriovenous fistula. When a fistula is located near the heart, the hemodynamic alterations and the potential for cardiac failure are increased; peripheral arteriovenous fistulae, located distally in an extremity, are less likely to cause congestive heart failure but are more likely to cause ischemia. Fistulae involving branches of the portal system have few systemic effects, perhaps because of the high outflow resistance offered by hepatic sinusoids.

An arteriovenous fistula may be considered in terms of the fistula itself, a proximal and distal artery and vein, and collateral arteries and veins. The resistance offered by the fistula depends on its diameter and length. Because a fistula markedly reduces resistance, flow in the proximal artery is greatly increased, especially during diastole, compared with flow in the normal artery. Blood flow in the proximal vein is also increased and becomes more pulsatile in nature. Blood pressure in the distal artery is always reduced. Blood flow in the distal artery will be in the normal peripheral direction if resistance of the fistula exceeds that of the distal vascular bed. In large, low-resistance fistulae, however, blood flow in the distal artery will be retrograde toward the fistula. Venous pressure distal to a large, chronic fistula tends to be elevated, and blood flow will be retrograde in the distal vein. A competent valve will prevent retrograde flow, but in chronic fistulae, valves become incompetent in the dilated distal veins.

Systemic effects of an arteriovenous fistula include a decrease in total peripheral resistance, an increase in cardiac output, expanded blood volume, an increase in heart rate and stroke volume, an increase in right and left arterial pressure, and an increase in heart size. Cardiac failure may develop when there is a large, traumatic arteriovenous fistula. Patients with congenital arteriovenous fistulae are less likely to have elevated cardiac output and seldom develop heart failure.

Treatment of an arteriovenous fistula may be accomplished by ligation of all arterial and venous branches that contribute to the fistula. This includes ligation of the proximal and distal artery and vein to exclude the low-resistance fistula completely from the circulation. The preferred treatment of a traumatic arteriovenous fistula entails division of the fistula and repair of the involved vessels.

References

1. Mitsias P, Welch KMA: Medical therapy for transient ischemic attacks and ischemic stroke. In Ernst CB, Stanley JC (eds): Current Therapy in Vascular Surgery, 3rd ed. St. Louis, Mosby, 1995, pp 24–29.
2. Stanley JC, Barnes RW, Ernst CB, et al: Vascular surgery in the United States: Workforce issues. Report of the Society for Vascular Surgery and the International Society for Cardiovascular Surgery, North American Chapter, Committee on Workforce Issues. J Vasc Surg 1996; 23(1):172–181.
3. Johnson WTM, Salanga G, Lee W, et al: Arterial intimal embrittlement: A possible factor in atherogenesis. Atherosclerosis 1986; 59(2):161–171.
4. McGrath MA, Verhaeghe RH, Shepherd JT: The physiology of limb blood flow. In Juergens JL, Spittell JA Jr, Fairbairn JF II (eds): Peripheral Vascular Diseases. Philadelphia, WB Saunders, 1980, pp 83–105.
5. Fry DL: Acute vascular endothelial changes associated with increased blood velocity gradients. Circ Res 1968; 22(2):165–197.
6. LoGerfo FW, Nowak MD, Quist WC: Structural details of boundary layer separation in a model human carotid bifurcation under steady and pulsatile flow conditions. J Vasc Surg 1985; 2(2):263–269.
7. Zarins CK, Giddens DP, Bharadvaj BK, et al: Carotid bifurcation atherosclerosis: Quantitative correlation of plaque localization with flow velocity profiles and wall shear stress. Circ Res 1983; 53(4):502–514.
8. Chisolm GM III, Penn SM: Oxidized lipoproteins and atherosclerosis. In Fuster V, Ross R, Topol EJ (eds): Atherosclerosis and Coronary Artery Disease. Philadelphia, Lippincott-Raven Publishers, 1996, pp 129–149.
9. Ross R: The pathogenesis of atherosclerosis: A perspective for the 1990s. Nature 1993; 362(6423):801–809.
10. Benditt EP: Implications of the monoclonal character of human atherosclerotic plaques. Am J Pathol 1977; 86(3):693–702.
11. Gotto AM Jr: Interactions of the major risk factors for coronary heart disease. Am J Med 1986; 80(2A):48–55.
12. Olin JW, Cressman MD, Hoogerwerf BJ, et al: Diagnosis and treatment of lipid disturbances. In Young JR, Graor RA, Olin JW, et al (eds): Peripheral Vascular Diseases. St. Louis, Mosby-Year Book, 1991, pp 161–177.
13. Krupski WC, Bass A: Smoking and vascular disease. In Ernst CB, Stanley JC (eds): Current Therapy in Vascular Surgery, 2nd ed. Philadelphia, BC Decker, 1991, pp 366–370.
14. Glantz SA, Parmley WW: Passive smoking and heart disease. Mechanisms and risk. JAMA 1995; 273(13):1047–1053.
15. Grundy SM: Cholesterol and coronary heart disease. A new era. JAMA 1986; 256(20):2849–2858.
16. Randomised trial of cholesterol lowering in 4444 patients with coronary heart disease: The Scandinavian Simvastatin Survival Study. Lancet 1994; 344(8934):1383–1389.
17. Sacks FM, Pfeffer MA, Moye LA, et al: The effect of pravastatin on coronary events after myocardial infarction in patients with average cholesterol levels. N Engl J Med 1996; 335(14):1001–1009.
18. Widmer LK, Greensher A, Kannel WB: Occlusion of peripheral arteries: A study of 6,400 working subjects. Circulation 1964; 30:836–842.
19. Haimovici H: Patterns of arteriosclerotic lesions of the lower extremity. Arch Surg 1967; 95(6):918–933.
20. Stemmer EA: Influence of diabetes mellitus on the patterns and complications of vascular occlusive disease. In Moore WS (ed): Vascular Surgery: A Comprehensive Review, 4th ed. Philadelphia, WB Saunders, 1993, pp 490–501.
21. Keagy BA, Schwartz JA, Kotb M, et al: Lower extremity amputation: The control series. J Vasc Surg 1986; 4(4):321–326.
22. Allen BT, Anderson CB, Walker WB, et al: Vascular Surgery. In Levin ME, O'Neal LW, et al (eds): The Diabetic Foot, 5th ed. St. Louis, Mosby-Year Book, 1993, pp 385–422.
23. LoGerfo FW, Gibbons GW, Pomposelli FB Jr, et al.: Trends in the care of the diabetic foot. Expanded role of arterial reconstruction. Arch Surg 1992; 127(5):617–621.
24. Taylor LM Jr, Porter JM: The clinical course of diabetics who require emergent foot surgery because of infection or ischemia. J Vasc Surg 1987; 6(5):454–459.

25. Abou-Zamzam AM, Edwards JM, Porter JM: Nonatherosclerotic vascular disease. In Moore WS (ed): Vascular Surgery: A Comprehensive Review, 5th ed. Philadelphia, WB Saunders, 1998, pp 111–145.

26. Olin JW, Young JR, Graor RA, et al: The changing clinical spectrum of thromboangiitis obliterans (Buerger's disease). Circulation 1990; 82(suppl IV):IV-3–IV-8.

27. McPherson JR, Juergens JL, Gifford RW Jr: Thromboangiitis obliterans and arteriosclerosis obliterans: Clinical and prognostic differences. Ann Intern Med 1963; 59:288–296.

28. Joyce JW, Hollier LH: The giant cell arteritides: Temporal and Takayasu's arteritis. In Bergan JJ, Yao JST (eds): Evaluation and Treatment of Upper and Lower Extremity Circulatory Disorders. New York, Grune & Stratton, 1984, pp 465–481.

29. Lupi-Herrera E, Torres GS, Marcushamer J, et al: Takayasu's arteritis: Clinical study of 107 cases. Am Heart J 1977; 93(1):94–103.

30. Joyce JW: The giant cell arteritides: Diagnosis and the role of surgery. J Vasc Surg 1986; 3(5):827–833.

31. Fortner GS, Thiele BL: Giant cell arteritis involving the carotid artery. Surgery 1984; 95(6):759–762.

32. Vazquez JJ, San Martin P, Barbado FJ, et al: Angiographic findings in systemic necrotizing vasculitis. Angiology 1981; 32(11):773–779.

33. Kawasaki T, Kosaki F, Okawa S, et al: A new infantile acute febrile mucocutaneous lymph node syndrome (MLNS) prevailing in Japan. Pediatrics 1974; 54(3):271–276.

34. Cogan DG: Syndrome of nonsyphilitic interstitial keratitis and vestibuloauditory symptoms. Arch Ophthalmol 1945; 33:144–149.

35. Cheson BD, Bluming AZ, Alory J: Cogan's syndrome: A systemic vasculitis. Am J Med 1976; 60(4):549–555.

36. Little AG, Zarins CK: Abdominal aortic aneurysm and Behçet's disease. Surgery 1982; 91(3):359–362.

37. Citron BP, Halpern M, McCarron M, et al: Necrotizing angiitis associated with drug abuse. N Engl J Med 1970; 283(19): 1003–1011.

38. Porter JM, Edwards JM: Occlusive and vasospastic diseases involving distal upper extremity arteries—Raynaud's syndrome. In Rutherford RB (ed): Vascular Surgery, 4th ed. Philadelphia, WB Saunders, 1995, pp 961–976.

39. Porter JM, Taylor LM: Limb ischemia caused by small artery disease. World J Surg 1983; 7(3):326–333.

40. Dagher FJ, Pais SO, Richards W, et al: Severe unilateral ischemia of the lower extremity caused by ergotamine: Treatment with nifedipine. Surgery 1985; 97(3):369–373.

41. Kemerer VF Jr, Dagher FJ, Pais SO: Successful treatment of ergotism with nifedipine. Am J Roentgenol 1984; 143(2):333–334.

42. Corrin LS, Sadok BA, Houser OW: Cerebral ischemic events in patients with carotid artery fibromuscular dysplasia. Arch Neurol 1981; 38(10):616–618.

43. Stanley JC, Fry WJ, Seeger JF, et al: Extracranial internal carotid and vertebral artery fibrodysplasia. Arch Surg 1974; 109(2):215–22.

44. Stanley JC, Gewertz BL, Bove EL, et al: Arterial fibrodysplasia: Histopathologic character and current etiologic concepts. Arch Surg 1975; 110(5):561–566.

45. Anderson CB, Butcher HR Jr, Ballinger WF: Mycotic aneurysms. Arch Surg 1974; 109(5):712–717.

46. Brown SL, Busuttil RW, Baker D, et al: Bacteriologic and surgical determinants of survival in patients with mycotic aneurysms. J Vasc Surg 1984; 1(4):541–547.

47. Bennett DE, Cherry JK: Bacterial infection of aortic aneurysms: A clinicopathologic study. Am J Surg 1967; 113(3):321–326.

48. Jarrett F, Darling RC, Mundth ED, et al: Experience with infected aneurysms of the abdominal aorta. Arch Surg 1975; 110(11):1281–1286.

49. Stoney RJ, Cheng SWK: Neurogenic thoracic outlet syndrome. In Rutherford RB (ed): Vascular Surgery, 4th ed. Philadelphia, WB Saunders, 1995, pp 976–992.

50. Rich NM, Collins GJ Jr, McDonald PT, et al: Popliteal vascular entrapment. Its increasing interest. Arch Surg 1979; 114(12):1377–1383.

51. Verta MJ Jr, Vitello J, Fuller J: Adductor canal compression syndrome. Arch Surg 1984; 119(3):345–346.

52. Lawson JA: Surgical treatment of radiation induced atherosclerotic disease of the iliac and femoral arteries. J Cardiovasc Surg (Torino) 1985; 26(2):151–156.

53. Flanigan DP, Burnham SJ, Goodreau JJ, et al: Summary of cases of adventitial cystic disease of the popliteal artery. Ann Surg 1979; 189(2):165–175.

54. Schmidt FE, Hewitt RL, Flores AA Jr: Aneurysms of anomalous right subclavian artery. South Med J 1980; 73(2):255–256.

55. DeLaurentis DA, Friedmann P, Wolferth CC Jr, et al: Atherosclerosis and the hypoplastic aortoiliac system. Surgery 1978; 83(1):27–37.

56. Hollier LH, Stanson AW, Gloviczi P, et al: Arteriomegaly: Classification and morbid implications of diffuse aneurysmal disease. Surgery 1983; 93(5):700–708.

57. Thomas ML: Arteriomegaly. Br J Surg 1971; 58(9):690–694.

58. Williams LR, Flanigan DP, O'Connor RJA, et al: Persistent sciatic artery: Clinical aspects and operative management. Am J Surg 1983; 145(5):687–693.

59. Lindenauer SM: Vascular malformation and arteriovenous fistula. In Greenfield LJ, Mulholland MW,

Oldham KT, et al (eds): Surgery: Scientific Principles and Practice, 2nd ed. Philadelphia, Lippincott-Raven Publishers, 1997, pp 1916–1933.

60. Crawford ES: Marfan's syndrome: Broad spectral surgical treatment cardiovascular manifestations. Ann Surg 1983; 198(4):487–505.

61. Sheiner NM, Miller N, Lachance C: Arterial complications of Ehlers-Danlos syndrome. J Cardiovasc Surg (Torino) 1985; 26(3):291–296.

62. Boers GHJ, Smals AGH, Trijbels FJM, et al: Heterozygosity for homocystinuria in premature peripheral and cerebral occlusive arterial disease. N Engl J Med 1985; 313(12):709–715.

63. Kakkar VV: Pathophysiologic characteristics of venous thrombosis. Am J Surg 1985; 150(4A):1–6.

64. Sumner DS: Essential hemodynamic principles. In Rutherford RB (ed): Vascular Surgery, 4th ed. Philadelphia, WB Saunders, 1995, pp 18–44.

65. Flanigan DP, Tullis JP, Stretter VL, et al: Multiple subcritical arterial stenosis: Effect on poststenotic pressure and flow. Ann Surg 1977; 186(5):663–668.

66. John HT, Warren R: The stimulus to collateral circulation. Surgery 1961; 49:14–25.

67. Rosenthal SL, Guyton AC: Hemodynamics of collateral vasodilatation following femoral artery occlusion in anesthetized dogs. Circ Res 1968; 23(2):239–248.

68. Sumner DS: Hemodynamics and pathophysiology of arteriovenous fistulae. In Rutherford RB (ed): Vascular Surgery, 4th ed. Philadelphia, WB Saunders, 1995, pp 1166–1191.

2

The Systemic Venous System: Basic Considerations

Michael J. Rohrer, MD

❧ · ❧

The primary function of the systemic veins is to provide for the return of blood to the right side of the heart. These veins, however, do not function merely as passive conduits for the flow of blood. Instead, venous hemodynamics are complicated by the presence of only low pressure within the system (as compared with the arteries), vein collapsibility, flow variation with respiration, the effect of gravity, and even retrograde pulse transmission from right heart contraction.[1] These considerations become even more complex when normal physiology is altered by venous obstruction or venous valvular incompetence.

Venous disease of the lower extremities is both a highly prevalent and highly morbid condition. Varicose veins affect about 15 percent of the adult population.[2] The chronic swelling, induration, and ulceration of the postphlebitic syndrome are frequently disabling. Pulmonary embolism resulting from deep venous thrombosis is a highly lethal condition and is the most common fatal pulmonary disease in the United States.[3] Venous disease in the upper extremities is not so prevalent, but is becoming more common as invasive procedures such as subclavian catheterization for intravenous access, hemodialysis, hyperalimentation, and invasive hemodynamic monitoring become more frequent and can lead to upper-extremity venous thrombosis.[4-7]

VENOUS ANATOMY

Microscopic Anatomy

The vein wall, like the arterial wall, is composed of three discrete layers, the intima, media, and adventitia, which are identifiable microscopically. The innermost layer, the *intima*, is composed of a confluent layer of endothelial cells that is in contact with the blood flowing within the lumen of the vein. These endothelial cells are metabolically active and produce important inhibitors of intravascular coagulation such as prostacyclin, plasmin, and endothelium-derived relaxing factor (i.e., nitric oxide).[8] In the larger veins of the body, a subendothelial layer of supportive tissue can be identified within the intimal layer.

The primary histologic difference between arteries and veins is found in the composition of the *media*, which, in general, is much thicker in arteries and accounts for the artery's firm and minimally distensible character. The media of the superficial veins of the extremities has walls composed primarily of smooth muscle that gives support and provides some resistance to dilation. The muscular component of the medial layer is able to hypertrophy in response to increased intraluminal pressure, a change frequently seen in the veins of the forearm after creation of an arteriovenous fistula for hemodialysis access as well as in the saphenous vein that is used as an arterial bypass conduit.[9] The deep veins, which are located within the muscular compartment of the extremity, are almost completely devoid of this smooth muscle.[10]

The outermost layer, the *adventitia*, is a thin layer of loose connective tissue surrounding the vein.

Macroscopic Anatomy

Unlike the arteries, the veins of the extremity possess valves along their length that ordinarily allow only unidirectional flow back to the heart. Each valve consists of two extremely thin-walled cusps that originate at opposite sides of the vein wall and oppose in the midline. Blood is able to flow in a proximal direction through the valve between the valve cusps. Reverse flow is prevented by the apposition of the two cusps when pressure above the valve is greater than below (Fig. 2–1).

The vein wall is slightly dilated behind each of the venous valve leaflets. Without this dilated area, the open valves would be closely approximated to the venous wall, which would inhibit prompt closure. Because flow is slower or stagnant in these small recesses, however, small thrombi tend to form in these locations and may become an initial site of thrombus formation, initiating deep venous thrombosis.[11]

The location of the venous valves within the venous system is variable. Several generalizations can be made, however. The valves are more numerous and more closely located

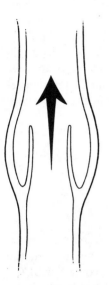
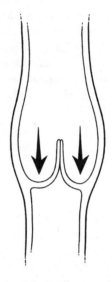

Figure 2–1. Schematic diagram of a normal venous valve in the open *(left)* and closed *(right)* positions. Reflux of blood is prevented when the valve is closed.

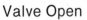

Valve Open   Competent Valve
                         Closed

in the smaller, more distal veins. Only a few valves are found in the femoral veins. The vena cava and common iliac veins are valveless.[12]

Gross Anatomy (Fig. 2–2)

The venous circulation of both upper and lower extremities is composed of a series of veins that course adjacent to the arterial circulation. There is a second, superficial venous system that runs in the subcutaneous tissue of the extremity. A series of veins known as communicating or perforating veins function to channel flow from the superficial to the deep veins.

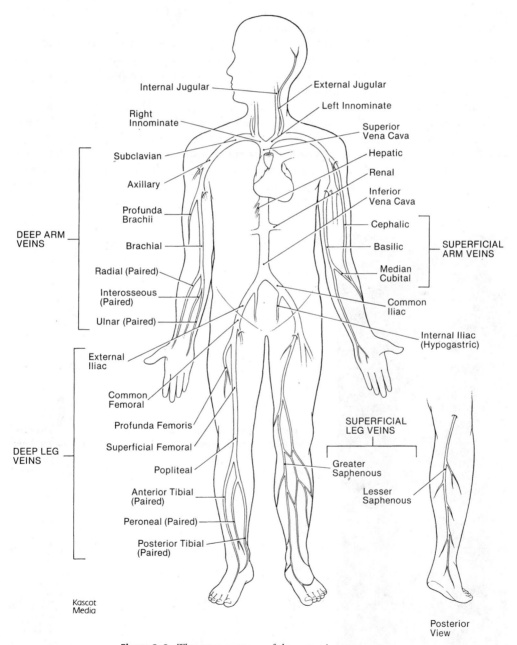

Figure 2–2. The gross anatomy of the systemic venous sytem.

The Lower Extremity.   The thin-walled deep veins of the lower extremities begin as sinusoids within the muscles of the calf. These veins coalesce into two anterior tibial veins, two posterior tibial veins, and two peroneal veins that accompany the arteries of the same name (Fig. 2–3). These veins become confluent at the popliteal vein, which is also occasionally paired.[13] The popliteal vein is renamed as the superficial femoral vein as it ascends through the hiatus of the adductor magnus muscle in the lower thigh. The profunda femoris vein, which drains the thigh, and the superficial femoral vein merge to create the common femoral vein at the groin (Fig. 2–4). The common femoral vein is renamed the external iliac vein as it crosses the inguinal ligament. The internal iliac vein (also called the hypogastric vein) provides venous drainage for the pelvis. It combines with the external iliac vein to become the common iliac vein, which joins the contralateral common iliac vein to form the inferior vena cava (Fig. 2–5). Numerous lumbar veins, a pair of renal veins, and several hepatic veins empty into the inferior vena cava within the abdomen before it ascends to the right atrium.

The left common iliac vein crosses beneath the right common iliac artery to reach the vena cava, where it may be compressed by the overlying artery. It is thought that this left iliac vein compression accounts for the greater than two-to-one preponderance of cases of left-sided deep venous thrombosis.[13, 14]

Congenital variations in venous anatomy are more common than in the arterial tree. Approximately 1 percent of the population have a simultaneous left- and right-sided vena cava, and a similar number have an isolated left-sided vena cava.[14, 15] This abnormal left-sided vena cava crosses over to its normal right-sided position at the level of the left renal vein, and then ascends to the right atrium in the normal retrohepatic position. Another anomaly of surgical significance includes the finding of a retroaortic position for the left

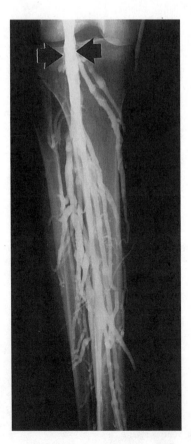

Figure 2–3. Normal ascending right leg venogram. The paired tibial veins empty into a single popliteal vein at the level of the knee *(arrows).*

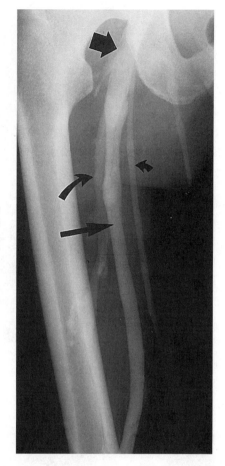

Figure 2–4. Normal venogram illustrating the veins of the right thigh. The profunda femoris vein *(long curved arrow)* and the superficial femoral vein *(long straight arrow)* converge to create the common femoral vein *(short thick arrow)*. The greater saphenous vein is imaged medially *(small curved arrow)*.

renal vein, which is usually found anterior to the aorta. This anomalous vein may be injured during abdominal aortic surgery.

The principal superficial veins of the lower extremity are the greater and lesser saphenous veins. The greater saphenous vein has a consistent origin just anterior to the medial malleolus at the ankle. From that point, it ascends in the subcutaneous tissue along the medial aspect of the leg and thigh and has numerous small tributaries. The greater saphenous vein joins the deep venous system at the common femoral vein through a defect in the fascia of the leg known as the foramen ovale. This point is consistently located just below the inguinal ligament and just lateral to the pubic tubercle.

The greater saphenous vein has considerable surgical significance. Its exceptional length combined with its strong muscular wall and easily accessible location make it an ideal conduit for coronary artery and lower-extremity arterial bypass procedures. Furthermore, its surgical removal is associated with minimal morbidity since the deep venous system remains intact to provide adequate venous drainage.

The lesser saphenous vein originates at the posterior border of the lateral malleolus and ascends along the posterior aspect of the leg. The lesser saphenous vein usually joins the deep venous system at the popliteal vein behind the knee.

There are between four and six major communicating or perforating veins that traverse the deep fascia of the leg and form a communication between the superficial and the deep venous circulation. Each of these communicating veins has venous valves that normally allow flow only from the superficial veins into the deep veins and prevent reflux of blood in the opposite direction. The major communicating veins are located at the area just superior to the medial malleolus, the medial calf, and the distal medial thigh.

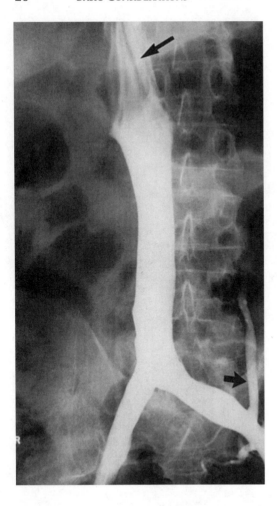

Figure 2–5. Normal venacavogram demonstrating the confluence of the two common iliac arteries into the vena cava. A prominent left gonadal vein is imaged *(short arrow)*. Nonopacified blood entering the vena cava from the two renal veins creates the streaming effect imaged in the suprarenal vena cava *(long arrow)*.

The Upper Extremity.   The veins of the upper extremities have an anatomic organization analogous to that in the lower extremity. The paired deep veins of the forearm are the radial, the ulnar, and the interosseous veins, which coalesce to form the paired brachial veins. These brachial veins join to become the axillary vein in the upper arm. At the lateral border of the first rib at the thoracic outlet the axillary vein is renamed the subclavian vein. The subclavian vein and the internal jugular vein on either side combine within the thorax to form an innominate vein. The two innominate veins combine to form the superior vena cava. The left innominate vein, which crosses the midline to get to the right-sided vena cava, is longer than the right innominate vein (Fig. 2–6).

The primary superficial veins of the upper extremity are the cephalic and the basilic veins. The cephalic vein courses along the lateral aspect of the forearm through the deltopectoral groove to join the deep venous circulation at the subclavian vein. The basilic vein runs along the medial border of the arm and joins the axillary vein in the mid upper arm. A median cubital vein is a consistent large branch between the brachial and cephalic veins that runs across the antecubital fossa, and is a common site of venipuncture.

Communicating veins are also present in the upper extremity to direct blood toward the deep circulation.

VENOUS PHYSIOLOGY

In many respects, venous physiology is much more complex than arterial physiology. Instead of high-pressure laminar flow in rather rigid conduits, as in the arterial tree, the

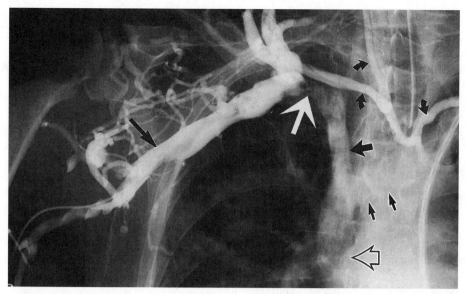

Figure 2–6. Right upper extremity venogram. The axillary vein *(long thin arrow)*, subclavian vein *(white arrow)*, and right innominate vein *(heaviest arrow)* are imaged. The obstruction in the right subclavian vein (imaged at the tip of the white arrow) has resulted in the filling of collateral veins *(small curved arrows)*, which cross the midline to fill the left innominate vein *(two small arrows)*. The superior vena cava is formed by the confluence of the two innominate veins *(open arrow)*.

physiology of the venous circulation deals with intermittent flow in collapsible tubes in a low-pressure system against the effects of gravity.

Compliance

Because veins are collapsible tubes, their shape, and therefore their volume, is determined by the transmural pressure, which is the difference in pressure between the intraluminal forces acting to expand the vein and the external pressures acting to compress the vein. The distensible nature of the vein wall means that it is able to increase its intraluminal volume a great deal with only minimal elevation in the venous pressure. For example, when venous transmural pressure is increased from 1 to 15 torr, the volume of the vein may increase by more than 250 percent.[16] This ability to accommodate large shifts in volume with only limited changes in venous pressure is known as compliance. The high degree of compliance demonstrated by the systemic venous circulation is a property that allows veins to serve as a reservoir for intravascular volume and allows the venous system to accept transfusions and intravenous fluids or blood loss and dehydration over a wide range of intravascular volume with only minimal change in the central venous filling pressure. Because of this high compliance, the venous system usually contains approximately 75 percent of the body's total intravascular volume at a pressure that is far below that of the arterial circulation.[16]

Normal Venous Hemodynamics

Venous hemodynamics differ significantly from the hemodynamics of the arterial circulation, where dynamic pressure—the pressure supplied by the contraction of the left ventricle—is the dominant force that typically provides a mean arterial pressure between 90 and 100 torr. On the venous side of the circulation the dynamic forces have been greatly dissipated by the passage of the blood through the high-resistance arteriolar-capillary bed, and the pressure typically averages only 5–10 torr at the level of the right atrium. Consequently, with the standing position, the hydrostatic pressure, that pressure created by the weight of the column of blood, greatly exceeds the dynamic pressure and acts to impede venous return.

With the recumbent position, the hydrostatic pressure exerted by gravity is eliminated. Venous flow becomes primarily phasic in nature and is in large part driven by the changes in abdominal and thoracic pressure induced by respiratory effort.[17] During inspiration, the intrathoracic pressure is decreased by the expansion of the chest and the lowering of the diaphragm. Simultaneously, the abdominal pressure is increased by the flattening of the abdominal wall muscles and the diaphragm, which both work to compress the abdominal viscera. The result of these pressure changes is an increased venous return to the heart from the veins within the chest, upper abdomen, and upper extremities. The increased intra-abdominal pressure during inspiration transiently slows or halts transit of blood from the lower extremities through the abdominal cavity. Lower-extremity flow is augmented during exhalation, when abdominal muscles relax and intra-abdominal pressure is lowered again.[11] These phasic changes are easily detected with a Doppler ultrasound device at the level of the femoral vein.

Venous hemodynamics become more complex in the upright position when the additional hydrostatic forces imposed by gravity must be overcome in order to return blood to the right heart. This driving force is provided by the musculovenous pump mechanism with energy provided from the contracting muscles of the legs. Pressures in excess of 200 torr can be generated when the calf muscles contract,[18] which is more than sufficient to provide energy for venous return. When the leg muscles contract around the intramuscular and deep veins of the leg, the blood is squeezed from the veins toward the heart. The venous valves play an essential role in the proper function of the musculovenous pump. The valves prevent the retrograde flow that would occur in a valveless system and direct the blood flow centrally back toward the heart in both the superficial and deep venous systems. Valves in the perforating veins allow blood to flow from the superficial veins into the deep veins, but escape of blood in the reverse direction does not occur when the venous valves are competent.

The presence of a functioning musculovenous pump results in a characteristic response of venous pressure to exercise. The compression of the veins and then prevention of retrograde flow by competent valves creates an effective mechanism of emptying the venous circulation, and causes a decrease in lower-extremity venous pressure (Fig. 2–7). Venous pressure, typically 80–90 torr at rest in the standing position, is rapidly decreased by walking to under 20 torr in as few as five steps.[11] After cessation of exercise, the venous pressure rises slowly to pre-exercise levels as the emptied veins refill through inflow from the arterial circulation.

Neural and Hormonal Influences

Although there is little, if any, parasympathetic innervation to the veins, the superficial venous system is richly supplied with sympathetic nerves that constrict with neurogenic stimulus.[19] This allows the superficial venous circulation to play an important role in the maintenance of temperature homeostasis. In cold surroundings, the thermoregulatory center at the hypothalamus directs sympathetic stimulation to the cutaneous veins, which constrict to redirect venous flow through the deep veins in order to reduce heat loss to the environment.

The deep veins have little or no sympathetic innervation, but, like the splanchnic venous bed and the cutaneous veins, they can be constricted by circulating catechol-amines.[19] Veins also constrict in response to epinephrine, norepinephrine, phenylephrine,

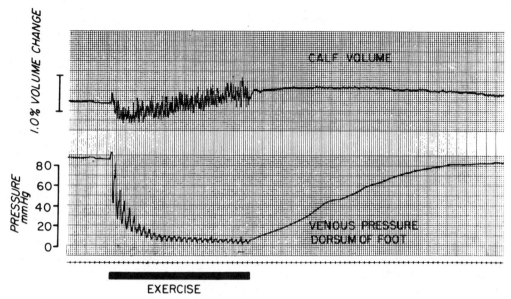

Figure 2–7. The musculovenous pump mechanism is responsible for the normal decrease in venous pressure associated with exercise. (From Strandness DE Jr, Sumner DS: Hemodynamics for Surgeons. New York, Grune & Stratton, 1975.)

serotonin, and histamine.[16, 19] Venous dilation is seen in response to barbiturates, reserpine, guanethidine, phenoxybenzamine, and phentolamine.[16] Most anesthetic agents also cause a venous dilation[16] that may lead to intraoperative hypotension, especially in the volume-depleted patient.

PATHOPHYSIOLOGY

The range of venous pathologic problems extends from the common and usually harmless condition of primary varicose veins to the deadly problem of pulmonary embolism, and from acute deep venous thrombosis to the chronic disabling postphlebitic syndrome. In spite of this broad spectrum of disease states, the scope of venous pathology is derived from only two basic pathophysiologic processes: obstruction of flow and venous valvular insufficiency.[9, 20]

Venous Obstruction

The acute obstruction of venous flow is most frequently caused by deep venous thrombosis (DVT), which involves the formation and propagation of thrombus within the lumen of the deep veins. Although typically manifested by leg swelling, dilated superficial veins, and calf and thigh tenderness, this is often an asymptomatic state.[21–23] DVT may be complicated by pulmonary embolization, in which case a part of the thrombus is dislodged from the deep venous circulation and travels through the chambers of the right heart to the pulmonary artery. There it obstructs blood flow to a segment of the lung, a potentially fatal occurrence.

The physiologic consequence of venous obstruction in the leg is an increased resistance to venous blood flow resulting in increased venous pressure. Normal venous pressures at the foot have been measured at 8 to 18 torr. Venous pressures in the setting of an acute iliofemoral thrombosis have been measured at an average of 50 torr.[24] The usual fall in venous pressure seen with exercise due to the function of the musculovenous pump is also absent in the setting of an acute DVT.[25] Due to the high intravenous pressures, collateral veins may become engorged, and are often observed clinically. Swelling also results from edema formation as fluid leaks from the high-pressure capillaries into the interstitial spaces.

Rarely, thrombosis of the venous circulation is so extensive that a near-total occlusion of venous outflow occurs. This produces rapidly rising venous pressure within the affected extremity, which eventually obstructs arterial inflow and can lead to gangrene. This entity, known as phlegmasia cerulea dolens, is both a limb- and life-threatening condition.[13]

DVT also occurs in the upper extremities, although with a lower frequency than in the lower extremities. Upper-extremity DVT is usually associated with an identifiable predisposing condition, such as a cervical rib or muscular band that causes venous compression, or following deep venous instrumentation.[4-6] The increasing use of central venous catheters for prolonged venous access, hyperalimentation, dialysis access, and hemodynamic monitoring has led to an increase in catheter-related central venous thrombosis.[4] Although upper-extremity DVT is only occasionally associated with pulmonary embolization,[26] it does lead to a high incidence of late sequelae of arm swelling and discomfort with exercise.[6]

Venous Valvular Insufficiency

The natural history of DVT of the lower extremities is gradual resolution of the venous occlusive process with recanalization of the venous lumen occurring in the vast majority of cases.[16, 27] There is, however, permanent damage done to the vein in the thrombotic process. Residual webs and bands may remain within the vein lumen and provide a partial venous obstruction. More important is the permanent damage that the thrombotic process has on the delicate venous valve, whose flow-directing function is usually irreversibly destroyed by the inflammatory reaction of the thrombotic process[13, 16] (Fig. 2–8). This venous valvular incompetence is permanent and progressive over the course of many years, with ongoing valvular fibrosis and increase in the degree of incompetence.[16]

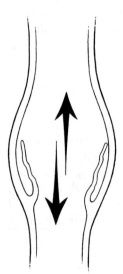

Figure 2–8. Following an episode of deep venous thrombosis, the venous valve is irreversibly damaged by a process of ongoing fibrosis. The result is an incompetent venous valve that is unable to prevent retrograde flow of blood.

Incompetent
Valve

The destruction of the deep venous valves allows the transmission of the hydrostatic pressure of the uninterrupted column of blood from the right atrium to the veins of the lower legs. This pressure is further transmitted to the communicating veins, which are also rendered incompetent, either by the original thrombotic process or by the increased venous distention and pressure. This high venous pressure is then further transmitted to the superficial venous circulation and surrounding skin and tissue. The result is development of varicose superficial veins. These are referred to as secondary varicose veins because the underlying pathology is unrelated to a primary defect in the saphenous vein.

The increased venous pressure in the tissue leads to skin changes characteristic of venous hypertension, with the brown discoloration and woody edema that are characteristic of the postphlebitic syndrome. Ulceration, typically along the medial malleolus overlying the area of the major perforating veins, is also common.

Venous pressure measurements in the postphlebitic state fail to show the characteristic decrease in pressure associated with the normally functioning musculovenous pump. Clinically, patients sometimes complain of a characteristic pain in the leg, described as an exploding or bursting pain, referred to as *venous claudication*. This sensation is attributed to the increased venous pressure and volume that are present during exercise with obstructed venous outflow and venous valvular incompetence.[28]

Isolated superficial venous valvular dysfunction is a common clinical occurrence and is the essential physiologic defect leading to the development of primary varicose veins. One author reports that 62 percent of normal, healthy people demonstrate some varicosities, although pronounced varicosities were found in only 4 percent of the subjects examined.[29] These varicosities are usually found in the greater saphenous system along the medial thigh, but approximately 12 percent of the time involve the lesser saphenous vein.[30]

Although the precise cause of primary varicose veins is unclear, the origin of this problem appears to be multifactorial. Absence of the valves in the common femoral vein and external iliac vein is an anatomic variant that seems to predispose one to the development of varicose veins.[12] This anatomic arrangement allows transmission of the hydrostatic pressure from the column of blood of the inferior vena cava and iliac veins to the most proximal saphenous valve. Subjected to this pressure for a prolonged period of time, this vein may dilate to preclude coaptation of the venous valve leaflets, which would allow reflux of blood distally in the saphenous vein.[2] Other authors have implicated an abnormally distensible vein wall that predisposes to saphenous dilation and loss of the normal valvular function.[16] Humoral factors present during pregnancy may increase venous wall compliance and create reflux and result in the venous varicosities associated with pregnancy.[13] Congenitally defective venous valves and an absence of the most superior greater saphenous valve are rare causes of varicose veins.[2, 13]

References

1. Strandness DE: Applied venous physiology in normal subjects and venous insufficiency. In Bergan JJ, Yao JST (eds): Venous Problems. Chicago, Year Book, 1976, pp 25–45.
2. Crane C: The surgery of varicose veins. Surg Clin North Am 1979; 59:737–748.
3. Wolfe WG, Sabiston DC Jr: Pulmonary Embolism. Philadelphia, WB Saunders, 1980.
4. Hoffman MJ, Greenfield LJ: Central venous septic thrombosis managed by superior vena cava Greenfield filter and venous thrombectomy: A case report. J Vasc Surg 1986; 4:606–611.
5. Warden GD, McDouglas WM, Pruitt BA: Central venous thrombosis: A hazard of medical progress. J Trauma 1973; 13:620–626.
6. Tilney NA, Griffith MD, Edwards EA: The natural history of major venous thrombosis of the upper extremity. Arch Surg 1970; 101:792–796.
7. Gloviczki P, Kazmier FJ, Hollier LH: Axillary-subclavian venous occlusion: The morbidity of a nonlethal disease. J Vasc Surg 1986; 4:333–337.
8. Shimokawa H, Takeshita A: Endothelium-dependent regulation of the cardiovascular system. Intern Med 1995; 34:939–946.

9. Hallet JW Jr, Brewster DC, Darling RC: Manual of Patient Care in Vascular Surgery. Boston, Little, Brown & Co, 1982.

10. Ludbrook J: Applied physiology of the veins. In Dodd H, Cockett FB (eds): The Pathology and Surgery of the Veins of the Lower Limb. Edinburgh, Churchill Livingstone, 1976, pp 50–55.

11. McCarthy WJ, Fahey VA, Bergan JJ, et al: The veins and venous disease. In Corry RJ, Perry JF (eds): Principles of Basic Surgical Practice. Philadelphia, Hanley & Belfus, 1987, pp 453–466.

12. Basmajian JV: Distribution of valves in femoral, external iliac and common iliac veins and their relationship to varicose veins. Surg Gynecol Obstet 1952; 95:537–542.

13. Sumner DS: Venous anatomy and pathophysiology. In Hershey FB, Barnes RW, Sumner DS (eds): Noninvasive Diagnosis of Vascular Disease. Pasadena, Appleton Davies, Inc, 1984, pp 88–102.

14. Dodd H, Cockett FB: The surgical anatomy of the veins of the lower limb. In Dodd H, Cockett FB (eds): The Pathology and Surgery of the Veins of the Lower Limb. Edinburgh: Churchill Livingstone, 1976, pp 18–49.

15. Giordana JM, Trout HH III: Anomalies of the inferior vena cava. J Vasc Surg 1986; 3:924–928.

16. Sumner DS: Hemodynamics and pathophysiology of venous disease. In Rutherford RB (ed): Vascular Surgery, 4th ed. Philadelphia, WB Saunders, 1995, pp 1673–1698.

17. Moneta GL, Bedford G, Beach K, Strandness DE: Duplex ultrasound assessment of venous diameters, peak velocities, and flow patterns. J Vasc Surg 1988; 8:286–291.

18. Ludbrook J: The musculovenous pumps of the human lower limb. Am Heart J 1966; 71:635–641.

19. Shepard JT: Reflex control of the venous system. In Bergan JJ, Yao JST (eds): Venous Problems. Chicago, Year Book, 1976, pp 5–23.

20. Kistner RL: Diagnosis of venous insufficiency. J Vasc Surg 1986; 3:185–188.

21. Wheeler HB, Rohrer MJ: Diagnosing and preventing venous thromboembolism. J Respir Dis 1988; 9:25–40.

22. Haeger K: Problems of acute venous thrombosis: 1. The interpretation of signs and symptoms. Angiology 1969; 20:219–223.

23. Heijbuer H, Ten Cate JW, Buller HR: Diagnosis of venous thrombosis. Semin Thromb Hemost 1991; 17(suppl 3):259–268.

24. DeWeese JA, Rogoff SM: Plebographic patterns of acute deep venous thrombosis of the leg. Surgery 1963; 53:99–108.

25. Husni EA, Ximenes JOC, Goyette EM: Elastic support of the lower limbs in hospitalized patients: A critical study. JAMA 1970; 214:1456–1462.

26. Campbell CB, Chandler JG, Tegtmeyer CJ, et al: Axillary, subclavian, and brachiocephalic venous obstruction. Surgery 1977; 82:816–826.

27. Killewich LA, Bedford GR, Beach KW, Strandness DE: Spontaneous lysis of deep venous thrombi: rate and outcome. J Vasc Surg 1989; 9:89–97.

28. Killewich LA, Martin R, Cramer M, et al: Pathophysiology of venous claudication. J Vasc Surg 1984; 1:507–511.

29. Widner LK, Mall T, Martin H: Epidemiology and sociomedical importance of peripheral venous disease. In Hobbs JT (ed): The Treatment of Venous Disorders. Lancaster, MTP Press, Ltd, 1977, pp 3–17.

30. Meyers TT: Varicose veins. In Allen EV, Barker NW, Hines EA Jr (eds): Peripheral Vascular Disease. Philadelphia, WB Saunders, 1962, pp 636–658.

3

Lymphedema

John J. Bergan, MD

⤳ · ⤳

The applicant stated that this enlargement of the extremities was a family characteristic which he had inherited from his mother.[1]

The patient with a swollen leg presents the physician with a diagnostic dilemma. It must be settled whether the problem is acute or chronic, whether it is due to a local problem or a generalized condition, whether it is related to the heart or the kidneys, hypoproteinemia, or salt-water imbalance. If the problem is localized to the extremity, is it a problem of the lymphatic or venous system? Furthermore, if one of those, is it congenital or acquired?

Fortunately, most of the answers to questions about the swollen leg can be obtained from the first visit of the patient to the physician, when a history and physical examination, combined with ancillary studies, will outline the nature of the problem and suggest the form of therapy to be employed. The purpose of this chapter is to provide information for the nurse to use to assist the patient by interpreting the findings of the physician and diagnostic studies, explaining the rationale for the therapy to be employed, and providing appropriate nursing care.

THE LYMPHATIC SYSTEM

Anatomy and Physiology

The lymphatic system consists of an extensive capillary network that collects lymph from the various organs and tissues and connects to an elaborate system of collecting vessels that transports the lymph to the blood stream (Fig. 3–1). Lymph nodes are placed like filters along the path of the collecting vessels and are an integral part of the system. Also, certain lymphatic organs that resemble lymph nodes, such as the tonsils, spleen, and thymus, are considered to be part of the system. Networks that collect lymph from the intercellular fluid constitute the beginnings of the lymphatic system. From these plexuses arise the lymphatic vessels that transport the lymph centrally through lymph glands to the thoracic or right lymphatic duct. Lymphedema occurs in the subcutaneous compartment, which is drained by the dermal plexus of lymphatics, collecting channels, and superficial lymphatic trunks. These superficial lymphatics are separate from the deep lymphatics, which drain the fascial compartments and the channels located near bone.

The superficial lymphatic system may be studied by lymphangiography, which shows that the lymphatic channels parallel the large superficial venous trunks, the greater and lesser saphenous veins of the lower extremity, and the basilic and cephalic veins of the

SIMPLIFIED LYMPHATIC ANATOMY

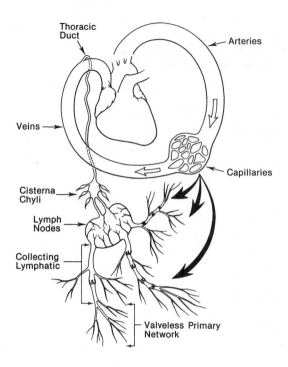

Figure 3–1. It can be seen in this diagram that tissue fluid exuded from capillaries is collected by a valveless primary lymphatic network, transported through valve-containing collecting lymphatics, filtered by lymph nodes, and collected by cisterna chyli and thoracic ducts and then returned to the circulation by way of major veins.

upper extremity. The lymph that is transported is an ultrafiltrate similar to plasma. This forms as a transudate from the relatively high hydrostatic pressure of the arterial system. Approximately 50 percent of circulating protein is lost from the arterial capillary system during a 24-hour period. While the vast majority of that is resorbed into venules by a combination of osmotic and hydrostastic forces, a small amount (0.1 percent) is not resorbed, and the lymphatic system returns this fraction to the venous system.

Lymph contains 0.1 to 0.5 g of total protein in each 100 ml, as compared with 6 g of protein in each 100 ml of blood. Lymph arises as an ultrafiltrate across a semipermeable membrane, which explains why there is a disproportionately high ratio of albumin to globulin in lymph, globulin having the higher molecular weight.

Valves in the lymphatics promote flow in a proximal direction, and lymph flow results from a combination of interstitial pressure, negative and positive fluctuation in the intra-abdominal and intrathoracic cavities, and the adjacent compression of muscular activity and arterial pulsations.

LYMPHEDEMA

Pathophysiology

Lymphedema has various definitions, but in all types there is impaired transcapillary fluid exchange and impaired transport of lymph. In failures of lymphatic transport, plasma proteins accumulate in the interstitial fluid and lead to an increase in interstitial fluid colloid osmotic pressure. Therefore, there is an increased movement of water into the interstitial space. The contact of lymph with subcutaneous tissue results in fibrosis and overgrowth of interstitial connective tissue. This is in response to the excess interstitial protein, particularly fibrinogen. This process is similar to chronic inflammation.

It is important to understand that, despite the fact that lymph contains less fibrinogen than plasma, lymph does clot. Although it clots more slowly than plasma, it contains virtually no fibrinolytic inhibitors. The coagulation properties of lymph and their role in pathogenesis of the thrombosed/obliterative type of lymphedema are not totally proven, but recognition of thrombosis in the pathogenesis of lymphedema is important.

Wolfe's description of pathogenesis of lymphedema is succinct and accurate[2]:

> Proximal lymphatic blockage can not only impede the outflow of lymph but also cause the initial lymphatics to dilate, opening the intercellular junctions by backflow. Lymphedema thus can occur when an abnormality consisting of too few, nonfunctional, or obstructed lymph pathways occurs, or when fluid overload overwhelms the functional capacity of the system. When either of these circumstances exists, a vicious circle is initiated in which retention of the high protein fluid concentration in the interstitial space further increases the tissue oncotic pressure, drawing more fluid into the extravascular space. The same high protein concentration also eventually sets off a chain of events leading to irreversible subcutaneous fibrosis.

Classification

All classifications of lymphedema are unsatisfactory, because the fundamental cause of lymphedema is unknown. However, because terms describing lymphedemas are in common use, they should be recognized and understood (Table 3–1). In one classification, three types of lymphedema are recognized: congenital, present at birth; praecox, presenting in early life up to age 35; and tarda, presenting in later life after age 35. Lymphedema secondary to removal of lymph nodes and/or radiation therapy would be termed *acquired lymphedema* (Fig. 3–2).

Kinmonth, who made the basic contribution of lymphangiography to clinical medicine, divided all causes into primary and secondary but gave no indication as to the cause of the primary variety. He further emphasized the ages of onset as being those already mentioned. He recognized that secondary lymphedema might be due to surgical excision of lymph nodes, radiation, or parasitic infestation by filariasis.

After lymphangiography had been firmly established in Kinmonth's clinic, he described three radiologic appearances: patients in whom no vessels were visualized (aplasia), those in whom a reduced number of vessels were seen (hypoplasia), and those in whom an increased number of dilated vessels were seen (hyperplasia). Although this classification is not useful, it remains in the literature.

Browse and Stewart have very logically suggested that primary lymphedema is caused

TABLE 3–1. **Simplified Classification of Lymphedema**

Primary lymphedema
  Congenital aplasia of lymphatics
  Congenital obliteration of thoracic duct or cysterna chyli
Secondary lymphedema
  Surgical excision of lymph nodes
  Radiation destruction of lymph nodes and lymphatics
Idiopathic fibrous obliteration of lymph nodes
Filariasis

Classification by time of onset includes:
  Congenital—at birth
  Praecox—under 35 years
  Tarda—over 35 years

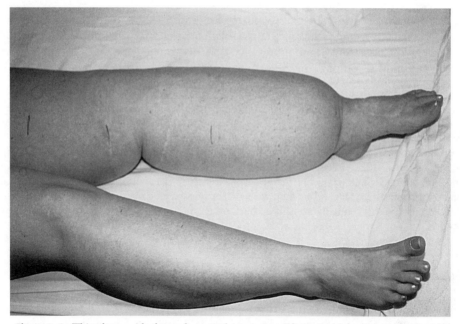

Figure 3–2. This photograph shows the typical appearance of acquired lymphedema of the calf, leg, and foot secondary to lymphadenectomy of the iliofemoral nodes. The additional radiation to this area, done in treatment of anal carcinoma with metastases to the groin, contributed to the massive calf swelling.

by an abnormality or disease of the lymph-conducting elements of the lymph vessels and lymph nodes.[3] They suggest that secondary lymphedema is caused by disease in the nodes or vessels that begins elsewhere, such as the trunk, or by the nonconducting elements of the lymph nodes, as in lymphoproliferative disorders. Also, secondary lymphedema follows surgical extirpation of lymph nodes or irradiation. Browse and Stewart point out that among the primary lymphedemas, some forms are caused by large-vessel abnormalities, such as congenital obstruction or aplasia of the thoracic duct and cysterna chyli. Also, primary lymphedema may be caused by congenital lymphatic valvular incompetence or congenital aplasia.

In lymphedema in which the underlying cause of the process is unknown, lymphangiography may reveal a reduced number of lymphatics. The age at onset helps to clarify some of these. Patients with this abnormality who present at or within a few years of birth can be considered to have been born with too few lymphatics, and this can be termed *true congenital aplasia* or *hypoplasia*. Those presenting at a later age have the histologic evidence of thrombosed or obliterated lymphatics. This would be an acquired, not a congenital, disease.

In monitoring patients with acquired or secondary lymphedema by lymphangiography, Kinmonth's group described gradual obliteration of proximal lymphatics in the presence of normal proximal lymph nodes. In the lower extremity, the normal lymph nodes were inguinal, and the obliterated lymphatics appeared in the thigh. Very little lymphangiographic contrast media appeared proximally in iliac vessels, but distal distention of lymphatics with a great deal of dermal backflow was seen. The distal lymphatic distention and pooling was occasionally massive, with extravasation of contrast demonstrated on the lymphangiograms.

This form of acquired lymphedema is poorly understood at present. However, it shows the greatest promise for discovery of the primary pathogenic process, with the hope that the condition can be understood and so brought under control, treated, or prevented.[3]

Summary of Classification

Another way of looking at a classification of lymphedema may eventually lead to directed treatment. There are four fundamental mechanisms of lymph drainage failure. These are reduced lymph-conducting pathways, poorly functioning lymphatics, obstructed lymphatics, and grossly incompetent lymphatics with reflux. Reduced lymph-conducting pathways may be caused by aplasia or hypoplasia of lymphatic vessels. Also, this may be caused by acquired obliteration of the lymphatic lumen due to lymph angiothrombosis or recurrent lymphangitis. Poorly functioning lymphatics may be described as those with contractility failure. Obstructed lymphatics may be caused by scarring from lymphadenectomy, radiotherapy, or infection. Finally, grossly incompetent lymphatics with reflux are seen on lymphangiography as megalymphatics or lymph vessel hyperplasia.

Clinical Presentation

Primary lymphedema may present in one of three ways. The most common presentation (in 80 percent of the cases) is mild edema of both ankles and legs in women, beginning at puberty or shortly after. The lymphedema is progressive but is not limiting. There may or may not be a family history. If lymphangiography is done (not recommended in every case), a total reduction in the number of distal lymphatic vessels will be seen, and normal ilioinguinal lymph nodes and vessels are demonstrated. Histologic examination showing obliterated lymphatics suggests that this is an acquired, not a congenital, abnormality, and it is therefore classified as a secondary lymphedema of unknown cause.

The second most common variety of presentation of lymphedema (10 percent) occurs in men and women at any age, may be unilateral, and usually involves the entire lower extremity. The condition may develop quickly, within 1 or 2 months, and may be associated with a minor event such as ankle sprain, insect bite, or episode of cutaneous infection. Lymphangiography, when it is done, reveals normal or dilated lymphatics in the foot, lower limb, and thigh but a reduced number of vessels and nodes in the inguinal and iliac region. In men, scrotal lymphedema may develop, and this will be associated with abnormalities of lymph nodes in the pelvis. Although this variety of lymphedema is also acquired, it appears to be caused by fibrotic obliterative changes within lymph nodes rather than in the lymph vessels. In this condition, an obliteration of the lymphatics occurs at the lymph nodes and progresses distally.

The third mode of presentation (10 percent) is true congenital lymphedema, affecting one or both limbs and present at birth or appearing at an early age. This may be associated with the appearance of vesicles on the skin. These vesicles leak lymph or chyle. The patient may have chylous ascites, chylothorax, or chyluria and may have other abnormalities such as a faint pink angioma of the skin, described by Milroy as "a slightly rosy hue extending around its (the leg's) whole circumference and involving the whole extremity, gradually disappearing near the knee."[1] Lymphangiography in this condition may show hyperplastic incompetent lymphatic vessels (megalymphatics). In this form of congenital lymphedema, swelling of the extremity may not appear at birth, but it develops later. Proximal chylous complications are dependent on involvement of preaortic and mesenteric vessels, as well as the thoracic duct itself. It is the form of familial, congenital, bilateral lymphedema resulting from absence of lymphatics that is truly called Milroy's disease.

True aplasia of the lymphatics may occur but is extremely rare.

Differential Diagnosis

The history and physical examination, taking into consideration those elements just described, are usually diagnostic. To repeat, the gradual onset of edema beginning at the dorsum of the foot and proceeding proximally over a period of several months, unassociated with other symptoms, is characteristic of lymphedema praecox or lymphedema tarda. The distinction between lymphedema and venous edema can be made on clinical evidence, because venous edema will be associated with cutaneous stigmata, including eczematoid dermatitis, ankle pigmentation with or without ulceration, and failure of skin healing. Lymphedema is not associated with cutaneous pigmentation or dermatitis. In major longstanding cases, however, hyperkeratosis of the skin, especially over the swollen toes, may occur (Fig. 3–3). Included in the elements of differential diagnosis is the fact that venous edema tends to improve rather rapidly upon leg elevation, whereas true lymphedema resolves not in hours but in days.

Few noninvasive studies are of value. However, isotope lymphography utilizing ^{99m}Tc-sulfur colloid has developed into a significant advance.[4] In this technique, the isotope is injected into the interdigital space and is quantitated in the ilioinguinal lymph nodes at 30 minutes, 1, 2, and 3 hours later. In diagnosis of lymphedema, the technique is 97 percent sensitive and 100 percent specific. Markedly decreased lymph flow is seen in lymphedematous limbs, and increased lymph flow is seen in those limbs with venous edema.[5, 6] The technique can be used in outpatients.

Lymphoscintigraphy has been used to select patients for microsurgical lymphatic reconstruction. Normal lymphatic flow is seen in patients with fat legs (lipedema) and in patients with idiopathic cyclic edema. However, in patients with lymphedema, these may be no flow, or dermal backflow, or large collateral flow as well as cross-over flow may be seen.

Newer imaging techniques reveal intrinsic architecture of the edema in swollen extremities.[7] In lymphedema, fluid collects in interstitial spaces, which become very prominent on computed tomography (CT) images. Chronic lymphedema reveals a honeycomb pattern seen in interstitial tissue as a result of fibrosis. In obesity, or lipedema, the subcutaneous fat layers are homogeneous but increased. Magnetic resonance (MR) imaging also reveals lymphedema in a fibrotic, honeycomb pattern and documents the increased circumferential size of the affected limb.[8] MR differentiates patients with lymphedema from those with deep venous thrombosis. Edema of leg muscles, particularly those in the posterior compartment, is characteristic of venous thrombosis.

Invasive studies, including lymphangiography and phlebography, may be used in special circumstances. Venography is informative in ruling out venous abnormalities; it is consid-

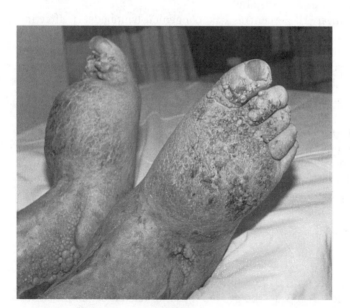

Figure 3–3. This clinical photograph shows the hyperkeratosis of lymphedematous toes associated with edema of the dorsum of the foot in a patient with acquired lymphedema. In this instance, the patient is a long-term survivor of the Charles procedure, and one can see the marked attenuation of tissue at the left ankle.

erably easier to perform and is more acceptable to the patient than is lymphangiography. The latter technique is tedious, difficult, and may even be hazardous.

When lymphangiography is performed, a concentrated dye (patent blue violet) is injected into the interdigital web spaces. It finds its way quickly by diffusion into the deep lymphatics. Once the superficial lymphatics are outlined by the dye, a transverse incision is made proximal to the site of injection, and the lymphatic channels are cannulated with a 27- to 30-gauge needle. Contrast material, such as ethiodized oil (Ethiodol), is injected slowly into the lymphatic system (Fig. 3–4). Multiple x-rays are obtained over the next 24 hours in order to visualize the lymphatics. Complications of lymphangiography are many, including ascending infection, lymphangitis, cellulitis, allergic reactions, and long-term staining of the extremity. The patient must be warned that the skin will turn blue. The procedure provides helpful information but should not be considered to be a routine diagnostic test.

Because lymphangiography is not without hazard, other methods of imaging have been developed. Among these are indirect lymphography, in which an intracutaneous injection of a water-soluble contrast medium is utilized. The contrast medium is administered through an infusion pump over a period of 10 minutes to create a depot of approximately 3 ml of solution. Intradermal and subcutaneous lymphatics are then seen by x-ray examination using the mammography film method. The technique is uncomfortable and produces rather limited visualization of lymph collectors. Also, the technique of fluorescence microlymphangiography has come into play. It uses vital microscopy in fluorescing macromolecules (FITC-Dextran, Sigma Pharmaceuticals). Subepidermal injection is utilized, and information regarding the morphology of the superficial lymphatic network distinguishes between Milroy's disease and other forms of primary lymphedema. Milroy's disease is characterized by total lymphatic aplasia. Obstructed lymphatics, which cause dermal backflow leading to formation of an extensive network in the dermis, can be visualized by this technique.

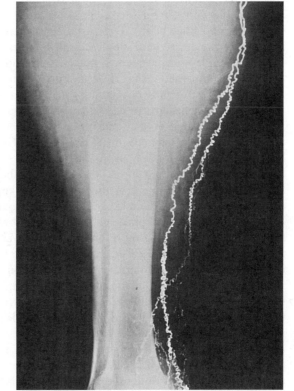

Figure 3–4. The characteristic picture of megalymphatic disease. The lymphangiogram typically shows elongated, tortuous, and varicose lymphatics without functioning valves distal to thrombosed lymphatics, fibrosed lymphatics, or fibrosed lymph nodes.

CT and MR imaging will reveal a characteristic honeycomb pattern in the subcutaneous portion of the limbs. Other edemas do not show this pattern. In venous insufficiency edema, for example, the muscle compartment deep to the deep fascia is enlarged but in lymphedemas it is unchanged or may show reduction in size of the muscle mass or hypertrophy due to the excessive forces required in moving a lymphedematous limb. MR imaging in particular may be more suitable than CT because of its ability to detect water. In general, the features are similar to those reported with CT, but MR techniques do not use radiation.

Nonsurgical Treatment

The objectives of treatment of lymphedema are to improve the cosmetic appearance of the extremity and to relieve limb heaviness by reducing lymphatic fluid. This, in turn, will decrease the tendency toward subsequent tissue fibrosis.

All of these objectives are achieved by external pneumatic compression. Such pneumatic compression may be obtained by a variety of pumps. Intermittent external pneumatic compression has proven to be effective in reducing limb girth. Patients without significant fibrotic reaction in subcutaneous tissue will have the best response, and conversely, those with the most subcutaneous fibrosis will have the least response to compression. In general terms, thigh and upper arm edema responds poorly to the low-pressure, single-compartment compression devices.

Because the single-compartment pressure devices distribute pressure distally as well as proximally, multicompartmental, high-pressure pneumatic compression devices have been developed.[9] Using a higher pressure (twice that of the unicompartmental devices) with a short cycle and distal-to-proximal milking action, greater reduction of lymphedema has been achieved.[10, 11] This form of therapy is expensive but does produce a high-pressure compression that does not cause cutaneous neurologic or muscular complications. The effect of the compression is achieved rapidly, and maintenance of reduction in lymphedema is achieved by very careful attention to skin care, prevention of infection, and the constant wearing of well-fitted elastic stockings. Best reduction in limb girth is achieved from long-term use of the device with supplemental treatments each day.

Patients undergoing sequential pneumatic compression, as well as those using unicompartmental compression, should be monitored very carefully so that lymphedema can be assessed and instructions on maintenance of compression therapy can be reinforced. If this is done, lymphedema in the vast majority of patients can be managed nonsurgically.

In addition, fitted elastic stockings apply external pressure when the limb is in the upright position to maintain beneficial effects of pumping. These stockings, in general, have been designed for venous disease; therefore, maximum pressure is applied at ankle level. Such stockings are crucial to good care but are limited in effectiveness simply because of the restrictions that they produce in knee movement and because of the low compression that is provided to the thigh of patients who have leg and thigh lymphedema.

In severe forms of lymphedema, as in severe forms of venous stasis edema, nonstretch support has proven to be more efficacious than elastic support. In venous insufficiency, the nonstretch bandage is called an Unna boot. In lymphedema, less prolonged bandaging is desirable. Therefore, multilayer bandaging is used for compression therapy and limb reduction. Layers of non-elastic, short-stretch bandages are applied. These generate little pressure at rest with the limb horizontal but apply high pressure during muscular contraction with the limb dependent. Short-stretch bandaging is combined with the use of foam rubber to distribute pressure more evenly, and the strategic positioning of the rubber pads irons out pockets of swelling and allows the shape of the leg to be maintained so that elastic hosiery worn subsequently will fit better. Unfortunately, multilayer bandaging, though effective, takes time to learn and time to perform.

If regular compression is neglected or abandoned, the swelling will slowly increase and will become progressively more difficult to control. O'Donnell has found that approximately 80 percent of patients treated by sequential pneumatic compression maintain a reduction in limb girth at greater than three levels of measurement. Success of sequential pneumatic compression is dependent on early application of the technique because the degree of subcutaneous fibrosis present at initiation of treatment greatly influences the results.[12]

Diuretics may be used in addition to pneumatic compression. They should be taken intermittently, especially in the premenstrual period.

Alternative Techniques

Popularity of massage therapy in other parts of the world has led to development of a particular therapy called *manual lymphatic drainage*. This was devised by Dr. Emil Vodder in Cannes in the early 1930s. Technologists were trained and many are in practice throughout Europe. The massage treatment portion of manual lymphatic drainage is combined with bandaging and compression and is supplemented by the use of made-to-measure elastic supports after optimal decompression is achieved. Information regarding this method of patient care can be obtained from Lymphedema Services at 360 East 57th Street, New York, NY 10022.

Attempts have been made to reduce excess protein in tissue fluid of lymphedema with benzopyrones. These have been extensively investigated, even using prospective, randomized, double-blinded, cross-over clinical trials.[13] As yet, these drugs have not been used extensively in the United States.

Surgical Therapy

When lymphedematous limbs are massively enlarged to the point that compression devices cannot be used nor elastic stockings worn, some form of surgical therapy may be employed. Surgical therapy of lymphedema may be classified as excisional or reconstructive.

Excisional Operations

Among the excisional operations is that described by Charles, in which all skin and subcutaneous tissue and deep fascia in the leg are removed (Fig. 3–5). The muscle that is left is covered by split-thickness skin grafting. Scarring in this operation is extreme, the grafts are easily injured, and the cosmetic appearance of the extremity is unsightly.

Staged subcutaneous excisions, leaving flaps of skin, have been described by Sistrunk and popularized by Homans. Symptomatic improvement is related to the amount of skin and subcutaneous tissue removed and the postoperative care given. Such operations do not cure the lymphedema, but do facilitate care by removing bulk from the limb. As much subcutaneous tissue and skin are removed as possible, while leaving enough tissue behind to effect primary wound healing (Fig. 3–6).

Although the initial treatment of lymphedema is nonsurgical, failures of such treatment require aggressive intervention. The most common surgical procedure is that advocated by Homans. The inner side of the calf and thigh is debulked in one operation and the lateral aspect of the limb operated upon a few months later. When the edema is gross and the skin infected, the Charles procedure is required.

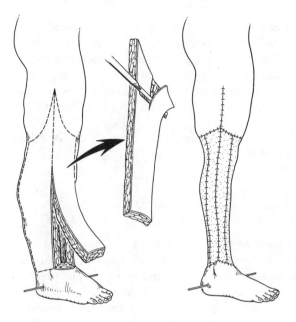

Figure 3–5. The Charles procedure. As shown in this diagram, the entire skin and subcutaneous tissue of the leg are removed surgically, with the limb held in place by a pin through the calcaneus. After removal of this tissue, skin grafts are taken from the excised tissue so as to cover the exposed muscles. Although the surgical result is cosmetically unappealing, the disability produced by intractable lymphedema can be reversed and the patient returned to an ambulatory life.

Reconstructive Lymphatic Operations

Experimental lymphaticovenous anastomoses have been performed since the early 1960s, and reports of use of this technique in treatment of lymphedema have been published since the 1970s (Fig. 3–7). The problems that attend such lymphovenous anastomoses include low lymph flow, differential between venous and lymphatic pressures, and the valvular incompetence that is present in lymphedema. A paradox exists in that, as lymphedema is decompressed by the lymphovenous anastomosis, lymph flow diminishes and thrombosis may occur, originating from the venous aspect of the anastomosis. Although normal lymphatics can maintain lymph flow against pressures as high as 50 mmHg, unfortunately, lymphatic pressure is not that high in chronic lymphedema.[14]

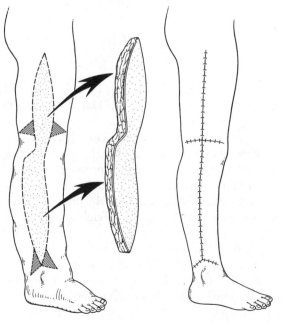

Figure 3–6. Excisional procedures, such as the one diagrammed here, produce more cosmetically satisfactory results than does the Charles procedure, but often must be performed in multiple stages in order to remove enough tissue to reverse the disability caused by lymphedema.

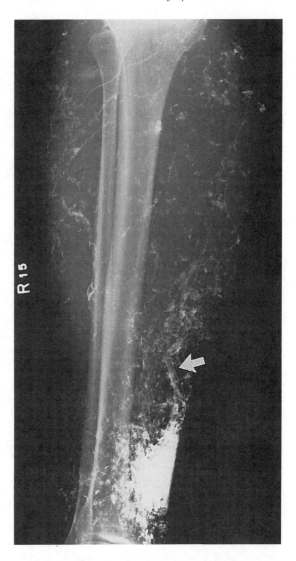

Figure 3–7. This photograph shows a patient 24 hours after lymphangiography was performed by injection of lymphatics in the foot with contrast medium. Note the extensive extravasation of contrast in the medial portion of the ankle and the outline of the saphenous vein proximal to this point, as indicated by the arrow. The perivenous lymphatics of the saphenous trunk are demonstrated and show the intimate relationship of veins and lymphatics. This relationship allows direct lymphaticovenous anastomoses to be made if large, obstructed lymphatics are visualized at the time of surgery.

Because of the difficulties of creating lymph flow through direct lymphaticovenous anastomoses, a more indirect technique has been developed by the group at St. Thomas' Hospital, London.[15] In this technique, lymphedema secondary to iliac lymph node and vessel obstruction was treated by construction of a bridge. The bridge consisted of intact mesentery draining a segment of bowel that had been opened and had its mucosa removed. Such bowel was then anastomosed to cut lymph nodes in the groin or along the external iliac axis. Sustained clinical improvement has been achieved in six of eight patients, and contrast lymphography has shown function of the enteromesenteric bridge in five of those six. Long-term patency of the bridge in transport of lymph has been demonstrated.

Direct microsurgical techniques to restore lymphatic flow have been the subject of worldwide investigations.[16–18] However, such treatment has not yet found acceptance among surgeons interested in routine treatment of lymphedema. Other attempts at increasing lymphatic transport such as implantation of omentum have also failed to achieve lasting acceptance.

Liposuction Debulking

Advent of liposuction after 1983 allowed this technology to be applied to debulking of lymphedematous limbs. The technique is now emerging as an alternative to ablative surgery with an average reduction in limb volume of 23 percent. Although in theory, application of interventional techniques such as liposuction should follow conservative therapy, in fact, experience using the reverse approach has shown no difference in results.[19] The most favorable results occur in those patients who are fitted with custom pressure support garments early following the surgical procedure.

Indications for intervention by liposuction are similar to those of surgical debulking. These include debility because of impaired mobility of the limb, pain, and esthetic deformity. A particular indication develops in those patients with radiation neuritis, in which muscle pump mechanisms used to propel lymphatic fluid are lost.[20] Although suction lipectomy can be used as primary and definitive treatment, it also can be applied to debulk a limb prior to surgical resection of skin and subcutaneous soft tissue.[21]

Nursing Intervention

Reducing Edema

Whether the patient is managed at home or in the hospital, the goal of basic treatment of lymphedematous extremity is to maintain an optimal edema-free state. To reduce edema, the affected extremity is wrapped with a snug elastic bandage from the digits to the trunk, and these wraps are removed and reapplied every 8 hours to maintain compression. A foam-rubber wedge may be applied to the bed and used during recumbency to elevate the leg steeply. Whenever intermittent pneumatic compression is used, the patient should return to the elevated limb position, and elastic bandages should be applied snugly to maintain the gains obtained during pumping. Maximal reduction in extremity edema can be achieved only by long periods of pneumatic compression. Failures of such pneumatic compression are frequently converted to success simply by doubling the pumping time.

Maintaining the Edema-Free State

When optimal size of the extremity has been reached, and this is detected by daily circumferential measurements at marked points on the extremity, then and only then is the extremity measured for continuous elastic support. For the upper extremity, the support will consist of a forearm and upper-arm sleeve with extension over the shoulder and across the trunk to maintain compression on the upper portion of the arm. A second and separate glove will be fitted to the fingers and hand.

For the lower extremity, the elastic support may extend to the knee when the thigh and leg are affected. In men, a scrotal support may be necessary as well. The elastic support is worn at all times when the patient is out of bed, but is removed at night for elastic bandaging and limb elevation during periods of sleep. Intermittent pneumatic compression pumps can be utilized in the home. These can be obtained from manufacturers on a lease or purchase basis.

Infection Control

Meticulous skin and foot hygiene aid in preventing invasive infection and subsequent cellulitis. It shoud be anticipated that episodes of invasive infection will occur, and these will stimulate erysipelas. Therefore, the patient should have in the home medicine chest an antibiotic chosen by the physician. At the earliest sign of infection, such as chills, fever, local tenderness, and/or ascending redness with streaks along lymphatic trunks, an antibiotic should be taken promptly. This antibiotic should be begun by the patient even before the physician is contacted, inasmuch as there may be delay in confirming the need for the antibiotic. Once the physician is contacted, antibiotic therapy may be continued for 5 to 10 days or can be monitored in other ways by the physician as desired. The objective of antibiotic therapy is to prevent ascending lymphatic destruction and/or thrombosis of lymphatics triggered by the infectious process.

Emotional Support

Whether conservative nonsurgical therapy, direct-excision surgical techniques, or direct lymphatic reconstruction is attempted, the most important aspect of care will be the nursing supportive management. This management will contribute to emotional support as well as counseling of the patient and the family. Since there is no cure for lymphedema and its conservative and surgical management is imperfect, it is imperative that the patient understand this disease and its chronic longstanding aspects, as well as the inadequacy of the palliative measures that help to control the chronic swelling.

All of the aforementioned measures may cause the patient to have anxiety regarding a change in body image and lifestyle. Nursing support must emphasize the need for a full and active life, limited only by the bulk of the lymphedematous limb. An optimistic view of the possibilities of controlling edema and improving lifestyles should be given to the patient.

Female patients, who make up the majority of those with lymphedema, will be concerned about passing the abnormality on to their offspring if they are of childbearing age. They will also be concerned regarding whether pregnancy will aggravate lymphedema. It can be said that, in the absence of a family history, lymphedema occurs sporadically and is not passed in an autosomal dominant manner. Pregnancy, because of its tendency toward fluid retention, may aggravate lymphedema. However, the palliative measures listed can be reinforced during pregnancy and usually control the lymphedema.

Patients, whether or not they are pregnant or considering pregnancy, should be reassured that selective athletic activity, including swimming, will help reduce edema by the milking action of muscular activity and enhanced arterial pulsations upon the lymphatic return mechanism. In nonwater sports, of course, the elastic supportive bandaging and stockings should be worn.

Additional nursing care is outlined in Table 3–2.

Postoperative Nursing Management

With all of the operations listed, and others that may be devised to improve the lymphedematous extremity, nursing management will play an important role in the immediate postoperative period. Increased swelling due to acute hematoma formation, external bleeding, and subsequent development of infection, are important factors to be noted by the nursing staff. These may require repeat surgical intervention at worst, or the administration of antibiotics at least. Antibiotics are administered to decrease the chance of infection.

Later in the healing phase of the postsurgical event, it will be necessary to maintain adequate compression of the extremity by application of elastic bandages, and, eventually, stockings. It may be that intermittent pneumatic compression will also be used, depending upon the operation chosen for therapy of the individual limb.

As stated above, the mainstay of reduction of edema in the lymphedematous extremity is the maintenance of extremity elevation. An exercise program to increase muscular

TABLE 3–2. **Nursing Care for Patients with Lymphedema**

POTENTIAL PROBLEM	NURSING INTERVENTION
Infection and impaired skin integrity	Monitor affected extremity for signs of infection, i.e., redness, warmth, tenderness, and fever. Teach patient and family signs of infection, and stress necessity of notifying the physician when noted. Administer antibiotics as prescribed, monitoring for signs of improvement. Maintain bed rest and leg elevation when infection occurs. Teach patient meticulous skin, nail, and foot care. A mild antiseptic soap should be used. The importance of properly fitting shoes to prevent trauma should be emphasized. Encourage the use of lotions such as lanolin and Eucerin that are free of potentially irritating perfumes.
Severe edema	Maintain bed rest. Elevate extremity above heart level. Assist with pneumatic pump devices as needed. Evaluate effectiveness of edema-reducing devices. Teach patient proper application of elastic support bandages or stockings, and proper use of pumping devices. Administer diuretics as prescribed, monitoring serum potassium level routinely. When patient resumes activity, walking and other exercise is good; standing still or sitting with the legs down promotes leg swelling.
Impaired physical mobility	Provide explanation for bed rest restriction. Encourage activities that will not interfere with bed rest. Emphasize the potential ability for sports and a normal lifestyle once the edema is controlled. Teach bed exercises that increase circulation, prevent venous stasis, and maintain muscle strength. Coordinate physical therapy consults when crutches or other devices are necessary for ambulation.
Disturbance in self-concept due to alteration in body image	Provide emotional support to patient and family. Encourage verbalization of feelings and questions. Encourage normal lifestyle and participation in selected activities and sports. Encourage normal growth and development in children. Discuss options for revisions in clothing or shoes. Offer opportunities to view before and after pictures of lymphedema following successful therapy or opportunity to meet another patient with lymphedema who is living a normal lifestyle or provide information about support group. Discuss prognosis, presenting an optimistic view of successful treatment.
Knowledge deficit about disease and course of treatment	Assess knowledge base of patient/family. Plan and implement teaching regarding the nature of the disease, diagnostic methods, prognosis, and treatment. Provide written material if available. Involve the patient and the family in the planning of care, and foster self-care when appropriate. If surgery is indicated, provide adequate preoperative teaching regarding the procedure, routines, visiting hours, expectations, recovery room, equipment, and restrictions and limitations.

activity and venous return and to promote pulse-pressure–induced lymphatic return will be beneficial to each patient.

Underlying all of the supportive nursing care in lymphedema is the understanding that the condition is not curable but is treatable. The challenges to long-term happiness may cause an alteration in lifestyle, but an open discussion of the treatment plan by the nurse with the patient will support the physician's suggestions to the patient and family members. Many of the unspoken fears and anxieties concerning lymphedema may be brought to the surface by the sympathetic nurse and, in being aired, can be alleviated.

References

1. Milroy WF: An undescribed variety of hereditary oedema. NY Med J 1982; 5:505.
2. Witte CL, Wolfe JH: Lymphodynamics and the pathophysiology of lymphedema. In Rutherford RB (ed): Vascular Surgery, 4th ed. Philadelphia, WB Saunders, 1995, pp 1889–1898.
3. Browse NL, Stewart G: Lymphoedema: Pathophysiology and classification. J Cardiovasc Surg 1985; 26:91–106.
4. Browse NL: The diagnosis and management of primary lymphedema. J Vasc Surg 1986; 3:181–184.
5. Stewart G, Gaunt JI, Croft DN, et al: Isotope lymphography: A new method of investigating the role of the lymphatics in chronic limb oedema. Br J Surg 1985; 72:906–909.
6. Vaqueiro M, Gloviczki P, Fisher J, et al: Lymphoscintigraphy in lymphedema: An aid to microsurgery. J Nucl Med 1986; 27:1125–1130.
7. Vaughan BF: CT of swollen legs. Clin Radiol 1990; 40:24–30.
8. Haaverstad R, Nilsen G, Myhre HO, et al: The use of MRI in the investigation of leg oedema. Eur J Vasc Surg 1992; 6:124–129.
9. Richmand DM, O'Donnell TF Jr, Zelikovski A: Sequential pneumatic compression for lymphedema: A controlled trial. Arch Surg 1985; 120:1116–1119.
10. Zelikovski A, Manoach M, Giler S, et al: A new pneumatic device for the treatment of lymphedema of the limbs. Lymphology 1980; 13:68–73.
11. Zelikovski A, Melamed I, Kott M, et al: The "Lympha-Press": A new pneumatic device for the treatment of lymphedema: Clinical trial and results. Folia Angiol 1980; 28:165–169.
12. O'Donnell TF Jr: The long-term results of compression treatment for lymphedema. J Vasc Surg 1992; 16(4):555–564.
13. Casley-Smith JR: The pathophysiology of lymphedema and the action of benzo-pyrones in reducing it. Lymphology 1988; 21:190–94.
14. Gloviczki P, et al: The natural history of microsurgical lymphovenous anastomoses: An experimental study. J Vasc Surg 1986; 4:148–156.
15. Hurst PAE, Stewart G, Kinmonth JB, et al: Long term results of the enteromesenteric bridge operation in the treatment of primary lymphodema. Br J Surg 1985; 72:272–274.
16. Baumeister RG, Siuda S: Treatment of lymphedemas by microsurgical lymphatic grafting: What is proved? Plast Reconstr Surg 1990; 85:64–74.
17. O'Brien BMcC, Mellow CG, Khazanchi RK, et al: Long-term results after microlymphaticovenous anastomoses for the treatment of obstructive lymphedema. Plast Reconstr Surg 1990; 85:562–572.
18. Gong-Kang H, et al: Microlymphaticovenous anastomosis for lymphedema of external genetalia in females. Surg Gynecol Obstet 1986; 162:429–432.
19. O'Brien BMcC, et al: Liposuction in the treatment of lymphoedema: A preliminary report. Br J Plast Surg 1989; 42:530–533.
20. Sando WC, Nahai F: Suction lipectomy in the management of limb lymphedema. Clin Plast Surg 1989; 16:369–373.
21. Louton RB, Terranova WA: The use of suction curettage as adjunct to the management of lymphedema. Ann Plast Surg 1989; 22:354–357.

Additional Readings

1. Browse NL: Single surgical procedures. A Colour Atlas of Reducing Operations for Lymphoedema of the Lower Limb, Vol. 39. London, Wolfe Medical, 1986.
2. Foldi M, Casley-Smith JR: Lymphangiology. Stuttgart, Schattauer, 1983.
3. Johnson HG, Pflug J: The Swollen Leg. London, Heinemann, 1975.
4. Kinmonth JB: The Lymphatics. London, Arnold, 1982.

5. Levick JR: An Introduction to Cardiovascular Physiology, 2nd ed. London, Butterworth Heinemann, 1995.

6. Mortimer PS: Investigation and management of lymphedema. Vasc Med Rev 1990; 1:1–20.

7. Roddie IC: Lymph transport mechanisms in peripheral lymphatics. News Physiol Sci 1990; 5:85–90.

8. Stewart G, Grant J, Croft DN, Browse NL: Isotope lymphography: A new method of investigating the role of lymphatics. Br J Surg 1985; 72:906–909.

9. Yoffey JM, Courtice JM: Lymphatics, Lymph and the Lymphomyeloid Complex. New York, Academic Press, 1970.

PART TWO

PERIOPERATIVE EVALUATION AND MANAGEMENT

4

Clinical Assessment of the Vascular System

Victora A. Fahey, RN, MSN, CVN

ᗧ · ᗤ

Despite new developments in noninvasive and invasive testing, the basic foundation for diagnosis in vascular disease remains a good history and physical examination. The assessment should also include an inquiry about regular health habits as well as changes in lifestyle necessitated by medical treatment. Such an assessment is one of the primary responsibilities of professional nursing. On the basis of the information obtained, appropriate interventions can be planned toward achieving optimal patient health.

In addition to the physical examination, patients' level of knowledge and attitude about their disease, their readiness to learn, as well as their psychosocial state, should be assessed. Because psychological factors strongly influence patients' adaptation to vascular disease, such information is essential to providing effective holistic treatment.[1] Patients' family members and/or significant others should be included in the assessment when necessary.

The history and physical examination provide an opportunity to establish a positive nurse-patient relationship. Achieving a good rapport will help increase the accuracy of the information gained and may improve and maintain the patient's health state.

This chapter will focus on the skills and techniques required in obtaining an accurate history and performing a physical examination of the peripheral vascular system. It is beyond the scope of this chapter to discuss every symptom and sign that may be present, but the significant features of arterial and venous disease are emphasized. More specific signs and symptoms and special examinations will be discussed in the appropriate chapters in this text. Characteristics and examination for lymphedema are discussed in Chapter 3. Because signs and symptoms of arterial and venous disease have specific characteristics, this chapter is divided into assessment of the arterial system and the venous system and further subdivided into body regions.

PREPARATION FOR HISTORY AND PHYSICAL EXAMINATION

An explanation of the history and physical examination to the patient prior to initiating the assessment should enhance the patient's willingness and ability to contribute pertinent information. Conditions that are essential to performing a good physical examination include good lighting in a warm, comfortable room, and full exposure of all extremities while preserving privacy. In addition to standard equipment, a portable Doppler ultrasound, stethoscope, and sphygmomanometer should be easily accessible to enhance efficiency of the examination. Gloves should be used when examining the patient.

A systematic order of assessment should be established. After a complete health history including the chief complaint is obtained, the physical assessment of the patient is then performed including inspection, palpation, and auscultation. Inspection elicits what is detectable visually, as well as information gained using the tactile (skin temperature and texture), olfactory (odor of necrotic tissue), and auditory (speech, voice) senses. Nonverbal communication exhibited by the patient can also reveal important information. Assessment should be performed bilaterally, always comparing one extremity or side with the contralateral one.

ASSESSMENT OF THE ARTERIAL SYSTEM

Atherosclerosis is a systemic process, and persons with peripheral arterial disease may also have significant cerebrovascular or coronary artery disease. Because of this, the initial patient evaluation should include an examination of the entire arterial system. Although the patient's cardiac status is significant, evaluation of this aspect of the cardiovascular system is not included in this chapter.

Patient History

Obtaining a comprehensive history is key to performing an accurate assessment. Components of a complete health history are included in Table 4–1. The disease may often be localized by history alone. The chief complaint is the reason the patient is seeking medical attention. Chief complaints will be discussed under each body region. It is important to listen and ask specific questions about these complaints.

Nurses play an important role in primary and secondary prevention of vascular disease. Obtaining risk factor information is an essential part of the history in order to plan appropriate intervention. Patients who smoke heavily have a more rapid progression of disease and worse prognosis.[2] Atherosclerotic disease is often accelerated in patients with diabetes.

Additional information to be gathered from the patient's history includes recent weight gain or loss, generalized weakness, problems with eating, gastrointestinal disturbances, and musculoskeletal problems. If significant malnutrition is suspected, a complete nutritional assessment should be performed. Protein-calorie malnutrition increases the risk of sepsis, delayed wound healing, pulmonary complications, and fluid and electrolyte imbalances.[3] Sepsis and delayed wound healing pose a serious threat of morbidity and mortality in vascular patients, especially when synthetic graft material has been used. Risk factors for the development of malnutrition are included in Table 4–2. Preoperative and postoperative nutritional supplements and correction of electrolyte imbalances will help decrease perioperative complications.

Vascular patients and their families vary greatly in their responses to the diagnosis and chronicity of vascular disease. It is important to evaluate these responses because psychosocial variables affect the ability to adapt to altered function and comply with the prescribed medical regimen. The goal of nursing intervention is to help the patient achieve the highest quality of life compatible with the illness. Nursing assessment should focus on the patient's perceived needs including social, financial, and safety issues.[4]

TABLE 4–1. **Components of a Complete Health History**

Chief Complaint/History of Present Illness
Location
Character (severity of symptoms)
Date of onset
Precipitating factors (stress, activity, medication)
Relief methods
Frequency of symptoms
Duration of symptoms
Progression of symptoms

Significant Medical-Surgical History
Cardiac history (angina, arrhythmias, myocardial infarction)
Hypertension—if yes, age at onset, severity, medications
Neurologic events or disorders: cerebrovascular or peripheral (loss of motor or sensory function,
    speech deficit, visual disturbances, dizziness, syncope, epilepsy, Parkinson's, multiple sclerosis)
Past injuries/spinal cord injury
Past surgeries
Infections
Renal disease/renal function
Malignancy
Diabetes
Collagen vascular disease
Clotting abnormalities (see Chapter 9)
Venous thromboembolism
Allergic reactions
Pregnancies
Present/past medication—Certain drugs can mimic or actually cause arterial occlusion. Inderal
    may increase patient's symptoms by decreasing cardiac output and systemic blood pressure.
    Ergot preparations for headache may cause arterial occlusion (see Chapter 1).

Family History
Arterial disease (cerebral, coronary, and peripheral or aneurysm disease)
Venous disease
Cholesterolemia
Clotting abnormalities

Psychosocial History
Occupational history: current and past—Use of vibratory tools; standing all day; professional
    athlete
Tobacco use
Drug abuse
Current activity level
Stress level
Dietary intake/obesity/weight loss
Alcohol intake
Emotional state
Activities of daily living/exercise program
Hygiene habits/foot care

Cerebrovascular Insufficiency

Chief Complaint

The patient may present with an asymptomatic bruit identified on physical examination. Clinical symptoms of cerebrovascular insufficiency may vary from a minor transient

TABLE 4–2. **Risk Factors for the Development of Malnutrition**

Inadequate nutritional intake	Cancer
Oral or gastrointestinal disturbances	Radiation therapy
	Chemotherapy
Sepsis	End-stage cardiac disease
Multiple surgical procedures	Excessive alcohol intake
Severe pulmonary disease	

neurologic event to a catastrophic stroke with paralysis and coma.[5] Symptomatic patients exhibit either carotid manifestations (hemispheric) affecting the anterior circulation or vertebrobasilar manifestations (nonhemispheric) affecting the posterior circulation (Table 4–3). Other nonspecific symptoms such as headache, seizures, or altered states of consciousness or cognition may occur. The symptomatology of cerebrovascular disease often mimics that of other neurologic entities. Classification of neurologic deficits is discussed in Chapter 13.

Inspection

A baseline neurologic assessment should be performed, including

- orientation with respect to person, place, and time;
- pupil size;
- reaction to light;
- grasp strength and equality;
- movement of all extremities;
- facial symmetry;
- tongue deviation; and
- the ability to communicate (speech) and swallow.

Inspect the carotid arteries for pulsation. Normally, carotid pulsation is not visible, although it may be visible at the base of the right neck with longstanding hypertension, with a tortuous carotid artery, and possibly with a carotid artery aneurysm or carotid body tumor.[6]

If the patient has experienced amaurosis fugax, an ophthalmoscopic examination should

TABLE 4–3. **Differentiation Between Carotid/Hemispheric Manifestations (Anterior Circulation) and Vertebrobasilar/Nonhemispheric Manifestations (Posterior Circulation)**

CAROTID/HEMISPHERIC	VERTEBROBASILAR/ NONHEMISPHERIC
Amaurosis fugax (fleeting monocular blindness)	Bilateral visual defects
Diplopia: no	Diplopia: yes
Contralateral motor and sensory deficits: weakness, tingling, numbness of extremity	Bilateral motor and sensory deficits: vertigo, syncope, dizziness, ataxia, dysphagia
Dysphasias (if dominant hemisphere is involved)	Drop attack/headache, confusion/memory loss

be performed. Bright, reflective spots may be seen in the retinal arteries. These are known as Hollenhorst plaques and represent cholesterol emboli from ulcerated plaque in the carotid or innominate arteries.[6] The fundi may also reveal evidence of severe hypertension, diabetes mellitus, or extensive atherosclerosis.[7]

Palpation

The common carotid pulse is palpated in the middle or lower neck between the trachea and the anterior border of the sternocleidomastoid muscle (Fig. 4–1). To palpate the carotid artery, feel the trachea and roll fingers laterally into the groove between it and the sternocleidomastoid muscle, which lies below and medial to the angle of the jaw. Each carotid artery should be palpated separately; massage or compression of the artery should be avoided to prevent reflex bradycardia or syncope related to carotid sinus manipulation. A palpable carotid pulse is not a significant finding, because even with a totally occluded internal carotid artery, a carotid pulse will be palpable if the external carotid artery is patent. The superficial temporal artery, a branch of the external carotid artery, can be palpated just anterior to the tragus of the ear. This suggests a patent external carotid artery.

The base of the neck and the supraclavicular fossa should be palpated for a pulsatile mass indicating an aneurysm or a carotid body tumor. The vertebral arteries are not readily accessible to palpation because they lie deep at the posterior base of the neck and are surrounded by cervical bone for most of their course.[6]

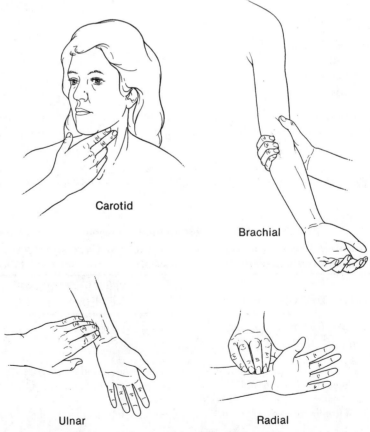

Figure 4–1. Palpation of the carotid, brachial, radial, and ulnar arterial pulses.

Auscultation

A bruit, the French word for noise, is an audible sound associated with turbulent blood flow created by a change in the diameter of the arterial lumen. While having the patient hold his or her breath, auscultate the carotid artery with the bell of the stethoscope from the base of the neck to the angle of the jaw. You are listening for a bruit, which usually signifies arterial stenosis at or proximal to the site of auscultation. Carotid bruits are usually loudest in the upper third of the neck in the area of the carotid bifurcation. If a bruit is heard, move the stethoscope toward the clavicle. If the sound intensifies, it probably originates in the heart or the subclavian artery; a diminished sound usually signifies the bruit originates in the carotid artery.

A totally or near-totally occluded artery, as well as an artery with a hemodynamically insignificant stenosis but an ulcerating plaque, may not produce a bruit. Thus, the absence of a bruit does not rule out a significant carotid lesion. If a carotid bruit was auscultated and then disappears at a later time, the carotid artery may have occluded during the interim. The severity of the stenosis cannot be determined by loudness of the bruit because a tight carotid stenosis may have minimal flow and a faint bruit.[6] To evaluate the hemodynamic significance of a carotid bruit, a carotid duplex scan is performed (see Chapter 5). The significance of carotid bruits is discussed in Chapter 13.

Upper-extremity blood pressures should be obtained bilaterally. This detects the presence of hypertension and arch vessel occlusive disease, most commonly affecting the left subclavian artery. Auscultation should be performed over the subclavian artery. An innominate artery stenosis produces a bruit in both the subclavian and carotid arteries; this should be differentiated from the bruit of aortic stenosis, which decreases in intensity on ascending the carotid artery. A vertebral artery bruit may be faint and is best heard over the tip of the shoulder.[8]

Upper Extremities

Chief Complaint

The most common symptoms exhibited with upper-extremity arterial insufficiency are acute onset of pain, chronic exertional muscle fatigue of the upper arm, and Raynaud's phenomenon (cold sensitivity). Acute arterial ischemia, characterized by severe pain, pallor, pulselessness, poikilothermia, and later paresthesias and paralysis, is usually the result of embolism, proximal thrombosis, or occasionally a subclavian artery aneurysm or an iatrogenic arterial injury (Table 4–4). Other symptoms of embolism are superficial skin lesions, petechia-like spots, and gangrene of the digits in the later stages of disease.

Muscle fatigue and discomfort occurring after prolonged use of the arm is similar to intermittent claudication of the lower extremity. The fatigue may be due to proximal arterial stenosis or occlusion, such as in the subclavian artery. Thoracic outlet syndrome can also produce fatigue, paresthesias, and numbness in the arm with activity. The

TABLE 4–4. **6 Ps of Acute Arterial Occlusion**

Pain
Pulselessness
Pallor
Poikilothermia
Paresthesias
Paralysis

symptoms are usually initiated by elevation or hyperabduction of the arm and result from neurovascular compression (see Chapter 14).

Intermittent hand coolness, pain, and numbness may accompany Raynaud's syndrome. It is characterized by episodic digital vasospasm associated with skin color changes precipitated by exposure to environmental cold, occupational exposure to specific types of vibratory equipment, and/or emotional stress.[9] Triphasic color changes of the digits occur; fingertips turn pale (white), then cyanotic (blue), then hyperemic (red) with accompanying pain and/or numbness. This most often occurs in the hands and fingers, but can also occur in the toes and feet.

Inspection

Examine the color of the extremity and fingertips. Check capillary refill. Note the time it takes to return to normal color; color should return within 3 seconds or less. With diminished blood flow, the return to normal color is delayed.

Inspect the size of the upper extremities, noting muscle atrophy, edema, fingertip lesions along the nail edge, skin ulceration, or gangrene (Fig. 4–2). Note the presence of needle tracks. If Raynaud's is suspected, inspect the fingers for tapering, a waxy appearance, joint mobility, and skin tautness or signs of scleroderma including shiny, atrophic skin. Observe for ulnar deviation of the hand, indicating possible rheumatoid arthritis.

Examine motor and sensory function of the hands and fingers, especially in the acutely ischemic limb. Have the patient flex and extend the fingers. Test sensory function with a dull object or light touch with a feather.

Palpation

Pulses should be palpated for their presence, rate, equality, regularity, and strength. However, the grading of pulses as normal, weak, or absent lacks precision.[10] Various scales are used by different institutions to evaluate pulse strength. Three such scales are listed in Table 4–5.

Because of the variety of scales, it is important to clarify which scale is used. Because

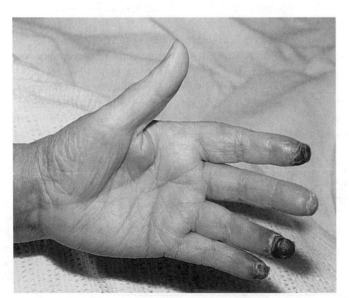

Figure 4–2. Ulceration and gangrene of the digits.

TABLE 4–5. **Scales of Pulse Examination**

(1) 0 = absence of pulses, 1 = marked impairment, 2 = moderate impairment, 3 = slight impairment, 4 = normal[14]

(2) 0 = absence, 1 = barely palpable, but definitely present, 2 = normal, 3 + = normal, easily palpable, and 4 + = abnormal, bounding (as in aneurysms)

(3) 0 = absent, 1 = diminished, 2 = normal, 3 = aneurysmal

grading of pulse strength is subjective, the simplest classification is either the presence or absence of a pulse.[6]

The presence or absence of peripheral pulses provides important information regarding the condition of the arteries and the level of disease. A diminished or absent pulse indicates the presence of an arterial stenosis or occlusion proximal to the site of examination. An abnormally strong pulse may suggest occlusion distal to the examination site or the presence of an aneurysm.

In the upper extremity, palpation of the axillary, brachial, radial, and ulnar artery pulses should be performed (see Fig. 4–1). The axillary artery is in the upper medial arm in the groove between the triceps and biceps muscle; the brachial artery is located medial to the biceps muscle at the antecubital fossa above the elbow; the radial artery is located at the lateral wrist over the distal radius; the ulnar artery may be palpated at the medial wrist over the distal ulna. Because of its anatomic location, the ulnar artery may be difficult to palpate. Doppler ultrasound may be used to assess arterial signals when pulses are not palpable. Postural changes may cause alterations in the pulse; therefore monitoring of the radial pulse in the various thoracic outlet maneuvers (see Chapters 5 and 14) should be performed.

The supraclavicular fossa should be palpated for a pulsatile mass (aneurysm) or a bony mass (cervical rib). The ulnar artery should be palpated for the presence of an aneurysm even in the palm. Skin temperature of the upper extremities can be palpated using the back of the hand. The temperature of the extremity becomes cool just distal to the arterial occlusion.

The radial and ulnar arteries are interconnected by two arches within the hand, which protects blood supply to the hands and fingers. Arterial patency of the palmar arch can be determined by performing the Allen test (Fig. 4–3), as follows: The patient holds the hand to be tested with the palm facing up. The radial artery of one wrist is compressed by the fingers of the examiner. The patient is asked to open and close the hand rapidly for 1 minute to squeeze the blood out of the hand, and then asked to extend the fingers quickly. When the hand is opened, the palm is mottled and pale. The radial artery is released and the hand is inspected for return of color and capillary refill. The response is normal if recovery of normal color is complete within a short period of time (less than 6 seconds). If pallor remains, incomplete continuity of the palmar arch is indicated, as well as occlusion of the radial artery; the hand is dependent on the ulnar artery for blood flow. This test should then be repeated with extended compression of the ulnar artery.[11] A positive Allen test is found in hypothenar hammer syndrome, in which repetitive trauma to the hand by either blunt or vibratory mechanisms can result from use of the palm of the hand in activities that involve pushing, pounding, or twisting.[12]

Auscultation

Auscultation of the upper extremity includes measurement of bilateral brachial blood pressure using a stethoscope or Doppler transducer. If more than 20 mmHg difference exists between arm pressures, it may indicate stenosis in the innominate, subclavian, or

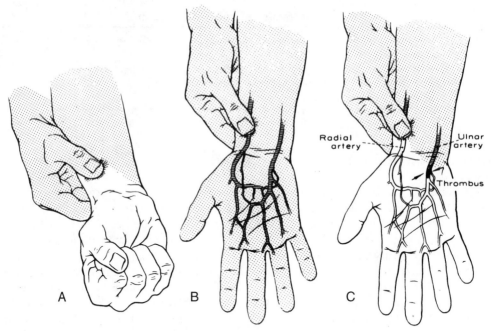

Figure 4–3. Allen test for patency of the palmar arch: **A,** Pallor induced by the clenched fist with radial artery compression. **B,** Return of the palm perfusion on relaxation of the hand with patent ulnar artery. **C,** Continued pallor of the hand due to ulnar artery occlusion. (From Fairbairn JF: Approach to the patient with peripheral vascular disease. In Fairbairn JF, Juergens JL, Spittel JA (eds): Peripheral Vascular Disease, 4th ed. Philadelphia, WB Saunders, 1972, p 27.)

axillary artery on the side of lower pressure. If such asymmetry of upper-extremity blood pressures is found, it is important to document in addition to informing the patient of this finding. This is significant not only from a vascular standpoint, but also because blood pressure medication may be given based on an inaccurate blood pressure.

A palpable distal pulse is usually only possible with a pressure of 70 mmHg or greater. When pulses are not palpable, the Doppler can be used to assess arterial signals. The Doppler is so sensitive it can pick up an arterial flow signal in a vessel that has only 20 mmHg pressure. However, a tone obtained using a Doppler does not equal a palpable pulse.[13]

The supraclavicular fossa should be auscultated for the presence of subclavian or innominate bruits. The presence of a bruit signifies arterial pathology of the proximal artery. Auscultation of the subclavian artery should be performed in a neutral position and in thoracic outlet maneuvers, noting the presence of a bruit (see Chapter 14). A bruit from aortic stenosis decreases in intensity on ascending the carotid artery.[8]

The Abdomen

Chief Complaint

The patient may be asymptomatic or may present with a pulsatile abdominal mass indicating an abdominal aortic aneurysm. Turbulent blood flow within the aneurysm may cause distal embolization, in which the patient presents with a blue toe (Fig. 4–4) or a painful toe. Although unusual, a large aneurysm may cause duodenal compression with weight loss and indigestion, or iliac vein compression resulting in lower-extremity edema.

A patient with a symptomatic aneurysm (leaking or ruptured) may present with abdomi-

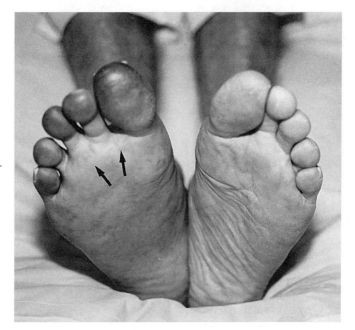

Figure 4–4. Blue toes *(arrows)* secondary to distal embolization.

nal pain radiating toward the back or groin, scrotal pain, syncope, shock, or hypotension. Tenderness of the abdomen may exist in the presence of inflammatory aneurysms. Discoloration of the abdomen, flank, or scrotum may occur due to extravasation of blood.

Intestinal angina may occur with mesenteric ischemia. A fear of food may develop due to pain that is experienced 15 to 30 minutes after eating, also known as postprandial pain. Because they avoid eating to prevent this discomfort, patients may experience significant weight loss. Acute intestinal ischemia may present as severe abdominal pain followed by vomiting and/or diarrhea (see Chapter 16).

Uncontrollable hypertension and new onset of renal failure may be indicative of renovascular hypertension (see Chapter 15).

In males, sexual impotence characterized by inability to maintain an erection is a complaint associated with aortoiliac occlusive disease (see Chapter 11). Impotence can also be a result of medications, psychological factors, or diabetes.

Inspection

The retroperitoneal position of the abdominal aorta and its branches limits the amount of information that can be obtained from the physical examination. Inspect the patient in a supine position, noting the contour of the abdomen, and the presence of obesity, ascites, pulsations, distention, or discoloration. Note incisions from previous surgery.

Palpation

The aorta bifurcates at the level of the umbilicus, and the aortic pulse may be palpated just above this in the nonobese patient. The normal size of the aorta approximates the width of a patient's thumb. To palpate, press fingers firmly deep into the abdomen to identify the aortic pulsation. If the pulse is prominent or feels wide, place the thumb along one side of the aorta and the fingers along the other side. An abdominal aortic aneurysm should be suspected if the width feels larger than 4–5 cm.[6] If the mass appears to extend to the xiphoid and costal margins, suspect a suprarenal or thoracoabdominal aneurysm. While palpating the abdomen, note any abdominal tenderness or referred pain; this may indicate rupture, leak, or inflammation. Iliac artery aneurysms of significant size may be palpable on rectal exam.

Auscultation

Bruits may be heard when significant occlusive disease of the aorta and its branches is present. Aortoiliac disease may cause bruits in the middle and lower abdomen. Renal artery bruits may be faint and localized in the upper abdominal quarter just lateral to the midline. Mesenteric artery stenoses are associated with epigastric bruits.[6] Although bruits may be detected, their significance is variable. Further diagnostic tests including ultrasound, computed tomography (CT) scan, and/or arteriogram are required to obtain the necessary information.

Lower Extremities

Chief Complaint

Although patients may be asymptomatic, a pulse deficit, a bruit, an abnormal pulsation, or an aneurysm may be found on routine physical examination. Symptoms may be disguised in patients whose activity levels are limited because of other health problems such as cardiac disease.

The most common presenting symptom in lower-extremity arterial disease is pain. The degree of pain depends on whether the problem has an acute or chronic onset, the severity of the disease (the extent of blood flow reduction), and the adequacy of collateral blood supply.

Chronic arterial insufficiency of the lower extremity causes two characteristic types of pain: intermittent claudication and ischemic rest pain. Claudication, derived from the Latin infinitive "to limp" (claudicare), is defined as cramping muscle pain brought on by walking a predictable distance and relieved by brief periods of rest.[14] The pain may vary from a slight ache to a severe, cramp-like pain. Claudication, similar to angina, indicates inadequate arterial blood supply to contracting muscles.

The location of muscle pain indicates the level of arterial occlusion (Fig. 4–5). The muscle groups affected will generally be one joint below the occlusive lesion. Arterial occlusive disease of the aortoiliac area causes buttock and thigh claudication, which the patient describes as a weakness or tiredness with exercise. Cramping calf pain usually results from a superficial femoral or popliteal artery stenosis or occlusion.

Pain in the legs brought on by exercise is a common complaint and not always due to arterial occlusive disease.[15] Patients with neurospinal compression or musculoskeletal disease may also present with pain while walking (Fig. 4–6).[16] Other causes of leg pain may be peripheral neuritis in diabetics, arthritis, sciatica, and reflex sympathetic dystrophy or minor causalgia, which is a burning pain in nature. Vascular intermittent claudication can be differentiated from neurogenic claudication if the following criteria for the vascular type are met:

1. The pain must start as a muscle cramp in the thigh, buttocks, or calf after walking a predictable distance.
2. The pain must be relieved by rest in a standing position after a predictable period of time.

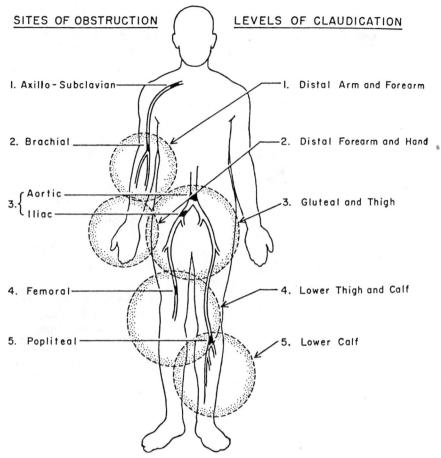

SITES OF OBSTRUCTION   LEVELS OF CLAUDICATION

1. Axillo-Subclavian   1. Distal Arm and Forearm

2. Brachial   2. Distal Forearm and Hand

3. { Aortic   3. Gluteal and Thigh
     Iliac

4. Femoral   4. Lower Thigh and Calf

5. Popliteal   5. Lower Calf

Figure 4–5. Sites of obstruction and corresponding levels of claudication.

3. The patient must then be able to walk a similar distance again, and again experience pain and then obtain relief after stopping for the same period as before.[17]

Calf cramps should not be confused with those that occur at night in older patients, some of whom may even have pulse deficits or other signs of arterial disease. Nocturnal muscle cramps have no known vascular basis; instead, they are thought to result from exaggerated neuromuscular response to stretching.[15]

Rest pain, which occurs with advanced arterial occlusive disease, is described as pain in the toes or metatarsal head area when the extremity is resting in a horizontal position. Rest pain initially occurs at night and interferes with the patient's sleep. Relief is obtained when the foot is placed in a dependent position, such as dangling it over the side of the bed.

Ischemic ulceration is caused by inadequate blood supply. The ulcer usually occurs at the tips of the toes and over pressure areas (Fig. 4–7) and occasionally between the toes (Fig. 4–8). Neurotrophic ulcers (Fig. 4–9) or interdigital ulcers in diabetics must not be confused with those due to severe ischemia (Table 4–6).

Tissue loss such as gangrene of the toes (Fig. 4–10) or forefoot in conjunction with rest pain represents the most severe form of ischemia. Superficial skin gangrene resulting from microembolization must not be confused with ischemic gangrene. In blue toe syndrome secondary to atherosclerotic debris, microemboli, or aneurysms, the digits are typically cold and painful (see Fig. 4–4). Gangrene of the toes may also be present in diabetics with palpable pedal pulses.

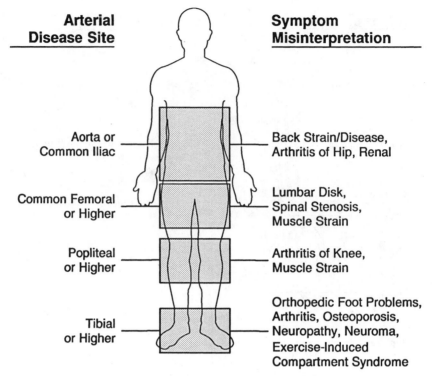

Arterial Disease Site		**Symptom Misinterpretation**
Aorta or Common Iliac		Back Strain/Disease, Arthritis of Hip, Renal
Common Femoral or Higher		Lumbar Disk, Spinal Stenosis, Muscle Strain
Popliteal or Higher		Arthritis of Knee, Muscle Strain
Tibial or Higher		Orthopedic Foot Problems, Arthritis, Osteoporosis, Neuropathy, Neuroma, Exercise-Induced Compartment Syndrome

Figure 4–6. Common misinterpretations of lower-extremity claudication, which often mimics neurologic or musculoskeletal disorders. Assessment of onset, precipitating factors, and relief methods is important for an accurate diagnosis.

Acute arterial occlusion of the lower extremities is characterized by the 6 Ps: sudden onset of pain, pallor, pulselessness, and poikilothermia (coolness) in the affected extremity; paresthesias and paralysis occur in later stages (see Table 4–4). These signs and symptoms may not be present in all patients.[14]

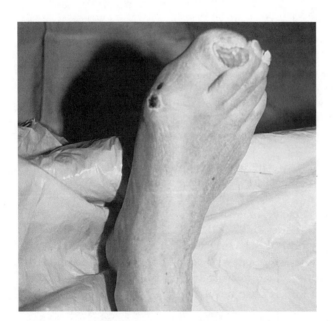

Figure 4–7. Ulceration over bony prominence.

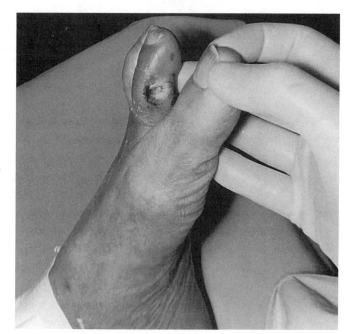

Figure 4–8. Ulcer between the toes.

Inspection

Color of the extremities should be examined with the patient in different positions. Elevate the patient's legs 30–45°. If arterial disease is significant, the legs become pale, a phenomenon known as "pallor with elevation"; the arterial system cannot pump adequate blood into the capillary system against gravity through the arterial blockages.

The patient should then hang his or her legs over the side of the bed. The legs should remain a healthy pink color. With arterial disease, a deep red color (dependent rubor)

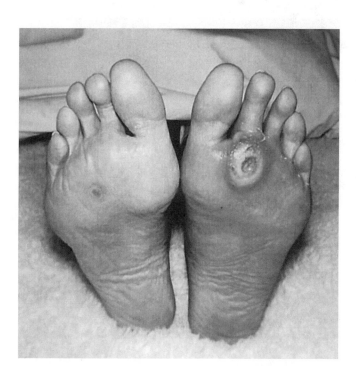

Figure 4–9. Neurotrophic ulcer.

TABLE 4–6. **Characteristics of Common Lower-Extremity Lesions**

CHARACTERISTIC	ISCHEMIC ULCER	VENOUS STASIS ULCER	NEUROTROPHIC ULCER
Onset	Traumatic or spontaneous	Traumatic or spontaneous	Spontaneous
Location	Toe, heel, dorsum of foot	Medial distal third of leg	Sole of foot under calluses or pressure points
Pain	Severe at night; relieved by dependency	Mild pain when infected; aching with dependency; relieved with elevation	None
Skin around ulcer	Atrophic; may be inflamed	Stasis dermatitis; pigmentation changes	Callous
Ulcer edge	Definitive	Uneven	Definitive
Ulcer base	Pale, eschar	Healthy	Healthy or pale
Pulses	Decreased or none	Normal	Normal
Associated signs	Trophic changes Gangrene may be present	Edema No gangrene	Neuropathy No gangrene Decreased sensation Diabetes

Data from Pousti TJ, Wilson SE, Williams RA: The clinical examination of the vascular system. In Veith FJ, Hobson RW, Williams RA, Wilson SE (eds): Vascular Surgery Principles and Practice. New York, McGraw-Hill Book Co, 1994, pp 74–89.

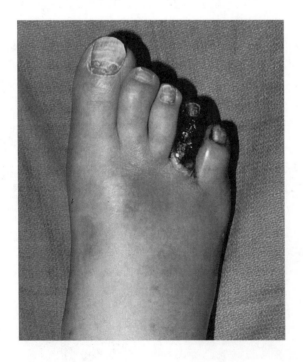

Figure 4–10. Gangrene of toe with cellulitis.

occurs as a result of blood pooling in the arterioles. The color changes reflect increased oxygen saturation and blood flow in the capillary venous plexus of the skin that occurs because of loss of the sympathetic reflex vasoconstriction normally found in dependency.[7] Areas of discoloration, petechia-like lesions on the toes or foot from microembolization (blue toe syndrome), should be noted. Capillary refill time, the time taken for a blanched area to "pink up," is a crude indication of blood flow. It can be checked by pressing on the tip of the toes or sole of the foot with a finger and then releasing pressure.

Inspect the extremities for trophic changes secondary to tissue malnutrition from arterial compromise. Trophic changes include:

- hair loss on the affected extremity;
- thin, smooth, shiny skin;
- thick, brittle nails with or without fungal infection (Fig. 4–11);
- tapering of toes or fingers; and
- any skin breakdown (possibly traumatic), ulceration, or gangrene.

Ischemic ulcerations are usually located over pressure points, i.e., heels, toes, and bony prominences, and on the dorsum of the foot and over metatarsal heads, especially I and V. Note the size and depth of the ulcer, color of the base (usually pale), and the presence and/or odor of drainage. Gangrene may be dry, mummified, blue-black eschar on toes, forefoot, or heel, or it may be moist (wet gangrene).

Inspect the extremities for size and symmetry, muscle atrophy, or edema that may be present secondary to the leg being in a dependent position or a potential compartment syndrome. Also note absence of a limb or digit or any scarring on the extremities from previous surgery or injury.

Acute ischemia reduces blood supply to distal nerve fibers and muscles; therefore, motor and sensory function may be diminished or absent. Motor function is evaluated by eliciting the movement of muscle groups whose blood supply is derived from arteries distal to the occlusion. Instruct the patient to perform digital flexion and extension as well as to move the extremity. Drop foot may be present with advanced ischemia. This condition requires urgent intervention.

Sensory function can be assessed by touch, pressure, or nailbed compression. Ask the patient to tell which toe is being touched while using a blunt-edged instrument such as a hemostat or paperclip. Invasive instruments such as safety pins should be avoided, to prevent a break in the skin. Diabetic neuropathy as well as previous surgery can contribute to impaired sensation.

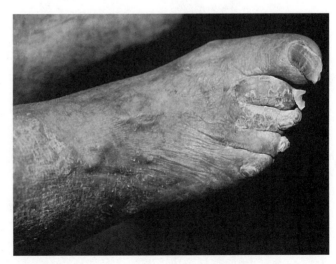

Figure   4–11. Thick,   deformed nails.

Palpation

One can determine the location of disease with examination of the pulses. Examination of the lower-extremity pulses includes palpation of the femoral, popliteal, posterior tibial, and dorsalis pedis arteries (Fig. 4–12). While palpating the pulses, note aneurysmal dilation. With the patient supine, the common femoral pulse can be palpated just distal to the inguinal ligament, mid-groin, between the pubic bone and the anterior superior iliac spine. It is difficult to palpate in an obese person. The examiner should stand on the side being examined and press deeply. The popliteal pulse is located deeply on the posterior medial aspect of the knee joint. With the patient's knee slightly flexed and calf muscles relaxed, cup both hands and press fingertips behind the knee against the flat surface of the tibia. If the pulse cannot be palpated in this position, have the patient lie on his or her abdomen and flex the knee 45°; then palpate again. If the popliteal pulse is easily palpated, a popliteal aneurysm should be suspected. The posterior tibial artery is found in the groove behind the medial malleolus of the ankle, one-third the distance from the malleolar prominence to the edge of the tendon. To palpate the left pulse, stand on the left side, with right fingertips curved behind the medial malleolus. The dorsalis pedis pulse, a continuation of the anterior tibial artery, is found on the dorsal midportion of the foot between the first and second metatarsals. Standing at the foot of the bed using the hand on the same side as that of the foot being palpated, place three fingers on the dorsum of the foot on an imaginary line drawn between the midpoint between the malleoli and the first web space. Because of anatomic variations, the posterior tibial and dorsalis pedis pulses may be absent in about 10 percent of the population.[15] If the dorsalis pedis

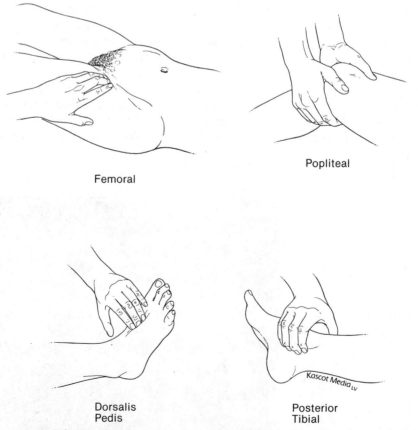

Femoral

Popliteal

Dorsalis
Pedis

Posterior
Tibial

Figure 4–12. Palpation of the femoral, popliteal, posterior tibial, and dorsalis pedis arterial pulses.

pulse is not palpable, the lateral tarsal artery, the terminal branch of the peroneal artery located laterally and in the midportion of the foot, should be palpated. Because the peroneal artery lies medial to the fibula behind the lateral malleolus, it is not usually palpable.

Patients with intermittent claudication may have superficial femoral artery disease and therefore have femoral pulses but absent distal pulses. Diabetics commonly have infrapopliteal disease and thus have palpable femoral and popliteal pulses but absent distal pulses. Intermittent claudication may occur in the presence of palpable pedal pulses; however, the pulse may disappear after exercise. The "disappearing pulse phenomenon," described by DeWeese, can be demonstrated by repeat palpation of pedal pulses after exercise.[18] The patient can rise up on the toes repeatedly or walk on a treadmill until claudication develops. Pulses disappear because of the marked decrease in vascular resistance that occurs in exercising muscle distal to an obstruction and because of the increased distribution of flow to muscle beds proximal to the obstruction.[8] The presence of normal pulses after exercise strongly suggests a nonarterial cause.[2] If a young person has a history of claudication with palpable pedal pulses, pulses should be rechecked during active plantarflexion or passive dorsiflexion. Popliteal artery entrapment syndrome may be present.

After completing the pulse evaluation, use the back of the hand to assess the skin temperature of the lower extremities. In addition to absent pulses, a temperature demarcation can be felt one skeletal segment below the site of arterial occlusion. Symmetric coolness usually indicates peripheral vasoconstriction; asymmetric coolness may represent arterial insufficiency.

Auscultation

The femoral artery may be auscultated for a bruit. The bruit occlusion test may help localize the stenosis, differentiating between iliac and superficial femoral artery disease. If the initial auscultation reveals a bruit, the examiner compresses the superficial femoral artery distal to the site of the stethoscope. If the bruit disappears or decreases in intensity, a stenosis in the superficial femoral artery is likely. Conversely, if no change or an increase in intensity occurs, the profunda femoris artery or another branch artery may be stenotic. By repeating this maneuver with the stethoscope placed above the inguinal ligament, the examiner may detect a stenotic lesion in the iliac artery.[7] Also, auscultation is important to confirm a suspected arteriovenous fistula, which is characterized by a continuous to-and-fro bruit.

By auscultating blood pressure measurements over the arteries in the leg, the examiner can determine the level and severity of disease. Normally, the systolic blood pressure at the ankle level is equal to or slightly higher than the brachial systolic pressure. To determine the percentage of blood supply to the extremity, the ankle pressure is divided by the highest brachial pressure.

$$\frac{\text{Ankle Pressure}}{\text{Brachial Pressure (Highest)}} = \text{Ankle-Brachial Index (ABI)}$$

Any decrease in pressure indicates arterial stenosis (Table 4–7). This is further discussed in Chapter 5. Diabetics may have an artificially elevated ABI as a result of calcified tibial arteries.

ASSESSMENT OF THE VENOUS SYSTEM

Venous disease, unlike arterial occlusive disease, is usually localized to one anatomic area and occurs most commonly in the lower extremities, although the upper extremities can

TABLE 4–7. **Ankle-Brachial Index**

No symptoms	= .7–1.0 or greater
Claudication	= .5–.7
Rest pain, ulcer, gangrene	= .3 or less

Data from Benjamin ME, Dean RH: Examination of the patient with vascular disease. In Dean RH, Yao JST, Brewster DC (eds): Current Diagnosis and Treatment in Vascular Surgery. Norwalk, CT, Appleton & Lange, 1995, pp 1–4.

be affected, especially with the increased use of central venous lines. Physical assessment of the venous system is less precise than the arterial system.

Head and Neck

Inspection

Dilated jugular veins may indicate an arteriovenous fistula, congestive heart failure, or venous occlusion proximal to the dilated veins. If both sides of the neck and both arms have dilated veins, a superior vena caval syndrome is suspected.[7]

Upper Extremities

When venous disease involves the upper extremity, acute or chronic obstruction of the axillary or subclavian vein is the most likely cause.[19] Acute deep venous obstruction usually results from subclavian vein catheterization for parenteral nutrition or intravenous therapy, thoracic outlet syndrome, or shoulder injury. Acute thrombosis following vigorous exercise, work, or lifting may be referred to as effort thrombosis. Chronic arm swelling may be the result of venous or lymphatic obstruction. Lymphatic obstruction is usually associated with history of a radical mastectomy, infection, or irradiation involving axillary lymph nodes (see Chapter 3).

Chief Complaint

Arm swelling, whether chronic or acute, is the chief complaint and may be accompanied by an aching pain. Intermittent swelling when in certain positions may indicate intermittent subclavian venous obstruction, especially when patients have the arm raised above the head or when they are unusually erect.[20]

With superficial thrombophlebitis, the patient may complain of localized tenderness or pain (dolor) along the course of the affected vein.

Inspection

Superficial Thrombophlebitis
Inspect the affected vein for erythema and swelling. Inspect the arm for any break in the skin, which is a potential source of cellulitis.

Deep Vein Thrombosis

Assess the extremities for symmetry. Unilateral swelling of the arm and the presence of dilated superficial veins around the shoulder may suggest subclavian vein thrombosis. Venous distention is not diminished when the arm is raised above the level of the heart. Note the color of the extremities, which may appear bluish or cyanotic in the acute stage (phlegmasia cerulea dolens).

Palpation

Palpation of the upper-extremity veins adds minimal information to the upper-extremity venous examination. If a superficial thrombophlebitis is suspected, however, a cord may be palpable along the affected vein with increased skin temperature.

Auscultation

Venous sounds are not usually audible with a stethoscope.[6] Patterns of abnormal venous flow in arms have not been as clearly defined as in the Doppler exam of the legs.[21] However, venous examination with Doppler ultrasound and duplex scanning is well recognized and discussed in Chapter 5.

A penetrating injury or surgery of the arm may cause an arteriovenous fistula. Auscultate over the affected area to detect the presence of a bruit.

Lower Extremities

Chief Complaint

The most common complaints of the lower extremities are related to superficial or deep venous thrombosis, varicose veins, and chronic venous obstruction.

Symptoms of superficial thrombophlebitis in the lower extremity include localized pain or aching and possible swelling over the affected vein.

With deep venous thrombosis (DVT), the most common symptom is complaint of sudden onset of unilateral edema or feeling of heaviness in the leg. Iliofemoral DVT may result in intense pain. However, with DVT, complaints may be absent or minimal depending on the size of the thrombus, the degree of obstruction, and the adequacy of collateral circulation. Reports state that only 50 percent of patients having a positive history and physical examination for DVT also had a positive venogram.[22] Thrombi in the leg veins are responsible for the majority of pulmonary embolism (PE) but are recognizable prior to death in less than 55 percent of patients with fatal PE.[20]

Patients with varicose veins complain of cosmetic disfigurement, unsightly veins with or without aching, cramping discomfort in their legs when standing, swelling in the evening, and possibly night cramps. Varicose veins are relieved by leg elevation. The pain may increase in severity prior to the menstrual period or during pregnancy.[20]

Patients with chronic venous insufficiency complain of swelling and aching discomfort in the legs when standing that is relieved by elevation of the legs above the heart. Swelling secondary to high venous pressure can be venous or cardiac in origin, with right-sided heart failure or tricuspid valvular insufficiency. Night cramps may be common but are unrelated. Ulceration may be present. Although related pain is uncommon, patients may complain of bursting pain in the calf after walking about 100–200 yards, which is slowly relieved by rest and elevation. This condition, known as venous claudication, is secondary to venous outflow obstruction.

Superficial Thrombophlebitis or Deep Vein Thrombosis

Inspection

With superficial thrombophlebitis, there is usually redness over a firm mass or cord with surrounding induration along the course of the affected vein (Fig. 4–13).

Inspect the lower extremities for unilateral edema in the calf, ankle, or thigh. Calf vein thrombosis may cause unilateral leg swelling below the knee. Iliac vein thrombosis may cause the entire lower extremity to swell and become pale. Extensive iliofemoral thrombosis is described further in Chapter 17. With unilateral leg swelling, the lower-extremity circumference should be measured to establish a baseline and evaluate the effectiveness of therapy. For the most reliable comparison, measure at the same level each time by marking the areas. Inspect for dilation of superficial veins in the legs or pelvis, and note the color of the extremity.

Palpation

Palpation for venous thrombosis of the lower extremities is the same as for upper extremities. Palpate the pelvic and femoral areas for a mass that may cause external venous compression.

Varicose Veins

Inspection

Patients who are being examined for varicose veins (Fig. 4–14) should stand to allow the long and short saphenous veins to fill. Inspect each leg for dilated, tortuous veins, usually located as tributaries to the greater saphenous vein. Note the location of the varicosities; any dilated suprapubic veins could be evidence of past iliofemoral or vena cava thrombosis. Mild edema may be present with uncomplicated varicose veins and rarely appears early in

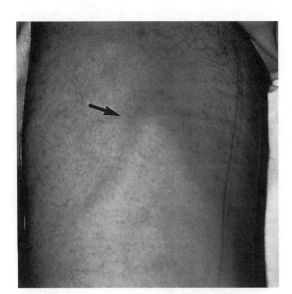

Figure 4–13. Superficial phlebitis of the lower extremity.

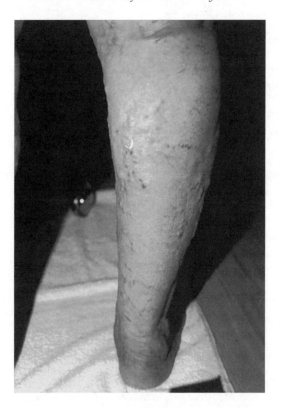

Figure 4–14. Varicose veins.

the day. Varicose veins that are a result of deep vein and perforator incompetence may result in similar signs and symptoms to chronic venous disease. Certain tourniquet tests are performed to diagnose valvular competence in the veins. These tests are discussed in Chapter 18.

Palpation

The examiner should palpate for fascial defects along the course of the affected vein representing the site of an incompetent perforator.[6]

Chronic Venous Insufficiency

Inspection

Inspect the patient's lower extremities for edema, cellulitis, and hyperpigmentation of the skin around ankle ulceration, resulting from breakdown of red blood cells into deposits of hemosiderin that stain the tissue a characteristic brownish color. Also note eczema, stasis dermatitis (dry scaling), induration and scarring from previous ulceration, and the color of the legs when dependent. Note the location of ulcers, their color, size, shape, and depth, and the presence of drainage or odor (see Table 4–6) (see Chapter 18).

Palpation

The examiner may palpate a fascial defect along the course of the affected vein representing the site of an incompetent perforator.

Auscultation

As in the upper extremities, auscultation with a stethoscope is not beneficial except in case of injury.

SUMMARY

The mainstay of diagnosis of vascular disease remains a good history and physical examination. Assessment of the vascular system is one of the fundamental activities of nursing practice. Its importance is paramount in providing quality nursing care as well as in initiating the nurse-patient relationship. In addition, the assessment provides the foundation of the nursing process: assessment, diagnosis, planning, implementation, and evaluation.

See Chapter 3 for assessment for lymphedema.

References

1. Ekers M: Psychosocial considerations in peripheral vascular disease. In Beaver BM, Wagner MW (eds): Nursing Clinics of North America: Peripheral Vascular Dysfunction. Philadelphia, WB Saunders, 1986, 255–263.
2. Benjamin ME, Dean RH: Examination of the patient with vascular disease. In Dean RH, Yao JST, Brewster DC (eds): Current Diagnosis and Treatment in Vascular Surgery. Norwalk, CT, Appleton & Lange, 1995, pp 1–4.
3. Casey J, Flinn WR, Yao JST, et al: Correlation of immune and nutritional status with wound complications in patients undergoing vascular operations. Surgery 1983; 93:822–827.
4. Ronayne R: Chronic illness. In Baumann A, Johnston WE, Antai-Otong D (eds): Decision Making in Psychiatric and Psychosocial Nursing. Toronto, BC Decker, 1990, pp 212–213.
5. Imparato AM: Carotid endarterectomy: Indications and techniques for carotid surgery. In Haimovici H (ed): Vascular Surgery: Principles and Techniques, 4th ed. Cambridge, Blackwell Science, 1996, pp 913–937.
6. Hallett JW, Brewster DC, Darling RC: Patient Care in Vascular Surgery, 2nd ed. Boston, Little, Brown & Co, 1987.
7. Young JR: Physical examination. In Young JR, Graor RA, Olin JW, et al: Peripheral Vascular Diseases. St. Louis, Mosby-Year Book, 1996, pp 18–32.
8. Pousti TJ, Wilson SE, Williams RA: The clinical examination of the vascular system. In Veith FJ, Hobson RW, Williams RA, Wilson SE, et al (eds): Vascular Surgery Principles and Practice. New York, McGraw-Hill Book Co, 1994, pp 74–89.
9. Porter JM, Edwards JM: Occlusive and vasospastic diseases involving distal upper extremity arteries—Raynaud's syndrome. In Rutherford RB (ed): Vascular Surgery, 4th ed. Philadelphia, WB Saunders, 1995, pp 961–975.
10. Nicolaides AN: Assessment of leg ischaemia. BMJ 1991; 303(11):1323–1326.
11. Allen, EV: Thromboangitis obliterans: Method of diagnosis of chronic occlusive arterial lesions distal to the wrist with illustrative cases. Am J Med Sci 1929; 178:237–244.
12. Conn J, Bergan JJ, Bell JL: Hypothenar hammer syndrome: Posttraumatic digital ischemia. Surgery 1970; 68:1122–1127.
13. Meacham PW, Dean RH, Smith BM: Vascular Physical Diagnosis: The Arterial System. Division of Vascular Surgery, Vanderbilt University School of Medicine, 1985.
14. Fairbairn JF: Clinical manifestations of peripheral vascular disease. In Juergens JL, Spittell JA, Fairbairn JF (eds): Peripheral Vascular Diseases, 2nd ed. Philadelphia, WB Saunders, 1980, pp 3–49.
15. Rutherford RB: The vascular consultation. In Rutherford RB (ed): Vascular Surgery, 4th ed. Philadelphia, WB Saunders, 1995, pp 1–10.
16. Callow AD: Clinical assessment of the peripheral circulation. In Callow AD, Ernst CB (eds): Vascular Surgery: Theory and Practice. Norwalk, CT, Appleton & Lange, 1995, pp 181–199.
17. Warren R: Two kinds of intermittent claudication [Editorial]. Arch Surg 1976; 111:739.
18. DeWeese JA: Pedal pulses disappearing with exercise. N Engl J Med 1960; 262:1214–1217.
19. Gloviczki P, Kaymier FJ, Hollier LH: Axillary-subcutaneous venous occlusion: The morbidity of a nonlethal disease. J Vasc Surg 1986; 4:333–337.

20. DeWeese JA: Clinical examination of patients with venous disesase. In Gloviczki P, Yao JST (eds): Handbook of Venous Disorders. London, Chapman & Hall, 1996, pp 63–80.
21. Yao JST: Non-invasive investigation of vascular disease. Curr Pract Surg 1989; 1:244–252.
22. O'Donnell TF, Abbott WM, Athanasoulis CA, et al: Diagnosis of deep venous thrombosis in the outpatient by venography. Surg Gynecol Obstet 1980; 150:69–74.

5

Noninvasive Vascular Testing

Donna R. Blackburn, RN, MS, RVT, and Linda Kennedy, RN, RVT

∽ · ∽

The past several decades have seen the emergence of noninvasive testing as a standard of care for the vascular patient. These techniques were designed to aid the clinician in the diagnosis and follow-up of peripheral vascular disease. Although not all-inclusive, the information provided in this chapter will familiarize the vascular nurse with the fundamentals of noninvasive testing.

INSTRUMENTATION

Instrumentation currently available in the vascular laboratory provides both hemodynamic and anatomic information about the peripheral vascular system. The methods employed are primarily diagnostic ultrasonography, including imaging, and several forms of plethysmography.

Ultrasonography

Sound travels in waves that, when they strike a surface, are reflected back. In the 1800s, Christian Doppler noted that there is a change in sound frequency in relation to a moving source.[1] This change can be noted in the whistle of a moving train as it approaches and passes.

Sound is the result of vibration. One complete vibration is known as a cycle, and the number of cycles per second is called frequency. Frequency is expressed in hertz (Hz). One hertz is one cycle per second. Ultrasound has a frequency greater than that detectable by the human ear (greater than 20,000 Hz). Most ultrasonographic instruments used in the vascular laboratory employ ranges of 2 to 10 MHz (million cycles per second).

Doppler Ultrasonography

Piezoelectric crystals are contained in the Doppler transducer. An electrical voltage applied to the crystal causes it to vibrate, producing ultrasound waves. When the transmitted waves strike moving red blood cells, sound is reflected back to the transducer. Ultrasound reflected from moving red blood cells is shifted in frequency in an amount proportional to the velocity of the moving blood. The difference in frequency between the transmitted and the received signals is the Doppler-shifted frequency. Flow moving toward the transducer reflects sound at a higher frequency than that transmitted. Conversely, lower frequencies than those transmitted are reflected from receding flow. The directional Doppler instrument has the capability of sensing flow direction by detecting these frequency changes.

Continuous-Wave Doppler Transducer. The continuous-wave Doppler transducer contains both a transmitting and a receiving crystal, which operate continuously. Flow at any point in the path of the sound beam will be detected with this device (Fig. 5–1).

Pulsed Doppler Transducer. One crystal acts as both a transmitter and a receiver in the pulsed Doppler transducer. Short pulses of sound are transmitted at regular intervals. The returning signal is received at specific times between transmissions (Fig. 5–2). The number of pulse repetitions per second can be varied with this system to allow sampling at a specific depth and site.

Signal Processing. Three methods are commonly used to process Doppler-derived signals: audible output, zero crossing technique, and spectrum analysis (Fig. 5–3).

Audio Analysis. The signal may be interpreted audibly with either a loudspeaker or earphones. This method is subjective and requires that the examiner be experienced in understanding normal and abnormal flow characteristics.

Zero Crossing Technique. The zero crossing technique converts the audio signal to an analog tracing. This method produces an output voltage proportional to that of the zero crossings of reflected ultrasound waves.

Spectrum Analysis. Spectrum analysis displays the entire frequency and amplitude content of the Doppler signal. Time is displayed on the horizontal axis, frequency on the vertical axis, and amplitude is represented by gray-scale brightness.

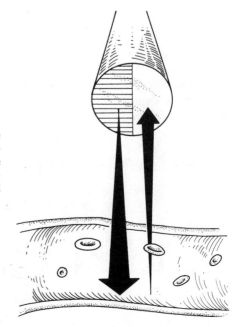

Figure 5–1. Schematic illustration of a continuous-wave Doppler transducer. One crystal continuously emits an ultrasound beam; the other crystal continuously receives the backscattered signal. (From Pomajzl JM: Real-Time Ultrasound Imaging and Pulsed/Gated Doppler Instructional Manual. Indianapolis, Biosound, Inc., 1984, p 35.)

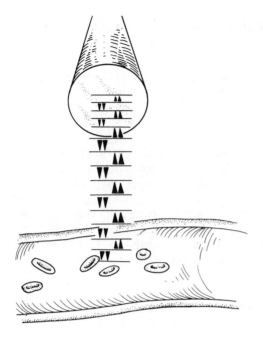

Figure 5–2. Schematic illustration of a pulsed Doppler transducer. The same crystal acts intermittently as both a transmitter and a receiver. (From Pomajzl MJ: Real-Time Ultrasound Imaging and Pulsed/Gated Doppler Instructional Manual. Indianapolis, Biosound, Inc., 1984, p 35.)

B-Mode Ultrasonography

B-mode (brightness mode) is a method of processing reflected ultrasound waves to produce a two-dimensional image. Ultrasound echoes reflected from tissue interfaces are displayed in shades of gray; the higher the density, the brighter the echoes. Because blood is a poor reflector of ultrasound, a blood vessel appears as an area of poor reflection surrounded by its walls, which are good reflectors. A rotating transducer within the scan head produces images in real time. Duplex systems combine real-time imaging and pulsed Doppler capabilities, thus providing both anatomic and physiologic information.

Color Duplex Imaging

Color imaging is actually a method of displaying Doppler-shifted frequencies with a pulse-echo technique. Echoes reflected from moving red blood cells are displayed with colors that correspond to direction of flow. Commonly, flow toward the transducer is displayed in red and flow away from the transducer is displayed in blue. As flow velocities increase at an area of stenosis, the color hue lightens, going from red to orange to yellow or from blue to aqua to white. Poststenotic turbulence is represented by a mosaic pattern of all

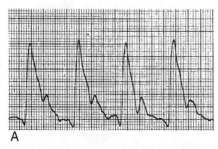
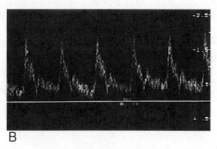

A   B

Figure 5–3. A, Output processed with the zero crossing technique. **B,** Spectrum analysis of the same signal.

colors. Color duplex systems superimpose color images on the standard gray scale image to provide simultaneous anatomic and hemodynamic information.

Plethysmography

Plethysmographs are used to directly or indirectly record volume changes in the limbs. The various plethysmographic devices available for use in the vascular laboratory differ in the type of transducer employed for assessing dimensional changes. Forms of plethysmography commonly used for limb volume measurement include air plethysmography and photoplethysmography (PPG).

Air Plethysmography

A pneumatic cuff is applied to the extremity and inflated to a relatively low pressure to assure skin contact. Volume changes within the limb result in pressure changes within the air-filled cuff.

Photoplethysmography

The PPG transducer contains a light-emitting diode and a phototransistor that detects back-scattered light. An infrared light beam is transmitted through the skin. Changes in cutaneous blood content alter the quantity of reflected light recorded by the photocell.

VENOUS TESTING: ACUTE

Noninvasive techniques can be used to detect obstruction in the venous system of both the upper and lower extremities. Venous imaging has shown excellent correlation with venography in the diagnosis of deep venous thrombosis.[2] In addition to furnishing hemodynamic information, scanning provides the added ability to visualize and localize thrombus.

The patient exhibiting acute unilateral extremity pain or edema is a candidate for venous testing.[3] Testing is also indicated if pulmonary embolus is suspected. Venous testing is routinely performed in patients at high risk for development of deep venous thrombosis.

Venous Imaging Technique: Lower Extremity

The examination is performed with the patient in a supine position. The transducer is placed in a transverse orientation over the common femoral vein. Light probe pressure is applied to determine if the walls of the vein compress against each other. The transducer is moved slowly down the common femoral, greater saphenous, superficial femoral, and popliteal veins, assessing for vessel compressibility every one or two centimeters. If calf swelling is present, the posterior tibial, gastrocnemius, and peroneal veins are also assessed; Doppler flow characteristics are evaluated at the common femoral, superficial femoral, and popliteal veins.

Interpretation

Characteristics evaluated include vessel size, compressibility, flow patterns, presence of thrombus, and valve function. The normal vein has thinner walls and is slightly larger than the corresponding artery. Vein diameter fluctuates with the respiratory cycle and vessel size is augmented by a Valsalva maneuver. Normal veins compress with light pressure with the transducer (Fig. 5–4A and B). In acute deep vein thrombosis, the vein usually appears dilated, soft echoes may be seen within the lumen of the vein, and the vein will not compress (Fig. 5–5). In very fresh thrombosis or in obstruction in a proximal vein, the vein may appear black (normal), but the vein does not compress. With chronic thrombosis, the vein does not appear dilated, and bright echoes can be seen along the walls of the vein. The vein is partially compressible, and respiratory variation is present.

The normal venous signal is spontaneous and phasic with respiration. Changes in intra-abdominal pressure caused by respiratory movement of the diaphragm create phasic variations in the venous signal in the extremity. In the presence of deep venous thrombosis, flow signals are continuous or absent. Pulsatility of the leg veins is an abnormal finding most commonly seen in patients with congestive heart failure or fluid overload.

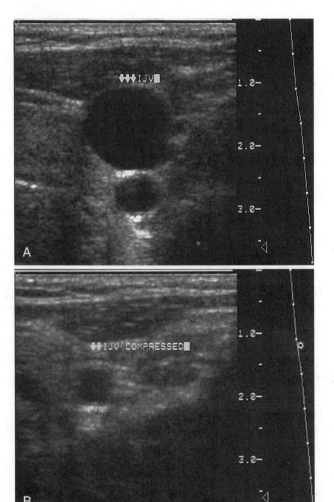

Figure 5–4. A, Duplex image of a normal internal jugular vein (IJV). **B**, Duplex image of the internal jugular vein with light probe pressure. Walls of the vein compress together, indicating a thrombus-free lumen.

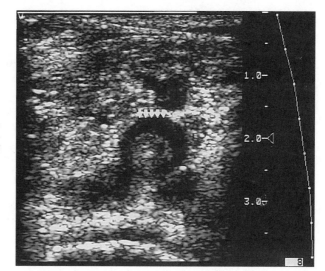

Figure 5–5. Venous image obtained with a duplex imager. The arrows indicate the venous wall. Thrombus *(speckled area)* is noted within the lumen.

Limitations

Scanning may be difficult in obese or extremely muscular patients, and small calf veins may not be easily visualized.

Venous Imaging Technique: Upper Extremity

Although deep venous thrombosis in the upper extremity is uncommon, routine use of central venous catheters has led to an increased incidence of upper-extremity venous thrombosis. Upper-extremity venous scanning is indicated in patients with edema of the arm or neck. The brachial, axillary, subclavian, and jugular veins are examined when thrombosis is suspected.

The patient is placed in a supine position with the head of the bed flat. The internal jugular, innominate, subclavian, axillary, and brachial veins are sequentially scanned. Doppler flow patterns are evaluated at all levels. Compression maneuvers are performed over all segments not lying beneath a bony prominence.

Interpretation

Interpretation criteria are the same as those used in the lower extremity except that the Doppler signals in the internal jugular, innominate, and subclavian veins are normally pulsatile due to their proximity to the heart.

Limitations

Central lines and bony structures make it difficult to evaluate clearly all portions of the venous system in the upper extremity.

VENOUS TESTING: CHRONIC

The veins are equipped with one-way valves that open to permit the flow of venous blood toward the heart. If the valves become damaged or the veins stretched, the valves may no longer close adequately and reflux flow will occur.

Venous refill after exercise normally occurs as a result of arterial inflow across the capillary bed and is thus prolonged. Reflux flow through incompetent valves results in rapid postexercise refilling times.

Photoplethysmographic techniques assess venous valve function by detecting changes in cutaneous blood volume. Changes in tissue opacity beneath the photocell result in a baseline shift when recorded on a strip chart.

Testing for venous valve function is indicated in the patient with stasis changes on the skin of the lower leg, varicose veins, nonhealing venous ulcers, or chronic lower-extremity edema after documented deep vein thrombosis.

Photoplethysmography

Technique

The patient is seated with the legs in a dependent, non–weight-bearing position. A PPG photocell is attached with double-faced tape to the skin just above the medial malleolus (Fig. 5–6). The patient is instructed to dorsiflex and plantarflex the feet five times and then to relax the limbs completely. If the patient is unable to exercise adequately, manual calf compression can be performed by the examiner. The superficial venous system may be occluded by application of a cuff or tourniquet at thigh or calf level, and the procedure repeated.

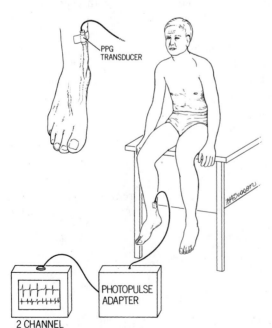

PPG
TRANSDUCER

PHOTOPULSE
ADAPTER

2 CHANNEL
RECORDER

Figure 5–6. The photoplethysmography (PPG) examination is performed with the patient's legs dangling and the transducer applied to the medial aspect of the ankle.

Interpretation

Recovery time is defined as the number of seconds required for the postexercise recovery curve to achieve a stable baseline (Fig. 5–7). A recovery time of 25 seconds or more is normal. Superficial incompetence is demonstrated by a recovery time of less than 20 seconds that normalizes after cuff application. A recovery time of less than 20 seconds both before and after tourniquet application indicates venous valve incompetence in the deep or perforating systems.[4]

Limitations

Probe placement may have to be altered in the patient with a stasis ulcer in the malleolar area.

Direct Venous Pressure Measurement

Although invasive in nature, direct venous pressure measurements are performed in the vascular laboratory. This procedure continues to be the most reliable method for evaluation of venous function in the lower extremities.

Technique

A dorsal vein in the foot is cannulated, and venous pressure is measured with the patient either standing or sitting with the legs hanging in a dependent position. The patient is then instructed to walk in place for 15 seconds if standing or to dorsiflex and plantarflex the foot five times if seated.

Interpretation

Normally, venous pressure drops by 50 to 100 percent with exercise, and the time for return to baseline pressure exceeds 20 seconds. In the patient with venous reflux, there will be a diminished pressure drop and a recovery time of less than 20 seconds. If venous occlusion is present, there will be no drop in venous pressure with exercise.

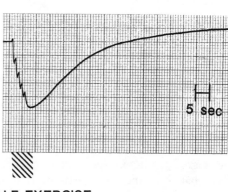

Figure 5–7. Normal photoplethysmography (PPG) curve. After exercise, there is a gradual refilling of the venous bed.

CALF EXERCISE

Limitations

The technique is a painful one, and frequently the veins of the foot cannot be easily cannulated. The procedure therefore has limited use in the clinical setting.

ARTERIAL TESTING

Noninvasive techniques have been developed to document the presence and evaluate the severity and location of arterial disease in the upper and lower extremities. These modalities provide physiologic information in contrast to arteriography, which provides anatomic information. Indications for arterial testing include screening patients for disease, defining severity of disease, and follow-up.

Screening

Palpation of pulses is one of the hallmarks of a vascular physical examination. Pulses may not be easily palpable, however, because of an examiner's inexperience or the presence of aberrant anatomy, edema, or arterial occlusive disease.

Definition of Severity of Disease

Noninvasive techniques provide a quantitative method to determine the severity of the disease process, especially with lesser degrees of disease, in which pulses may be diminished, and in patients whose distal pulses are absent.

Follow-up

Serial examinations provide assessment of graft patency and disease progression in surgically treated patients. This is especially helpful in patients with multilevel disease, in whom pulses may not reappear after surgery at one level. Serial examinations also allow evaluation of medical or exercise regimens and evaluation of the development of collateral circulation.

Doppler-Derived Analog Waveforms

A continuous-wave bidirectional Doppler transducer is coupled with a zero crossing detector. The audible signals are processed so that a permanent record is generated.

Technique

By examining the arterial system at various sites, one can locate the diseased segment. Examination of the lower extremities is performed with the patient supine. The vessels assessed are the common femoral, popliteal, dorsalis pedis, and posterior tibial arteries.

Interpretation

The normal arterial signal has a sharp systolic component and one or more diastolic components (Fig. 5–8A). This waveform implies relatively normal flow in an elastic, unobstructed artery. Minor degrees of stenosis do not usually alter this waveform significantly.

As the vessel becomes narrowed, the diastolic components disappear and the systolic component becomes wider (Fig. 5–8B). In the occluded vessel, the systolic component of the waveform becomes blunted and there are no diastolic components (Fig. 5–8C). An abnormal signal indicates disease proximal to the site at which that signal was obtained. In the patient with iliac disease, waveforms and signals will be abnormal at all levels (Fig. 5–9). With a superficial femoral artery occlusion, the common femoral artery will be normal and the popliteal and distal sites will be abnormal. The degree of abnormality will depend on the collateral flow and the state of the distal vessels. When multilevel disease is present, there will be a change in the waveform from one level to the next.

Sequential Volume Plethysmography

Pneumatic cuffs are placed at various levels on an extremity. A standardized quantity of air is used to slightly inflate the cuff. Volume changes that occur beneath the cuff are detectable and are converted to pulsatile pressure changes. These changes are recorded for analysis.

Technique

With the patient supine, a small cushion is placed beneath the heels. A large thigh cuff is placed on the thigh as far proximally as possible. Smaller cuffs are placed around the calf and at the ankle. Cuffs are inflated one level at a time to a pressure of 65 mmHg. Volume recordings are made at each site for five or six cardiac cycles.

Interpretation

Strandness described the changes that occur in the volume pulse recordings with occlusive disease (Fig. 5–10)[5]:

1. Normal—sharp systolic peak; prominent dicrotic wave.
2. Mildly abnormal—sharp systolic peak; absent dicrotic wave; downslope bowed away from baseline.
3. Moderately abnormal—flattened systolic peak; upslope and downslope nearly equal; dicrotic wave invariably absent.

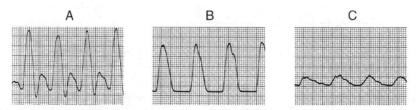

Figure 5–8. Analog recordings obtained over normal **(A)**, stenotic **(B)**, and occluded **(C)** vessels.

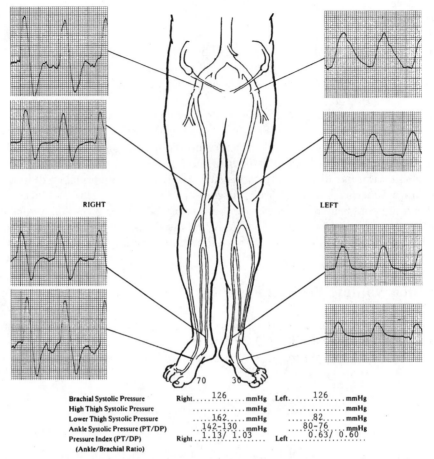

Brachial Systolic Pressure	Right......126......mmHg	Left......126.....mmHg
High Thigh Systolic Pressure	..............mmHg	..............mmHg
Lower Thigh Systolic Pressure	......162.....mmHg	......82......mmHg
Ankle Systolic Pressure (PT/DP)	...142-130...mmHg	...80-76...mmHg
Pressure Index (PT/DP)	Right 1.13/ 1.03	Left 0.63/ 0.60
(Ankle/Brachial Ratio)		

Figure 5–9. Analog tracings and systolic pressures obtained in a patient with a left iliac occlusion. The right side is normal.

4. Severely abnormal—pulse wave of very low amplitude or entirely absent; if present, equal upslope and downslope time.

Analysis of the volume pulse recordings from the different levels can determine the location of the diseased arterial segment and provide an estimate of the severity of the disease process.

Segmental Pressures

Measurement of segmental pressures using a Doppler instrument is the most frequently used means of quantifying arterial flow.[6] Coupled with Doppler analog waveform analysis

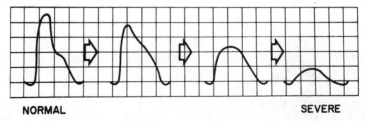

NORMAL   **SEVERE**

Figure 5–10. Volume pulse recordings illustrating progression of disease from normal to severe. (From Kempczinski RF, Yao JST (eds): Practical Noninvasive Vascular Diagnosis. Chicago, Year Book, 1987, p 141.)

or volume plethysmography, this method provides a thorough, concise examination in the vascular laboratory. Alone, these pressures are helpful to the practitioner in evaluation of the arterial system in an office, recovery room, or nursing unit.

Technique

With the patient supine and in a resting state, segmental cuffs are applied and systolic pressure measurements are recorded. A standard arm cuff is placed immediately above the ankle to procure measurements at the dorsalis pedis and posterior tibial arteries (Fig. 5–11). A standard thigh cuff is placed around the thigh to obtain a popliteal pressure. Bilateral brachial pressures are taken and the higher pressure is used for comparison.

Interpretation

Normally, the systolic pressure in the leg is equal to or slightly higher than the systolic arm pressure. This is due to the highly resistant vascular bed in the lower extremity. With occlusive disease, the systolic pressure drops proportionately to the severity of disease. The ratio of the segmental pressure to the systolic arm pressure provides a method of quantifying the severity of disease.[7] This can be applied to all pressures; however, most frequently used is the ankle-brachial pressure index (ABI). In addition, this index is necessary for comparison with the previous studies because the systemic pressures will vary from one examination to another. This ratio is proportional to the degree of ischemia present (Table 5–1).

ABI changes within a 0.15 range are considered to be within normal limits because of changes in pressures and examiners. A change in ABI greater than 0.15 indicates a significant improvement or deterioration. Importantly, ankle pressures obtained postoperatively that do not increase by at least 0.15 indicate no improvement in arterial perfusion.[8]

A difference in pressure of more than 30 mmHg between segments indicates disease. The popliteal pressure is especially useful in predicting healing in patients undergoing

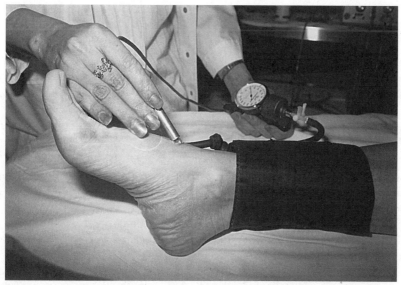

Figure 5–11. Measurement of ankle pressure with the Doppler probe placed over the dorsalis pedis artery.

TABLE 5–1. **Ankle-Brachial Pressure Ratio (ABI): An Index of ABI Disease Severity**

Normal	1.0–0.95
Mildly abnormal	0.95–0.80
Claudicant	0.75–0.40
Ischemic	<0.40

amputation. If the thigh pressure exceeds 60 mmHg, the probability is high that a below-knee amputation site will heal.

Limitations

Calcification of the arterial wall prevents accurate pressure measurements. Pressures can be falsely elevated (frequently to above 300 mmHg) because of an incompressible vessel. This condition is most frequently seen in patients with diabetes and chronic renal failure. A prosthetic distal graft, if tunneled through soft tissue, will be incompressible. Pressure measurements in these patients are invalid, and diagnosis must be based on waveform signal analysis.

Toe Pressure Measurements

Technique

Great toe measurements are frequently performed to assess distal arterial flow. This is especially useful in diabetics in whom calcification of the larger vessels is present. A 2.5 × 9 cm cuff is placed proximally on the toe. The distal arterial signal is obtained with a Doppler transducer or a plethysmograph. A systolic pressure is then obtained.

Interpretation

The normal toe pressure is 60 mmHg.[9] The toe pressure is useful in predicting healing of toe and forefoot wounds and toe amputation sites. If the toe pressure exceeds 30 mmHg, chances that a forefoot wound or amputation site will heal are high.

Stress Testing

Stress testing is indicated when resting flows are not grossly abnormal, when symptoms do not correlate with the resting flows, and in cases of back disturbances that may simulate claudication (neurogenic claudication).

Two methods of evaluating flow after stress are in standard use. The optimal method of stress testing involves performance of the activity associated with the patient's symptoms (i.e., walking). However, because of the average patient's older age, concomitant cardiac disease, and other associated diseases (arthritis, hypertension, etc.), exercise testing cannot be performed in all cases in which it is indicated. Reactive hyperemia testing may be performed in those patients who cannot undergo standard exercise testing. Whenever possible, exercise is the choice for stress testing. Because of the high percentage of concomitant cardiac disease, cardiac monitoring during exercise is strongly recommended.

Exercise Testing

Technique

After resting studies are performed, the patient is asked to walk at a standardized speed and grade (1.4 mph at a 10 percent grade) until disabling claudication occurs. A maximal walking time of 5 minutes is standard. After exercise, the ankle pressure (measured over the dorsalis pedis or posterior tibial artery) is recorded in each limb at 1-minute intervals until pre-exercise levels are reached. Measurements are terminated if resting levels are not reached in 10 minutes.

Interpretation

Normally flow increases with exercise. In the diseased state, flow and pressure decrease distal to a stenosis. This pressure drop is proportional to the severity of the disease and will be of the greatest magnitude with multilevel disease.

Reactive Hyperemia

Technique

A cuff is positioned around the thigh and inflated to a suprasystolic level. This pressure is maintained for 3–5 minutes. Ankle pressures are measured immediately after cuff release and every 30 seconds until preocclusion levels are reached.

Interpretation

Because the limb is totally ischemic during cuff occlusion, normal subjects will exhibit a slight drop in distal pressure in the immediate postocclusion period. However, they will show a return to preocclusion levels within 1 or 2 minutes. In the diseased patient, it will take more than 2 minutes for preocclusion pressures to be reached.

Peripheral Arterial Scanning

Images generated from the duplex scanner provide anatomic as well as hemodynamic information and can precisely locate diseased segments. Duplex imaging is most commonly used as a guide in localizing and grading the severity of stenosis in patients with known peripheral vascular disease. The technique should be used in conjunction with standard analog waveforms and segmental pressures.

Technique

A 5-MHz linear transducer is used to evaluate the upper and lower extremities. A low-frequency abdominal probe is required for examination of the aortoiliac segment. Each vessel is interrogated along its entire length. Doppler velocity samples are recorded before stenosis, at the stenosis, and after stenosis.

Interpretation

A greater than 100 percent increase in velocity between the proximal and stenotic segments or a peak systolic velocity of more than 100 cm/sec is consistent with a 50–99 percent reduction in diameter.

Arterial Graft Assessment

Duplex imaging provides a means for determining the patency and hemodynamics of arterial bypass grafts.

Indications

Bypass grafts should be examined in the immediate postoperative period and at least yearly thereafter. Imaging is also indicated if there is a drop in ABI values, new claudication has developed, or a bruit or thrill is noted over the graft.

Technique

The graft is examined in the longitudinal plane from the proximal to distal anastomosis. Doppler velocity recordings and vessel diameter measurements are made throughout the length of the graft and in both the inflow and outflow vessels.

Interpretation

A focal increase in peak systolic velocity in association with spectral broadening is indicative of diameter reduction in the graft.

Upper Extremity

Many of the same principles and techniques used for assessing the lower extremity are applied to the arm. Indications for upper-extremity evaluation include decreased or absent distal pulses, a pressure gradient of more than 20 mmHg between arms, pain on exercising, frank ischemic changes (pallor, cyanosis, pregangrenous or gangrenous changes), and nonhealing wounds.

Techniques and Interpretation

Doppler waveforms are recorded at the axillary, brachial, radial, and ulnar arteries. Pressures are taken over the brachial, radial, and ulnar arteries. There should be no more than 30 mmHg difference between segments of the same arm or between segments of one arm and like segments of the opposite arm. Normal and abnormal waveforms are analyzed in a manner similar to that used in the lower extremity.

The palmar arch is assessed by means of a modified Allen test. The Doppler probe is placed in the flexion crease of the palm to locate the signal over the palmar arch. Alternate radial and ulnar artery compressions are then performed.

Normally the palmar arch is supplied by both the ulnar and radial arteries. With compression of one artery, a signal remains in the palmar arch. If the arch is totally dependent on one vessel, the signal in the palmar arch will obliterate with compression. Although an incomplete arch (supplied by only one vessel) is present in 20 percent of normal subjects, it is an important finding.[10] Thus arterial punctures of the dominant artery should never be performed. It is important to inform the patient of this finding, should an arterial puncture be required in the future.

Digital Pressures

Technique

A digital cuff is placed proximally on the finger, and the distal arterial signal is obtained with a Doppler device or plethysmograph. Systolic pressures are recorded in this manner on each digit.

Interpretation

The digital pressure should be equal to that of the next proximal recording point. There should be less than 20 mmHg difference between digits and between the next proximal recording point. With proximal disease, all digits will have equal reductions in pressure. In digital arterial occlusions, the affected digits will have relatively lower pressures (Fig. 5–12).

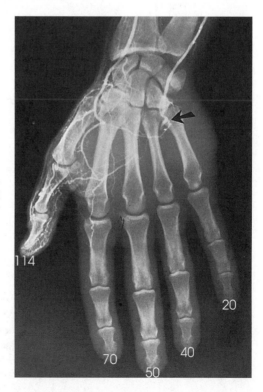

Figure 5–12. Upper-extremity arteriogram demonstrates distal ulnar artery occlusion *(arrow)*. No digital arteries are visualized in the fingers, and all finger pressures are abnormal.

Cold Sensitivity

Cold-sensitivity testing may be added to the upper-extremity examination in those patients whose presenting symptom is hypersensitivity to cold. A standard upper-extremity examination, including digital pressures, should be performed to exclude an organic cause of these symptoms. If the standard examination is normal, testing for Raynaud's disease is indicated.

Technique

Thermistor sensors are attached to the distal portion of each finger. Baseline temperatures are recorded in each digit. The hands are then submerged in ice water for 20 seconds. Temperatures are taken immediately after the ice bath and every 5 minutes thereafter until pre-ice temperatures are regained.

Interpretation

Normal digits will rewarm in 20 minutes or less. In the patient with Raynaud's disease, digital temperatures will remain below pre-ice bath levels for more than 20 minutes (Fig. 5–13). In those with Raynaud's disease, all fingers are usually affected. In patients with digital artery occlusion, only the affected digits will have a prolonged recovery time.

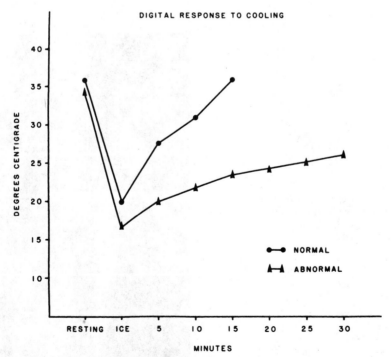

Figure 5–13. Digital temperature recovery times in normal subjects and in those with cold sensitivity. (From Bartel P, Blackburn DR, Peterson LK, et al: The value of noninvasive tests in occupational trauma of the hands and fingers. Bruit 1984; 8:15–18.)

Thoracic Outlet Evaluation

Arterial compression at the thoracic outlet may cause pain, pallor, and pulselessness in the upper extremity. Although obliteration of arterial flow with the arm in an exaggerated position occurs in a percentage of the population, it rarely produces symptoms.

Indications

Patients with complaints of pain and paresthesia in the upper extremity are candidates for thoracic outlet testing. In addition, young patients with ischemia of the hand should be evaluated for the presence of thoracic outlet syndrome. Aneurysms of the subclavian artery caused by the intermittent arterial compression in thoracic outlet syndrome may develop. Frequently, the first symptom is digital ischemia caused by embolization from the aneurysm.

Technique

The study is conducted with the patient in a sitting position. A photoplethysmograph is placed on one finger of each hand, and a tracing of the arterial pulse is made. The arms are then moved to a 90° horizontal position, then to directly over the head (180°), and then to an exaggerated military position, with the arms bent at the elbow and the shoulders thrust back. Tracings are obtained in each position. The patient is also asked to put the arms in the position that causes symptoms.

Interpretation

Obliteration of the arterial pulse in any position indicates compression of the artery and is considered positive. Diminution of the arterial pulse is not considered a positive result.

Limitations

Although arterial compression may not occur, the vein or nerve may be compressed, resulting in symptoms. This procedure documents the presence or absence of only arterial compression at the thoracic outlet.

Cavernosal Duplex Imaging

Duplex imaging is employed to directly image and assess flow characteristics in the cavernosal arteries to determine the cause of impotence. Erectile dysfunction can be caused by arterial insufficiency, venous leak, nerve dysfunction, psychogenic causes, or a combination of these.

Technique

A color duplex system with a high-frequency transducer is used to obtain vessel diameter measurements and flow velocities both before and after an intracavernosal injection of 30 mg of papaverine or 10 μg of prostaglandin E_1.

Interpretation

Normally, vessel diameter will increase after injection by 50 percent, peak systolic velocities will increase 100 percent and are greater than 25 cm/sec, and the end-diastolic velocities are below 5 cm/sec.

Arterial insufficiency is demonstrated by the fact that diameter does not increase by 50 percent and the peak systolic velocities do not increase by 100 percent and do not reach 25 cm/sec. A venous leak is indicated when the vessel diameter increases by 50 percent, the peak systolic velocities increase by 100 percent and are above 25 cm/sec, but the end-diastolic velocities are greater than 5 cm/sec.[11]

Splanchnic System

Indications

Indications for mesenteric scanning include postprandial abdominal pain (intestinal angina), unexplained weight loss, or an abdominal bruit.[12]

Technique

Patients should receive nothing by mouth at least 8 hours before examination. It is preferable for patients to have these studies early in the morning after an overnight fast. A low-frequency transducer, usually 3 MHz, is required to examine the deep abdominal vessels. With the patient in the supine position, the scan head is placed just below the xyphoid process; the supraceliac aorta is identified, and Doppler velocity signals are recorded. The celiac trunk is the first visceral branch of the aorta. The superior mesenteric artery (SMA) arises anteriorly from the aorta just distal to the celiac trunk (Fig. 5–14). These vessels are interrogated, and Doppler velocity samples are obtained. After the fasting examination, stress testing may be performed on patients with equivocal studies. A high-calorie liquid meal (8 oz Ensure Plus or an equivalent product) is ingested by the patient. The celiac trunk and the SMA are restudied 30–40 minutes postprandially.

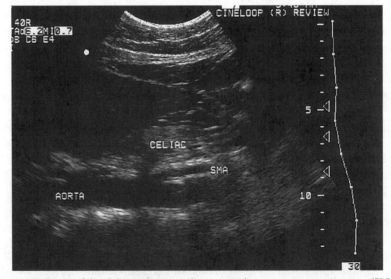

Figure 5–14. Image of the abdominal aorta, celiac axis, and superior mesenteric artery (SMA).

Interpretation

The normal celiac signal demonstrates forward flow throughout diastole with a window below the spectral wave. Both systolic and diastolic flow velocities will normally increase after a test meal. A peak systolic velocity of more than 200 cm/sec is indicative of a stenosis of 70 percent or more.

The normal SMA signal in a fasting patient is biphasic or triphasic. Postprandially, both systolic and diastolic flow velocities will increase and the signal will convert to a lower resistance pattern because of peripheral vasodilation in the gut. A peak systolic velocity of more than 275 cm/sec in a fasting patient indicates a greater than 70 percent stenosis of the SMA.[13]

Limitations

Studies may be inadequate because of obesity, excessive bowel gas, and/or recent abdominal surgery.

Renovascular System

Indications

Renal artery imaging is indicated in patients in whom renovascular hypertension is suspected.

Technique

Patients should maintain at least an 8-hour fast before examination. The procedure is performed with a low-frequency transducer while the patient is in the supine position. The juxtarenal aorta is identified, and flow velocities from both renal arteries are recorded while a 60° angle of insonation is maintained.

Interpretation

The renal artery Doppler signal normally demonstrates continuous flow throughout diastole, like that seen in the internal carotid artery. Vessel stenosis causes an increase in flow velocity. A ratio of the peak systolic velocity (PSV) in the renal artery and the aorta is calculated.

$$\frac{\text{PSV renal artery}}{\text{PSV aorta}} = \text{Renal/aortic ratio}$$

A ratio greater than 3.5 indicates a greater than 60 percent renal artery stenosis.[14]

CEREBROVASCULAR EXAMINATIONS

Noninvasive studies that examine the extracranial carotid artery are divided into two groups: those that examine the carotid artery directly and those that assess flow through the carotid artery indirectly by examination of its distal branches. By far the most common diagnostic study is duplex imaging. Indirect testing is rarely done.

Carotid testing is indicated in patients with hemispheric symptoms of stroke; transient ischemic attacks; amaurosis fugax; and nonhemispheric symptoms, including dizziness, loss of memory, drop attacks, and blurred vision; and in patients with an asymptomatic bruit. These procedures are helpful in the detection of operable lesions and disease progression in medically treated patients. Routine follow-up examinations after endarterectomy permit early detection of restenosis of the carotid artery.

Cerebrovascular Duplex Examination

The most accurate way to detect disease in the extracranial carotid and vertebral arteries is by direct assessment of the vessels.[15] Duplex imaging provides direct visualization of the vessels and Doppler assessment of flow characteristics. The images themselves provide anatomic information. High-resolution images allow for definition of plaque morphology. Soft versus calcified plaque can be defined and smooth plaque can be differentiated from irregular plaque and ulcerative lesions. Aberrant anatomy and vessel tortuosity can be defined. Because both vessel wall and residual lumen can be visualized, the percentage of diameter reduction can be accurately measured.

Technique

The examination is performed while the patient is in a supine position with the neck extended. The Doppler transducer is placed as low on the neck as possible, and a signal from the common carotid artery (CCA) is located. The probe is slowly advanced up the neck to the carotid bifurcation (approximately at the level of the thyroid cartilage). The signals from the internal carotid artery (ICA) and the external carotid artery (ECA) are located and recorded. These vessels are followed up to the level of the jaw. Following examination of the carotid vessels, the vertebral artery is evaluated by moving the transducer laterally from the CCA until the vertebral bodies are visualized. Flow signals are recorded in the vertebral artery between the vertebral bodies. The vessel should be examined from the upper neck to its origin at the subclavian. A Doppler signal is then recorded in the subclavian artery. The contralateral side is then evaluated in a similar fashion.

Interpretation

Normally, the intima is visualized throughout the common, internal, and external carotid arteries (Fig. 5–15). Normal flow signals are obtained in all vessels. In diseased states, plaque is identified and classified (Fig. 5–16). Diameter reduction is measured, and flow signals are evaluated.

Spectrum Analysis

Interpretation

Normal flow in an artery is laminar. Higher frequencies are found in the center of the vessel, whereas lower frequencies are found along the wall. This creates a parabolic curve (Fig. 5–17A). Frequencies will be similar throughout the vessel, creating a narrow band.

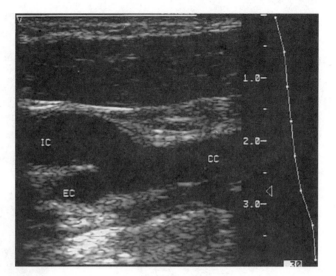

Figure 5–15. B-mode image of a normal carotid bifurcation. CC, common carotid artery; EC, external carotid artery; IC, internal carotid artery.

On the spectral display, there is an area of black (under this band). This is called the acoustic "window" and implies relatively normal flow (Fig. 5–17B). In lesser degrees of stenosis, the band of frequencies will be wider, showing more varying frequencies, but the window will still be present. In higher degrees of stenosed segment, many frequencies are present within the vessel. At the point of narrowing, the blood jets through the stenosed segment, creating high frequencies. In addition, just distal to the area of narrowing, flow becomes turbulent as the red blood cells bounce off the walls of the artery. This creates flow in many directions, and virtually all frequencies of sound can be found in this area (Fig. 5–17C). The spectral display will show high frequencies and loss of the acoustic window because of the many low and mid frequencies that are present (Fig. 5–17D). Frequencies and turbulence increase in proportion to the degree of stenosis. With total occlusion, no signal can be obtained in the vessel.

The ICA, ECA, and CCA all have individual normal flow characteristics. The ICA supplies a low-resistance vascular bed (the brain). The signals from the ICA, therefore, show constant flow, even in diastole. The ECA supplies a high-resistance bed (the scalp, face, and skin). Therefore the flow signal in the ECA sounds very much like that of a peripheral artery, where there is reversal of flow in diastole. The CCA has a combination

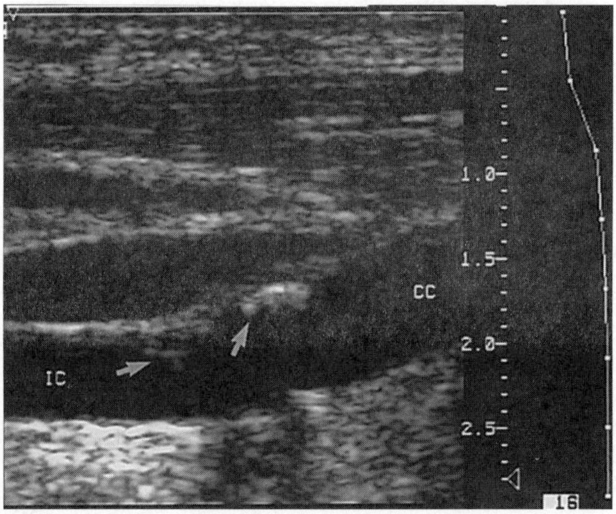

Figure 5–16. B-mode image of the internal carotid artery (IC) demonstrating plaque formation *(arrow)*. CC, common carotid artery.

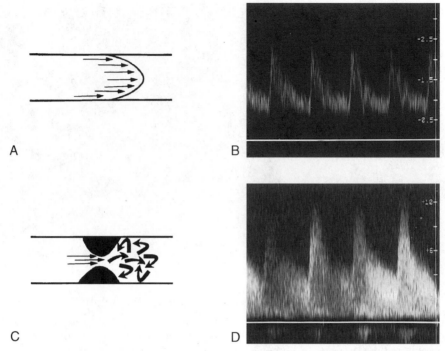

Figure 5–17. A, Normal parabolic curve. **B,** Normal spectral band with acoustic window present. **C,** Flow characteristics through and distal to a stenotic segment. **D,** Spectral display indicating severe stenosis. Frequencies are markedly elevated, and there is total loss of the acoustic window.

of the ICA and ECA flow characteristics. Table 5–2 shows the criteria for interpreting flow signals obtained in the ICA, with use of a 5-MHz pulsed Doppler instrument.

Limitations of Direct Testing

1. The accuracy of direct testing is dependent on technique of the examiner.
2. Aberrant anatomy can present problems; a skilled technologist can reduce these.
3. If the bifurcation is high in the neck, the ICA and the ECA may not be easily or adequately evaluated.
4. Technical difficulties may prevent adequate visualization of the vessels.
5. Direct testing is able to detect disease only below the angle of the jaw.

Transcranial Doppler Examination

The transcranial Doppler examination is one of the newer modalities.[16] It uses a low-frequency (2-MHz) pulsed Doppler transducer to assess the intracranial arteries. Duplex imaging may be used to assess these arteries.

Indications

Transcranial Doppler examination is used to assess the following:

1. Intracranial stenosis.
2. Collateral circulation in patients with ICA occlusions.
3. Vertebrobasilar insufficiency.
4. Cerebral vasospasm after subarachnoid hemorrhage.

TABLE 5–2. **Criteria for Interpreting Internal Carotid Artery (ICA)
Flow Signals Recorded with 5-mHz Pulsed Doppler**

Normal	Peak frequency is not in excess of 2 times the peak frequency in the common carotid artery. Normal acoustic window.
Less than 60% stenosis	Peak frequency is more than 2 times the common carotid peak frequency.
	Spectral band is widened.
	Acoustic window is present. End-diastolic frequency is less than 2.5 kHz.
60–80% stenosis	Peak frequency is more than 2 times common carotid artery peak frequency. Peak systolic frequency is >9.0 kHz.
	Loss of acoustic window (turbulent flow).
	End-diastolic frequency > 2.5 kHz but < 4.5 kHz.
81–99% stenosis	Peak frequency is more than 2 times common carotid artery peak frequency.
	Loss of acoustic window.
	End-diastolic frequency is above 4.5 kHz.
Total occlusion	Absence of signal in ICA.
	Common carotid artery is more resistant, when compared with the contralateral artery, because it is supplying only the external carotid artery. Signal may show reversal of flow in diastole, which is normally seen only in the external carotid artery.

Technique

Because ultrasound does not penetrate bone very well, several acoustic "windows" are used where the skull is thin (Fig. 5–18). The transtemporal window is used in assessing the middle cerebral artery, the anterior cerebral artery, and the posterior cerebral artery. The orbital window is used in evaluating the ophthalmic artery and the carotid siphon. The foramen magnum is used in evaluating the distal vertebral arteries and the basilar artery.

Interpretation

See Table 5–3.

QUALITY CONTROL

The noninvasive modalities discussed in this chapter have undergone extensive research regarding accuracy rates of the various examinations. These results are documented in the literature. Because most examinations are subjective and rely on the expertise of the examiner, these statistics should be used as a guideline for the examiner and the interpreter. The limitations of each examination should be understood. Each laboratory needs to evaluate its own results. Regular conferences in which laboratory results are compared with the "gold standard" are mandatory. Accuracy rates in each laboratory for each

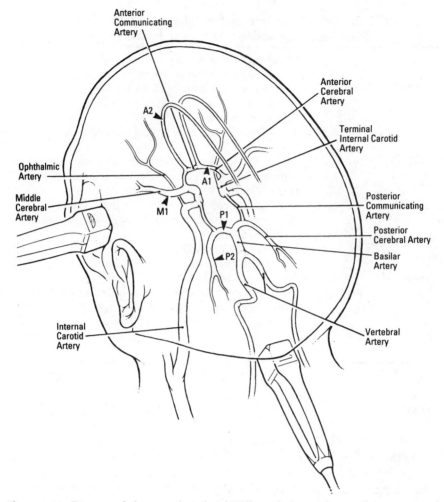

Figure 5–18. Diagram of the normal circle of Willis and the window used in transcranial examination. (From Advanced Technology Laboratories, Bothell, WA: Vascular Scanning Protocols, 1992.)

Table 5–3. **Normal Values and Flow Direction for Transcranial Examination**

VESSEL	MEAN VELOCITY (cm/sec)	DEPTH FROM PROBE	FLOW DIRECTION
MCA (M1)	62 ± 12	40–60 mm	Towards
ACA (A1)	50 ± 12	65–75 mm	Away
ICA	Varies	65 mm	Towards
PCA (P1), (P2)	42 ± 10	65–75 mm	Towards/away
Vertebral	36 ± 10	60–85 mm	Away
Basilar	39 ± 10	>85 mm	Away

MCA = middle cerebral artery; ACA = anterior cerebral artery; ICA = internal carotid artery; PCA = posterior cerebral artery.

From Advanced Technology Labs, Bothell, WA: Vascular Scanning Protocols, 1992.

procedure should be assessed; if these rates vary from those reported in the literature, re-examination of technique or interpretation must be made. Such evaluations will enhance the examiner's knowledge and improve the quality of these noninvasive procedures.

References

1. Doppler C: Abh K Bohm Ges Wiss 1842; 2:465.
2. Zwiebel WJ, Priest DL: Color duplex sonography of extremity veins. Semin Ultrasound CT MR 1990; 11:136–167.
3. Fowl RJ, Strothman GB, Blebea J, et al: Inappropriate use of venous duplex scans: An analysis of indications and results. J Vasc Surg 1996; 23(5):881–885.
4. Abramowitz HB, Queral LA, Finn WR, et al: The use of photoplethysmography in the assessment of venous insufficiency: A comparison to venous pressure measurements. Surgery 1979; 86:434–441.
5. Strandness DE: Peripheral Arterial Disease—A Physiologic Approach. Boston, Little, Brown & Co, 1969.
6. Aburahma AF, Khan S, Robinson PA, et al: Lower extremity arterial evaluation: Are segmental arterial blood pressures worthwhile? Surgery 1995; 118:496–503.
7. Lijmer JG, Hununk MG, van den Dungen JJ, et al: ROC analysis of noninvasive tests for peripheral arterial disease. Ultrasound Med Biol 1996; 22(4):391–398.
8. Yao JST, O'Mara CS, Flinn WR, et al: Postoperative evaluation of graft failure. In Bernhard VM, Towne JB (eds): Complications in Vascular Surgery. Orlando, Grune & Stratton, 1980, pp 1–19.
9. Ramsey DE, Manke DA, Sumner DS: Toe blood pressure: A valuable adjunct to ankle pressure measurement for assessing peripheral arterial disease. J Cardiovasc Surg 1983; 24:43–48.
10. Coleman SS, Anson BJ: Arterial patterns in the hand based upon a study of 650 specimens. Surg Gynecol Obstet 1961; 113:409–424.
11. Kadioglu A, Erdigru T, Karoidag K, et al: Evaluation of penile arterial system with color Doppler ultrasonography in nondiabetic and diabetic males. Eur Urol 1995; 27(4):311–314.
12. Flinn WR, Rizzo RJ, Park JS, et al: Duplex scanning for assessment of mesenteric ischemia. Surg Clin North Am 1990; 70:99–107.
13. Moneta G, Yeager RA, Dalman R, et al: Duplex ultrasound criteria for diagnosis of splanchnic artery stenosis or occlusion. J Vasc Surg 1991; 14:511–520.
14. Olin JW, Piedmonte MR, Young JR, et al: The utility of duplex ultrasound scanning of renal arteries for diagnosing significant renal artery stenosis. Ann Intern Med 1995; 122:833–838.
15. Moneta GL, Edwards IM, Papanicolaou G, et al: Screening for asymptomatic internal carotid artery stenosis: Duplex criteria for discriminating 60–99% stenosis. J Vasc Surg 1995; 21:989–994.
16. Aaslid R, Nornes H: Non-invasive transcranial Doppler ultrasound recording of flow velocity in basal cerebral arteries. J Neurosurg 1982; 57:769–774.

Additional Reading

Bernstein EF (ed): Vascular Diagnosis, 4th ed. St. Louis, CV Mosby, 1993.
Edelman S: Understanding Ultrasound Physics. Woodlands, TX, ESP, 1994.
Strandness DE: Duplex Scanning in Vascular Disorders. New York, Raven Press, 1993.
Talbot SR, Oliver M: Techniques in Venous Imaging. Pasadena, Appleton Davies, 1992.
Taylor KJW, Burns PN, Wells PNT (eds): Clinical Applications of Doppler Ultrasound. New York, Raven Press, 1988.
Zwiebel WJ: Introduction to Vascular Ultrasonography, 3rd ed. Philadelphia, WB Saunders, 1992.

6

Percutaneous Vascular Intervention and Imaging Techniques

Robert L. Vogelzang, MD

ᗉ · ᗂ

The imaging and percutaneous treatment of vascular disease has undergone exceptionally rapid change in the last 10 years and without much doubt will change even more in the next 5 as a result of the maturation of technologies that began in the 1970s. Up to that time, the radiographic identification and characterization of vascular disease were confined to conventional arteriography and venography. These techniques were strictly diagnostic, and the radiologist served in an adjunctive role in the treatment of these patients. It was in the early part of the 1970s that angioplasty and other techniques, which are now widely used, began to be taught and applied. These methods included angioplasty, transcatheter infusion for vascular thrombosis, and embolization for treatment of hemorrhage and control of tumor growth. Simultaneous with the development of these innovative percutaneous methods, imaging techniques such as computed tomography (CT), magnetic resonance imaging (MRI), and high-resolution digital subtraction angiography (DSA) were invented and disseminated. These advances enabled the interventional radiologist to see anatomic structures with significantly more clarity than had previously been possible. They also permitted complex interventions to be undertaken with far more confidence and assurance.

All these developments, however, essentially set the stage for the introduction of the metallic endoluminal stent, which in the 10 or so years since its approval for use in humans has revolutionized the field of vascular therapy. The stent has markedly expanded the range of vascular beds that can be effectively treated with percutaneous techniques including some such as the carotid artery that were strictly off-limits prior to this development. The addition of stent coverings to make stent-grafts has had an even greater impact so that aortic aneurysms are now treated without open surgery.

The addition of these new methods demands that appropriate indications be understood so that tests and treatments are not duplicated. With newer transcatheter intervention, different complications occur, sometimes with greater frequency than with conventional arteriography. This chapter addresses the indications for and techniques, complications, and results of these procedures, emphasizing the role of nursing in preprocedural assessment, periprocedural care, and postoperative management.

OVERVIEW OF INTERVENTIONAL RADIOLOGY NURSING

As interventional radiology has evolved as a specialty and as more complex procedures are performed on larger numbers of patients (many of whom are critically ill), the need for skilled, dedicated periprocedural nursing care has grown. As a result, a new nursing discipline has emerged. An interventional radiology nurse has a number of responsibilities, some of which are new to the field and others that involve the essential skills of nursing practice. On a personal level, the nurse has a responsibility toward ensuring personal radiation safety. The basic requirements involve wearing film monitoring badges and protective lead aprons. From a patient care perspective, nurses must be aware of the potential hazards of ionizing radiation to their patients, in particular women of childbearing age. The basic nursing responsibilities of comfort, reassurance, support, and preservation of patient dignity must remain foremost in the nurse's role. The presence of "high tech" machinery and long waiting periods in an unfamiliar, busy department may create an apparently hostile environment to which the nurse must orient the patient.

The nurse should discuss the procedure with the patient and help allay any anxieties he or she may have. In addition, specific nursing needs such as the presence of urinary catheters, surgical dressings, or central venous lines should be noted; patients may require special attention for a variety of reasons including recent surgery, chronic disabilities, and/or medical conditions, all of which affect the conduct of the procedure.

During the procedure, nursing needs are intensive and include such activities as starting intravenous lines, preparing and directing the puncture site, and, most importantly monitoring the physiologic status of the patient. Basic monitoring includes electrocardiographic recording of rate and rhythm, measurement of blood pressure and respiration at regular intervals (every 5 to 10 minutes), continuous monitoring of oxygen saturation via fingertip pulse oximetry, and peripheral circulation. In many interventional radiology procedural areas, nurses are responsible for administering intravenous sedatives and narcotics to assure a pain-free, comfortable condition for the patient. The use of newer short-acting, rapidly metabolized agents such as fentanyl and midazolam is preferred for intraprocedural medication. These drugs also provide the added benefit of production of retrograde amnesia about the procedure. Safe induction of conscious sedation must be accompanied by accurate documentation of level of consciousness, vital signs, and oxygen therapy periprocedurally.

After the procedure, the interventional radiology nurse will assess the patient's suitability for transfer to the floor and provide a written nursing summary on the chart. An oral report to the patient's nurses on the nursing unit from the interventional radiology nursing team prior to transfer is extremely beneficial. This exchange will ensure that any specific conditions requiring special attention are highlighted. This may include issues as diverse as the insertion of a urinary catheter during the procedure, or a notation about a stable hematoma which needs to be monitored.

ARTERIOGRAPHY

Indications

The indications for arteriography have narrowed since the 1950s and 1960s, when arteriography was used not only for the detection of vascular disease but also for identification and characterization of many tumors throughout the body. The introduction of CT, ultrasound, and MRI has markedly reduced the use of arteriography in tumor detection and in most cases eliminated it altogether. In the 1990s, arteriography is now mainly used for the identification of abnormalities confined to the vessel itself or for intravascular therapy. Current indications for arteriography include vascular disease and access for transcatheter therapy.

Vascular Disease

The most common indication for the performance of arteriography is the presence of occlusive vascular disease in the extremities, extracranial or intracranial circulation, or visceral arteries for renovascular hypertension or intestinal ischemia. Patients with aneurysms of the aorta or extremities also may undergo arteriography.[1, 2]

Arteriography is *not* a screening technique; a patient with symptoms of peripheral or cerebrovascular disease should first have a thorough physical examination, including palpation of pulses and arterial auscultation as well as a detailed clinical history. In addition, these patients require appropriate screening with noninvasive techniques such as Doppler and real-time ultrasound imaging of the affected vessels. Magnetic resonance arteriography is now increasingly substituted for arteriography because it produces extremely good depiction of vessels throughout the body

If vascular disease of sufficient severity is detected on clinical examination and noninvasive testing, arteriography is obtained in patients considered candidates for arterial surgery or transluminal angioplasty. Other candidates for arteriography include postoperative patients with suspected graft occlusion or pseudoaneurysm formation.

Tumor Detection

Arteriography has been used extensively in the past for the detection of tumors in solid organs such as the liver or kidney. In order to identify these tumors, catheterization and injection of the vessel supplying the organ is performed, and the radiologist searches for changes produced by the tumor. These changes, including displacement of vessels, the presence of abnormal tumor vessels, and vascular occlusions, may allow differentiation between benign and malignant masses. In general, however, arteriography is used only to define the vessels supplying the tumor before surgery.

Access for Transcatheter Therapy

The most common transcatheter therapies now performed for vascular disease are percutaneous transluminal angioplasty (PTA) and stenting. PTA/stenting may be performed at the time of initial arteriography if an amenable lesion is identified or may be deferred to the following day if a different arterial access site is required or if contrast dose limits have been exceeded. Transluminal angioplasty requires careful patient selection to determine which lesions can and should be treated because long-term results vary depending on the lesion characteristics and location.

Transcatheter therapy may also be used to lyse clot within a vessel or graft due to embolism or thrombosis.[3, 4] Transcatheter fibrinolysis is usually most effective when performed early after the occluding episode, but chronic thrombosis within a graft or (more commonly) within a native artery may also be treated by this means. The utilization of fibrinolytic therapy should be approached carefully since the complication rate is higher than that for angioplasty or arteriography.

The arteriographic catheter may also be used to occlude vessels as well as open them. Therapeutic transcatheter embolization involves injection of occluding materials such as surgical gelatin, particulate matter, liquids, or steel coils to occlude the vascular supply to a selected region. The technique may be performed to control hemorrhage in a patient who cannot undergo surgery or whose bleeding site is obscure or not readily located surgically.[5] Embolization may also be used primarily to control congenital arteriovenous malformations by selectively catheterizing feeding vessels and injecting particles or liquids that occlude the central vascular mass.

Technique

Virtually all arteriography and interventional radiologic procedures are performed using the so-called Seldinger technique, which was invented by Sven Ivar Seldinger in 1953.[6] The method, elegant in its simplicity, involves needle puncture of the artery followed by placement of a wire through the needle into the lumen of the vessel. Over this wire, a catheter may be safely placed within the vessel, with the wire acting as a "guide" to the catheter (hence the designation of the wire as a *guidewire*). The guidewire is then withdrawn and the catheter can be directed to a specific location and an injection made.[7] The guidewire technique also allows numerous and repetitive changes of a catheter to be performed without excessive trauma to the vessel wall. The technique is summarized graphically in Figure 6–1.

In order to be used to gain access to the arterial system, a vessel to be punctured must meet the following requirements: (1) it should be readily accessible; (2) it should be sufficiently large that the catheter does not occlude the vessel; and (3) it should not be diseased.[8] Three arteries that generally meet these qualifications are the common femoral artery, the axillary artery, and the brachial artery.[9–11]

The *transfemoral* approach is the most widely used, safest, and most effective route for arteriography (Fig. 6–2). If the femoral artery is not available for catheterization due to prior surgery, arterial stenosis, or occlusion, alternate routes for arteriography include the brachial approach, in which puncture is made in the brachial artery at or just above the antecubital fossa, and the axillary approach, in which the proximal brachial artery is punctured near the axilla. The choice of arterial access sites depends on many factors; each site has advantages and disadvantages and may be used in different circumstances. The brachial or axillary route is used in patients with aortoiliac occlusive disease and a minimally palpable or nonpalpable femoral pulse, or in those patients with previous femoral or aortic grafts, although graft puncture is not definitely contraindicated.[12] If a patient has had a prior history of stroke, the brachial or axillary route may be contraindicated because the proximity of the catheter to the cerebral vessels increases the risk of stroke following the examination. The axillary approach also has major disadvantages, such as the risk of hematoma formation with brachial plexus compression, which can result in long-term morbidity. This complication occurs because the artery is punctured near the axilla, where it is enclosed in the axillary sheath together with the nerves supplying the upper extremity. Even small amounts of bleeding into this sheath can cause compression and ischemic injury of the brachial plexus. The clinical sequelae can range from small sensory deficits to major motor deficits. The angiographer's goal is to select the approach that provides the best diagnostic films with the least amount of risk to the patient.

Variously shaped catheters for specific purposes and vessels may be placed into the vascular system during a procedure. The most commonly used catheter in lower-extremity vascular disease is the "pigtail" catheter, which allows injection of a large amount of contrast material with minimal risk. These catheters are usually placed in the aorta, where contrast injection can be made with the blood flow carrying the material into the lower extremities for subsequent filming. Branches of the aorta and their subdivisions are selectively catheterized via the use of an appropriately shaped catheter designed to "seek" the vessel to be examined (Fig. 6–3).

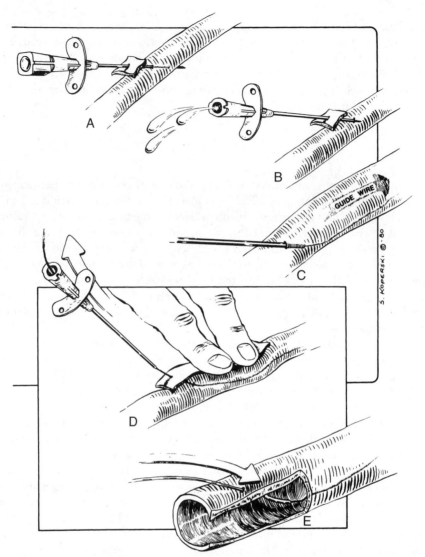

Figure 6–1. Seldinger technique for arterial catheterization. **A,** The artery is percutaneously punctured. Note that the needle punctures both walls of the artery. **B,** The inner sharpened stylet is removed and the outer cannula withdrawn until it lies within the arterial lumen and there is free return of blood. **C,** The guidewire is advanced into the artery through the cannula. **D,** After full advancement of the guidewire into the artery, the cannula is withdrawn and pressure is applied over the arterial puncture site to prevent bleeding. **E,** A catheter is threaded over the guidewire and advanced into the artery. (From Neiman HL: Techniques of angiography. In Neiman HL, Yao JST [eds]: Angiography of Vascular Disease. New York, Churchill Livingstone, 1985, p 5.)

Although many catheters exist, an angiographer generally will use only a small number of catheters with which he or she is familiar. Other highly specialized catheter shapes may be made by forming the catheters under steam in the angiographic laboratory. Guidewires also have specific functions and have different shapes for various requirements. They come in sizes ranging from 12 thousandths (.012) of an inch to 38 thousandths (.038) of an inch, with the majority in the .035- and .038-inch sizes. Catheter sizes usually range from 4 French to 7 French, although there is occasional need for catheters as small as 2 French and as large as 10 French. (One French equals one-third of a millimeter.) Most radiologists now use a vascular sheath, which allows multiple catheter exchanges to be made with less arterial damage and less risk of bleeding.

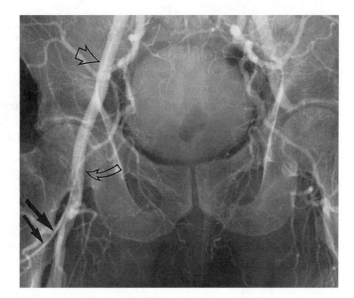

Figure 6–2. Catheterization of the common femoral artery. Catheter *(arrows)* enters the right common femoral artery *(curved arrow)* and passes up the external iliac artery *(open arrow)*. The left femoral artery is occluded.

After proper placement of the catheter, contrast material is injected using a pressure injector that is programmed for the appropriate flow rate and total volume to be given. For example, average flow rates and volumes for arteriography of the abdominal aorta (aortography) would be approximately 15–25 ml/sec, for a total of 30–50 ml of contrast material. In aortic branches, injection rates are usually decreased, with volumes adjusted for the capacity of the vessel in question. Renal artery injections average 6 ml/sec for a total of 9 ml, whereas injection into the superior mesenteric artery averages 8–10 ml/sec, for a total of 50–70 ml. Because of the renal toxicity of contrast agents, the total dose for an exam should not usually exceed 350 ml, although in extended procedures larger amounts can be used.

Due to the potentially thrombogenic nature of the catheter, heparinized flush solution is constantly used to keep the catheter free of clot. The guidewire has a heparin coating

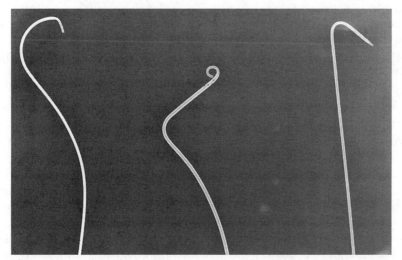

Figure 6–3. Various catheter shapes designed for different purposes. A "cobra" shape *(left)* is used for injection into branches of the aorta. A catheter with a small "pigtail" at the tip *(middle)* is used for pulmonary arteriography. Its right-angle bend is designed to aid passage of the catheter through the right atrium and right ventricle. The catheter on the right is a simple bent catheter for entry into branches of the aorta.

and the catheter materials are designed to be of low resistance, with relatively little friction. In addition, the position of the catheter is crucial, so that blood flow can occur around the catheter and not be occluded by it. The catheter and guidewire combination is never forced into a narrowed area or placed directly adjacent to an area of disease unless a therapeutic intervention is being performed. Following the arteriogram, the catheter is withdrawn and manual compression of the artery that has been punctured is applied to prevent hematoma formation. After an appropriate period of time, usually 15–20 minutes, pressure is released; if no bleeding occurs, the patient is transferred back to the hospital room.

Complications

The interventionist is concerned with the safe conduct of the examination. Complications of arteriography for which the patient is carefully monitored during and after the examination are listed in Table 6–1.

Nursing Management

Nursing care of the patient undergoing diagnostic arteriography includes patient education, preangiographic preparation, and periprocedural and postangiographic monitoring. The nursing care process begins with accurate assessment of the patient's overall condition upon arrival in the department. Specific nursing diagnoses relevant here are anxiety, knowledge deficit, pain, impaired gas exchange, potential for aspiration, potential for infection, potential for fluid/electrolyte imbalance, altered tissue perfusion, and altered coagulation.

Routine orders and restrictions vary according to each institution and radiologist. Preprocedural preparation and orders usually include the following:

1. An accurate appraisal of renal function by blood urea nitrogen (BUN) and serum creatinine determinations; this is significant because contrast material is potentially nephrotoxic and postprocedure monitoring of the renal function requires a baseline test.
2. Assessment of coagulation parameters by measurement of partial thromboplastin time (PTT), prothrombin time (PT), and platelet count.
3. Adequate hydration with intravenous fluids and oral intake; good hydration is essential in order to prevent the occurrence of renal failure induced by contrast material.
4. No solid foods after midnight of the day before the procedure.
5. Discontinuation of heparin or other anticoagulation.

After the procedure, careful monitoring of distal pulses is vital because a change in the pulse status may indicate a complication such as arterial thrombosis or embolism. Prompt detection of vascular occlusion is a high priority in preventing further complications. The nurse must monitor the patient for the development of a puncture-site hematoma (nonpulsatile mass), false aneurysm (pulsatile mass), contrast reaction, and contrast-induced renal failure. Some difficulties in postprocedural assessment may arise; for example, a hematoma at a puncture site may be confused with simple fullness or fleshiness. This sometimes-confusing distinction can often be made by comparing the opposite groin and remembering that hematomas are generally firm and not soft. The findings and appropriate therapies for many of the complications of diagnostic and therapeutic arteriography are listed in Table 6–1.

Routine postprocedural orders include:

TABLE 6–1. **Complications of Arteriography**

COMPLICATION	FINDINGS	SYMPTOMS	MONITORING REQUIRED	THERAPY
Puncture site hematoma	Stable or expanding swelling at puncture site and or pulse loss	Pain, swelling, paresthesia, coolness of extremity, sensory and motor loss (in axillary or brachial artery punctures)	Pulse, blood pressure, pulse character, sensory and motor function, size and rate of expansion of hematoma	Direct pressure, cold pack, surgery
Pseudoaneurysm	Firm, pulsatile mass over puncture site	Pain, swelling, arterial compromise	Size and rate of expansion, vital signs, distal pulses	Ultrasound-guided compression, surgery
Local arterial occlusion (thrombosis)	Cool, pulseless extremity	Pain, sensory and motor loss	Vital signs, sensory and motor function, pulses	Heparinization, surgery, transcatheter fibrinolysis
Embolism	Loss of a distal pulse	Pain, coolness, sensory and motor loss	Vital signs, sensory and motor function, pulses	Heparinization, surgery, transcatheter fibrinolysis
Contrast-induced allergy and/or anaphylaxis	Urticaria, wheezing, dyspnea, cardiac arrhythmias, cardiac arrest (reactions may be immediate or delayed)	Itching, flushing, hives, nausea, shortness of breath, respiratory stridor	Vital signs, cardiac status, respiratory status	IV fluids, intravenous epinephrine, respiratory support
Contrast-induced renal failure	Anuria/oliguria	Few	Urine output, creatinine	Fluid management, diuretics, dialysis
Neurologic complications	Aphasia, confusion, unconsciousness, hemiparesis	Blurred vision, speech deficit, motor or sensory deficits	Vital signs, neurologic status	Heparinization, CT or MRI scan, careful monitoring

CT = computed tomography; MRI = magnetic resonance imaging.

1. Frequent checks of vital signs, neurologic function, and pulses in both extremities with particular attention to the extremity that has been catheterized (q 15 minutes × 4, and q 1 hour × 2).
2. Assessment of the puncture site for hematoma and the appearance of the extremity distal to the puncture site.
3. Bed rest for 6–8 hours, with the punctured extremity kept straight.
4. Intravenous hydration continued for 6–8 hours.
5. BUN and creatinine levels assessed the next day. A complete blood count should be obtained if a translumbar approach has been used.
6. Resumption of preprocedural dietary and medication orders. If a patient has been on heparin, the drug is not resumed for a minimum of 4 hours.

VENOGRAPHY

Indications

Venography is used to demonstrate venous abnormalities in the lower and upper extremities, as well as in the vena cava and its branches such as the hepatic or renal vein.[13, 14]

Ascending venography is usually performed to assess patency of the deep venous system and presence of deep venous thrombosis[15]; the test is indicated when noninvasive studies are indeterminate or negative in the face of a strong clinical suspicion of thrombotic occlusion. Venography allows differentiation between acute thrombosis and chronic venous occlusion, and can accurately assess venous anatomy prior to surgical procedures. Venography can also distinguish intrinsic thrombus formation from that secondary to venous compression, and can evaluate congenital venous anomalies. *Descending venography* is used in the lower extremity to assess venous valvular competence, rather than to define venous anatomy.[16]

Technique

The technique for ascending venography involves placement of the patient in a 45° upright position, with the leg to be examined in a non–weight-bearing position. Contrast material is injected into a distal foot vein to fill the entire venous system of the extremity. Fluoroscopy and filming then allow the detection of flow patterns and of venous occlusion. Thrombus is identified as a filling defect within the vein (Fig. 6–4). If visualization of larger veins such as the vena cava is required, puncture of a centrally located vein such as the femoral or antecubital vein may be performed with catheter placement into the appropriate location. Serial filming then takes place after rapid injection of contrast material.

Descending venography is performed by directly catheterizing the femoral vein and injecting contrast with the patient upright. The contrast, which is heavier than blood, descends to the venous valves, which, if competent, do not permit its passage. When the valves are diseased and incompetent, they allow contrast to flow distally.

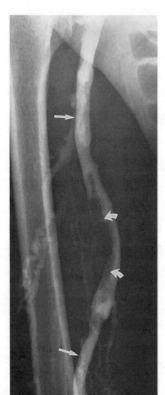

Figure 6–4. Venogram of the femoral vein *(straight arrows)* demonstrates a "filling defect" *(curved arrows)* within the vein, diagnostic of thrombosis.

Other techniques include transcatheter venous pressure monitoring, which is useful in obstructive diseases of the veins such as portal hypertension. Selective catheterization of veins such as the renal or hepatic vein can allow samples to be withdrawn for analysis of specific products, such as renin in the evaluation of renovascular hypertension.[17] Selective venography may also be performed.

Complications

The main complication associated with venography is thrombophlebitis. Contrast material has been shown to injure venous endothelium and induce clot formation. As a preventive measure, all contrast material should be flushed from the venous system using heparinized saline. Despite these measures, however, postvenographic thrombosis can and does occur.

Extravasation of contrast medium at the injection site may cause inflammation and even lead to skin necrosis; this complication is fortunately quite rare and usually is seen only in patients with compromised blood flow in the area of extravasation. Hypersensitivity (allergic) reactions to contrast may also occur.

Nursing Management

Nursing care is directed toward patient education because the procedure may involve multiple attempts at finding and puncturing a vein, detection of complications at the injection site, monitoring for the presence of contrast-induced thrombophlebitis, and maintaining adequate hydration. The patient is usually on clear liquids for 3–4 hours prior to the procedure. The patient is to remain at bed rest for 2 hours after the procedure if the femoral vein in the groin is used for puncture.

TRANSLUMINAL BALLOON ANGIOPLASTY AND STENTING

Transluminal angioplasty has had a major impact on the treatment of vascular disease. The technique was invented by Charles Dotter of the University of Oregon in 1964[18] and popularized in Europe. The original Dotter technique dilated vessels by the passage of progressively larger catheters through an area of arterial blockage or narrowing. Lower-extremity arteries, such as the iliac and femoral vessels, were amenable to this therapy, but branch arteries such as the renal or coronary vessels could not be dilated. In 1974, Andreas Gruntzig devised a usable balloon dilating catheter that provided increased safety and broader range of application.[19] The technique has been successfully used in every major artery in the body, including lower-extremity, renal, coronary, and brachiocephalic vessels.[20–25]

Balloon angioplasty, however, has major limitations. Principal among the limitations is a relatively high rate of recurrence after angioplasty (as much as 50 percent recurrence or restenosis at 1 year).[25] Other problems include the failure of angioplasty to effectively treat long-segment arterial occlusions and/or occlusions and stenoses in the majority of patients with femoropopliteal disease. These drawbacks led many investigators to devise and use different methods and devices such as catheters that removed plaque mechanically or via lasers. In the 1980s a large number of these atherectomy and laser devices were invented and investigated, of which very few proved to show improved results over conventional balloon angioplasty.[26–28]

The invention of vascular stents, however, radically changed the face of vascular intervention. These endoluminal metallic devices were rapidly proven to be not only useful but also a significant improvement over angioplasty in many vascular territories, and stent placement has become the preferred method of treating occlusive arterial lesions (Fig. 6–5).[29, 30] The availability of these stents has also broadened the range of vessels and lesions treatable with these techniques.[31–33]

From a nursing standpoint, all vascular recanalization procedures are quite similar in that the patients are essentially identical to those undergoing balloon angioplasty. Postprocedural nursing care will thus concentrate on assessment of the treated limb or organ and the puncture site. In this section, we will discuss transluminal balloon angioplasty and stenting as a general model for this group of procedures and later briefly describe differences between these newer therapies and balloon angioplasty from a nursing and technical (procedural) standpoint.

Indications

In the lower extremities, transluminal angioplasty and stenting are indicated for treatment of arterial occlusive disease. In general, angioplasty is used in the treatment of segmental (less than 10 cm in length) stenoses and occlusions of the aortoiliac, femoropopliteal, and tibial arteries. Balloon dilatation of lesions more than 10 cm long has been shown to give less durable results, and in the iliac circulation, stents are now quite routinely placed for long-segment occlusions and stenoses. In the femoropopliteal vessels, angioplasty of long lesions is still undertaken in patients with ischemia who are not operative candidates. Angioplasty of long areas of disease may allow limb salvage or convert the need for a proximal amputation to a more distal one. In diabetic patients with ischemia and a nonhealing foot ulcer, angioplasty of less-than-ideal lesions may often permit adequate wound healing. Routine stenting of femoral and popliteal artery lesions is still controversial

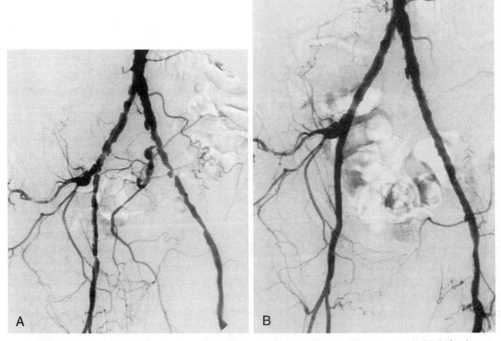

Figure 6–5. Treatment of bilateral diffuse iliac artery disease with extensive stenting. **A,** Multifocal bilateral disease. **B,** Excellent result after bilateral stenting with Wallstents.

and many interventionists still reserve the use of stents for acute failures of angioplasty[34] (Fig. 6–6). The tibial arteries are very rarely treated with stenting.

Angioplasty and stenting also frequently serve an adjunctive role to surgery. For example, a patient with an iliac stenosis proximal to a femoral artery occlusion may benefit from dilatation or stenting of the iliac stenosis prior to femoral artery bypass surgery. Improved iliac artery inflow is a prerequisite to the femoral surgery and PTA/stenting may help to avoid a proximal surgical procedure.

Renal artery angioplasty and stenting are indicated for the nonoperative treatment of renovascular hypertension in those patients with amenable lesions, including (1) patients with fibromuscular dysplasia or atherosclerosis of the main renal artery (angioplasty is generally the treatment of choice for fibromuscular dysplasia); (2) patients with segmental lesions of the proximal branches; (3) patients with renal transplants who develop stenoses at the arterial anastomosis[20, 35] (Figs. 6–7 and 6–8).

Brachiocephalic artery angioplasty and/or stenting is indicated in specific lesions of the subclavian, innominate, vertebral, and/or carotid arteries such as fibromuscular disease of the common or internal carotid artery and atherosclerotic lesions of the proximal subclavian and/or innominate artery (Fig. 6–9). Recently there has been a great deal of enthusiasm and interest in primary treatment of common carotid artery atherosclerotic lesions with stenting, a trend that is likely to continue based on the limited data available.[36] Many other vascular sites may be dilated or stented successfully. Some of the most common include stenoses of hemodialysis access fistulae and stenoses of veins caused by trauma, malignancy, or old thrombosis (Fig. 6–10). Postoperative arterial anastomotic stenoses and/or bypass vein graft stenoses can also be dilated successfully.

Technique

The techniques for angioplasty and stenting are similar to those used for arteriography, with the exception that the catheter and guidewire are maneuvered across areas of

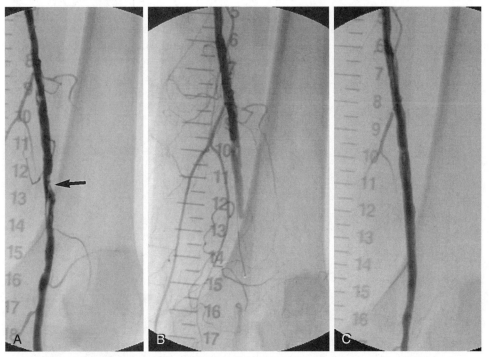

Figure 6–6. Treatment of femoropopliteal angioplasty failure with stent. **A,** Initial lesion *(arrow)* was treated with angioplasty, with subsequent dissection and occlusion **(B).** After placement of Palmaz stent, there was an excellent result **(C).**

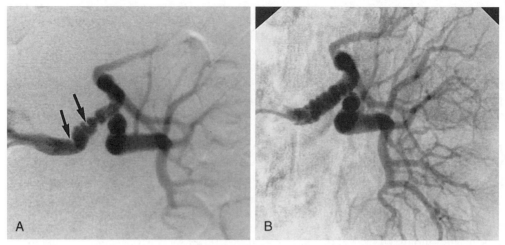

Figure 6–7. Renal angioplasty for renal artery stenosis in a 42-year-old woman with severe refractory hypertension. **A,** Left renal arteriogram shows so-called "string of beads" appearance of main renal artery *(arrows)* characteristic of dysplasia. **B,** After balloon angioplasty, considerable luminal widening is noted, with elimination of stenoses. The patient had excellent clinical response; she was normotensive and was able to discontinue all medications following the procedure.

narrowing or occlusion. Additionally, larger holes are made in the punctured artery by these larger devices and the vascular sheaths needed to introduce them. After the blockage has been passed with a wire, an angioplasty catheter with an attached balloon of appropriate diameter is placed across the lesion. The dilating catheter is a double-lumen catheter that has an inflatable but nondistensible balloon at the tip. It has a distal end-hole that permits monitoring of pressure or infusion of contrast material or medication during the procedure. Typical balloon lengths are between 2 and 6 cm, with balloon diameters of between 4 to 15 mm. Balloons of smaller and larger sizes may occasionally be used for specialized circumstances.

After the catheter is positioned across the lesion, heparin is given to prevent thrombosis of the distal vessel while flow is temporarily occluded during balloon inflation. A vasodilator, such as nitroglycerin, is frequently administered intra-arterially at a dose of 200 μg. The balloon is inflated in the diseased segment for 30 seconds; contrast material is used to inflate the balloon so that it may be seen fluoroscopically. Radiopaque metallic markers

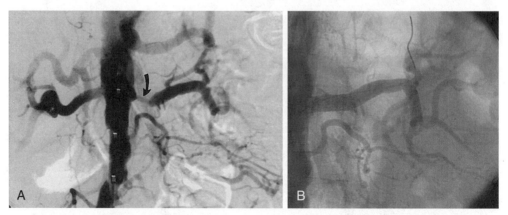

Figure 6–8. Stenting for renal artery stenosis. **A,** Initial high-grade left renal artery stenosis *(curved arrow)* was treated with angioplasty with a poor result. **B,** Palmaz stent was placed, and an excellent anatomic result was achieved.

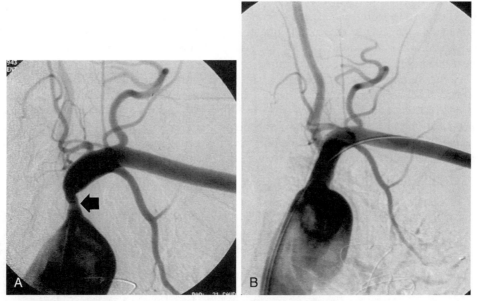

Figure 6–9. Treatment of subclavian artery stenosis with stenting. **A,** Proximal left subclavian artery stenosis *(arrow)* was responsible for posterior fossa symptoms related to subclavian steal. **B,** After placement of Palmaz stent, there was an excellent result with good filling of the left vertebral artery *(arrow)*. Symptoms resolved.

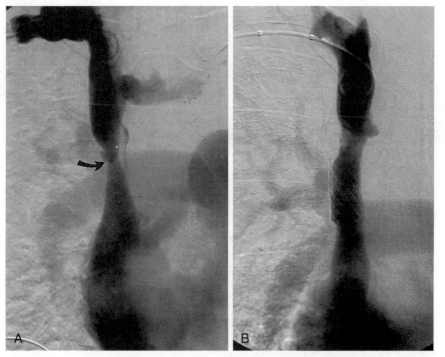

Figure 6–10. Stenting for treatment of superior vena cava (SVC) syndrome in a 52-year-old woman with a high-grade SVC stenosis. **A,** The stenosis *(arrow)* was secondary to chronic central venous catheterization. **B,** Following stenting, significant symptoms disappeared.

are also located at both ends of the balloon to allow precise localization in the stenotic area (Fig. 6–11). After dilatation, the catheter is withdrawn proximal to the dilated segment and an angiogram is obtained to assess the success of the procedure. If an adequate result is not accomplished (persistent stenosis or residual pressure gradient), repeat dilatation or stenting is performed.

Arterial stenting is conducted in a similar manner to angioplasty except that the operator has two basic stent types and a number of available products from which to choose. The two types of stents are self-expanding (e.g., Schneider Wallstent) and balloon expandable (e.g., Palmaz stent), and the benefits and disadvantages of each are taken into account by the operating physician. For instance, renal arteries are usually recanalized with Palmaz balloon expandable stents whereas iliac and femoral arteries are often best treated with self-expanding stents.[20, 31]

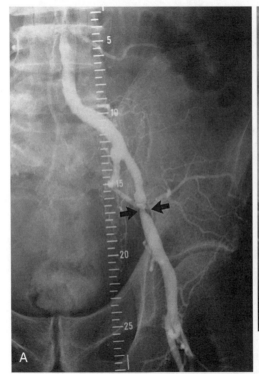

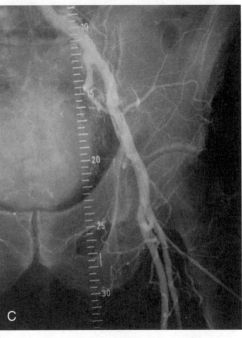

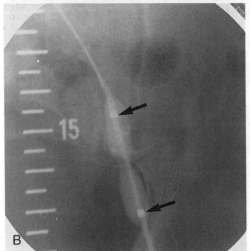

Figure 6–11. Dilatation of an external iliac stenosis. **A,** Preangioplasty arteriogram performed via the femoral route shows a short left external iliac stenosis *(arrows).* Radiopaque ruler allows localization of the stenosis at fluoroscopy. **B,** After insertion of balloon catheter across stenosis, the balloon is inflated with dilute contrast material. Notice narrowing of the balloon in the region of stenosis as the dilatation takes place. Small radiopaque markers *(arrows)* allow localization of the balloon prior to inflation. **C,** Post-angioplasty arteriogram shows disappearance of stenosis.

After successful completion of the angioplasty or stenting, the catheter is withdrawn. Because heparin has generally been given, the vascular access sheath is not usually withdrawn until the effects of heparinization have been reversed by protamine or wear off on their own.

Complications

Complications of angioplasty/stenting occur in 2–4 percent of patients but most are minor and do not require intervention. Complications requiring surgical or radiologic intervention occur in about 1 percent. Complications that can occur include distal embolization of fragments from the treated site with resultant ischemia, arterial dissection, or occlusion at the dilatation site from local trauma, arterial thrombosis and occlusion, and hematoma or false aneurysm formation at the catheter insertion site.[37] These complications can require surgical treatment with the exception of small or moderate-sized hematomas at the puncture site. Most occur in the periprocedural period, which emphasizes the need for attentive nursing care.

Nursing Management

Both preprocedural nursing care and the complications from PTA/stenting are similar to those in routine diagnostic arteriography (Table 6–1). Postprocedural care requires astute observational skills and aggressive nursing care because these complications may be more severe than in routine arteriography. Puncture site hematoma and pseudoaneurysm are of greater concern in these patients because of the use of heparin and the larger size of the puncture hole. The degree of fullness at the puncture site should be noted upon the patient's arrival on the nursing unit and any changes carefully noted. If a hematoma is initially present, its borders should be marked on the skin to allow quantification of change. Peripheral pulses must be monitored at 15-minute intervals ($\times 4$) followed by checks at half-hour intervals ($\times 2$) and 1 hour ($\times 2$) to observe for arterial thrombosis or embolization. Sensation and neurologic status of the limb should also be assessed. Aspirin and other antiplatelet agents are also administered after angioplasty.

TRANSCATHETER THROMBOLYSIS

It has been known for many years that certain enzymes can accelerate the normal processes by which intravascular clot is lysed. These substances, mainly urokinase, have been administered systemically for the treatment of pulmonary embolism and coronary thrombosis, but clinical trials led to the conclusion that the complication rate was excessive. In an attempt to take advantage of these substances' lytic action against thrombosis but reduce their toxicity, lower doses of the enzymes were infused directly through a catheter into occluded vessels, with very encouraging results. Transcatheter dissolution of intravascular clot is now an accepted therapy in the treatment of vascular disease.

Indications

Transcatheter fibrinolysis may be used as an alternative to surgical thrombectomy in patients with acute thrombosis of a bypass graft or native artery. Particular efficacy of fibrinolytic agents has been found in grafts and emboli to native arteries.[38, 39] Other indications for transcatheter fibrinolytic therapy include use when thrombotic or embolic complications occur during angioplasty. Iliac, femoral, popliteal, and subclavian deep venous thrombosis and pulmonary embolism have also been treated with local infusions[40] (Fig. 6–12). Contraindications to the use of these agents include recent surgery, hemorrhage, or trauma. Patients with a new stroke may also be at risk for the bleeding complications of this therapy.

Technique

Transcatheter thrombolysis is probably the most labor- and time-intensive procedure done in interventional radiology. It differs considerably from other procedures in that an arterial infusion catheter is left in place for extended periods of time (as long as 72 hours) as clot lysis progresses (Fig. 6–13). During this period of time, major demands are placed upon nursing personnel for monitoring of the drug infusion, catheter entry site, and the extremity under treatment. These added patient care requirements can be met properly only in an intensive care unit setting.

The technique of transcatheter thrombolysis involves insertion of a catheter directly into the thrombosis or embolus.[38] In general, the catheter for lower-extremity occlusions is inserted in the opposite common femoral artery and passed around the aortic bifurcation, but other sites including the femoral artery on the same side or the brachial artery may be used. During the procedure systemic anticoagulation with heparin is used to prevent thrombosis around the catheter or in the slowly flowing blood within the treated artery or graft. The procedure may also be combined with angioplasty if clot lysis uncovers a causative stenosis, or if there is a complication of angioplasty (Figs. 6–14 and 6–15).

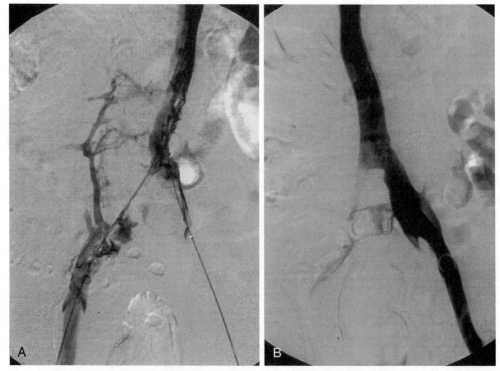

Figure 6–12. Treatment of iliocaval thrombosis with local infusion of urokinase. **A,** Extensive iliocaval thrombophlebitis was treated with 72 hours of bilateral urokinase infusion, with complete elimination of thrombus and disappearance of severe lower extremity swelling and cyanosis **(B).**

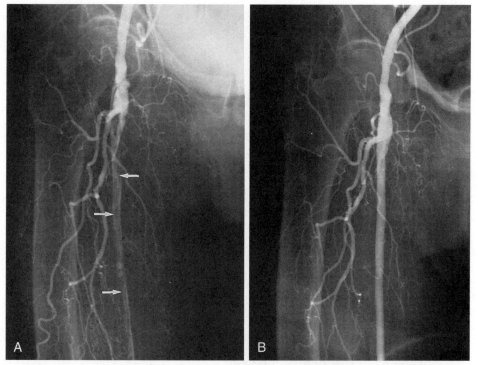

Figure 6–13. Transcatheter lysis of thrombosed graft. **A,** Arteriogram prior to therapy shows multiple radiolucent filling defects within a previously placed femoral-popliteal synthetic graft (*arrows*). **B,** After 12 hours of transcatheter infusion of streptokinase, the graft is free of clot; distal pulses were restored.

Some physicians will attempt to accelerate the clot lysis by forcefully injecting high doses of urokinase into the clot.[39]

Complications

The major complication rate of transcatheter thrombolytic therapy ranges between 2 and 10 percent. Most of the complications are hemorrhagic, with bleeding occurring at the catheter site or elsewhere. Other events that may occur include loosening of clot with distal embolization, and formation of new clot around the indwelling catheter. Puncture site hematomas and pseudoaneurysms are also more frequent with this therapy.[38]

Nursing Management

As indicated above, thrombolytic therapy is the most nursing-intensive vascular interventional procedure performed. Postprocedural orders reflect that complexity. A typical example of routine orders for thrombolysis is reproduced in Table 6–2. There are four major areas of nursing concern during this therapy. They include:

1. *Catheter site management.* Catheter position is critical to this therapy, thus the catheter is carefully secured and an adhesive dressing is placed. Despite these precautions, flexing of the thigh and other movements may dislodge the catheter; avoidance of such movements is thus mandated. Patients will, however, require shifting and movement for bed linen changes and use of a bedpan; these should be

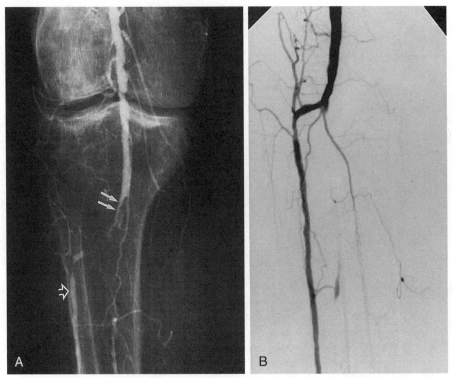

Figure 6–14. Lysis of spontaneous arterial thrombosis. The patient was an 82-year-old woman suffering from acute onset of right lower extremity rest pain. **A,** Initial angiogram showed occlusion of the distal popliteal artery by filling defect *(arrows)*, with collaterals reconstituting the anterior tibial *(open arrow)*. **B,** Following overnight infusion of urokinase at the site of occlusion, there was complete opening of the popliteal and anterior tibial arteries, with excellent clinical results.

TABLE 6–2. **Urokinase Infusion Nursing Protocol**

1. Monitor vital signs, distal pulses, affected limb temperature, sensory and motor function, and puncture sites _____ q 15' × _____; q 30' × _____.
2. Monitor closely for signs of hemorrhage from any area of the body.
3. No arterial punctures/avoid unnecessary venipunctures.
4. Strict bed rest with _____ hip extended/arm rest.
5. Patient may be log rolled side to side.
6. Head of bed elevated _____°.
7. Ensure that dressings are intact; do not manipulate catheter.
8. Follow-up angiogram scheduled on: _____.
9. Notify SERVICE and INTERVENTIONAL RADIOLOGY FELLOW (include phone numbers) for:
   • Fibrinogen level <100 mg/100 ml.
   • Change in vital signs; decreased or absent pulses; urine output <200 ml/8 hrs; change in color, temperature, or sensation in either lower/upper extremity; bleeding or hematoma at puncture site (apply pressure to site); presence of pain in any area of the body. Do not apply sandbags over puncture site at any time.
10. Time urokinase infusion started: _____ hrs on (date) _____.
    • Rate started at _____ units/min.
    • Infuse at above rate for _____ hrs.
    • Then infuse at _____ units/min for _____ hrs.
11. Start heparin infusion at _____ units/hrs.
12. PT, PTT, fibrinogen, FDP at _____ and at every _____ hr(s).

PT = prothrombin time; PTT = partial thromboplastin time; FDP = fibrin degradation products.

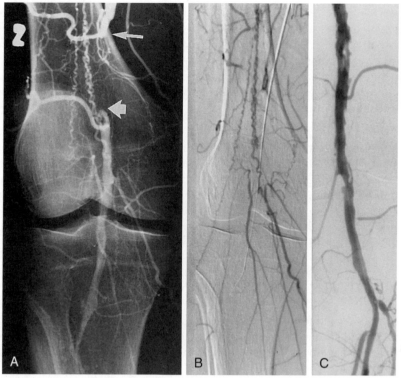

Figure 6–15. Use of thrombolysis to treat a thrombotic complication of transluminal angioplasty. The patient was a 56-year-old man with right lower extremity claudication. **A,** The original arteriogram demonstrated a short segment occlusion of the popliteal artery *(arrows)*. **B,** Following dilatation, complete thrombosis of the femoral popliteal artery was observed. **C,** Urokinase was infused overnight with restoration of patency.

accomplished with assistance. The catheter insertion site must also be monitored for the development of bleeding or hematoma formation, complications that occur with increased frequency in light of the concurrent use of heparin. Minimal catheter site oozing is typically seen and generally is controlled by light pressure. Repeat angiography is also frequently performed. During the repeat visits to the radiology suite (when the concealing dressings are likely to be removed), careful checking of the catheter insertion site for hematoma should be made.

2. *Drug management.* Doses of intra-arterial urokinase are usually in the range of 1 to 4,000 IU per minute. A typical protocol may be to give 4,000 IU per minute for 4 hours, followed by 2,000 IU per minute for the remainder of the procedure for therapy. Careful calculation of drug concentration and infusion flow rates, always administered by infusion pump, is thus critical to avoid potentially catastrophic dosing errors. In addition, anticoagulation with intravenous heparin is used and must be monitored by maintaining the partial thromboplastin time (PTT) at 1½ to 2 times control value.

3. *Hematologic monitoring.* Thrombolytic therapy can and does cause major alterations in systemic coagulation and hemostasis. Careful observation of the patient for signs and symptoms of local or remote hemorrhage including gastrointestinal or intracranial bleeding is thus mandated. Oozing from intravenous puncture sites may be seen; unnecessary punctures should be avoided because of the patient's altered clotting parameters. Also, laboratory values such as fibrinogen, platelets, PT, and PTT must be monitored at 4- to 6-hour intervals. The fibrinogen level should not fall below a value of 100 mg per 100 ml.

4. *Monitoring of the limb under treatment.* Thrombolytic therapy is generally used for ischemic conditions of the extremity. As lytic therapy progresses, changes in the perfusion of the limb can be expected to occur. Certainly, if therapy is successful, return or strengthening of distal pulses may be auscultated or palpated. Color and temperature of the extremity can be expected to improve as well. These changes may occur gradually or rather suddenly depending on the nature of the occlusion and the efficacy of therapy.

During thrombolytic therapy, an acute worsening of the extremity's vascular status manifested by pain and/or loss of pulses can result from "showering" of distal embolization of fragmented clot distally. Although this may be initially alarming, the sudden development of ischemic signs and symptoms should be correctly identified as progress and therapy continue because the signs and symptoms will generally resolve with continued infusion. Side effects of the fibrinolytic agent may include generalized body shaking, anxiety, impaired gas exchange, fever, and hypertension. The reaction is generally short-term and the patient is usually continued on the drug.

TRANSCATHETER EMBOLIZATION

Arteriography can be used to diagnose areas of hemorrhage and to identify tumors. The same catheter used to diagnose can also be used to occlude the blood supply to tumors and site of hemorrhage by injecting materials that block the blood supply to those areas.

Indications

Transcatheter occlusion of vessels is indicated as definitive therapy in patients who are not candidates for surgery, or in certain conditions such as arteriovenous malformations. Transcatheter occlusion can also be a useful adjunct to surgery. In these patients, preoperative embolic occlusion of the vascular supply to neoplasms may reduce surgical blood loss considerably. Additionally, malignant liver tumors not amenable to surgery are also now being effectively treated. When performed appropriately, these catheter techniques may be lifesaving and provide levels of occlusion not obtainable surgically. This is most dramatically seen in the treatment of arteriovenous malformations, which may be difficult to excise or control surgically. Transcatheter therapy may obliterate these lesions without surgery (Fig. 6–16); however, multiple procedures may be required to progressively occlude the malformation. Control of gastrointestinal, postsurgical, or posttraumatic hemorrhage is also possible (Fig. 6–17).[41–43]

Technique

In this technique, the catheter is positioned in the vessel to be occluded. Once catheter position is obtained, the vessel may be occluded with a variety of substances, including particles such as pieces of surgical gelatin (Gelfoam) or small plastic bits. Other substances used include liquids such as alcohol or tissue adhesive (bucrylate); devices for large vessel occlusion include steel coils and inflatable detachable balloons.

Complications and Nursing Management

The main complications associated with transcatheter embolization therapy are local catheter entry site problems and, most important, inadvertent occlusion of vessels outside

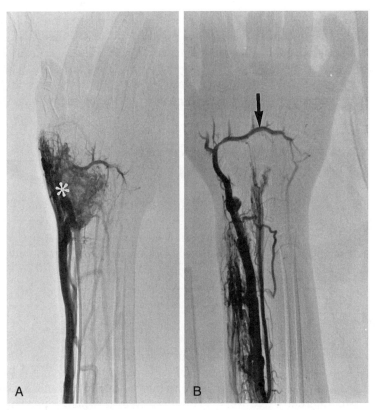

Figure 6–16. Transcatheter treatment of an arteriovenous malformation. **A,** Injection into the radial artery shows an enlarged radial artery feeding an extremely hypervascular mass (*) on the thenar eminence. The patient had developed high-output congestive failure as a result of this congenital arteriovenous malformation. **B,** After embolization with tissue adhesive, arteriogram demonstrates complete occlusion of the malformation and good filling of the arterial arch *(arrow)* supplying the hand. The patient was stabilized hemodynamically by the procedure and was relieved of the chronic pain that had accompanied the lesion.

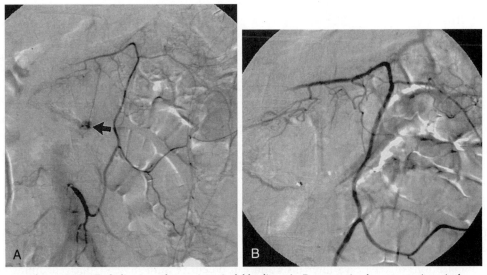

Figure 6–17. Embolization of gastrointestinal bleeding. **A,** Postoperative lower gastrointestinal (GI) bleeding was documented by contrast extravasation on inferior mesenteric arteriography *(arrow)*. **B,** After embolization with microcoils and surgical gelatin pledgets, bleeding and contrast extravasation are no longer evident.

the target area. Pain may commonly be seen after an embolization; this is related to ischemia produced in the intended area of embolization and should not be seen as a complication. In general, good medication management can eliminate this problem, which is seen most intensely in the first 24 hours. Postoperative care also requires careful assessment of distal pulses, as well as constant monitoring of the patient for signs of infarction of other organs or tissues, depending on the location of embolization.

PERCUTANEOUS INFERIOR VENA CAVA FILTER REPLACEMENT

Vena cava filters have been in wide use for about the last 20 years, primarily in the form known as the Greenfield vena cava filter, which was implanted operatively through a venotomy. Recently, however, a new generation of smaller filters that have proven to be as effective and as safe as the Greenfield filter has been introduced; these devices are now placed percutaneously by interventional radiologists.[44-46]

Indications

Pulmonary embolism (PE) is a life-threatening complication of deep venous thrombosis. It is estimated that about 30 percent of patients will die of the disease if it is left untreated. Treatment usually consists of anticoagulation therapy with heparin and warfarin sodium, which reduces the mortality rate for PE considerably to less than 5 percent. There are, however, a number of patients in whom anticoagulation therapy cannot be used usually because of a bleeding tendency, anticipated surgery, or a history of recurrent PE despite adequate anticoagulation. Other patients may not be able to tolerate any further episodes of PE because of reduced cardiac or pulmonary capacity or may be at risk for massive embolism from a large clot in the vena cava or iliac veins. These selected individuals are candidates for placement of a vena cava filter in order to prevent pulmonary embolism.

Technique

Vena cava filters are placed through the right internal jugular or the right femoral venous approach. The procedure itself is simple and straightforward in that catheterization of the vena cava is performed under local anesthesia. A venacavogram is first done to identify any abnormalities and to ensure that no clots are present in the vessel. If the angiographic appearance is unremarkable, the filter is deployed in the infrarenal segment of the vena cava below the renal veins through a sheath ranging from 9 French to 15 French in diameter, depending on the device used (Fig. 6–18). Following filter deployment, the catheter is withdrawn, hemostasis is achieved, and the patient is returned to the hospital room.

Complications

Complications of vena cava filter insertion can be either immediate or delayed. Immediately, improper deployment or positioning of the filter may reduce filtering efficiency. Perforation of the vena cava with retroperitoneal bleeding has also been very rarely described. Late complications of vena cava filter placement include movement or migra-

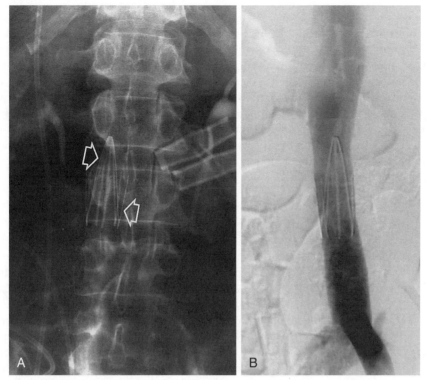

Figure 6–18. Vena cava filter. **A,** Plain film of the abdomen showing the Vena-Tech filter in position *(arrows)*. Note the inverted cone design similar to the Greenfield filter. This filter, however, adds stabilizing legs to center the device properly. **B,** Venacavogram performed after filter insertion. Note the well-centered position of the Vena-Tech filter.

tion of the filter, with some filters rarely migrating to the heart or pulmonary artery. Occlusion of the vena cava can also occur when a large embolus is trapped.[46]

Nursing Management

Nursing management for insertion of vena cava filters involves several areas. Frequently, these patients are quite ill and may have a number of other coexisting medical conditions that require nursing management. Deep venous thrombosis with attendant leg swelling may often be present or there may be a recent episode of PE that produced cardiovascular or pulmonary instability. The filter insertion is relatively straightforward and not painful; however, postprocedural management should concentrate mainly on observation for hematoma or venous thrombosis at the site of insertion and any signs or symptoms of filter migration. Follow-up with plain abdominal x-ray is usually obtained 1 to 2 days after a filter insertion to ensure that the filter is sufficient. In rare circumstances, the patient may be continued on anticoagulation. In these cases, the anticoagulation should not be begun for at least 4 hours after the insertion of the filter and withdrawal of the deployment sheath.

TRANSJUGULAR INTRAHEPATIC PORTOSYSTEMIC SHUNTS (TIPS)

Introduction and Indications

Portal hypertension, usually caused by parenchymal liver disease relating to viral or alcoholic hepatitis, is a major cause of morbidity and mortality in the United States.

Portal hypertension, defined as increased pressure in the portal vein, results from progressive scarring and fibrosis within the liver parenchyma. As a result of this scarring, increased resistance to portal flow develops and a large number of portal venous collateral channels are formed, including collateral veins around the stomach and gastroesophageal junction. These veins can bleed massively, which is the cause of many of the problems caused by portal hypertension. Therapeutic options in the past have included endoscopic sclerotherapy, in which injection of sclerosing liquids into the varices prevents bleeding, and surgical shunting of the obstructed portal vein into the vena cava by the use of a portacaval shunt. Unfortunately, surgical mortality is very high in the patients who are actively bleeding and who have the poorest liver function. Surgical mortality in this group (Child's class C) may be greater than 50 percent.

Technique

A new interventional radiologic therapy has been devised and perfected that allows nonsurgical placement of a large-caliber shunt between the portal vein and the hepatic vein (the outflow vein of the liver). The procedure is performed under local anesthesia and intravenous sedation. A large steerable needle is placed through the right internal jugular vein into the hepatic vein, and a passage made between the hepatic vein and the portal vein, which lies a short distance (2–4 cm) away from the hepatic vein. After entry of the portal vein, a guidewire is passed and the tract through the liver dilated. The tract is then held open by placement of a metallic vascular stent (Fig. 6–19). The procedure provides a large decompressive shunt that reduces flow in the varices, permitting cessation of bleeding. The shunt operation is effective and has been performed in several hundred patients around the United States; it promises to improve markedly the therapy of portal hypertension. The procedure has been very well received by liver transplant surgeons because it provides a portacaval shunt without the need for an operation. The shunt allows stabilization of the patient; an operation can then be performed under much better circumstances in a nonoperated abdomen.[47-49]

Complications and Nursing Management

Patients with cirrhosis and portal hypertension present complex nursing management difficulties. These patients may be actively bleeding, with many associated hemodynamic problems. The patient is usually in the intensive care unit and generally requires nursing management during the entire procedure, such as fluid management, cardiovascular and respiratory management, and appropriate sedation. Following the procedure, careful observation of the patient for continued bleeding and/or complications of the procedure such as hepatic encephalopathy or high-output cardiac failure is necessary.

ULTRASONOGRAPHY

Indications

Ultrasound examination of the vascular system is widely used because it is accurate, inexpensive, and noninvasive. Indications include the evaluation of abnormalities of blood flow using Doppler and frequency analysis and direct depiction of anatomic abnormalities, such as aneurysm and plaque disease. Ultrasound evaluation is useful in screening for the presence of aneurysms of the aorta and of the femoral or popliteal arteries, as well as the detection and treatment of postcatheterization femoral artery pseudoaneurysms. It can

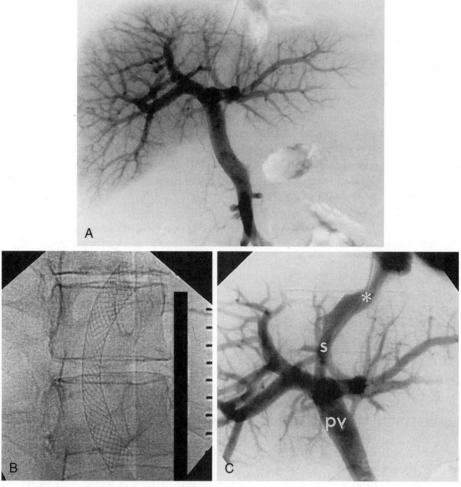

Figure 6–19. Transjugular intrahepatic portosystemic shunt (TIPS). A patient with progressive portal hypertension and variceal bleeding underwent the transjugular procedure. **A,** After placement of a catheter from the hepatic vein through the hepatic parenchyma into the portal vein, a portal venogram was performed. **B,** After balloon dilatation of the tract, a metallic shunt was placed, which causes shunting of blood between the portal vein and hepatic vein. **C,** Portal venogram following the procedure shows contrast in portal vein (pv) with flow-through shunt (s) directly into hepatic vein (*).

readily differentiate hematoma from pseudoaneurysms. Ultrasound can also detect the presence of fluid, hematomas, seromas, and perivascular abnormalities. Detection of intra-abdominal masses or fluid collections in the postoperative vascular patient is another important indication for diagnostic ultrasound.

Technique

The body part to be examined is scanned using any of a variety of transducers utilizing various frequencies. In general, lower frequencies such as 3 MHz (3 million cycles/sec) are used for imaging of deeper structures such as the retroperitoneum and abdomen. Higher-frequency transducers, such as 7 MHz, provide more detail and are best used for more superficially located structures, such as the gallbladder. Ultrahigh-frequency transducers up to 10 MHz usually provide a small field of view and substantially reduced penetration (a few centimeters), but provide exceptional detail of small superficial structures such as the thyroid gland, as well as of superficially located vessels and grafts. Sound waves generated by the transducer penetrate the body part and are reflected, refracted, or absorbed. Those sound waves are reflected and refracted by the structures beneath the transducer and are detected by the same transducer that is sending the signals. These returning sound waves are then converted to images and displayed on a television monitor. In most cases, "real-time" ultrasound is used, which allows detection of motion as well as blood flow.

Ultrasound does have several limitations. In the abdomen, the image may be degraded or blocked by gas and/or fat, which cannot be penetrated by sound waves. Obese patients or patients with excessive bowel gas may not be candidates for complete ultrasound evaluation. Bowel gas can be eliminated by the ingestion of liquid by mouth or the introduction of a water enema for reduction of gas artifact from the colon. Bowel gas may also be shifted in the abdomen by having the patient assume different positions.

Ultrasound-guided compression of postcatheterization femoral artery pseudoaneurysms has been particularly useful. This technique has eliminated the need for surgical repair of 90–95 percent of catheter-related femoral artery pseudoaneurysms. The procedure is simple in that the same transducer that has been used to demonstrate flow within the pseudoaneurysm is used to directly compress the pseudoaneurysm at the point of communication with the underlying artery. Manual compression by the examiner takes place until flow ceases within the pseudoaneurysm and thrombosis occurs. Several cycles of compression of up to 10 minutes each may be necessary to accomplish thrombosis of the pseudoaneurysm unless there is an underlying coagulopathy or the pseudoaneurysm is chronic.[50]

Complications and Nursing Management

Complications of diagnostic ultrasound are essentially nonexistent. Nursing care is directed toward patient education and preparation for the examination, which is relatively simple. For evaluation of the abdominal organs, the patient is usually on NPO status (nothing by mouth) 8 hours prior to testing to reduce gas and to distend the gallbladder maximally. Water may also be administered orally during the examination. Postexamination care is minimal because contrast is not given.

Ultrasound-guided compression of pseudoaneurysms is generally very well tolerated. The patient may experience some pain during forceful compression of the pseudoaneurysm, which might require sedation or injection of local anesthesia at the site of compression. After ultrasound-guided compression obliterates the pseudoaneurysm, careful monitoring of the site for the return of a pseudoaneurysm should be performed clinically because occasionally these may recur. Typically, the patient is monitored with a repeat ultrasound study at 24 or 48 hours to ensure that no pseudoaneurysm remains. The limb under examination should be monitored during and after compression therapy to ensure that all the distal pulses are intact and that there has been no change in the perfusion of the extremity due to the forceful compression of the common femoral artery.

COMPUTED TOMOGRAPHY

Introduction and Indications

Computed tomography (CT) is a powerful imaging tool in vascular disease. CT scanning is routinely used for accurate staging of abdominal aortic aneurysms, as well as in complex postoperative problems such as graft infection, repetitive graft occlusion, hemorrhage, or abscess.[51–54] In addition, CT can be used for guidance of biopsy procedures. All of these developments in CT have been made possible by the technical improvements in the machines available for clinical use. Initially, body scanning was performed with an 18-second scan time and a small number of x-ray detectors. Current scanners are capable of completing a scan in 2 seconds, which substantially reduces motion artifact.[49] These machines also possess an increased number of x-ray detectors, which improves image quality and resolution. The major advantage of CT over other imaging modalities, including arteriography, is that CT allows direct depiction of the arterial wall, and accurately defines processes and structures around the vessel wall that are indicators of disease (e.g., fluid, air, and hematoma).

Technique

Computed tomography produces axial slices of the body, so that anatomy is depicted in cross-section. This sectioning of the body is performed by placing the patient in a circular gantry around which are arrayed an x-ray tube and multiple x-ray detectors. The tube moves around the body while emitting x-rays that are confined to a very narrow beam or slice. The rays pass through the body and are detected on the opposite side by the detectors. The information from the detectors is then processed by high-speed computer and an image is generated. Various sections are obtained by moving the patient through the gantry. The thickness of the slice taken can also be varied between 2 and 10 mm.

For the majority of cases, contrast is administered orally or intravenously. Oral contrast allows identification of bowel and avoids confusion with pathologic masses. Intravenous contrast administration causes enhancement of vessel lumens and allows them to be distinguished from processes such as thrombus in the peripheral portion of an aneurysm, vessel, or graft (Fig. 6–20). It also allows determination of whether a graft or vessel is occluded. Intravenous contrast administration also causes many parenchymal organs, such as the kidney, liver, and spleen, to enhance or become denser. This aids in the detection of benign and malignant masses, which usually do not enhance to the same degree as seen with normal parenchyma.

Biopsies and drainage procedures are also frequently performed under CT guidance, which allows precise localization of masses and fluid collections. A needle, catheter, or guidewire can be placed into collections or masses, using CT to avoid overlying structures. In this manner, postoperative abscesses are drained and deep masses are biopsied.

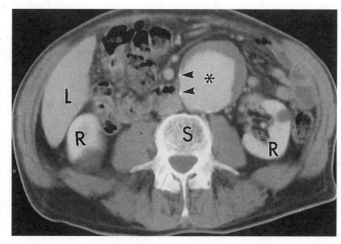

Figure 6–20. Computed tomography of an abdominal aortic aneurysm. Large abdominal aneurysm (*) is identified. Intravenous contrast has opacified (whitened) the lumen of the aneurysm, and thus enables differentiation from unopacified peripheral lower-density thrombus. Notice exquisite anatomic detail that is obtained, including demonstration of minimal calcifications (*arrowheads*) in aortic wall and kidneys (R). Low-density areas within the kidneys represent cysts. Also note liver (L) and spine (S).

Complications and Nursing Management

Complications in CT are minimal because the technique is noninvasive. Patients may experience contrast-induced renal failure or reactions, so urine output and creatinine must be monitored and the patient should be observed for contrast reactions. Additionally, biopsy or drainage procedures performed under CT guidance may rarely have hemorrhagic or septic complications. Nursing care for CT thus revolves primarily around adequate patient preparation, which includes the need for good hydration, because of the use of contrast.

MAGNETIC RESONANCE IMAGING

Indications and Technique

Magnetic resonance imaging (MRI) has now become an accepted imaging tool for vascular disease because of its ability to demonstrate vessels in multiple projection and because conventional intravenous contrast need not be used to demonstrate the vascular lumen. Magnetic resonance angiography (MRA) shows great promise in reducing or even eliminating altogether the need for a number of examinations that were previously performed by conventional arteriography, including evaluation of the carotid bifurcation and detection of lower-extremity vascular disease and abdominal aortic aneursyms. MRA is replacing a significant amount of routine diagnostic angiography procedures in many institutions. CT continues to be used very commonly for evaluation of the thoracic and abdominal aorta. However, MRA is now the technique of choice at many hospitals.

MRI is a simple examination in that no intravenous contrast is given, but not all patients are suitable for the examination. In particular, patients with pacemakers (particularly older varieties that have not been shielded from magnetic resonance frequencies) cannot be scanned due to interference with the pacemaker.

Metallic devices such as implanted surgical clips or vena cava filters, as well as joint replacements, can produce large artifacts that distort or obscure the image. In these patients, CT may be the only technique available. Patients who have had recent intracranial surgery with clips or aneurysm clipping should also not be scanned with MRI because of the possibility that clip movement may occur. Finally, critically ill patients who require life support devices such as respirators (which are made of metal) cannot be scanned using MRI because of the need for absence of any ferromagnetic objects in the room. The reason for their prohibition is simple: The extremely powerful magnet used in MRI can literally pull these devices toward the magnet, potentially causing bodily harm; thus, they are prohibited from being placed anywhere in the scanning room. For these individuals, CT will continue to be the imaging technique of choice.[55] MRI has also been used preliminarily as a guidance system for interventional procedures.[56]

Complications and Nursing Management

Complications in MRI are minimal because the technique is noninvasive. As indicated above, conventional intravenous contrast is not given; therefore, the technique is ideal for patients with renal failure or those who are allergic to contrast. Magnetic resonance contrast is used, but these agents have essentially no renal toxicity or allergic problems. Probably the main issue surrounding nursing care of these patients is the fact that patients must lie relatively motionless during production of the scans, which generally take longer than CT (which usually takes 1–2 seconds per image). However, ultrafast imaging is rapidly being developed, and these techniques make it much easier to obtain diagnostic information in most patients. For individuals who are not able to hold still or who are anxious, appropriate sedation is vital to enable production of good-quality diagnostic scans. Some patients may also become somewhat claustrophobic in the scanner because the gantry completely surrounds the body. In these individuals, reassurance and/or sedation may alleviate the problem.

References

1. Polak JF: Femoral arteriography. In Baum S (ed): Abrams Angiography, 4th ed. Boston, Little, Brown, & Co, 1997, pp 1697–1742.
2. Hallisey MJ, Maranze SG: The abnormal abdominal aorta: Arteriosclerosis and other diseases. In Baum S (ed): Abrams Angiography, 4th ed. Boston, Little, Brown, & Co, 1997, pp 1052–1072.
3. Ouriel K, Shortell CK, DeWeese JA, et al: A comparison of thrombolytic therapy with operative revascularization in the treatment of acute peripheral arterial ischemia. J Vasc Surg 1994; 19:1021–1030.
4. McNamara TO, Fischer JR: Thrombolysis of peripheral arterial and graft occlusions: Improved results using high-dose streptokinase in the treatment of arterial occlusions. AJR 1985; 144:769–775.
5. Feldman L, Greenfield AJ, Waltman AC, et al: Transcatheter vessel occlusion: Angiographic results versus clinical success. Radiology 1983; 147:1–5.
6. Seldinger SI: Catheter replacement of the needle in percutaneous arterography: A new technique. Acta Radiol 1953; 39:368–371.
7. Braun MA, Nemcek AA Jr, Vogelzang RL (eds): Interventional Radiology Procedure Manual. New York, Churchill Livingstone, 1997.
8. White RI: Fundamentals of Vascular Radiology. Philadelphia, Lea and Febiger, 1976.
9. Kandarpa K, Aruny JE (eds): Handbook of Interventional Radiologic Procedures, 2nd ed. Boston, Little, Brown, & Co, 1996.
10. Roy P: Percutaneous catheterization via the axillary artery: A new approach to some technical roadblocks in selective arteriography. AJR 1965; 94:1018–1024.
11. Crain MR, Mewissen MW: Abdominal aortography. In Baum S (ed): Abrams Angiography, 4th ed. Boston, Little, Brown, & Co, 1997, pp 1013–1023.
12. Smith D, Grabvle G, Shipp D: Safe and effective catheter angiography through prosthetic vascular grafts. Radiology 1981; 138:487–488.
13. Lea Thomas M, Browse NL: Venography of the lower extremity. In Neiman HL, Yao JST (eds): Angiography of Vascular Disease. New York, Churchill Livingstone, 1984, 421–480.
14. Beckmann CF, Abrams HL: Renal venography: Anatomy, technique, applications, analysis of 132 venograms and a review of the literature. Cardiovasc Intervent Radiol 1980; 3:45–51.
15. Lea Thomas M, McAllister V, Tonge K: The radiological appearance of deep venous thrombosis. Clin Radiol 1971; 22:295–305.
16. Herman RJ, Neiman HL, Malave S, et al: Descending venography: A method of evaluating lower extremity venous valvular function. Radiology 1980; 137:63–69.
17. Marks LS, Maxwell MH: Renal vein renin: Value and limitations in the prediction of operative results. Urol Clin North Am 1975; 2:311–318.
18. Dotter C, Judkins M: Transluminal treatment of arteriosclerotic obstructions: Description of a new technique and a preliminary report of its applications. Circulation 1964; 30:654–670.
19. Gruntzig A, Kumpe DA: Technique of percutaneous transluminal angioplasty with the Gruntzig balloon catheter. AJR 1979; 132:547–522.
20. Tegtmeyer CJ, Matsumoto AH, Johnson AM: Renal angioplasty. In Pentecost M, Baum S (eds): Abrams Angiography Interventional Radiology. Boston, Little, Brown, & Co, 1997, pp 294–325.
21. Frieman DG, Ring EJ, Oleaga JA, et al: Transluminal angioplasty of the iliac, femoral, and popliteal arteries. Radiology 1979; 132:285–288.
22. Gruntzig AR, Senning A, Siegenthalar WE: Nonoperative dilatation of coronary artery stenosis. N Engl J Med 1979; 301:61–70.
23. Motarjeme A, Keiffer JW, Zuska AJ: Percutaneous transluminal angioplasty of the brachiocephalic arteries. AJR 1982; 138:457–560.
24. Rholl KS: Percutaneous aortoiliac interventions in vascular disease. In Pentecost M, Baum S (eds): Abrams Angiography Interventional Radiology. Boston, Little, Brown, & Co, 1997, pp 225–261.
25. Becker GJ, Katzen BT, Dake MD: Noncoronary angioplasty. Radiology 1989; 170:921–940.
26. Kim D, Gianturco LE, Porter DH, et al: Peripheral atherectomy: 4-year experience. Radiology 1992; 183:773–778.

27. McCarthy WJ, Vogelzang RL, Nemcek AA Jr, et al: Excimer laser-assisted femoral angioplasty: Early results. J Vasc Surg 1990; 13:607–614.
28. Douek PC, Leon MB, Geschwind H, et al: Occlusive peripheral vascular disease: A multicenter trial of fluorescence-guided, pulsed dye laser-assisted balloon angioplasty. Intervent Radiol 1991; 180:127–133.
29. Gunther RW, Vorwerk D, Antonucci F, et al: Iliac artery stenosis of obstruction after unsuccessful balloon angioplasty: Treatment with a self-expandable stent. AJR 1991; 156:389–393.
30. Long AL, Page PE, Raynaud AC, et al: Percutaneous iliac artery stent: Angiographic long-term follow-up. Radiology 1991; 180:771–778.
31. Murphy TP, Webb MS, Lambiase RE, et al: Percutaneous revascularization of complex iliac artery stenoses and occlusions using Wallstents: 2-year experience. J Vasc Interv Radiol 1996 7:21–27.
32. Palmaz JC, Laborde JC, Rivera FJ, et al: Stenting of the iliac arteries with the Palmaz stent: Experience from a multicenter trial. Cardiovasc Intervent Radiol 1992; 15:291–297.
33. Hausegger KA, Lammer J, Hagen B, et al: Iliac artery stenting: Clinical experience with the Palmaz stent, Wallstent, and Strecker stent. Acta Radiol 1992; 33:292–296.
34. Henry M, Armor M, Ethevenot G, et al: Palmaz stent placement in iliac and femoropopliteal arteries: Primary and secondary patency in 410 patients with 2–4 year follow-up. Radiology 1995; 197:167–174.
35. Tegtmeyer CJ, Kellum CD, Ayers C: Percutaneous transluminal angioplasty of the renal arteries: Results and long term followup. Radiology 1984; 153:77–84
36. Roubin GS, Yadav S, Iyer SS, et al: Carotid stent-supported angioplasty: A neurovascular intervention to prevent stroke. Am J Cardiol 1996; 78(3A):8–12.
37. Levy JM, Hessel SJ: Complications of angiography and interventional radiology. In Baum S (ed): Abrams Angiography, 4th ed. Boston, Little, Brown, & Co, 1997, pp 1024–1051.
38. Cragg AH, Smith TP, Corson JD, et al: Two urokinase dose regimens in native arterial and graft occlusions: Initial results of a prospective long term randomized clinical trial. Radiology 1991; 178:681–686.
39. Valji K, Roberts AC, Davis GB, Bookstein JJ: Pulsed-spray thrombolysis of arterial and bypass graft occlusions. AJR 1991; 156:617–621.
40. Dake MD, Semba CP: Thrombolytic therapy in venous occlusive disease. J Vasc Intervent Radiol 1986; 6:73S–77S.
41. Zuckerman DA, Bocchini TP, Birnbaum EH: Massive hemorrhage in the lower gastrointestinal tract in adults: Diagnostic imaging and intervention. AJR 1993; 161:703–711.
42. Lang EK: Transcatheter embolization of pelvic vessels for control of intractable hemorrhage. Radiology 1981; 140:331–339.
43. Vogelzang RL, Yakes WF: Vascular malformations: Effective treatment with absolute alcohol. In Pearce WH, Yao JST (eds): Arterial Surgery: Management of Challenging Problems. Appleton & Lange, 1996, pp 553–550.
44. Dorfman GS: Percutaneous inferior vena caval filters. Radiology 1990; 174:987–992.
45. Murphy TP, Dorfman GS, Yedlicka JW, et al: LGM vena cava filter: Objective evaluation of early results. J Vasc Interv Radiol 1992; 2:107–115.
46. Ferris EJ, McCowan TC, Carver DK, et al: Percutaneous inferior vena caval filters: Follow-up of seven designs in 320 patients. Radiology 1993; 181:851–856.
47. Richter GM, Noeldge G, Palmaz JC, et al: Transjugular intrahepatic portacaval stent shunt: Preliminary clinical results. Radiology 1990; 174:1027–1030.
48. Haskal Z: Interventions in portal hypertension. In Pentecost M, Baum S (eds): Abrams Angiography Interventional Radiology. Boston, Little, Brown, & Co, 1997, pp 525–546.
49. Zemel G, Becker GJ, Bancroft JW, et al: Technical advances in transjugular intrahepatic portosystemic shunts. Radiographics 1992; 12:615–622.
50. Fellmeth BD, Roberts AC, Bookstein JJ, et al: Postangiographic femoral artery injuries: Nonsurgical repair with US-guided compression. Radiology 1991; 178:671–675.
51. Larsson EM, Albrechtsson U, Christenson JR: Computed tomography versus aortography for preoperative evaluation of abdominal aortic aneurysm. Acta Radiol Diagn 1991; 25:95–100.
52. Anderson PE, Lorentzen JE: Comparison of computed tomography and aortography in abdominal aortic aneurysms. J Comput Assist Tomogr 1983; 7:670–673.
53. Mark A, Moss AA, Lusby R, et al: CT evaluation of complications of abdominal aortic surgery. Radiology 1982; 145:409–414.
54. Williams LR, Flinn WR, Yao JST, et al: Extended use of computerized tomography in the management of complex aortic problems: A learning experience. J Vasc Surg 1986; 4:264–271.
55. Vogelzang RL, Fitzgerald SW: Magnetic resonance imaging of venous disorders. In Yao JST, Pearce WH (eds): Technologies in Vascular Surgery. Philadelphia, WB Saunders, 1992, pp 106–125.
56. Wildermuth S, Debatin JF, Leung DA, et al: MR-guided intravascular procedures: Initial demonstration in a pig model. Radiology 1997; 202:578–583.

7

Intraoperative Nursing Care of the Vascular Patient

Carol Cox, RN, and Lynn M. Borgini, RN

∽ · ∽

Beyond the "Surgery—No Admittance" signs is a technologically advanced world of highly skilled professionals who work in unison to provide care to a wide and varied surgical population. The team consists of two nurses (a circulating nurse and a scrub nurse), the surgeon and his or her assistants, an anesthesiologist, and ancillary personnel.

Health care workers and patients alike frequently perceive the operating room (OR) as a mysterious and threatening environment. Because of a lack of exposure to the OR during the formal education process, health care workers may be unfamiliar with OR protocols. They may also be intimidated by the many restrictions and strict adherence to technique that guide OR practice. The anticipation of surgery is a very stressful time for the patient and the family, resulting in high anxiety levels. Patients scheduled for surgery are sedated with drugs that have an antianxiety and amnesic effect. As a side effect of these drugs, the patient's recall of events during the perioperative phase is severely diminished or lost.

The information presented in this chapter is pertinent to the nurse who cares for the patient before and after surgical intervention as well as the perioperative nurse. The purpose of this chapter is to familiarize all nurses with the nursing process of assessment, planning, intervention, and evaluation and its application in the vascular OR suite. In addition, it will provide the novice vascular OR practitioner with the advanced knowledge and expertise necessary to aid the vascular patient through this operative phase of his or her illness.

The nurse plays a significant role in the vascular OR suite. He or she must have a thorough knowledge of vascular anatomy and physiology as well as expertise in the technical component. It is an exciting role that continues to expand and challenge the vascular OR nurse.

INTRAOPERATIVE NURSING CARE

Intraoperatively, vascular patients require a multidisciplinary approach. Good communication skills are an essential priority within the specialty of perioperative nursing. The scrub and circulating nurses have an ongoing communication process throughout the operative phase. The circulating nurse works closely with the anesthesiologist, vascular nurse clinician, surgical intensive care unit, and ancillary departments. This collaborative effort among health team members is vital for a successful outcome.

Aseptic Technique

It is the dual responsibility of the scrub and circulating nurses to create, maintain, and monitor surgical asepsis to reduce the potential for infection. A safe and aseptic environment is achieved through careful observance of the principles of asepsis throughout all phases of the operative procedure. The principles of sterilization, disinfection, decontamination, and environmental monitoring are used in maintaining a surgically clean environment.

Equipment

To maintain an efficient, safe intraoperative environment, the scrub and circulating nurses must have a thorough working knowledge of all specialized equipment. They must coordinate and organize equipment and supplies on the basis of patient needs and type of surgical procedure. These items are selected in an organized, timely, and cost-effective manner. The nurse must make sure this equipment is in proper working order and readily available for the procedure. All supplies to be used on the operative field must be inspected for sterility. Package integrity and expiration date must be noted before placement on the sterile field (Fig. 7–1). The scrub nurse is responsible for the preparation and organization of all instruments and supplies on the sterile field and for the efficient handing of instruments to the surgeon and the surgeon's assistants throughout the procedure. The nurse anticipates the need for additional instruments and supplies due to unplanned changes in the surgical procedure. Both nurses count sponges, needles, blades, and instruments (according to hospital policy). The counts must be documented on the

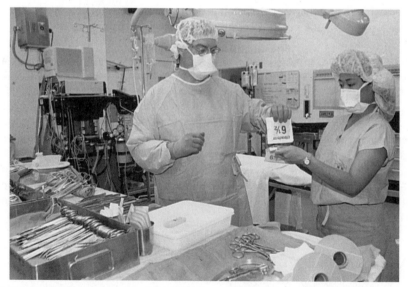

Figure 7–1. Scrub and circulating nurses following aseptic technique when handling sterile items on the surgical field.

patient's operative record (Fig. 7–2). Counts are performed before the first incision and before closure of the incision sites.

Patient Care

The nurse's health assessment of the patient consists of the identification of physiologic, psychologic, and psychosocial data. Interpretation of this information assists the nurse in forming a plan of care and in identifying individual patient problems (Table 7–1).

The nurse assesses the patient's coping mechanisms, expectations of care, and knowledge of the proposed procedure and the specific operative site. The nurse reinforces what the surgeon has explained to the patient regarding the procedure, making sure that he or she has a clear understanding of the operative event.

The circulating nurse has multiple responsibilities. The nurse must perform a thorough assessment of the patient in the preoperative holding area. After introducing herself to the patient, the nurse verifies the patient's name and hospital number through analysis of the patient's addressograph plate and identification bracelet (Fig. 7–3). If blood products have been ordered, the patient's name and identification number on the blood band bracelet are confirmed with that on the blood products.

Results of laboratory tests, coagulation profile, electrocardiogram, and chest radiograph are verified. Completed and signed operative and anesthesia consent forms, allergy and NPO (nothing by mouth) status are confirmed. The presence of any valuables such as dentures, eyeglasses, jewelry, or contact lenses should be documented and the valuables returned safely to the nursing unit or a family member.

In the preoperative holding area, the anesthesiologist interviews and assesses the patient. The various forms of anesthesia available, depending on age and concurrent medical conditions, are discussed. Intravenous and arterial lines are inserted; a Swan-Ganz catheter may be inserted in the OR suite if indicated.

In the OR suite, the circulating nurse and the anesthesiologist coordinate the safe

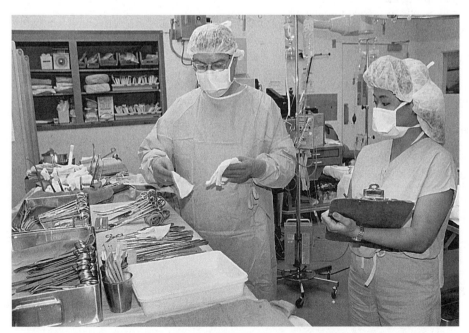

Figure 7–2. Scrub and circulating nurses counting Raytec sponges before surgical procedure. The circulating nurse documents these counts on a separate count sheet and the operative record.

TABLE 7–1. **Nursing Diagnoses and Interventions**

Anxiety
Nursing Intervention
Assess patient's anxiety level.
Assess patient's knowledge and understanding of procedure.
Reinforce preoperative teaching.
Explain all procedures and preoperative preparation.
Discuss patient's questions and concerns in the preanesthetic area.
Provide comfort/security measures as needed (e.g., warm blankets, holding hand) during induction.
Introduce patient to personnel responsible for his/her care.
Maintain a quiet environment in the operating room suite.
Maintain patient dignity.
Maintain patient confidentiality.

Impairment of Skin Integrity
Nursing Intervention
Document presence of allergies.
Assess and document condition of patient's skin preoperatively, e.g., skin turgor, elasticity, rashes, bruises, or reddened areas.
Provide a preoperative wet shave in the holding room to prevent breaks in patient's skin integrity.
Move patient slowly and gently onto the operating room bed.
Document type of skin preparation used for preoperative scrub.
Provide adequate padding to all bony prominences, protecting nerve pathways.
Provide ongoing assessment of pressure points and relieve pressure as identified.
Place electrocautery dispersive pad on muscular body parts, avoiding bony prominences.
Document on the operative record all equipment and positioning devices.

Infection
Nursing Intervention
Visibly inspect room for cleanliness prior to opening sterile supplies.
Provide sterile skin preparation to operative site.
Inspect sterile items for package integrity, expiration date, and sterilization process indicator.
Create effective barriers to transmission of microorganisms through proper gowning, gloving, and draping procedures.
Maintain aseptic technique throughout the procedure.
Initiate corrective action when break in technique occurs.
Limit traffic in the vascular suite during procedure.
Apply sterile dressings at end of procedure.
Administer antibiotics per physician's order.
Open prosthetic grafts as close to time of insertion as possible.

Hypothermia
Nursing Intervention
Assess patient's weight, height, and age.
Place warming blanket and check correct temperature settings.
Increase room temperature before the patient enters vascular suite.
Place warm blankets on patient when entering vascular suite.
Limit exposure of patient during surgical preparation.
Provide warm intravenous fluids for anesthesia (i.e., provide blood warmer).
Provide warm fluids for irrigation of the surgical field.

TABLE 7–1. **Nursing Diagnoses and Interventions** *Continued*

Surgical Intervention

Nursing Intervention

Assess and document preoperative level of consciousness.

Assess preoperative vital signs.

Assess preoperative laboratory values.

Anticipate potential blood loss.

Confirm and document availability of blood products for transfusion.

Implement use of blood salvage machine and/or rapid infusion when indicated.

Document amount of irrigation used on surgical field.

Retained Foreign Body

Nursing Intervention

Follow established policy and procedures for sharp, sponge, and instrument count.

Confine and contain all discarded sponges, sharps, and instruments. Do not remove counted items or trash from the operating room suite after initiation of surgical count.

Notify attending surgeon when surgical counts are incorrect. Document corrective action and persons notified on incident form for risk management.

Document results of surgical counts on operative record.

Perform surgical count during change of shift and document on surgical count sheet.

transfer of the patient onto the OR bed. To ensure the patient's safety, a safety belt attached to the bed is applied above the knees. Monitoring equipment, a blood pressure cuff, a pulse oximeter, an arterial line, and electrocardiogram leads are applied.

This can be a very stressful time for the patient, who is surrounded by unfamiliar faces and equipment that can appear frightening. The circulating nurse continues to provide emotional support, comfort, and a quiet atmosphere. These measures can minimize stress during this time.

The temperature of the OR is quite cool, between 68° and 70° Fahrenheit. This cool temperature, as well as a low humidity setting, is used to prevent the growth of

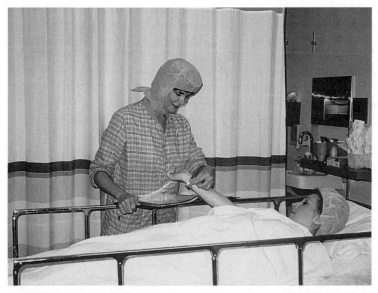

Figure 7–3. Circulating nurse performing a preoperative assessment of the patient in the preoperative holding area.

microorganisms. A warming blanket, warm intravenous fluids, and irrigation solutions are used throughout the procedure to prevent hypothermia.

The patient is anesthetized and an indwelling Foley catheter is inserted into the bladder if the procedure dictates. The endotracheal tube and monitoring and infusion lines are secured and easily accessible to the anesthesiologist. The circulating nurse places the dispersive pad for the electrocautery unit in a dry, well-padded area (usually the buttocks).

Positioning of the patient is a collaborative effort on the part of the surgeon, the circulating nurse, and the anesthesiologist. The circulating nurse obtains and arranges all equipment necessary for patient positioning before the patient is admitted to the OR. Positioning is performed slowly and carefully to provide maximal exposure of the surgical site without compromising respiratory, neurologic, and vascular function. All bony prominences and areas of potential circulatory compromise are padded.

Preparation of the operative site consists of a one-step prep consisting of iodophor (0.7 percent iodine) and 74 percent isopropyl alcohol. It provides rapid, long-lasting microbicidal action against a broad spectrum of microbes. The scrub nurse assists the surgical team in applying sterile drapes around the operative site. Equipment and supplies needed for the procedure (i.e., cautery, suction) are passed off the field by the scrub nurse. The circulating nurse connects the equipment to the appropriate unit and confirms any power settings with the surgeon.

CAROTID ENDARTERECTOMY

Carotid endarterectomy is performed for arteriosclerotic occlusive disease of the carotid artery. A carotid endarterectomy surgically removes the occluding atheroma, and eliminates the source of emboli. Transient ischemic attacks (TIAs) and stroke are embolic or thrombotic in origin. As a result of potential atheromatous debris, emboli may arise from the carotid bifurcation and lodge in the ipsilateral cerebral hemisphere, or the internal carotid artery may occlude as a result of atheroma and/or thrombosis of the carotid artery.

Indications include severe asymptomatic stenosis of the carotid artery, a TIA, stroke, and recurrent carotid artery disease. A bruit, caused by turbulent blood flow through a narrowed artery, can often be auscultated in persons with carotid artery disease. This turbulence, which takes the form of vibrations, is transmitted to the skin surface. A TIA can cause motor and sensory deficits of the extremities on the side opposite the diseased carotid artery. Speech impairment may occur if the dominant hemisphere (speech center) is involved. Patients often ignore these symptoms because of rapid recovery. If these symptoms are ignored, a subsequent TIA can lead to a stroke.[1]

Cerebral perfusion occurs via collaterals and the circle of Willis when the carotid artery is clamped. Intraoperative surveillance of cerebral blood flow may be performed continuously with an electroencephalogram (EEG) monitor during carotid endarterectomy. Acute cerebral ischemia can be immediately assessed, as can the efficacy of any corrective actions. EEG monitoring also provides a permanent record of the adequacy of anesthesia and information about any complications.[2] An EEG monitoring cap is placed on the patient's head perioperatively in the holding area by an EEG technician (Fig. 7–4).

After the induction of anesthesia, the patient remains supine on the OR bed with a blanket roll under the shoulders. The patient's head is placed on a foam ring for support. This position allows for slight hyperextension of the neck for adequate surgical exposure of the carotid vessels (Fig. 7–5).

A light touch is used during the surgical preparation to avoid dislodging atheromatous plaque in the carotid artery. A neck incision approximately 4 inches in length is made parallel to the sternocleidomastoid muscle. The incision begins medially and extends posteriorly under the lobe of the ear. Nerve injuries are caused by inadvertent transection or surgical retractors. The hypoglossal nerve (twelfth cranial nerve) must be identified

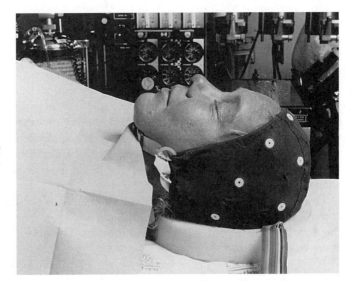

Figure 7–4. Patient with electro-encephalogram (EEG) monitoring cap before carotid endarterectomy.

and preserved. Injury to this nerve can result in deviation of the tongue to the operative side, with difficulty in speech and mastication.

The surgeon proceeds by dissecting down to the carotid sheath. The common facial vein that runs across the carotid artery is identified and divided. The carotid sheath is opened, and the common, internal, and external carotid arteries are identified and isolated with vessel loops. At this time the patient may experience bradycardia or hypotension as a result of manipulation of the carotid sinus. In this event, the surgeon injects into the carotid sinus 0.5–1.0 ml of local anesthetic (1 percent lidocaine), which the scrub nurse has prepared on the surgical field.

The surgeon orders heparin to be given intravenously by the anesthesiologist approximately 5 minutes before clamping of the arteries. Heparin is given to prevent thromboemboli while the carotid arteries are clamped.

In addition to EEG monitoring, internal carotid artery back-pressure (stump pressure) is used to assess the adequacy of cerebral perfusion. Stump pressure is measured with a 21-gauge needle attached to a 4-foot pressure line. The needle is inserted into the common carotid artery. The opposite end of the line is passed to the anesthesiologist and

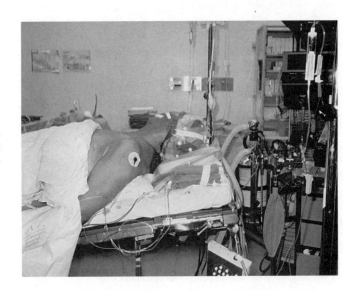

Figure 7–5. Patient on the operating table positioned for carotid endarterectomy with EEG monitoring cap.

attached to the arterial line. A pressure measurement is obtained before clamping of the common carotid artery. The common carotid artery is clamped with a vascular clamp, and a second pressure measurement is obtained. A stump pressure greater than 35 mmHg (mean) is usually adequate for proper cerebral perfusion.

If the stump pressure is below 35 mmHg and/or EEG changes occur with carotid clamping, an intraluminal shunt is used to provide temporary cerebral perfusion. The shunt permits blood flow to the brain via the internal carotid artery. The shunt consists of silicone elastomer with stainless steel spring reinforcements to minimize kinking and occlusion of the cannula lumen. The ends of the shunt have cone-shaped bulbs to facilitate fixation of the shunt in the vessel (Fig. 7–6). These shunts come in different diameters to adapt to the patient's anatomy.

Once the stump pressure has been measured, vascular clamps are placed on the common, external, and internal carotid arteries. The arteriotomy (surgical incision into the artery) is made with a No. 11 knife blade. The arteriotomy is extended with angled Potts vascular scissors.

If an intraluminal shunt is indicated, the distal end of the shunt is inserted into the common carotid artery; the proximal end of the shunt is inserted into the internal carotid artery. The previously placed vascular clamps are removed from the common and internal carotid arteries as each end of the shunt is inserted. A specialized clamp replaces each vascular clamp to secure the shunt.

The surgeon performs the endarterectomy around the shunt. The plaque is carefully peeled off the intima layer of the artery with a blunt instrument. The plaque is sent to the pathology department for examination and documentation. Before the artery is closed, the arteriotomy site is irrigated with heparin-saline solution to remove any small atheromatous debris left behind. Before complete closure of the arteriotomy, the three arteries are reclamped and the shunt is removed. The arteriotomy is closed and completed with monofilament polypropylene suture material.

In some cases (i.e., with reoperative carotid endarterectomy and in patients with small arteries), a patch graft of autogenous vein or prosthetic material is used in reconstruction of the artery. Placement of such a patch, known as a patch graft angioplasty, prevents compromise in arterial diameter or blood flow. Before wound closure, hemostasis is

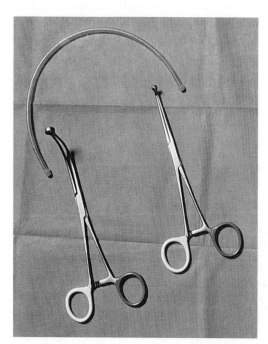

Figure 7–6. Carotid shunt with cone-shaped bulbs to facilitate fixation of the shunt in the carotid artery. The shunt is held in place with specialized clamps.

achieved at the arteriotomy site and small bleeders are cauterized. Muscular, subcutaneous, and skin layers are closed and a dressing is applied.

The patient is awakened in the OR for assessment of neurologic function. Assessment is performed by asking the patient to follow simple commands, such as moving the fingers and toes contralateral to the affected carotid. Extremity strength is assessed by having the patient grasp the surgeon's hand. Then the patient is discharged to the recovery room.

Postoperative complications include perioperative stroke, hypertension, hypotension, hematoma, and operative death. Neurologic deficit is caused by intraoperative cerebral embolism or insufficient cerebral blood flow during carotid clamping. Factors contributing to hematoma formation include aspirin administered preoperatively, heparin given intra-operatively, coughing and straining during extubation, and technical factors. Hematomas should be treated aggressively because they can cause tracheal compression with airway compromise.

AORTIC SURGERY

The majority of patients undergoing surgery of the aorta are seen because of aneurysm or arterial occlusive disease. Risk factors for occlusive disease and aneurysm are similar: smoking, hypertension, age, diabetes mellitus, and genetics.

Occlusive disease occurs as a result of atherosclerosis. A combination of changes in the intima and media layers of the artery results in atherosclerosis. Intimal plaque enlargement can produce lumen stenosis. However, atherosclerosis is associated with artery dilation in the major arteries such as the aorta. As a result, aortic repair for occlusive disease is seen less frequently.[3]

Aneurysms are irreversible dilations of the arterial wall involving all layers. They are usually caused by one of four conditions: degenerative, mycotic, traumatic, or inherited. Recent clinical observations and research suggest that pathogenesis of aneurysms may be more complex than initially believed and is probably multifactorial in origin.

The size of the abdominal aortic aneurysm is a vital indicator in the decision for operative intervention. Symptoms of a leaking or ruptured aneurysm are the sudden onset of back and abdominal pain accompanied by hypotension.

Preoperative Evaluation

The major cause of death after surgery of the aorta is myocardial infarction. Before surgery it is essential to assess cardiac and pulmonary status by means of an electrocardiogram, a radiograph of the chest, routine blood work, and, if indicated, a dipyridamole-thallium scan and cardiac catheterization. Such an assessment can significantly reduce the morbidity and mortality of the elective procedure.

A computed tomography scan provides an accurate determination of the size and level of the aneurysm. An arteriogram delineates the renal, mesenteric, iliac, and lower-extremity arteries.

Elective treatment of an abdominal aortic aneurysm involves resection of the aneurysm and replacement with a synthetic graft. Treatment of arterial occlusive disease involves replacement with a synthetic graft or occasionally an aortic endarterectomy. These synthetic grafts can be straight (tube) or bifurcated, extending to both iliac or femoral arteries. The disease process may dictate that one limb of the bifurcated graft extend to the iliac artery and the second limb to the femoral artery.

Monitoring lines inserted preoperatively include an arterial line and, if indicated, a Swan-Ganz catheter. General endotracheal anesthesia is induced and a Foley catheter is inserted. The abdomen is prepared from the nipple line to the knees. A midline incision is made from the xyphoid to the symphysis pubis. The abdomen is explored for other pathologic conditions (i.e., malignant disease). If such conditions are found, the elective procedure may be cancelled so that these subsequent findings can be addressed. A self-retaining retractor holds the abdomen open. A nasal gastric tube is inserted by the anesthesiologist, and its placement is checked by the surgeon. The bowels are lifted out of the abdominal cavity. Moist towels or lap sponges are placed over the bowels to eliminate exposure and provide protection.

Proximal control of the aorta is obtained by placement of a large vessel loop around the aorta. When required, the iliac and femoral arteries are also controlled with vessel loops. Before the vessels are clamped, heparin is given systemically by the anesthesiologist and allowed to circulate for 5 minutes. The iliac vessels are clamped first to prevent dislodgment of atheromatous debris into the legs. The proximal aorta is clamped, usually below the renal arteries in 90–95 percent of the cases. Clamping above the renal arteries for approximately 30–45 minutes is usually tolerated by the kidneys. An arteriotomy is made in the aorta with a No. 11 knife blade and extended with scissors. In aneurysmal disease, the thrombus is evacuated and lumbar arteries are ligated within the aneurysm. Blood loss is suctioned into the cardiotomy reservoir of a blood salvage machine for reinfusion by the anesthesiologist (see section on "Blood Salvage").

The lumen of the aorta is sized by the surgeon for proper selection of a synthetic graft. The circulating and scrub nurses confirm graft size before placement on the surgical field. The end-to-end anastomosis between native aorta and graft is performed proximally. A straight tube graft is used if the iliac and femoral arteries are free of disease. If the iliac and/or the femoral arteries are diseased, a bifurcated graft is used. The graft is flushed with arterial blood to remove thrombus and debris that might otherwise embolize to the distal limbs.

The proximal clamp is slowly released to prevent hypotension. The rate of declamping is determined by continuous monitoring of the patient's blood pressure. If hypotension is detected, the aorta is temporarily reclamped and additional fluids are given by the anesthesiologist.

Hemostasis at the anastomotic suture lines is achieved to prevent postoperative hematoma formation. The old aneurysm wall is sutured over the synthetic graft. Closure of the retroperitoneum is essential to prevent erosion of the bowel into the synthetic graft and a resultant aortoduodenal fistula. At this time the first sponge and needle count is performed by the scrub and circulating nurses.

The midline incision is closed with a heavy suture. A second sponge and needle count, as well as an instrument count, is performed. A final sponge and needle count is performed at the time of skin closure. The incisions are covered with sterile dressings, and the drapes are removed. Continuity of sterility of instrumentation is maintained by the scrub and circulating nurses until the patient leaves the OR. This is mandatory in the event of immediate reoperation. The femoral and pedal pulses are assessed before the patient is extubated.

RUPTURED ABDOMINAL AORTIC ANEURYSM

An aortic rupture is usually characterized by the escape of blood into the space between the wall of the aorta and the periaortic sheath. The patient will experience a sudden onset of pain and a transient drop in blood pressure. This hematoma may be confined to the periaorta for a few hours or much longer. If the hematoma breaks through into the retroperitoneum and peritoneal cavity, hypovolemic shock occurs. It is crucial that these patients be transported to the OR and the aorta cross-clamped without delay.

Nursing Care

Intraoperative nursing care of the patient undergoing elective repair of an abdominal aortic aneurysm differs from that of the patient with a ruptured abdominal aortic aneurysm. In the latter, time is of the essence to control aortic bleeding and save the patient's life. In this short span of time, multiple demands are placed on the OR nursing staff, and the knowledge and skills they bring to the task are of critical importance. It is essential that the scrub and circulating nurses be capable of prioritizing these responsibilities. An emergency abdominal vascular cart with instruments, supplies, and suture material should be available in the vascular OR suite at all times.

The OR nurses receive notification from the emergency room that a patient is being admitted directly to the OR. On arrival, the patient is taken directly to the vascular OR suite, where preparations to administer an anesthetic and to open the abdomen can proceed simultaneously. The circulating nurse opens the supplies while the scrub nurse gowns and gloves only. Time does not permit scrubbing the hands and arms before gowning and gloving. It is important for nurses and physicians to maintain sterility while circumventing some steps practiced in an elective procedure.

The circulating nurse is responsible for the availability of the blood salvage machine and all blood products. If the blood salvage technician is not readily available, the circulating nurse is responsible for the partial set-up of the blood salvage machine.

Emergency Blood Salvage — Partial Set-up

Supplies

Blood salvage machine
Cardiotomy reservoir
1 L 0.9 percent sodium chloride
40,000 U heparin
2 blood salvage suction tubings
1 standard suction tubing

Instructions for Set-up

Open cardiotomy reservoir and place into the ring on blood-salvage machine.

Hang 1-L bag of 0.9 percent sodium chloride with 40,000 U heparin from the intravenous pole on the machine.

Open two blood salvage suction tubings on the sterile field.

Place one end of the standard suction tubing to the wall suction and the other end to the cardiotomy reservoir.

The blood salvage suction tubing has one end consisting of an intravenous spike and suction port. This end is handed off the sterile field by the scrub nurse to the circulating nurse. The circulating nurse connects the spiked end to the liter of heparinized saline solution and the suction port to the cardiotomy reservoir.

Allow 100 ml of heparinized solution to run into the cardiotomy reservoir, reducing flow to keep an open rate.

Partial set-up is complete.

TABLE 7–2. **Mayo Stand Instrumentation
for Abdominal Aortic Aneurysm**

1	No. 10 knife blade
2	Hemostats
2	Boettcher hemostats (tonsil)
2	Vascular Mixter (fine tip)
2	Short DeBakey tissue forceps
2	Long DeBakey tissue forceps
1	7″ Potts-Smith scissor (Richter)
1	9″ Potts-Smith scissor (Richter)
2	Boettcher hemostats with 4-0 nonabsorbable suture pass points
1	Boettcher hemostat with 2-0 nonabsorbable suture pass points
1	2-0 nonabsorbable suture ligature to ligate lumbar arteries
2	Large DeBakey vascular clamps
1	Aortic compressor

In addition:

1	Self-retaining retractor (Grieshaber)
2	Blood salvage suction tubings
2	Wet towels
2	Glass retractors
1	Large Deaver retractor

Trained ancillary personnel may be needed to assist the circulating nurse in emergency care of the patient. They can access necessary blood products, notify emergency personnel, and provide additional support staff for nurses, the surgeon, and the anesthesiologist. This allows the circulating nurse to provide immediate, direct, intraoperative care to the patient.

Time does not permit an instrument or sharp count. However, lap sponges must be counted. It must be noted on the OR medical record that an instrument and sharp count was not performed due to an emergency. The surgeon must be notified and an incident report filed with risk management.

Before intubation by the anesthesiologist, a germicidal solution is painted over the patient's abdomen from nipple line to knees. The surgeon gowns and gloves only. Sterile drapes are applied.

The instruments for elective and emergency operations on abdominal aortic aneurysms are virtually the same. Instrumentation will be specific to each institution. Initial, emergency instrumentation on the Mayo stand is listed in Table 7–2.

For control of rupture, the aortic compressor is placed on the proximal end of the aorta and the aorta is clamped proximally and distally with large DeBakey clamps (Fig. 7–7).

Hypothermia is most often a clinically important problem during prolonged operations

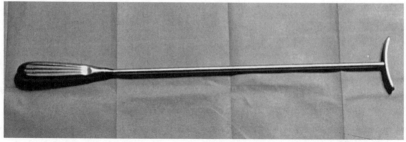

Figure 7–7. The surgeon places the aortic compressor proximal to the point of aortic rupture to control hemorrhage.

that require a large surgical incision and large volumes of intravenous fluids. Heat loss is common in all patients during general anesthesia because anesthetics alter thermoregulation. An adverse effect of hypothermia is postoperative shivering. This is a risk, particularly in the elderly, because it increases the basal metabolic rate. Oxygen consumption increases, placing additional demands on the cardiac and pulmonary systems. In the elderly, if either of these systems cannot compensate, arterial hypoxemia may result.

All intravenous fluids should be kept warm by means of fluid warmers. A warmer supplied with saline irrigation and various intravenous fluids may be useful. The circulating nurse keeps these fluids readily available for when they are needed by the anesthesiologist and the scrub nurse. Warmth reduces blood viscosity and improves tissue blood flow. A warm OR at the outset of the procedure is beneficial until the patient is draped. Control of OR temperature throughout the procedure limits radiant heat loss from surgical incisions.

The patient will be discharged to the recovery room or directly to an intensive care unit. If the patient is to remain intubated and dependent on a ventilator, the circulating nurse receives ventilator settings from the anesthesiologist. The nurse then informs the intensive care nurse of the patient's direct admission, ventilator settings, and any other pertinent information. Additional responsibilities of the circulating nurse for patient transfer include availability of an Ambu bag, an oxygen tank, and an electrocardiogram monitor.

Improved operative techniques, better monitoring in the intensive care unit, and improved preoperative and postoperative management have reduced the risks associated with repair of the abdominal aortic aneurysm. A successful outcome of this procedure depends on careful operative technique, close attention to anesthetic technique, and highly skilled perioperative nursing care.

Retroperitoneal Approach

Indications for a retroperitoneal approach to the aorta include pulmonary or cardiac insufficiency, multiple previous abdominal surgical procedures, and obesity. There are several advantages to retroperitoneal exposure of the aorta over the standard transperitoneal approach. The intestines are not exposed or manipulated with this approach. As a result, patients may resume oral intake sooner, body temperature is easier to maintain, and operative stress is decreased. A flank incision also causes less respiratory compromise than a midline abdominal incision. These are important factors in patients with significant heart disease and obstructive pulmonary disease. As a result of multiple abdominal procedures, adhesions form within the abdominal cavity. Adhesions require lysis with the standard midline abdominal incision; the retroperitoneal approach avoids these adhesions, which decreases incidence of bowel perforation.

Endovascular Approach to the Abdominal Aortic Aneurysm

Nursing care of the patient undergoing an endovascular graft replacement presents a new and challenging role for the vascular nurse.

The endovascular graft is wound tightly in a catheter that is introduced through a skin incision into the femoral artery (Fig. 7–8). The catheter is then advanced to a level above the aortic aneurysm but below renal arteries. The graft is then released from the catheter and attached into the aorta above the aneurysm with a series of hooks. The catheter is pulled back to a point below the aneurysm and attached in the same way.

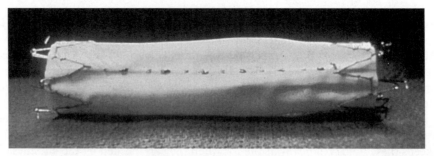

Figure 7–8. Endovascular graft.

These procedures are performed in collaboration with interventional radiology in the OR setting. The vascular surgeon and the interventional radiologist work together using technology that involves fluoroscopic imaging, balloon catheter insertion, and guidewire manipulation. The OR suite used for these procedures must be large enough to accommodate the necessary radiographic equipment as well as two back-table set-ups (Fig. 7–9).

The femoral artery exposure is performed on the side with the least amount of vessel tortuosity and atherosclerosis. A puncture is made in the artery with an 18-gauge needle followed by insertion of a guidewire, dilator, and sheath. Further manipulations are made through the sheath with fluoroscopic guidance. A femoral arteriotomy is required for the larger sheath that accommodates the endovascular graft. To prevent clot formation in the sheath, pressurized bags of 1,000 ml 0.9 percent sodium chloride with 2,000 U of heparin are continuously infused.

A large single basin with 1,000 ml NaCl and 5,000 U of heparin should be included in

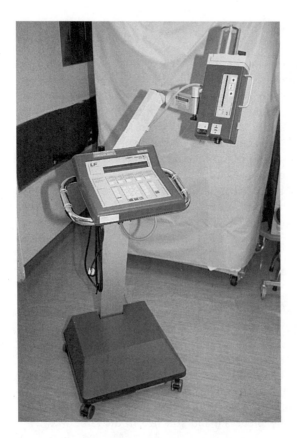

Figure 7–9. A power injector is a pump for controlled injection of radiographic contrast material of specific volumes at specified rates.

the set-up. The numerous guidewires and catheters can be coiled loosely and stored in this basin.

After the endovascular graft is deployed, intravascular ultrasound is used. The ultrasound can assess how well the graft is seated in the aorta and the graft's proximity to the renal and/or hypogastric arteries and can identify any kinks in the graft. The ultrasound can also assess for atherosclerotic flaps or stenosis of the native artery.

The surgeon repairs the arteriotomy site and achieves hemostasis. The femoral incision is closed in layers using the standard wound closure technique.

The complications of this procedure can include aneurysm rupture, peripheral embolization, and misdeployment of the graft, which all require emergency surgical intervention. As, a result, the vascular OR nurses involved in an endovascular graft procedure must be ready for its immediate conversion to an open procedure.

The same abdominal vascular instrumentation used in the standard open approach is used in the endovascular approach. All instrumentation is counted initially in the event that immediate conversion to an open procedure is necessary.

Blood Salvage

The patient's own red cells, which were previously lost to wall suction and discarded, can now be salvaged with use of the blood salvage machine. This salvaged blood can be washed of coagulation factors (heparin, tissue, clots, and other debris) and returned to the patient in the form of packed red cells.

Autologous transfusion is not a new concept. Reinfusion of shed blood was employed as early as 1818 by James Blundell of Guy's Hospital in London. Preoperative blood donation was advocated by Bernard Fantus in 1937, the year he established the first blood bank in the United States. The primary stimulus for the rapid growth of autologous transfusion programs has been the fear of transfusion-transmitted disease, particularly acquired immunodeficiency syndrome (AIDS).[4] Increasing scarcity of banked blood and the risks of transfusion reactions and hepatitis are additional reasons.

The blood salvage machine is a fast, simple, and economical system. The hardware of the machine consists of a 2,200-ml cardiotomy reservoir with filter, a waste bag, a blood transfer pouch, and a 225-ml cone-shaped centrifuge bell. All are interconnected by tubing system to form a closed, sterile unit.

The blood loss from the surgical field is collected in the cardiotomy reservoir via sterile suction tubing. The fluid and blood are heparinized in the sterile suction tubing and cardiotomy reservoir by way of a heparinized drip solution. A roller pump transports the filtered, heparinized blood from the reservoir to the centrifuge bell. The cellular components are deposited onto the wall of the centrifuge bell at a rate of 5,650 rpm. When the erythrocyte sediment has reached the curved level of the bell, it is filled. In a second step, the erythrocyte sediment is rinsed with a normal saline solution until a clear rinse solution appears in the waste bag. The final step is the subsequent reversal of the roller pump transporting the washed erythrocyte concentration into the blood transfer pouch. Once in the transfer pouch, the packed cells can be retransfused immediately to the patient.

A trained, dedicated team is essential for intraoperative blood salvage. Regulation and selection of cycling parameters, determination of the amount of anticoagulant, vacuum level adjustment, waste bag disposal, and documentation of the procedure are all responsibilities of the operator of the blood salvage machine. This team has 24-hour accountability for elective and emergency cases that require blood salvage (Fig. 7–10).

Before blood salvage became possible, numerous units of blood bank blood were required. Blood salvaging has decreased the number of units of blood bank blood required for the patient, thus reducing cost to the patient. However, the patient is charged for the use of the blood salvage machine. The cost includes the expense of the hardware and the

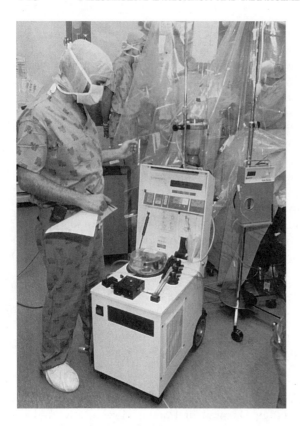

Figure 7–10. Member of the blood salvage team reprocessing salvaged blood for reinfusion.

operation of the machine. Each institution should decide on the use of banked blood versus blood salvage in terms of patient cost and patient safety.

VASCULAR PROSTHETIC GRAFTS

To replace large-caliber arteries, the surgeon will select a polyethylene terephthalate (Dacron) graft or a polytetrafluoroethylene (PTFE) prosthetic graft. Dacron grafts were among the earliest synthetic materials to be used. Dacron is a polymer made into fibers or threads that are then fabricated, with the use of textile technology, into a graft. There are three types of Dacron grafts: woven, knit, and knitted velour. Compared with knitted grafts, woven ones are more tightly constructed, less porous, and stiffer and, therefore, do not handle as well. However, most woven grafts have greater structural integrity than knitted grafts and are less likely to dilate after they are implanted in the patient. A Dacron graft can be lined with a microloop pile on the exterior or interior surface or on both surfaces. This is called a velour lining. Adding a velour to the construction of the graft increases the ease with which the graft is preclotted. The need for preclotting a graft can be eliminated if the graft is preclotted with albumin or collagen.[5]

Knitted and loosely woven grafts must be preclotted by the surgeon before systemic heparinization of the patient. The surgeon preclots the graft before it is implanted by soaking it in the patient's nonheparinized blood. The graft is then stretched several times to ensure that blood fills the fabric interstices and then is "milked" to remove excessive thrombus. Exposure of the blood-soaked graft to air activates the blood's clotting mechanism.[5]

Low-porosity grafts are very stiff, having a porosity of 50 cc, and they do not require preclotting. These grafts are used in procedures in which blood loss must be kept to an absolute minimum, such as repair of a thoracoabdominal aneurysm.

In 1976, expanded PTFE grafts were released for clinical use and became the preferred prosthetic conduit in femoropopliteal reconstructions. Surgeons prefer the PTFE graft because of its ease of handling and tight interstices that do not require preclotting. Accordingly, the use of Dacron for femoropopliteal reconstructions has declined.[5] Dacron prosthetic grafts have been the standard for use in the abdomen. In 1980, however, PTFE grafts were released for use in the abdomen.[5]

FEMORAL ARTERY RECONSTRUCTION

Areas of atherosclerosis within the arterial wall become covered with fibrous tissue, forming plaque. As the plaque enlarges within the artery, the lumen of the artery is reduced, resulting in decreased blood flow. When a patient has pain at rest, nonhealing lower-extremity ulcers, or gangrene of the toes or foot, arterial reconstructive surgery is indicated to increase blood flow to the lower extremity and prevent amputation.

Anatomy

The abdominal aorta bifurcates into the common iliac arteries, each of which divides into the internal iliac artery and the external iliac artery (see Chapter 11). The external iliac artery becomes the common femoral artery as it passes under the inguinal ligament into the leg. The common femoral artery gives rise to the superficial femoral artery and the deep femoral artery. The superficial femoral artery becomes the popliteal artery in the distal thigh and gives rise to the anterior tibial artery below the knee. Distal to the anterior tibial artery are the posterior tibial artery and the peroneal artery. The posterior tibial artery continues medially down the leg, passing behind the medial malleolus into the foot. The anterior tibial artery lies in the anterior compartment of the leg and continues on to the dorsum of the foot as the dorsalis pedis artery. The peroneal artery courses through the center of the leg and terminates in the distal part of the leg. Two branches from the peroneal artery serve as collaterals to the pedal arch.

Diagnosis

Once the diagnosis of arterial insufficiency has been demonstrated by noninvasive testing, angiography is performed. This is the most precise diagnostic tool for the assessment of arterial anatomy in the lower extremity, outlining the location and extent of arterial obstruction. Complete evaluation requires depiction of the aorta, iliac, femoral, popliteal, and tibial arterial segments. The common femoral artery is the most common site of angiographic access (see Chapter 12).

Femoral Artery Bypass Surgery

At the onset of the operation, the surgeon determines the proper bypass by selecting the best proximal site for inflow and the best distal site for outflow. Arterial bypass surgery may be done with a two-team approach. One team of surgeons makes the proximal incision on the upper thigh over the inguinal ligament where the femoral artery and saphenous vein are close together and can be easily dissected. The second team of surgeons makes an incision distally to expose the vessel of choice (i.e., popliteal, tibial, or peroneal artery).

An arteriogram just before arterial bypass may be indicated when the tibial vessels are poorly visualized on the preoperative arteriogram. The arteriogram is performed after the femoral artery is first exposed through a groin incision. A 16-gauge angiocatheter is inserted into the femoral artery; the artery is then clamped proximal to the angiocatheter. The femoral artery is then injected with approximately 50 ml of contrast material. This enables the surgeon to visualize the tibial vessel with the least disease and best outflow to the foot. That vessel should be selected for the distal anastomosis.

The patient's own saphenous vein remains the graft of choice for arterial bypass surgery. The saphenous vein provides the best patency rate and can be reversed for use as an arterial bypass graft, allowing blood to flow unobstructed through the vein valves. The saphenous vein is removed from the leg, and the small end of the vein is anastomosed to the common femoral artery. The large end of the vein is anastomosed to the popliteal or tibial artery. The disadvantage of this technique is the size mismatch of the saphenous vein to the native vessel.

An alternative technique was developed to use the saphenous vein in its natural position without reversal. This technique is known as an in situ saphenous vein bypass. This procedure requires interruption of the valves within the saphenous vein. An advantage of the in situ bypass is the anastomotic size match of both ends of the saphenous vein to the native arteries. This technique may decrease ischemic damage to the vein graft wall because the saphenous vein is never entirely removed from the leg and therefore retains its adventitial blood supply.[6]

Preparation of the saphenous vein for use in situ entails exposure of the saphenous vein in the subcutaneous region of the affected leg. The proximal end of the saphenous vein is anastomosed to the common femoral artery. This produces arterial pressure within the vein graft and distends the vein to the most proximal vein valve. Side branches of the saphenous vein are dissected and ligated with ties of nonabsorbable suture material and stainless steel ligating clips. These venous branches are ligated to prevent arteriovenous fistulae when the vein is arterialized. The valve cusps are rendered incompetent through the use of a stainless steel valvulotome (Figs. 7–11 and 7–12). The valvulotome, which

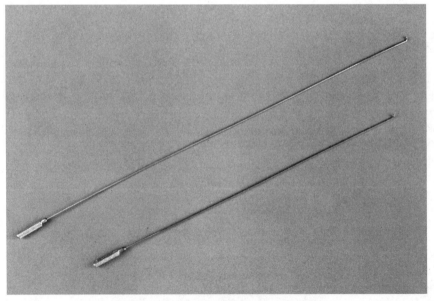

Figure 7–11. Rigid stainless steel valvulotome.

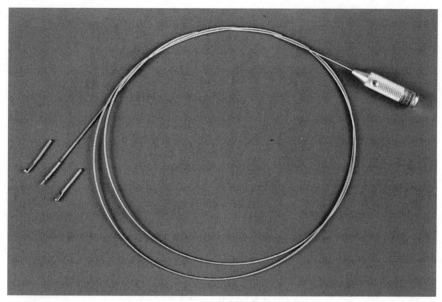

Figure 7–12. Flexible stainless steel valvulotome.

has a sharp blade, is placed into the vein through a venous side branch. The surgeon makes the valve incompetent by sharp division of each valve cusp while preventing damage to the inner surface of the vein. The distal end of the saphenous vein is anastomosed to the distal vessel of choice (i.e., tibial or peroneal artery).[6]

If the saphenous vein has been removed for use in another operation or is not long enough or large enough, a synthetic graft is used. The synthetic graft most widely accepted is the PTFE graft. PTFE anastomosed to the tibial vessels has a decreased patency rate; therefore, every effort should be made to use a venous reconstruction.

On completion of the bypass, an intraoperative arteriogram is performed to assess technical competence of the arterial reconstruction, particularly the distal anastomosis. It also provides documentation of the distal runoff anatomy, which is valuable in future therapeutic decisions. If a technical error is detected by arteriogram, it can be corrected immediately. If the results of the arteriogram are acceptable and adequate flow is confirmed, hemostasis is achieved at all incision sites. An absorbable suture material is used to close incision sites. The surgical drapes are removed and dressings are applied.

As in all vascular procedures, it is important that the scrub and circulating nurses maintain the sterility of all instruments until the patient leaves the OR suite. Before the patient is awakened, the surgeon confirms the presence of dorsalis pedis and posterior tibial artery pulses with Doppler ultrasonography indicating adequate blood flow through the bypass graft. When the surgeon is satisfied with these pulses, the patient is awakened and transported to the recovery room.

THROMBOLYTIC AGENTS

Urokinase is the thrombolytic agent used to treat acute arterial occlusion, arterial graft thrombosis, or distal embolization. Urokinase is isolated from human urine or fetal kidney cells, it is not a foreign protein, and therefore causes fewer allergic reactions. Urokinase is usually infused via direct intra-arterial infusion into a catheter through the femoral artery. Thrombolysis is designed to open up the arterial tree of occluding thrombus. Intraoperatively, a bolus of 250,000 U of urokinase in 50 ml of 0.9 percent sodium chloride may be injected into the affected limb through a 16-gauge angiocatheter. This bolus is injected intra-arterially prior to the closure of the distal limb anastomosis.

VASCULAR ENDOSCOPY

Angioscopy is a safe, accurate technique for intraoperative assessment and monitoring of distal revascularization procedures. It provides the surgeon with a real-time, three-dimensional view of the reconstructed vessel. Angioscopy is used to identify previously unrecognized intraluminal details, thus reducing the possibility of reocclusion; to visualize arterial plaque and/or thrombus within the native vessel or previous arterial bypass graft; to inspect anastomotic suture lines after bypass surgery; and to provide direct visualization of valve cutting in the in situ vein graft (Fig. 7–13A–D). These findings ultimately may affect long-term patency of the graft, and clinical application of angioscopy may contribute to the understanding of graft failure.

ANGIOSCOPY FOR FEMORAL-DISTAL BYPASS SURGERY

A bypass graft is performed with a reverse saphenous vein graft, an in situ saphenous vein graft, or a synthetic graft. The surgeon chooses an angioscope that is of the appropriate size for the bypass graft. The circulating nurse gives the sterilized angioscope and video

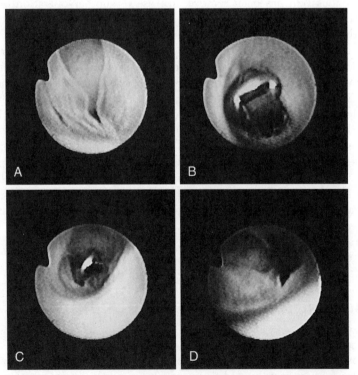

Figure 7–13. View through an angioscope. **A,** Partially closed valve. **B,** Valvulotome above valve. **C,** Valve incision. **D,** Completed valvulotomy. (From Pearce WH, Baxter BT, Almgren CC, et al: The use of angioscopy in the saphenous vein bypass graft. In Yao JST, Pearce WH [eds]: Technologies in Vascular Surgery. Philadelphia, WB Saunders, 1992, p 291.)

camera to the scrub nurse. The video camera is sterilized with ethylene oxide for initial use. When subsequent use is required, a sterile plastic camera drape is employed.[8]

The vascular OR should have dedicated video equipment for angioscopy. This will ensure 24-hour availability of the equipment when requested by the surgeon. At the start of the procedure, the surgeon usually requests the angioscope. OR nurses trained in angioscopy can set up the equipment in 10 minutes; therefore, the occasional unexpected use of the angioscope does not present a problem.[8]

The circulating nurse prepares 1 L of 0.9 percent sodium chloride with 2,000 units heparin for use with the irrigation pump. This nurse is also responsible for assembling and priming the irrigation pump tubing. The scrub nurse hands the ends of the video camera cord and the light source cord off the sterile field to the circulating nurse, who then inserts the ends into the camera unit and light source. One end of the irrigation pump tubing is passed off the sterile field to the circulating nurse, who connects it to the previously primed irrigation pump.[8]

The surgeon inserts the disposable angioscope into the vein bypass graft or synthetic bypass graft. The angioscope can also be inserted into the vein bypass graft through a side branch of the vein. The surgeon or the scrub nurse attaches the camera to the angioscope. The primed irrigation tubing is connected to the irrigation channel on the angioscope. A vascular clamp helps maintain occlusion of arterial inflow throughout the procedure.[8]

The irrigation pump is capable of delivering high- and low-volume flow rates. Typical rates are 50 ml/minute low and 150 ml/minute high. Surgeons using the irrigation pump should determine standards of irrigation that best meet their visual needs (Fig. 7–14).[8]

The irrigation pump is controlled by digital input and a bimodal foot pedal. One action of the foot pedal provides a high flow rate to initially clear the vessel of blood. The low flow rate is used to maintain clarity during the procedure. The key to successful angioscopy is the maintenance of a blood-free field. The smallest amount of blood flowing into the field significantly blurs the image on the monitor.[8]

The irrigation pump provides a continuous readout on total volume infused. Through-

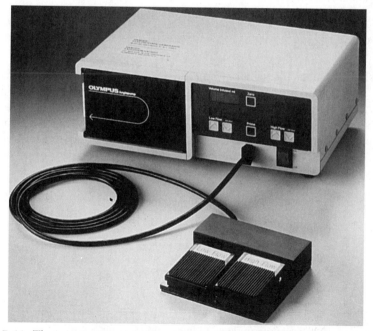

Figure 7–14. The irrigation pump used in angioscopy. (Courtesy of Olympus Corporation, Lake Success, NY.)

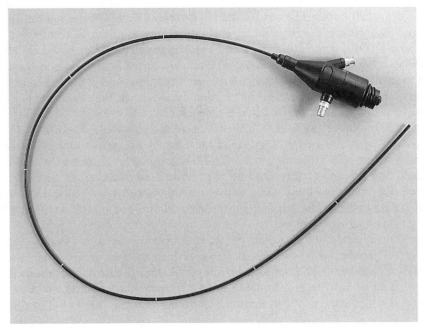

Figure 7–15. 2.8-mm angioscope. (Printed with the permission of Baxter Healthcare Corporation, Vascular Systems Division.)

out the procedure, the circulating nurse informs the anesthesia staff regarding total fluid volume infused. This irrigation solution remains in the patient's vascular system and becomes part of the total fluid volume received by the patient intraoperatively.[8]

The image from the angioscope is transferred directly to a high-resolution color monitor, which allows simultaneous viewing by the surgical team. The procedure can be recorded with the video cassette recorder. This information can be reviewed later for teaching and documentation.

Set-up of Equipment

The OR nurses are responsible for the set-up and preparation of all angioscopy equipment. They should have a working knowledge of this equipment to facilitate an efficient and diagnostically accurate procedure.

The disposable angioscopes come in three sizes: a 1.5-mm, 100-cm; a 2.3-mm, 80-cm; and a 2.8-mm, 80-cm with irrigation channels (Fig. 7–15). Equipment required for angioscopy is listed in Table 7–3. Equipment used in vascular surgery organized by type of procedure is listed and pictured in Table 7–4.

TABLE 7–3. **Equipment Required
for Angioscopy**

1. Video monitor
2. Combined video camera unit, light source
3. Video cassette recorder
4. Irrigation pump
5. Irrigation pump tubing
6. 1000 ml of warm 0.9% sodium chloride containing
   2,000 U heparin for use with the irrigation pump

TABLE 7–4. **Operating Room Trays for Vascular Procedures**

Peripheral Vascular Basic Tray (tray on left)

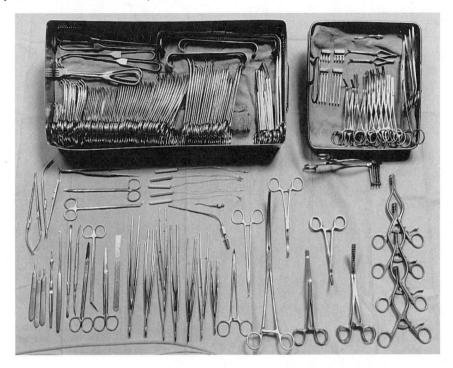

14	Towel clip
12	Mosquitoes, 5″ curved
6	Mosquitoes, 5″ straight
16	Hemostat, Kelly, curved
2	Allis, 6″
12	Péan, curved, 6″
2	Péan, curved, 8″
2	Sponge forceps, Foerster, 9 1/2″
2	Mixter, petit point
4	Mixter, Adson, curved
1	Mixter, regular, 7 3/4″
4	Boettcher, 7″ (tonsil hemostat)
3	Needle holder, Ryder, 7″ (regular)
4	Needle holder, Mayo-Hegar, 6 1/4″
2	Needle holder, Mayo-Hegar, 7″
2	Scissor, Potts-Smith, angled 60°
1	Scissor, Potts-Smith, 5 1/2″ (Richter)
3	Scissor, Potts-Smith, 7″ (Richter)
2	Scissor, Mayo, straight, 6 3/4″
4	Diamond tissue forceps, 7″
3	Gerald tissue forceps, 7 3/4″
4	DeBakey tissue forceps, 7 3/4″
2	Carmody tissue forceps, fine, 7 3/4″
2	Adson tissue forceps, 4 3/4″
1	Ruler, 6″
1	Blunt hook, Adson (nerve hook)
1	Suction tip, Frazier with stylet, #2
1	Clamp, aortic, DeBakey, 19″ (for tunneling grafts)

Table continued on following page

TABLE 7–4. **Operating Room Trays for Vascular Procedures**
Continued

2	Retractors, rake, 4-prong, sharp, 7 3/4"
2	Retractors, vein, straight, 10 1/2"
2	Retractors, Cushing, 10 1/2"
2	Retractors, ribbon, Sistrunk, small
2	Retractors, ribbon, large
2	Retractors, Richardson, double-ended, small
2	Retractors, Richardson, double-ended, large
2	Retractors, Army/Navy
2	Freer elevator
2	Knife handles, #3, 5 1/2"
2	Knife handles, #7, 7"
2	Sling, Silastic, small
2	Sling, Silastic, large

Peripheral Vascular Clamp Tray (tray on right)

1	Edwards spring applicator (bulldog applier)
2	Henley clamps
2	Deep-angled Cooley clamps (patent ductus)
2	Curved Cooley clamps
2	Straight Cooley clamps
7	Pediatric Cooley clamps
	1 spoon-shaped jaws
	2 60° angled
	2 30° angled
2	Gregory bulldogs, angled, short
2	Baby "J" clamps (Dennis anastomosis clamps)
2	Profunda clamps
4	Weitlaner retractors, medium
1	Henley retractor with:
	2 short blades
	2 medium blades
	2 long blades
2	Webster cannulas, short

Microvascular Tray

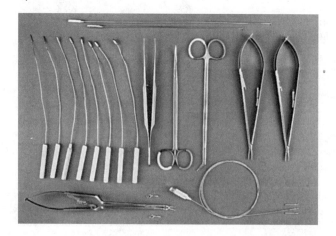

TABLE 7–4. **Operating Room Trays for Vascular Procedures**
Continued

6	Castroviejo needle holders
1	Mills saphenous vein tissue forceps
1	Baby Potts scissors
1	Fine dissecting scissors
8	Coronary dilators, size 1 mm through 4.5 mm

Abdominal Vascular Basic Tray (tray on left)

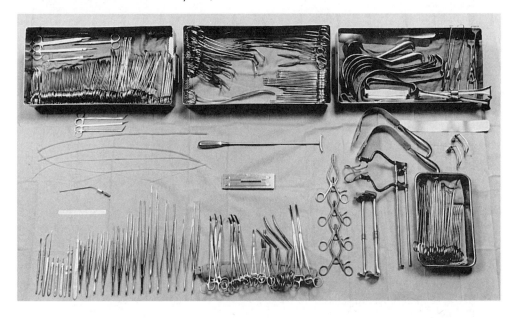

8	Towel clips, 5 1/2"
12	Mosquitoes, curved
6	Mosquitoes, straight
16	Hemostats, Kelly, curved
10	Kocher, 6 1/4"
12	Péan, 6" curved
2	Péan, 8" curved
4	Kocher, 8"
4	Sponge forceps, Foerster
2	Mixters, petit point
4	Mixter, Adson
2	Mixters, 7 3/4"
6	Boettcher (tonsil hemostats)
2	Scissors, Potts-Smith, angled 60°
3	Scissors, Potts-Smith, 7" (Richter)
2	Scissors, Potts-Smith, 9" (Richter)
1	Scissors, Mayo, heavy, 9" curved
1	Scissors, Mayo, 6 3/4" curved
2	Scissors, Mayo, 6 3/4" straight
2	DeBakey tissue forceps, 12"
3	DeBakey tissue forceps, 9 1/2"
4	DeBakey tissue forceps, 7 3/4"
3	Potts-Smith tissue forceps, 9"
2	Gerald tissue forceps, 7"

Table continued on following page

TABLE 7–4. **Operating Room Trays for Vascular Procedures**
Continued

4	Diamond tissue forceps, 7"
1	Smooth tissue forceps, 12"
2	Potts-Smith tissue forceps, 10 1/4"
2	Tooth tissue forceps, short
2	Adson tissue forceps with teeth
2	Elevator, Freer
2	Knife handle, #3
2	Knife handle, #7
1	Knife handle, long #3
1	Ruler
1	Blunt hook, Adson (nerve hook)
1	Suction tip, Frazier with stylet, #2

Abdominal Vascular Clamp Tray (tray in middle)

3	Mayo-Hegar needle holder, 8"
3	Mayo-Hegar needle holder, 7"
3	Mayo-Hegar needle holder, 6"
2	Sternal needle holder
6	Ryder needle holder, 9"
3	Ryder needle holder, 7"
1	Deep-angled Cooley clamp
2	Patent ductus clamps, straight
7	Pediatric Cooley clamps
	1 spoon
	2 curved jaws
	2 60° angle
	2 30° angle
2	Baby "J" clamps (Dennis anastomosis)
2	Profunda clamps
1	DeBakey aortic clamp, "S" curved
3	DeBakey aortic clamp, large
2	DeBakey aortic clamp, small
1	DeBakey angled aortic clamp
4	Satinsky vena cava clamps
3	Harken clamps (#1, #2, #3)
2	Henley clamps
2	Wylie hypogastric clamps
2	Fogarty clamps, short
2	Fogarty clamps, long
1	Edwards spring applicators (bulldog appliers)
1	Aortic compressor
2	2-cc glass syringe
2	Webster cannula, short
4	Small slings, Silastic
4	Large slings, Silastic

Abdominal Vascular Retractor Tray (tray on right)

2	Retractor, vein, straight
2	Retractor, Cushing
2	Retractor, Richardson-Eastman, large, double-ended
2	Retractor, Richardson-Eastman, medium, double-ended
2	Retractor, Deaver, wide
2	Retractor, Deaver, medium
2	Retractor, Deaver, narrow

TABLE 7–4. **Operating Room Trays for Vascular Procedures**
Continued

1	Retractor, Mayo
2	Retractor, Glass
1	Retractor, Harrington
4	Retractor, Weitlaner, medium
2	Retractor, Parker, large
2	Retractor, Sistrunk
1	Retractor, malleable, 2″ curved
1	Retractor, malleable, 1 1/2″ curved
1	Retractor, malleable, 1 1/4″
2	Retractor, rake, 6-prong, sharp
1	Retractor, extra-wide, Grieshaber with 2 long blades and 2 short blades

Abdominal Vascular Long Instruments (front right tray)

6	Boettchers, 7 1/4″
1	Scissors, Potts-Smith, 11″ (Richter)
2	Long Babcock, 10 1/2″
2	Needle holder, diamond jaw, 10 3/4″
2	Needle holder, Ryder, 10 1/2″
2	Hemostats, deep bridge, curved, extra-long, 22 3/4″
2	Mixters, right angle, extra-long, 20 3/4″
2	Hemoclip appliers, large
2	Hemoclip appliers, medium
1	Base clip

Omni Retractors

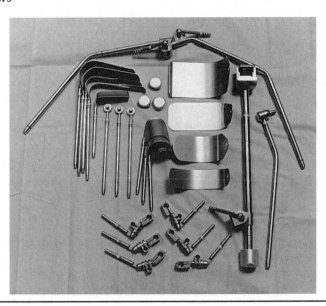

Risks

The risks of angioscopy include the potential for endothelial trauma related to the mechanical passage of the angioscope through a graft and into the native artery. It is important that the smallest angioscope be used to avoid this risk. Another risk is that of fluid overload owing to the amount of irrigation fluid used. The amount of fluid volume infused is usually 800 ml to 1000 ml. A significant amount of irrigation fluid is lost through the open distal vein.

CONCLUSION

The knowledge and skills required of the vascular OR nurse cover a broad spectrum, ranging from the elective minor procedure, to the ruptured aortic aneurysm to an injury to a major blood vessel in a trauma patient. The nurse must continually strive to remain abreast of new technology. This knowledge allows for optimal intraoperative care of the patient.

Acknowledgments

We thank Drs. James Yao, Walter McCarthy, William Pearce, and Jon Matsumura for their appreciation and recognition of our expertise in the perioperative care of their patients; and our vascular nursing colleagues Ann Guerrero, Robert Johnson, Melanie Gongaware, Charmaine Reid, and Paula Majewski for their contribution and knowledge in the care of the vascular patient.

References

1. American Heart Association: Guidelines for Carotid Endarterectomy. A Multidisciplinary Consensus Statement from the Ad Hoc Committee. Circulation 1995; 991:566–579.
2. van Alphen HAM, Polman CH: The value of continuous intra-operative EEG monitoring during carotid endarterectomy. Acta Neurochir 1988; 91:95–99.
3. Yao JST, Pearce WH (eds): Aneurysms New Findings and Treatments. Norwalk, CT, Appleton & Lange, 1994.
4. Stehling L: In Stehling L (ed): Perioperative Autologous Transfusion: Transcribed Proceedings of a National Conference. Arlington, VA, American Association of Blood Banks, 1991, p xi.
5. Pevec WC, Abbott WM: Femoropopliteal Dacron graft: Five- to ten-year patency. In Yao JST, Pearce WH (eds): Long-Term Results in Vascular Surgery. Norwalk, CT, Appleton & Lange, 1993, pp 273–277.
6. Pearce WH, Baxter BT, Almgren CC, et al: The use of angioscopy in the saphenous vein bypass graft. In Yao JST, Pearce WH (eds): Technologies in Vascular Surgery. Philadelphia, WB Saunders, 1992, pp 289–294.
7. Goodman GR, Laurence PF: Intraoperative thrombolytic therapy. In Yao JST, Pearce WH (eds): Technologies in Vascular Surgery. Philadelphia, WB Saunders, 1992, pp 475–491.
8. Borgini L, Almgren CC: Peripheral vascular angioscopy: Performance, equipment, technique. AORN J 1990; 52:543–550.
9. Moore W: Endovascular repair of abdominal aortic aneurysm: An update on the Multicenter Endovascular Graft System Trial. In Yao JST (ed): Progress in Vascular Surgery. Norwalk, CT, Appleton and Lange, 1997, pp 141–146.

8

Medications Used in Vascular Patients

Janice D. Nunnelee, PhD(C), RN, CVN, ANP

There are many facets of the armamentarium in the treatment of vascular disorders. One of these facets is the array of medications available to the practitioner for treatment of the disease. Nurses must administer drugs safely and educate patients in their usage, and advanced practice nurses may prescribe. Thus nurses need to be aware of current medications—their purpose, actions, dosages, and side effects—and the educational needs of the patient related to these medications.

This chapter discusses anticoagulants, thrombolytic agents, antiplatelet agents, and various miscellaneous medications in current usage as well as those under investigation.

ANTICOAGULANTS

Heparin

Heparin was first isolated and described as an anticoagulant in 1916.[1] Its use in prevention of thromboembolism in the postoperative period was not evident until Murray's research in 1937.[2] It was not until the mid-1960s that mini-dose heparin was introduced for prophylaxis against deep venous thrombosis (DVT). Heparin is now one of the most widely employed drugs used in vascular patients and the indications are included in Table 8–1. Contraindications are seen in Table 8–2.

Heparin, which is synthesized by the mast cell, is a complex heterogeneous polysaccharide (molecular weight 3000 to 30,000) with a strong negative charge.[6, 9] Unfractionated and low-molecular-weight heparin act indirectly to accelerate antithrombin (heparin cofactor, previously known as antithrombin III) in its interaction with thrombin and activated factor Xa. The majority of heparin's action is a result of a pentasaccharide that has a high affinity for antithrombin.[6, 9] Heparin, when given in adequate amounts, prevents extension and embolization of thrombi. It does not dissolve thrombi but helps to prevent recurrence. Because of its large molecular size, it does not cross the placental barrier and this allows its use in pregnancy.[7] The chief disadvantage of heparin is the fact that it must be given parenterally.

Unfractionated or low-molecular-weight heparin is often administered alone in the presence of an active thrombotic process. However, time constraints currently in force secondary to Medicare and Diagnosis Related Groups (DRGs) usually dictate that warfarin

TABLE 8–1. **Indications for Heparin**

Preoperative and postoperative prophylaxis for deep venous thrombosis (DVT)
Treatment of acute arterial (or graft) occlusions
Intraoperative use
Postoperative prophylaxis for patients with synthetic grafts
Flushing of various invasive lines
Angiography
DVT and pulmonary embolism (PE)
Cerebrovascular embolic disorders
Distal emboli (blue toe syndrome)
Venous thrombotic events during pregnancy (warfarin is contraindicated in
    pregnancy)[3]

be initiated immediately if it is planned at discharge. Unfractionated heparin is given until oral anticoagulants have produced their therapeutic effect. Low-molecular-weight heparin may be initially given in the hospital and then in the outpatient setting, or may be administered solely on an outpatient basis.[6, 8–10] In other cases, heparin is given until the cause of embolism is surgically treated and no outpatient anticoagulation planned.

Unfractionated Heparin

Various methods of assessing coagulation levels are available. The most widely used test in the United States is the activated partial thromboplastin time (PTT or APTT). Other laboratory tests include the Lee-White clotting time, plasma clot time, and the activated clotting time. A PTT of 2–2½ times control is considered indicative of adequate anticoagulation levels.

Response to heparin varies among individuals and can also vary greatly in the same individual. Close monitoring is necessary to avoid unnecessary complications. If possible, a baseline PTT should be obtained before initiation of therapy, but a prothrombin time is unnecessary.[10] Daily measurement of the PTT is the minimum assessment of a patient who is stable on intravenous heparin. The half-life of heparin is 60–90 minutes after intravenous injection. When continuous intravenous therapy is given, the anticoagulant

TABLE 8–2. **Contraindications/Precautions**
With Heparin

Contraindications

Active or suspected bleeding (e.g., intracranial hemorrhage, decreasing
    hematocrit levels)
Known coagulation disorders (e.g., hemophilia, antithrombin III deficiencies)
During or following ophthalmic or neurosurgical procedures
Endocarditis
Threatened abortion
Heparin sensitivities
Heparin-induced thrombocytopenia[4, 5, 8]

Use Caution in the Presence of:

Severe liver or kidney disease
Open wounds
Increased capillary permeability
Postoperative epidural catheter[9]

effect should be measured at 4–6 hours after initiation of the drug (three half-lives), at which time levels should be stabilized.[10] Variability in response to unfractionated heparin is secondary to the individual differences in plasma-binding proteins. In the first few days of therapy the effect of heparin must be measured several times a day because doses may need altering. Later in therapy, particularly for deep venous thrombosis (DVT), the coagulation process will be slower and smaller amounts will be needed. Fewer measurements of the effect will be necessary.

Heparin must be measured according to a biologic standard of anticoagulant effectiveness, expressed in international units (IU). This is due to the fact that each source of heparin produces different strengths if measured by weight or volume. Preparations are available in concentrations ranging from 1000 to 40,000 units/ml.

Heparin is administered parenterally. There are three accepted means of heparin administration: continuous intravenous infusion, intermittent (pulse) intravenous injection, and subcutaneous injection in an aqueous solution. Because of erratic absorption and the risk of hematoma formation at the injection site, heparin should not be given intramuscularly. With continuous intravenous infusion, the preferred route of administration for treatment of thromboembolic phenomena, heparin is diluted in a saline solution. Prior to continuous infusion, a bolus injection may be given to introduce an immediate effect. The heparin is then delivered via an accurate infusion pump so that a known quantity of heparin is administered over a given time. Bolus amounts are determined by both the patient's weight and the extent of the clot. With large thrombi or pulmonary emboli, the bolus may be large, and up to 1800 units/hour may be given initially. The dose varies among physicians. Some centers now have clinical pathways for anticoagulation for DVT or for prophylaxis of DVT. These pathways also vary. Continuous therapy offers the advantage of constant blood levels of heparin once the circulating volume is stabilized. Therefore, a PTT should be accurate at any time that it is drawn. If the infusion is interrupted at any time in the hours before obtaining the PTT, the health care provider should be notified when the result is called. Disadvantages of constant infusion are the limitation of the patient's activity due to an intravenous line and potential for bleeding from the catheter insertion site. Other studies indicate that the cost of the hospital stay may not be justified.[6, 8, 9]

For intermittent (pulse) intravenous injection, heparin is given in an undiluted form via heparin lock, venipuncture, or a port in the intravenous tubing. Heparin is given at 4- to 6-hour intervals to maintain proper levels of circulating heparin. Dosage in this method is approximately 5000 units at each injection. Complications of this particular method of injection include infection and thrombophlebitis from constant venipuncture or invasion of an indwelling line. This type of therapy has been shown in some studies to create more frequent bleeding complications than other methods even with close monitoring.[12] PTTs are checked just prior to dose administration to assess the minimal heparin level for anticoagulant effectiveness. Although this method is rarely used today, it was often used in the past.

Subcutaneous heparin is rarely administered for DVT. It is often given for prophylaxis against DVT, especially in high-risk patients. Subcutaneous heparin given for venous thrombosis is administered at 4- to 12-hour intervals in doses of 5000–15,000 units. Absorption of the drug is erratic and control is difficult during the treatment of any form of thrombosis. In the pregnant patient who receives intravenous heparin for treatment, the regimen for the duration of the pregnancy is administration of a dose sufficient to keep the PTT at 1.5–2.0 times normal. The dose may be administered every 8–12 hours. PTT is assessed 6 hours after injection.[7]

When heparin is given by this route for prophylaxis of DVT, heparin inhibits factor X, thus preventing the activation of prothrombin. Two hours prior to surgery 5000 units of heparin are given and this is followed by doses every 8–12 hours until the patient is fully ambulatory. One problem frequently encountered with this method is pain and ecchymoses at the injection sites.

Low-Molecular-Weight Heparin

Low-molecular-weight heparin (LMWH) was developed after the discovery that the antithrombotic effect of LMWH was the same as that of unfractionated heparin, but that LMWH produced fewer complications.[6] LMWH is prepared by a chemical cracking process and has a longer biologic half-life. The half-life is approximately two to four times that of unfractionated heparin.[10] LMWH strands are shorter than those of unfractionated heparin and do not have enough sites for binding both antithrombin and thrombin.[6, 10] Because of this characteristic, LMWH primarily acts on factor Xa. This action on factor Xa results in a longer half-life due to the more rapid clearance of longer heparin chains.

The anticoagulation action of LMWH is more predictable than that of unfractionated. This predictability is secondary to the better bioavailability, longer half-life, and dose-dependent clearance of LMWH. Therefore, in contrast to unfractionated heparin, LMWH does not require monitoring of the PTT except in renal patients or patients weighing less than 50 kg or more than 80 kg. The PTT may not accurately reflect the anticoagulant efficacy of the medication.

LMWH has been given with safety in the outpatient setting for DVT and has not resulted in increased mortality or morbidity.[3, 8, 6, 13] A fixed-dose LMWH has been found to be as effective as unfractionated heparin in treatment of DVT with or without pulmonary emboli. In addition, LMWH has the advantage of home administration and lack of the need for laboratory monitoring.[6, 13]

Heparin Administration

Subcutaneous heparin must be injected into adipose tissue. The most common site is the abdomen, but the posterior arm, lateral thigh, and fat pad of the scapula may be used. Some centers have encountered problems with hematoma formation if injections are given within a few inches of an abdominal incision, so these areas should be avoided. The fat fold should be one inch when it is pinched between the thumb and the forefinger and should be free of induration or ecchymoses. A short needle (one half to five eighths of an inch) should be inserted at a 45 to 90° degree angle. Backflow should not be checked; a rotation chart should be made of injection sites. To avoid hematoma formation, the injection site should not be massaged.

Heparin Complications

The most frequent complication of heparin therapy is bleeding. Other uncommon complications of heparin are found in Table 8–3. Bony defects secondary to ascorbic acid deficiency can be enhanced by heparin; therefore, this deficiency is a relative contraindication to heparin treatment.

Heparin-induced thrombocytopenia is an unusual yet extremely serious occurrence in heparin therapy, and its seriousness warrants further discussion. It appears to be rare in LMWH but does occur. Most reports place the incidence of this disorder in unfractionated heparin therapy at approximately 3 percent.[14, 15] The etiology of this complication seems to be related to the biologic source of the heparin, with use of bovine preparations producing a higher incidence than porcine solutions.

TABLE 8–3. **Uncommon Complications of Heparin Therapy**

Hypersensitivity and anaphylaxis (rare)
Bronchoconstriction
Cutaneous necrosis
Urticaria
Alopecia
Osteoporosis (seen only with long-term therapy such as in pregnancy)
Pathologic features[3,12]

Mild forms of thrombocytopenia generally are noted on the second to fifth day of heparin therapy and usually are accompanied by few serious complications.[4] The platelet count rarely falls below 100,000 K/UL and no treatment is necessary. Cessation of the drug causes a return to a normal state rather rapidly. The more severe form of heparin-induced thrombocytopenia (HIT) occurs in 5–6 percent of patients on heparin and is often accompanied by thrombosis and rarely hemorrhage (Fig. 8–1). Thrombosis may include stroke, myocardial infarction, graft occlusion, or DVT. This type may occur at any time during treatment but is most common between days 4 and 15. The platelet count drops precipitously below 100,000 K/UL. A drop from baseline of 40 percent or more in the platelet count is considered diagnostic of HIT.

The cause of HIT is believed to be an immune-mediated response.[4, 16–18] Antibodies cause a secretion of adenosine diphosphate and thromboxane A, resulting in thrombocyte consumption (and bleeding) and/or activation of the coagulation cascade (and thrombosis). Both platelet counts and duration or amount of heparin therapy have been unrelated to the severity of either response.

Nursing Responsibility With Heparin

Nursing responsibility with any patient on heparin therapy begins with ensuring that the proper tests (PTT, platelet counts, and so on) are performed as ordered, and are then

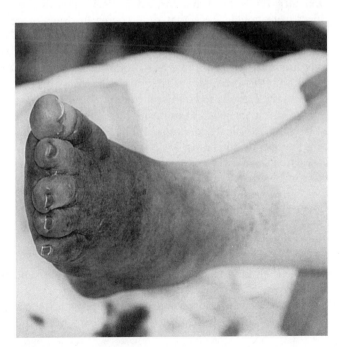

Figure 8–1. Lower extremity arterial thrombosis secondary to heparin-induced thrombocytopenia.

reported to the physician or vascular nurse. It is important to inform the responsible clinician if heparin therapy is interrupted at any time, because interruption would influence laboratory results. When the nurse contacts the clinician for further orders, it is helpful to have readily available the test result, the previous result, the present heparin dose, and the previously adjusted dose, if applicable. Additionally, it is the nurse's responsibility to ensure that unnecessary tests are not performed if the patient is on LMWH.

Heparin is reversed by protamine sulfate. An intravenous dose of 1–1.5 mg per 100 units of heparin will reverse the effect.[19] The action of protamine is thought to be due to its binding with heparin to prevent its reaction with antithrombin. If large amounts of heparin are being administered, a "heparin rebound" may occur requiring additional protamine. Other side effects of protamine sulfate are hypotension, bradycardia, and dyspnea. These effects can be reduced by slow injection. Research in a new protamine variant is being performed; this form holds promise for fewer side effects than with standard protamine.[20]

Nurses must observe for signs of bleeding and also educate the patient about these signs. Unusual ecchymoses, bleeding from mucous membranes, melena, hematemesis, hematuria, or cutaneous necrosis should be explained in lay terms and written instructions given to the patient. Menstruating women should report any radical changes in flow, and pregnant women should immediately report any vaginal bleeding or severe abdominal pain.

Instructions on proper technique of self-administration, site rotation, and appropriate disposal of biohazardous waste are part of a complete discharge instruction plan. Reassurance to the patient and significant others regarding the ability to administer the medication is helpful. If alopecia occurs, the patient should be aware that this is temporary. Complications can best be avoided by strict attention to dosages, adequate determination of anticoagulation effects, and proper staff and patient education. In the patient with previous heparin therapy requiring hospitalization, the use of LMWH in the outpatient setting may require additional information and reassurance.

Oral Anticoagulants

Oral anticoagulants were identified in 1941 when the coagulation effects of spoiled sweet clover were noted. Since that time coumarin drugs (warfarin, bishydroxycoumarin) have been synthesized and indanedione derivatives (diphenadione, phenindione) were made available. Warfarin is the drug of choice in the United States for oral anticoagulation. Indications are seen in Table 8–4. Long-term use of oral anticoagulants (with or without aspirin) after vascular reconstruction varies with surgeons.[21]

Contraindications to coumarin therapy are similar to those of heparin. Caution should be used in the presence of drainage tubes, malabsorption syndromes, dietary deficiencies, gastrointestinal ulcers, or impaired hepatic or renal function. Pregnancy is an absolute contraindication to the use of coumarin compounds. During pregnancy, coumarin compounds can cause teratogenic effects, especially if taken in the first trimester. Because these medications cross the placental barrier, the fetus may suffer from bleeding complications either before birth or during labor or delivery.[7]

Warfarin sodium is absorbed in the gastrointestinal tract and binds to albumin. The unbound portion, approximately 3 percent, is responsible for the anticoagulant effect of the drug.[22] The binding property of warfarin is partly responsible for its long half-life (range, 1.5 to 2.5 days; average, 36 hours).[23] The half-lives of the four vitamin K–dependent clotting factors range from 6 to 90 hours and therefore it may take 3–5 days for therapeutic values to be reached.

The advantage of coumarin drugs is their oral form, and their disadvantage is prolonged action time. These medications should be discontinued 2–3 days prior to surgical proce-

TABLE 8–4. **Indications for Oral Anticoagulants**

Following heparin or thrombolytic therapy for:
  Deep venous thrombosis (DVT)
  Pulmonary embolism
  Arterial thrombosis
  Embolism
  Arterial or venous graft failures
Presence of a prosthetic valve
Valvular heart disease with subsequent embolism
Chronic or intermittent atrial fibrillation (to prevent
  embolism)
Inherited coagulation disorders
Cerebrovascular or extracranial carotid artery disease who
  are poor surgical risks (controversial)

dures to ensure normal clotting. If surgery precludes the use of oral anticoagulants, interim coverage with heparin or mechanical interruption of the vena cava may be necessary (see Chapter 17).

There has been much controversy regarding the initiation of coumarin therapy; however, with constraints of managed care, it is generally begun the same time as heparin therapy. Controversy still exists over the duration of therapy. Most physicians advise a 3- to 6-month course of therapy after initial heparin therapy. The dose of coumarin should be approximately 10 mg with smaller doses for the elderly, debilitated, or nutritionally impaired patient.[23] A loading dose offers no advantage and without protection from further thrombosis may even lead to bleeding complications.[24]

In the United States the prothrombin time (PT, or Pro X) and the International Normalized Ratio (INR) are the most commonly employed tests to monitor coumarin therapy. The prothrombin time has been available for over 40 years and is both rapid and reliable. Values of 1.4–2 times control are considered therapeutic. The prothrombin time has largely been replaced by the INR. The INR was devised in 1982 by the World Health Organization to provide a universal application to the monitoring of oral anticoagulation. It was not used extensively in the United States until the early 1990s. The INR is calculated by dividing the patient's prothrombin time by the mean prothrombin time, multiplied by the sensitivity index of the thromboplastin. The sensitivity index is a comparison of the batch of thromboplastin to the international reference thromboplastin (value 1).[24] Desired levels of INR are seen in Table 8–5. The INR is the most accurate measure of anticoagulant control.

On the basis of the increase or decrease in test levels, the dosage is adjusted accordingly. Doses may vary from 1 mg daily in extremely sensitive patients to as high as 15–20 mg in others. The physician or vascular nurse monitoring the dosage will determine the

TABLE 8–5. **Desirable International Normalized Ratio (INR) Values**

2.0–3.0	2.5–3.5
Treatment of deep venous thrombosis (DVT)	Acute myocardial infarction
Prevention of DVT	Valvular heart disease
Prevention of systemic embolism	Atrial fibrillation
Treatment after pulmonary embolism	Recurrent systemic embolism
	Mechanical prosthetic valves

frequency of blood tests. In some patients the frequency may be every 2–4 weeks in long-term therapy, but in others more careful monitoring may be necessary. Studies have shown that monitoring of anticoagulation can be easily performed by a nurse clinician, specialist, or nurse practitioner.[25]

Complications during coumarin therapy are similar to those during heparin treatment. Bleeding is the most common problem. Other side effects, which include gastrointestinal complaints and dermatitis, are infrequent.

A rare complication of coumarin therapy is skin necrosis. This has been reported to occur after one dose but is most common after 3–10 days of therapy. It occurs most frequently in females and more often in patients who are being treated for a venous thrombosis rather than for cardiac or cerebrovascular disease.[27] The sites affected initially are commonly the breasts, thighs, buttocks, and legs.[26–31] Some studies link the presence of a carcinoma to the presence of skin necrosis.[31, 32] Studies by several authors point to a connection between a protein C or S or antithrombin III deficiency and skin necrosis.[33, 34]

The skin lesions that occur typically begin with intense pain, localized erythema, and petechiae. Swelling in the tissues follows, with color changes to a dark cyanotic appearance. Large blisters then develop over the area (Fig. 8–2). Necrosis may extend into subcutaneous or fat tissue. The tissue sloughs with resultant ulceration. The occurrence of skin necrosis is unrelated to dosage or elevated INR. The few pathology specimens from early changes point to a microvascular injury with fibrin deposition in small capillaries and veins.[27]

Treatment for this complication includes cessation of the drug, increase or reinstitution of heparin therapy, and comfort measures. Some early studies recommended the use of steroids, hypothermia, and administration of vitamins C and K. These measures have proven ineffective.[27, 28, 33] Surgical debridement, topical antibacterial ointments (especially sulfa compounds), and skin grafting may be necessary. If necrosis is extensive, amputation may be required.

When an elevated INR occurs without hemorrhage, simply omitting a dose or several doses of the drug may correct the problem. The drug should then be restarted at a lower dose with close monitoring of effects for some time. If there is bleeding or the time is exceptionally prolonged (INR >5.0), then vitamin K (10 mg orally, or 2.5–10 mg intramuscularly or intravenously) is used to reverse the drug. With hemorrhage, 10–15 mg is given intravenously and repeated every 4 hours if necessary.[23] The reversal occurs in approximately 6–12 hours. If rapid reversal is needed, 5 mg of vitamin K is given intravenously along with fresh frozen plasma. The INR should be reassessed after all of these measures and the clinician controlling the dosage should be notified. Vitamin K should always be available for parenteral use in an emergency.

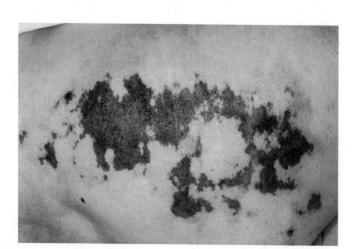

Figure 8–2. Skin necrosis that occurred after 5 days of coumarin therapy. Note large dark blisters.

TABLE 8–6. **Some Medications That Affect Warfarin (Coumadin)***

Decreases INR	Increases INR
Barbiturates	Aspirin
Rifampin	Heparin
Estrogens	Nonsteroidal anti-inflammatory drugs
Cholestyramine	High-dose penicillins
Griseofulvin	"Mycins"
Itraconazole (Sporanox)	Ticlopidine
Tamoxifen	Thyroxine
Quinidine	Cephalosporins
	Sulfa compounds
	Steroids
	Indomethacin
	Fluconazole
	Cimetidine

* Any medications that affect the cytochrome P-450 affect warfarin.
INR = international normalized ratio.

Many medications can alter the actions of coumarin. This effect can occur because of alteration in the clearance of the drug or rate of intestinal absorption. A partial list is seen in Table 8–6. For a complete list or information on a particular drug, a pharmacist or medication reference book should be consulted.

Nursing responsibility at discharge begins with an assessment of the patient's level of comprehension. The patient and a significant other must be aware and capable of recalling dose, side effects, precautions, and medical follow-up. In addition, the nurse should assess for a potential for falling, which might make oral anticoagulation dangerous outside of the hospital.

A flow sheet in simple form may assist the patient in recording and recalling coumarin doses and the times for PT determination. If the patient is incapable of traveling to a laboratory, arrangements should be made for home care to perform the test. Third-party payers will generally cover regulation of anticoagulants and patient compliance for a period of time. If the patient has trouble determining the tablet strength, a simple routine of 2-mg tablets (and no mixture of strengths) may be suggested to the physician. In addition, a daily dose packet may be made up by the discharge nurse and then the patient or family member. Simplicity of dosage increases compliance in some studies.[34]

The patient should understand that the INR must be obtained as ordered. Instruct the patient to call the clinician's office personally if no call is received with instructions following the test. The patient should be given an instructions sheet (Table 8–7). In addition to the written sheet, verbal directions from the nurse and community dietitian may assist in patient comprehension.

Documentation of instructions to the patient and the family is essential. Each piece of information given should be recorded in the hospital or home care record. Documentation of the assessment of level of understanding is crucial. Failure to document patient education carries significant medical-legal risks.

ANTIPLATELET AGENTS

Antiplatelet agents such as aspirin, dipyridamole (Persantine), and nonsteroidal anti-inflammatory drugs have been employed for many years to reduce the risk of platelet

TABLE 8–7. **Warfarin Discharge Instructions**

Make sure you understand the correct dose of medication.

Take your pills at the same time each day. If you miss a dose, do not double it the next day. Call your health care provider for instructions.

Get your blood tests as ordered. If you do not get instructions on what dose to take soon after the test, call your health care provider.

Do not take over-the-counter medication, especially aspirin or ibuprofen, without consulting your health care provider.

Do not take new prescription medications without notifying the provider who is controlling your warfarin.

Watch for signs of bleeding: blood in stools (red or black and tarry), blood in the urine, bleeding gums, joint or back pain, swollen joints, coughing up blood, severe nosebleed, vomiting "coffee grounds." If any of these happens, do not take your medicine until you check with your health care provider.

Carry a card or wear a bracelet that notes you take warfarin.

Inform all of your health care providers including your dentist that you take warfarin.

Use an electric razor.

Do not walk barefoot.

Do not play contact sports.

If you cut yourself, apply pressure for 10 minutes without pausing to look. If it continues to bleed, continue pressure and call your health care provider.

Do not take vitamins that contain vitamin K.

Get regular dental checkups to avoid unnecessary dental work.

Eat a balanced diet and avoid crash diets. Changes in dietary habits may affect your response to warfarin.

Use alcohol in moderation.

Notify your health care provider if any skin changes occur anywhere on your body (especially toes), such as hair loss, itching, or rash. Blue or purple spots on the toes or fingers should be reported immediately.

aggregation and thrombus formation. Earlier it was believed that the combination of two medications decreased platelet activity better than the use of one drug alone. It has since been shown that aspirin alone produces the same results and dipyridamole adds no additional benefit.

Ticlopidine (Ticlid) is a relatively new platelet aggregation inhibitor that is used for cerebrovascular disease, and in some institutions for intermittent claudication and sickle cell disease.[22] Clopidigrel is a new antiplatelet agent approved for use.

Antiplatelet agents are indicated for prevention of transient ischemic attacks, stroke, thromboembolic complications associated with artificial valves, myocardial infarction (post infarction and for primary prevention), graft occlusion in coronary or peripheral arterial bypass surgery, and following carotid endarterectomy. Aspirin has been studied for the prevention of DVT and has not proved effective.[36]

Contraindications to antiplatelet agents include known sensitivity to the drugs or active gastric ulcers. Aspirin is contraindicated in pregnancy and should be used with caution if the patient is anticoagulated.

Aspirin inactivates the enzyme cyclooxygenase in the platelet, resulting in inhibition of the synthesis of thromboxane A2. It also blocks the synthesis of prostacyclin in the vascular endothelium. Both are strong platelet aggregators and vasoconstrictors.[36] Aspirin has no direct effect on the coagulation cascade and is not used for treatment of active venous or arterial thrombosis.

The dosage of aspirin ranges from 1 baby aspirin to 4 adult (5 grain) aspirins a day. Some studies indicate higher doses are not necessary and may in fact be harmful. Side effects are most frequently gastrointestinal (e.g., nausea, vomiting, epigastric distress, possible ulcers, gastrointestinal bleeding). Other possible effects are prolonged bleeding time, anemia, and dizziness. Aspirin can cause confusion, neurologic disturbances, convulsions, acid-base disturbance, and tinnitus. Aspirin toxicity occurs at high doses. Nonsteroidal anti-inflammatory drugs frequently cause minor upper gastrointestinal upsets (such as nausea or heartburn) but may cause ulcers and severe gastrointestinal bleeding without warning symptoms. Side effects of all of these drugs are decreased if the drug is administered with a meal.

Instructions to the patient must include information regarding side effects. The patient must be informed in lay terms to watch for hematuria, melena, ecchymoses, hematemesis, abdominal pain, or dizziness. Alcohol should be consumed in moderation. It should be emphasized that the purpose of the medication is to prevent transient ischemic attacks and/or decrease the risk of thrombus formation. Daily compliance should be emphasized.

ANTITHROMBOTIC AGENTS

Therapy for extensive venous or arterial thromboses was traditionally anticoagulation, arterial thrombectomy, or embolectomy or arterial bypass surgery. Since the advent of thrombolytic enzymes, other methods of treating these disorders are available and are increasingly being used. Depending on the institution and the physician, these agents are used in varying degrees in the treatment of vascular disease.

Urokinase (UK), streptokinase (SK), and tissue plasminogen activator (t-PA) are thrombolytic agents in current use. They may be indicated in a number of situations (Table 8–8). Some physicians are studying the effectiveness of thrombolytic therapy in acute stroke and it is promising.[43, 44] Strong medical contraindications to surgery and surgically inaccessible clots are also possible indications for thrombolytic therapy.

The purpose of these medications is to restore venous or arterial blood flow with minimal damage to the pulmonary vascular bed, venous valves, or graft material. It is believed that thrombolytic agents can reduce the risk of subsequent venous disease in the lower extremities or the risk of pulmonary hypertension.[37]

Contraindications to therapy include those seen in Table 8–9. Caution should be used when patients have these relative contraindications. Urokinase does not form antibodies and can be used repeatedly.[46] The costs of UK and t-PA are much greater than SK.[41]

Urokinase is an enzyme produced by the kidneys and excreted in the urine. It is mass-produced from kidney tissue cultures. It acts directly to break the plasminogen molecule and yields plasmin. Streptokinase is a nonenzymatic protein produced by group C beta streptococci.[41, 46] It works by reacting with plasminogen to produce an activator complex that converts plasminogen to the lytic enzyme plasmin. t-PA is a naturally occurring

TABLE 8–8. **Indications for Thrombolytic Agents**

Acute massive pulmonary embolism
Recent extensive deep venous thrombosis
Acute arterial graft occlusion
Central venous catheter occlusion
Superior vena cava syndrome
Acute arterial thrombosis and coronary artery occlusion following myocardial infarction
Identification of a cause of thrombosis so repair may be performed
To decrease the level of amputation if the clot cannot be removed completely
Prevention of arterial wall damage from thrombectomy
Acute arterial occlusion

Data from references 38–45.

TABLE 8–9. **Contraindications to Thrombolytic Therapy**

Absolute

Recent surgical procedures (less than 10 days)
Arteriogram
Lumbar puncture
Paracentesis
Renal or liver biopsy (less than 14 days)
Recent trauma (including cardiopulmonary resuscitation)
Pregnancy (including 10 days postpartum)
Visceral carcinoma
Ulcerative colitis
Severe hypertension (200 mmHg systolic or 110 mmHg diastolic)
Ulcerative wounds
Active tuberculosis
Defective hemostasis
Central nervous system surgery (2 months)
Gastrointestinal bleeding (6 months)
Allergic reaction

Relative

Endocarditis
Atrial fibrillation (danger of bleeding into an unknown area of cerebral infarction)
Antibody formation—streptokinase only (such as after a recent streptococcal infection)

enzyme that converts plasminogen to plasmin. The plasmin dissolves the clot by specifically working on the fibrin network.

Thrombolytic therapy works best in lesions of less than 7 days of age and in vessels that are not too small.[41, 46] Massive thrombus requires a longer time to lyse than do smaller clots. If endogenous inhibitors are abnormally elevated, the fibrinolytic system may not activate adequately.

All three agents are fast acting and are rapidly cleared. The half-life of UK is approximately 16 minutes and of t-PA, 5–8 minutes; SK has two half-lives, 18 and 83 minutes. All are given intravenously or intra-arterially and are excreted in the urine.[38, 41]

For systemic therapy these drugs are given via peripheral vein (because it is compressible). For intra-arterial use they are administered via angiographic catheter, inserted as close to the clot as possible. Urokinase is "laced" into the clot by pushing the angiogram catheter into the clot and infusing the drug as it is pulled back to the beginning of the clot.

Streptokinase and urokinase are given intra-arterially for 12–16 hours but may be given longer. Streptokinase may be given for 24–72 hours and UK for up to 48 hours, depending upon the application. t-PA is given for shorter periods: 1 hour for cerebrovascular accidents, approximately 90 minutes in intracoronary applications, and 2 hours for pulmonary emboli.[38] The systemic loading dose for SK is 250,000 units/hour over 30 minutes followed by 100,000 units/hour. Intra-arterial doses may be smaller, with a bolus of 20,000 units and a continuous infusion of 5000–10,000 units/hour. Intra-arterial UK is administered with a dose of 250,000 units to lace the clot, 250,000 units over the next 2 hours, and then the dose adjusted to 10,000–60,000 units/hour until the clot is lysed. Some centers administer 100,000 units/hour after the initial dose.[37] Systemic UK (for pulmonary emboli) is started with a loading dose of 4400 units/kg for 10 minutes, followed by 4400 U/kg/hr for 12–24 hours.[37] The t-Pa dose varies with use as does that of UK and may range from 80 mg in intracoronary use to 50 mg/hr in pulmonary emboli.

These drugs are administered at a fixed dose, unlike heparin and coumarin drugs. Heparin is given in conjunction with thrombolytic therapy. Thrombin times and/or fibrinogen levels may be ordered to be certain that the thrombolytic system has been activated. It is important to remember that no blood test is directly correlated to complications, and they may occur despite acceptable test results. The major complication of thrombolysis is bleeding. Some have suggested that febrile reactions to thrombolytic therapy may be due to contaminants with bacterial endotoxins or to the release of catabolic products of thrombolysis. Mild reactions to these drugs do not necessitate discontinuance of therapy. t-PA has no antigenic properties because it occurs naturally in the body.

Nursing implications in thrombolytic therapy are very complex and are related to the stage of therapy—preinfusion, intrainfusion, and postinfusion. In the preinfusion state, the patient may be moved to a monitored area. Blood work should be performed to establish a baseline PTT, PT, hematocrit, white blood cell count, platelet count, thrombin time, and plasminogen level. These tests provide evidence of normal hemostasis and coagulation. If these results are abnormal for an *unknown* reason, the physician should be notified. If the bleeding time is greater than 15 minutes, therapy should not be instituted. Cross-matched blood should be available in case of bleeding. Aminocaproic acid (Amicar) is the antidote for use if bleeding occurs. The thrombolytic solution must be administered via volumetric pump whose flow rate is not dependent on drop size.

In the pretherapy assessment of the patient, a good history is essential. Recent streptococcal infection may diminish the drug's effects. Ingestion of anticoagulant or antiplatelet drugs should be recorded. Baseline pulses and/or pressures in each extremity must be obtained, using a Doppler transducer if necessary.

During infusion, vital signs are closely monitored in addition to extremity perfusion. Observation of the stool, urine, emesis, or dressings for bleeding is important. The nurse must be alert for hematoma formation, back pain, swelling, flank pain, and a falling hematocrit. If bleeding does occur, direct pressure is applied, infusion stopped, and the physician notified. Sandbags may be employed if necessary. Whole blood, fresh frozen plasma, or aminocaproic acid may be administered. Corticosteroids may be necessary for allergic reactions.

No intramuscular injections should be given within 24 hours of infusion and no new medications initiated during therapy. No medications may be mixed with the thrombolytic drugs. Anticoagulants, antiplatelet agents, dextran, and phenylbutazone should be used with caution.

Invasive procedures may not be performed during therapy. If arterial blood gases are absolutely indicated, pressure must be applied to the site for 30 minutes and the site frequently observed for bleeding. A flow sheet of all doses and laboratory data should be kept. Thrombin times should be elevated 2–5 times and fibrinogen level should be approximately 100 mg/dl.

Postinfusion, direct pressure by hand or sandbag should be applied to the infusion site. The patient should be on bed rest with the extremity immobile in straight alignment. Heparin is continued postinfusion and the usual precautions for heparin therapy apply.

Patient education regarding thrombolytic agents should include the purpose of therapy, possible side effects, and expected activity level both during and after therapy. Emotional support is essential. Patients are in a crisis situation and must be reassured that procedures are normal. It is important that the patient and the family be informed before the patient is transported to the radiology unit that if thrombolytic therapy is started, the patient will be transferred to the intensive care unit or a monitored unit.

Pain is common in patients receiving thrombolytic therapy. Assessment of pain before initiation of therapy is essential, and the source must be determined. Accurate assessment of pain to determine if distal embolization has occurred is essential. Pulse rate and ankle-brachial index determination are standard measures of arterial flow; color, capillary return, and temperature may also be assessed. If pain becomes worse with reperfusion, analgesia must be given. Back pain from bed rest is common but must be differentiated from severe pain caused by retroperitoneal bleeding.

MISCELLANEOUS DRUGS

Dextran

Dextran is a polysaccharide first introduced as a plasma expander, for use when blood or blood products were not available. Its antithrombotic effect was a secondary finding and has been demonstrated in subsequent studies. This effect may be due to several factors: (1) increased blood volume; (2) decreased blood viscosity; (3) reduced platelet adhesiveness; (4) altered fibrin polymerization; and (5) interference with factor VIII antigen and the von Willebrand cofactor.[46]

One indication for dextran is prophylaxis against venous thrombosis. This is especially indicated in the patient at risk who, in addition, needs volume replacement. Controversy exists over its effectiveness.

Contraindications for dextran include known bleeding disorders, anuria, hypervolemic state, and drug-induced cardiac decompensation.[22] Care should be exercised in administering dextran to patients with cardiac or renal insufficiency or while heparin is administered. It is unknown whether the drug crosses the placental barrier, and therefore dextran is not recommended in pregnancy.[22]

Dextran is given intravenously. Doses of dextran are begun with 10 mg/kg just prior to surgery and then increased to 500 ml/day for 2–3 days. It may be continued for up to 3 weeks with a dose of 500 ml every 2–3 days.[23]

Dextran must be given slowly in patients with cardiac insufficiency. Central venous pressure must be monitored carefully. Oliguria or anuria should be reported to the physician. Complications of dextran include fluid overload, bleeding, decreased urine output, and anaphylactic reactions. Fluid overload and pulmonary edema can be avoided by limiting rate and volume in elderly patients or in patients with renal insufficiency. It is important to reassure the patient that urinary output problems are generally temporary. Anaphylaxis is a rare complication but occurs immediately after infusion. For this reason the initial dose should not be given while the patient is under general anesthesia. Anaphylaxis is not related to a previous infusion history. Anaphylactoid reactions can be avoided with an intravenous injection of 20 ml of monovalent dextran.

Pentoxifylline

Pentoxifylline was introduced in the United States in the early 1980s. It is indicated for intermittent claudication or in high-risk patients with rest pain. This latter group might benefit from any improvement in blood flow, but the medication does not solve the problem of rest pain or gangrenous lesions. Pentoxifylline is contraindicated in patients with a history of intolerance to caffeine, theophylline, or theobromine.[22] Additionally, it should be used with caution in patients with coronary artery disease or impaired renal function.

Pentoxifylline is absorbed in the gastrointestinal tract, metabolized in the liver and excreted in the urine. Its action is a result of improved erythrocyte flexibility, reduction in blood viscosity, and improved tissue oxygen concentration.[22, 47] Therapeutic effects occur after 4–8 weeks of therapy. Patients must be aware that results will not be noticeable for up to 2 months. Otherwise, they may become discouraged.

Dosage of the medication is 400 mg three times a day with meals. If stomach upset occurs, it may be reduced to twice a day. Most common side effects are nausea, heartburn, dizziness, headache, and tremor. These are usually mild. Pentoxifylline may increase the effect of antihypertensives.[22]

Controversy exists as to whether pentoxifylline actually increases exercise tolerance or whether a planned program of exercise is more effective (see Chapter 10). Studies have been performed that support both arguments.[47, 48]

OTHER MEDICATIONS

Research continues to discover medications to assist the vascular patient. Antihypertensive medications, lipid-lowering agents, and diabetic medications are beyond the scope of this chapter but continue to be important in the management of these patients.

Hirudin is being investigated for use as an anticoagulant. Hirudin is the thrombin inhibitor found in the saliva of the leech. Evaluation continues to determine whether hirudin is efficacious as an anticoagulant drug.[49]

SUMMARY

The nurse who is knowledgeable about the drugs most commonly used in vascular patients can monitor as well as educate the patient adequately. With advanced practice laws, nurses with advanced training can prescribe medication in all states except Illinois. Knowledge of medications is essential for this group of nurses. All nurses must cooperate to decrease medication complications and to increase adherence to the prescribed routine.

References

1. McLean J: Thromboplastin action of cephalin. Am J Physiol 1916; 41:250.
2. Murray D, Jacques L, Perrett T, et al: Heparin and the thrombosis of veins following injury. Surgery 1937; 2:163–187.
3. Rosenfeld J, Estrada F, Orr R: Management of deep venous thrombosis in the pregnant female. J Cardiovasc Surg 1990; 31:678–682.
4. Fahey V: Heparin induced thrombocytopenia. J Vasc Nursing 1995; 13:112–116.
5. Matula P: Management of patients undergoing vascular surgery who are receiving epidural analgesia. J Vasc Nurs 1993; 11(4):104–107.
6. Nunnelee J: Low molecular weight heparin. J Vasc Nursing 1997; 15:94–96.
7. Falter H: Deep vein thrombosis in pregnancy and the puerperium: A comprehensive review. J Vasc Nurs 1997; 15(2):58–62.
8. Koopman M, Prandoni P, Piovella F, et al: Treatment of venous thrombosis with intravenous unfractionated heparin administered in the hospital as compared with subcutaneous low molecular weight heparin administered at home. N Engl J Med 1996; 334:682–687.
9. Lensing A, Prins M, Davidson B, Hirsch J: Treatment of deep venous thrombosis with low molecular weight heaprins—a meta analysis. Arch Intern Med 1995; 155:601–607.
10. Weitz JI: Low-molecular-weight heparin. N Engl J Med 1997; 337(10):688–698.
11. Erban S, Kinman J, Schwartz JS: Routine use of the prothrombin and partial thromboplastin times. JAMA 1989; 262:2428–2432.
12. Hyers T, Hull R, Weg J: Antithrombotic therapy for venous thromboembolic disease. Chest 1989; 95(suppl):37s–51s.
13. The Columbus Investigators: Low molecular weight heparin in the treatment of patients with venous thromboembolism. N Engl J Med 1997; 337(10):657–662.
14. Harrington L, Hufnagel J: Heparin induced thrombocytopenia and thrombosis syndrome: A case study. Heart & Lung 1990; 19:93–98.
15. AbuRahma A, Boland J, Witsberger T: Diagnostic and therapeutic strategies of white clot syndrome. Am J Surg 1991; 162:175–179.
16. Warkentin TE, Levine MN, Hirsch J, et al: Heparin induced thrombocytopenia in patient treated with low molecular weight heparin or unfractionated heparin. N Engl J Med 1995; 332:1330–1335.
17. Aster R: Heparin induced thrombocytopenia and thrombosis. N Engl J Med 1995; 332:1374–1376.
18. Visentin G, Ford S, Scott J, Aster R: Antibodies from patients with heparin induced thrombocytopenia/thrombosis are specific for platelet factor 4 complexed with heparin or bound to endothelial cells. J Clin Inves 1994; 93:81–88.

19. Wheeler H, Anderson F: Prophylaxis against venous thromboembolism in surgical patients. Am J Surg 1991; 161:507–511.
20. Hulin, M, Wakefield T, Andrews P, et al: A novel protamine variant reversal of heparin anticoagulation in human blood in vitro. J Vasc Surg 1997; 26:1043–1048.
21. Clagett GP, Krupski WC: Antithrombotic therapy in peripheral arterial occlusive disease. Chest 1995; 108(4):431S–443S.
22. Hodgson B, Kizior R: Saunders Nursing Drug Handbook. Philadelphia, WB Saunders, 1998, pp 1062–1064.
23. Hirsh J, Dolan J, Deykin D, et al: Oral anticoagulants. Chest 1992; 102(suppl):312s–326s.
24. Kurgan A, Nunnelee J: Upper extremity venous thrombosis. J Vasc Nurs 1995; 13(1):21–23.
25. Knaus V, Davis K, Burton S, et al: Vascular nurse practitioner: A collaborative practice role in the acute care setting. J Vasc Nurs 1996; 14(2):40–44.
26. Comp P, Elrod J, Karzenski S: Warfarin induced skin necrosis. Semin Thromb Hemost 1990; 16:293–298.
27. Cole M, Mimifee P, Wolma F: Coumarin necrosis: A review of the literature. Surgery 1988; 103:271–277.
28. Kandrotas R, Detering J: Genital necrosis secondary to warfarin therapy. Pharmacology 1988; 3:351–354.
29. Leath M: Coumarin skin necrosis. Tex Med 1983; 79:62–64.
30. Heaton R, Wright L, Hargraves R, et al: Coagulopathy and warfarin associated breast necrosis in a patient with a primary brain tumor. Surg Neurol 1990; 33:395–399.
31. Everett R, Jones F: Warfarin induced skin necrosis: A sign of malignancy: Postgrad Med 1986; 79:97–103.
32. Konrad P, Mellblom L, Berquist D, et al: Coumarin associated skin necrosis. Vasa 1988; 17:208–215.
33. Conlan M, Bridges A, Williams E, et al: Familial type II protein C deficiency associated with warfarin induced skin necrosis and bilateral adrenal hemorrhage. Am J Hematol 1988; 29:226–229.
34. Conn V, Taylor S, Kelley S: Medication regimen complexity and adherence among older adults. Image: J Nurs Scholarship 1991; 23:231–235.
35. Clagett GP: Prevention of postoperative venous thromboembolism: An update. Am J Surgery 1994; 168:515–522.
36. DeWeese M: Nonoperative treatment of acute superficial thrombophlebitis and deep femoral venous thrombosis. In Ernst CB, Stanley JC (eds): Current Therapy in Vascular Surgery II. Philadelphia, BC Decker, 1991, pp 951–961.
37. Apple S: New trends in thrombolytic therapy. RN 1996; 59(1):30–34.
38. Butler L, Fahey V: Acute arterial occlusion of the lower extremity. J Vasc Nurs 1993; 11(1):19–22.
39. Crouch M: Urokinase therapy in mesenteric venous thrombosis: A case study. J Vasc Nurs 1993; 11(4):99–103.
40. Ronayne R: Acute lower limb ischemia: A case study. J Vasc Nurs 1992; 10(3):14–19.
41. Anderson K: Thrombolytic therapy for treatment of acute peripheral arterial occlusion. J Vasc Nurs 1992; 10(3):20–24.
42. Gwynn M: TPA in acute stroke: Risk or reprieve? J Neurosci Nurs 1993; 25(3):180–184.
43. Hacke E, Kaste M, Smith T, et al: Intravenous thrombolytics with recombinant tissue plasminogen activator for acute hemispheric stroke. JAMA 1995; 224(13):1017–1019.
44. Kumpe D, Cohen M: Angioplasty/thrombolytic treatment of failing and failed hemodialysis sites: Comparison with surgical treatment. Prog Cardiovasc Diseases 1992; 34(4):263–278.
45. Weitz J, Byrne J, Clagett P, et al: Diagnosis and treatment of chronic arterial insufficiency of the lower extremities: A critical review. Circulation 1996; 94(11):3026–3049.
46. Nehler MR, Taylor LM, Moneta GL, Porter JM: Natural history, nonoperative treatment and functional assessment in chronic lower extremity ischemia. In Moore WS (ed): Vascular Surgery: A comprehensive review. Philadelphia, WB Saunders, 1998, pp 251–265.
47. AbuRahma AF, Woodruff BA: Effects and limitations of pentoxifylline therapy in various stages of peripheral vascular disease of the lower extremity. Am J Surg 1990; 160:266–270.
48. Williams LR, Ekers M, Collins PS, et al: Vascular rehabilitation: Benefits of a structured exercise risk factor modification program. J Vasc Surg 1991; 14:1636–1639.
49. Chesbro J: Hirudin: A specific thrombin inhibitor. J Vasc Surg 1990; 12:201–202.

9

Thrombotic Disorders in Vascular Patients

Przemyslaw Twardowski, MD, and David Green, MD, PhD

Normally, blood is maintained in a fluid phase while it circulates through the vascular system. Upon injury to the blood vessel, a coagulum (blood clot) is formed to prevent exsanguination. This process is defined as hemostasis. Thrombosis refers to the abnormal formation of thrombi within the closed vasculature. Blood vessels, platelets, coagulation proteins, inhibitors of coagulation, and activators and inhibitors of fibrinolysis interact with one another in one of the most intricate and tightly controlled of biologic systems.

The basic mechanism of hemostasis is divided into four phases:

1. Primary hemostasis, involving the formation of a platelet thrombus that, within seconds, plugs the rent in the blood vessel wall.
2. Activation of the coagulation cascade, leading to formation of fibrin that reinforces the platelet plug and creates the mature thrombus.
3. The regulation of the extension of the thrombus by coagulation factor inhibitors and the fibrinolytic (blood clot dissolving) system.
4. The remodeling and repair of the injury site after arrest of bleeding.

The blood vasculature forms a circuit lined by a continuous layer of endothelial cells. Injury to endothelial cells exposes subendothelial supporting structures and adhesive proteins (collagen, von Willebrand factor, fibronectin, vitronectin) that provide binding sites for platelets. Platelets adhere to subendothelial proteins through specific receptors, become activated, and aggregate together to form a platelet plug.

Injury of the blood vessel endothelium and activation of platelets initiates the coagulation cascade that ultimately leads to the formation of fibrin, which constitutes a major portion of the mature clot. The coagulation system is composed of a series of serine proteinases and their cofactors, which react on the phospholipid surfaces of platelets and damaged endothelial cells. The coagulation cascade is divided into an extrinsic pathway triggered by tissue factor–factor VII interaction and an intrinsic pathway initiated by surface contact factors. Recent evidence suggests that the extrinsic pathway is physiologically more relevant in the initial generation of fibrin.[1]

Coagulation processes are balanced by an elaborate system of naturally occurring inhibitors, including tissue factor pathway inhibitor, antithrombin III, protein C, and protein S, that prevent excessive propagation of thrombus. Deficiencies in these anticoagulants, or interference with their normal functioning, may increase the risk for the development of thrombosis. In this review, we will focus on hypercoagulability and thrombosis in vascular disease.

INHERITED THROMBOTIC DISORDERS

A number of genetic disorders predispose to thrombotic problems either in the newborn period or later in life. Table 9–1 lists the more common of these disorders.

Antithrombin Deficiency

Antithrombin (AT III) is a circulating anticoagulant that inhibits several coagulation proteases including activated factors XI, X, IX, thrombin, and the tissue factor–factor VIIa complex. Its activity is greatly enhanced in the presence of heparin. Deficiency of AT III is inherited in autosomal dominant fashion. All clinically recognized patients are heterozygous for this disorder; homozygosity is probably lethal in utero. Type I deficiency refers to a quantitative reduction in the level of AT III, and type II deficiency describes qualitative abnormalities that reduce the functional activity of the molecule. It is estimated that the lifetime risk for the development of venous thromboembolism in AT III–deficient individuals is about 50 percent.[2] Thrombotic episodes can occur spontaneously, but in 60 percent of patients they are associated with a predisposing risk factor such as surgery, trauma, pregnancy, or the use of oral contraceptives.[3] Patients with known AT III deficiency should undergo aggressive antithrombotic prophylaxis in high-risk situations, for example, in the immediate postoperative period. Treatment of an established thrombosis is accomplished with intravenous heparin followed by warfarin. Occasionally, very high doses of heparin are required to achieve adequate anticoagulation.[4] In selected situations commercially available AT III concentrate can be infused to restore normal levels of this anticoagulant.

Protein C Deficiency

Protein C is converted to its active form when thrombin is generated during clotting. The thrombin binds to an endothelial protein called thrombomodulin, and the thrombin-thrombomodulin complex activates protein C. Activated protein C inactivates clotting factors V and VIII; the reaction is greatly enhanced by a cofactor designated protein S. The synthesis of protein C and protein S requires vitamin K. Type I and type II deficiencies of protein C have been described. The gene for the protein is located on chromosome 2; if mutant genes are inherited from both parents, the child is homozygous for this disorder and the levels of protein C are less than 1 percent of normal. Necrotizing

TABLE 9–1. **Inherited Disorders Predisposing to Thrombosis**

Antithrombin (AT III) deficiency	Factor V Leiden mutation
	Prothrombin 20210A
Protein C deficiency	mutation
Protein S deficiency	Homocysteinemia

skin and muscle lesions—purpura fulminans—appear shortly after birth, and the child will die unless protein C is provided.

Patients who are heterozygous for protein C deficiency generally experience the first episode of thrombosis in early adulthood, and are more likely to have venous thrombosis than arterial thrombosis. Approximately 70 percent of episodes of thrombosis develop spontaneously, and 30 percent are associated with known predisposing risk factors. Thromboses in patients with protein C deficiency are managed with heparin and warfarin, but the duration of warfarin therapy is unsettled; most clinicians would continue treatment for 6 to 12 months after a first episode of thrombosis and indefinitely in patients with recurrent thrombosis. Patients with protein C deficiency who have never had thrombotic events are not routinely given anticoagulants but should receive antithrombotic prophylaxis when they undergo surgery or are exposed to other risk factors for thrombosis.

Protein C deficiency predisposes to an important complication called warfarin-induced skin necrosis. This syndrome occurs because of the presence of a transient hypercoagulable state that develops after initiation of warfarin therapy. Because the half-life of protein C is shorter than that of several of the vitamin K–dependent procoagulants (factors II, IX, X), its levels fall more quickly than those of these procoagulants, creating an imbalance in favor of thrombosis during the first 24 hours of warfarin administration. This may cause skin and muscle necrosis, similar to that occurring in purpura fulminans. About 30 percent of patients with warfarin-induced skin necrosis have an underlying protein C deficiency.[5] Treatment of this complication includes prompt discontinuation of warfarin, intravenous heparin, and injection of vitamin K. In severe cases, infusion of plasma can rapidly restore levels of protein C.

Protein S Deficiency

Protein S acts as a cofactor for protein C. The gene for this protein is found on chromosome 3, its synthesis by the liver requires vitamin K, and it circulates both free and bound to the C4b-binding protein. Only the free form is active as the cofactor for protein C. The clinical manifestations and management of deficiency states are similar to those described for AT III and protein C. An association with thrombotic strokes has also been reported.[6]

Factor V Leiden Mutation

The factor V Leiden mutation is found most often in patients with inherited thrombophilia. It is caused by a single mutation in the factor V gene that results in substitution of glutamine for arginine at position 506 of the protein. This substitution renders factor V partially resistant to inactivation by activated protein C.[7, 8] The prevalence of this trait is approximately 5 percent in persons of European extraction and is between 20 and 50 percent in various cohorts of patients with venous thrombosis. This is much more common than deficiencies of AT III, protein C, and protein S, which combined are detected in only 5–10 percent of patients with thrombosis.

The risk of thrombosis for heterozygous carriers of factor V Leiden is estimated at 1.0 per year between the ages of 20 and 50, which is about 10 times higher than in the general population. The risk in women who are pregnant or on oral contraceptives is increased about 30-fold. The risk of thrombosis in individuals with mutations of both genes for factor V (homozygotes) is 30–140-fold that in normal persons.[9, 10]

Patients with the factor V Leiden mutation have similar clinical manifestations to those in patients with deficiencies of antithrombin, protein C, or protein S. While venous thrombosis is generally observed, there is an increased risk for stroke in the very young[11] and myocardial infarction in persons with additional risk factors such as cigarette smoking.[12]

Acute thrombotic episodes are treated with heparin and warfarin. Studies[13] have shown about a twofold increased risk for recurrence of thrombosis if warfarin is discontinued within the first 6 months of thrombosis, but whether patients need to remain on treatment for longer than 6 months is unclear. Prophylaxis with adjusted doses of heparin, low-molecular-weight heparin, or warfarin is required at the time of increased risk for thrombosis such as during the perioperative period, while on prolonged bed rest, or pregnancy. Patients with recurrent or life-threatening thrombosis may need indefinite anticoagulant therapy.

Prothrombin 20210A Mutation

A mutation in the regulatory elements of the prothrombin gene leads to overproduction of this molecule and an increase in the risk of venous thrombosis.[14] This mutation is observed in 18 percent of patients with a personal and family history of thrombosis. The thrombotic tendency is closely related to the level of plasma prothrombin; most affected patients have prothrombin concentrations in excess of 1 U/ml. The relative risk for thrombosis in persons with this mutation has been estimated at 2.8.[15]

Inherited Homocysteinemia

Homocysteine is an amino acid that is formed during the course of folate metabolism. It undergoes enzymatic conversion to methionine and cystathionine in a series of reactions requiring several enzymes as well as folic acid, vitamin B_{12}, and pyridoxine. In the rare disorder homocystinuria, the activity of the enzyme cystathionine synthase is decreased, and high concentrations of homocysteine are present in blood and urine. More commonly, a thermolabile form of the enzyme methylene-tetrahydrofolate reductase is inherited, leading to mild homocysteinemia.[16] More severe increases occur if there is concomitant deficiency of folic acid or vitamin B_{12}. Elevated homocysteine concentrations injure the endothelium, decrease protein C activation, and enhance the binding of lipoprotein (a) to fibrin.[17, 18] Hyperhomocysteinemia has been found in association with deep vein thrombosis and arterial occlusion, leading to stroke, myocardial infarction, and limb ischemia.[19–22] In patients with elevated levels of this amino acid, a trial of treatment with folic acid and/or vitamin B_{12} should be undertaken,[23] although investigations to document a beneficial effect on vascular disease are still in progress.[24]

ACQUIRED THROMBOTIC DISORDERS

Acquired (noninherited) factors that predispose to thrombosis are age over 40, obesity, and cancer.[25] With regard to the last, thrombosis occurs three to five times more frequently in cancer patients than in other patients undergoing surgery.[26] Multiple mechanisms are at play that predispose the cancer patient to thrombosis. Because of poor nutrition, the plasma concentrations of the anticoagulant proteins C and S are often decreased, and stress-related procoagulants such as fibrinogen and factor VIII are increased, thereby shifting the coagulation balance in favor of thrombosis. A potent inhibitor of fibrinolysis, plasminogen activator inhibitor–1, is another stress-related factor that is increased in cancer, enhancing clot formation over clot dissolution. Cancer cells may also activate clotting by exposing tissue factor and releasing specific cancer procoagulants. Lastly, tumor cells may injure endothelium and activate platelets and monocytes, encouraging thrombosis.

In patients with arterial thrombosis, the plasma lipid profile is usually examined; some fractions of low-density lipoproteins are particularly vasculopathic and promote thrombosis. In addition, lipoprotein (a) should be specifically measured. This lipid competes with plasminogen for binding sites on fibrin and is therefore thrombogenic.[27] Accelerated atherosclerosis in diabetes or renal failure may also predispose to arterial thrombosis.

Conditions associated with either venous or arterial thrombosis include the antiphospholipid antibody syndrome, hyperhomocysteinemia, myeloproliferative disorders, and heparin-induced thrombocytopenia with thrombosis (HITT) syndrome. These conditions are listed in Table 9–2.

The Antiphospholipid Antibody Syndrome

The antiphospholipid antibody syndrome is defined by two principal components: a positive laboratory test for an antiphospholipid antibody and certain characteristic clinical findings. These latter include venous and/or arterial thrombosis, neuropsychiatric disorder, valvular heart lesion, thrombocytopenia, and recurrent fetal deaths due to placental infarcts. There are two forms of the syndrome: autoimmune and alloimmune.[28] The autoimmune form may be primary (idiopathic) or secondary to systemic lupus erythematosus or other connective tissue diseases, or associated with drugs such as chlorpromazine. The alloimmune form occurs after infections or in association with malignancies.

The antiphospholipid antibodies are thought to arise because of an event that exposes anionic (negatively charged) membrane phospholipids.[29] These phospholipids are normally located on the inside of cell membranes. When exposed to the flowing blood, they may initiate coagulation. To protect against thrombosis, circulating phospholipid-binding proteins such as β_2-glycoprotein-1 form complexes with negatively charged phospholipids. In genetically susceptible persons, these complexes act as antigens and elicit the formation of antibodies. The antibodies cross-react with complexes of cardiolipin and β_2-glycoprotein-1 and are designated anticardiolipin antibodies (ACA). Antibodies may also develop to complexes of phospholipid and clotting factors (i.e., prothrombin), and these are called lupus anticoagulants (LA). Thus, ACA and LA are distinct entities.

The mechanism of the thromboses in this syndrome is under intensive investigation. Most evidence favors the hypothesis that the antiphospholipid antibodies interfere with the protein C–protein S system. Protein C binds to the lipid bilayer of cell membranes and is activated by a complex of thrombin and membrane-bound thrombomodulin. With protein S as a cofactor, activated protein C inactivates factors Va and VIIIa. Resistance to

TABLE 9–2. **Acquired Conditions Predisposing to Thrombosis**

Age over 40
Obesity
Malignancy
Thrombogenic lipid disorders
Antiphospholipid antibody syndrome
Hyperhomocysteinemia
Myeloproliferative disorders
Heparin-induced thrombocytopenia with thrombosis

activated protein C manifested by impaired inactivation of factor Va has been observed in patients with lupus anticoagulant and one or more episodes of thrombosis.[30, 31]

Other thrombogenic actions of antiphospholipid antibodies include the formation of immune complexes of antibody and phospholipid-binding protein. These may bind to and cross-link platelet F_c receptors, resulting in platelet activation. Activated platelets promote thrombosis and are consumed, resulting in thrombocytopenia. Another mechanism for thrombosis is related to the effects of the antiphospholipid antibodies on endothelial cells. The antibodies impair the release of prostacyclin, a potent endothelial cell inhibitor of platelet function.[32] Effects on AT III and fibrinolysis have also been described.[33]

A variety of clinical manifestations of the syndrome have been recorded. Most prominent among these is thrombosis, involving either arterial or venous vessels, or, rarely, both. Men and women are affected equally, and often the thrombi appear before age 40. In patients with the lupus anticoagulant, the risk of thrombosis is increased 9.4-fold, whereas in patients with high titers of anticardiolipin antibody, it is only increased 1.9-fold.[34] A typical patient will have recurrent strokes, peripheral arterial occlusion, and myocardial infarction. Others may present with repeated deep vein thromboses and pulmonary emboli. Livedo reticularis is a manifestation of thrombosis in superficial skin arterioles, and has the appearance of tiny serpiginous lines in a map-like pattern. It may be seen on the back, arms, or legs, and often occurs in association with stroke (Sneddon's syndrome). Other neurologic manifestations are episodes of transient blindness (amaurosis fugax), retinal artery occlusion, and psychoses.

The antiphospholipid antibody syndrome is often suspected in women who have recurrent miscarriages, typically in the second trimester. Examination of the placenta may disclose thrombosed vessels and placental infarcts. Another manifestation of the syndrome in these women is thrombocytopenia. In patients with systemic lupus erythematosus, fibrin thrombi may be detected on heart valves using the technique of echocardiography. In a series of 35 patients, Asherson and associates[35] detected venous thrombosis in 37 percent, arterial thrombosis in 29 percent, recurrent abortions in 17 percent, livedo reticularis in 37 percent, and valvular heart lesions in 65 percent.

The diagnosis of the antiphospholipid antibody syndrome depends on a characteristic clinical picture combined with a positive test for either the lupus anticoagulant or another antiphospholipid antibody such as anticardiolipin. Detection of the lupus anticoagulant relies on the prolongation of a phospholipid-dependent test of coagulation. Often, the patient has a prolonged partial thromboplastin time that is not correctable with normal plasma but shortened by the addition of platelets or phospholipids.[36] However, to detect this, it is necessary that fresh patient plasma be doubly centrifuged or filtered to remove residual platelets because these may mask the effect of the lupus anticoagulant. Low-titer lupus anticoagulants may not prolong the partial thromboplastin time; it is often necessary to use a sensitive, phospholipid-dependent test such as the diluted Russell viper venom time to recognize them.[37] In patients who are being treated with heparin or warfarin, test results for lupus anticoagulants are altered; the laboratory must be informed of these treatments so that the testing can be modified.

Anticardiolipin antibodies are detected by enzyme-linked immunosorbent assays that are unaffected by patient treatment with anticoagulants. Antibodies of the IgG, IgA, and IgM class are detected and quantified using phospholipid (PL) units. Thus, IgG antibodies would be recorded in GPL units, and IgM antibodies in MPL units. Antibody titer is important, because low antibody titers are found in 2 percent of blood donors and up to 12 percent of healthy elderly persons.[38] High titers predict the development of deep vein thrombosis,[39] and titers in excess of 30 GPL units are found in association with deep vein thrombosis.[40] Protein S concentrations decrease in patients with thrombosis and have been noted to vary inversely with the level of anticardiolipin antibody, with the lowest values in patients with the highest antibody titers.[41]

The treatment of patients with the antiphospholipid antibody syndrome is unsatisfactory. Despite the use of heparin and warfarin, patients often experience recurrent strokes and peripheral artery occlusion, resulting in progressive loss of function and disability. Repeated miscarriages despite intensive interventions are also common. Current therapeutic recommendations are mostly based on clinical experience rather than randomized, controlled trials.

Given these reservations, it has been suggested that acute thromboses be treated with heparin in full therapeutic doses, followed by warfarin to maintain the international normalized ratio (INR) at 3–4,[42] or warfarin plus acetylsalicylic acid (ASA) for an INR of 2–3 (the latter regimen is easier to manage and may pose less risk of bleeding). Although the risk of recurrence is high in patients with lupus anticoagulants, a significant difference was not observed after discontinuation of warfarin when those who were anticardiolipin-positive were compared with those who were anticardiolipin-negative.[40] Although an early study suggested that steroids be used to prevent recurrent miscarriages,[43] only small numbers of patients were evaluated; more recent experience indicates that steroids may be associated with an increased rather than a decreased rate of miscarriage.[44] Most authorities currently recommend the use of aspirin, 80 mg daily combined with heparin, 5,000–10,000 U given subcutaneously every 12 hours.[45]

Hyperhomocysteinemia

As described earlier, hyperhomocysteinemia is a risk factor for venous and arterial thrombotic disease, with odds ratios ranging from 2 to 13.[46] About 12 percent of the population have elevated levels of homocysteinemia, making this one of the more common risk factors. Patients having hyperhomocysteinemia as well as factor V Leiden, or other risk factors, are especially predisposed to thrombosis. Poor nutritional status associated with deficiencies of folic acid, pyridoxine, or vitamin B_{12} increases homocysteine levels; supplementing the diet with these vitamins decreases homocysteine blood levels and may slow the progression of vascular disease.

Myeloproliferative Disorders

These conditions are defined by an increase in one or more of the blood elements: red cells (polycythemia), white cells (myeloid leukemia), or platelets (thrombocythemia). Thrombosis may be a presenting manifestation of these disorders, although in some patients bleeding is more prominent. Patients often have an enlarged spleen and almost always an abnormal blood count. Once the diagnosis is established, appropriate management is imperative especially if an operative procedure is contemplated. For example, in patients with polycythemia, decreasing the hematocrit by phlebotomy may prevent intraoperative hemorrhage. Perioperative thrombosis in persons with chronic myelogenous leukemia or essential thrombocythemia may be avoided by preoperative treatment with hydroxyurea, a drug that decreases leukocyte and platelet counts. Thus, it is always important to review the preoperative blood count and, if it is abnormal, obtain a hematology consultation before surgery.

Heparin-Induced Thrombocytopenia with Thrombosis Syndrome

The HITT syndrome occurs in about 1 percent of patients receiving heparin therapy.[47] In patients treated with heparin for longer than 5 days, or in patients re-exposed to heparin, antibodies may develop to a complex of heparin and platelet factor 4 clustered on the surface of the platelet. These complexes trigger the platelet to form microparticles, which promote platelet aggregation, thrombus formation, and thrombocytopenia.[48] Venous thrombosis is more common than arterial thrombosis, and thrombi may occur in the deep veins of the legs, in the pulmonary arteries, and in the axillary, internal jugular, and subclavian veins. Other manifestations are limb gangrene, anaphylactoid reactions, and skin necrosis at sites where heparin has been injected. The HITT syndrome is significantly less frequent with low-molecular-weight heparin than with unfractionated heparin, but once the syndrome develops, there is a high degree of cross-reactivity to low-molecular-weight heparins.[49, 50] The diagnosis is suspected in patients receiving heparin who experience new thromboses during treatment or whose platelet counts acutely decline by 50 percent or more, and is confirmed by performing tests to detect the presence of heparin-platelet antibodies. Suspicion of HITT should trigger an immediate discontinuation of heparin in all forms and by all routes, including Hep-Locks and heparin flushes. Platelet transfusions worsen thrombosis and are contraindicated. Patients with evidence of thrombosis should receive prompt treatment with an antithrombotic agent such as lepirudin, which does not cross-react with heparin antibodies.[51] Lepirudin is a recombinant hirudin (leech anticoagulant) that is a direct thrombin inhibitor. It is given parenterally and monitored with the activated partial thromboplastin time. Warfarin therapy should be delayed until the patient is stable and the platelet count is rising.

PREOPERATIVE EVALUATION FOR HYPERCOAGULABILITY

Screening for hypercoagulability is indicated when there is strong clinical suspicion that a patient is at risk for thrombosis. Screening should not be performed indiscriminately, because the laboratory tests are expensive, test abnormalities require expertise in interpretation, and an abnormal result may stigmatize a patient, prejudicing future insurance coverage. However, persons with the risk factors shown in Table 9–3 should be further evaluated.[52] Thrombosis in the young, especially when it is recurrent, demands explanation. Similarly, a patient with thrombosis of mesenteric, dural, or retinal veins needs evaluation. Many thrombotic disorders are inherited, and family studies are helpful in localizing the cause of the index patient's event. Recurrent fetal loss is often associated with the antiphospholipid antibody syndrome.

Questions often arise about performing surgery in patients with a previous thrombotic event. Screening is probably not indicated if a thrombosis occurred in association with trauma or surgery and completely resolved with anticoagulant therapy. On the other hand, if the prior thrombosis was not associated with a precipitating event, screening is advisable.

In patients with a family history of venous thrombosis, molecular studies for factor V Leiden should be requested; if not available, the activated- protein C resistance test may

TABLE 9–3. **Characteristics of Patients with Hypercoagulable States: Indications for Further Investigation**

Venous thrombosis under age 45	Familial thrombosis
Recurrent venous thrombosis	Unexpected neonatal thrombosis
Thrombosis at unusual sites	Recurrent fetal loss
Arterial thrombosis under age 30	

be substituted.[53] In addition, laboratory tests of proteins C, S, and antithrombin should be obtained, because deficiency of one of the naturally occurring anticoagulants may occur either in isolation or in combination with factor V Leiden. If all of the above are negative, testing for abnormalities of fibrinogen, plasminogen, or deficiency of heparin cofactor II may be warranted.

In evaluating abnormal laboratory tests, it is important to consider the clinical setting. Thus, patients with underlying liver disease will have decreased levels of proteins C and S and antithrombin because these factors are synthesized by the liver. In persons with the nephrotic syndrome, protein C and antithrombin may be lost in the urine, and the plasma levels of these proteins are decreased. Patients who are pregnant or taking oral contraceptives usually have protein S levels below the normal range. Finally, intravascular clotting per se, manifested as pulmonary emboli, deep vein thrombosis, or disseminated intravascular coagulation (DIC), may be accompanied by a decrease in all of the anticoagulant proteins due to consumption of these factors. For example, a low value for protein S recorded in a patient with a pulmonary embolus should not be interpreted as evidence of inherited protein S deficiency. In most patients, repeating the test during convalescence will reveal normal values.

Other factors that may affect laboratory tests are the use of anticoagulants and the nutritional status of the patient. Heparin therapy alters most clotting tests, including antithrombin levels (usually slightly below the normal range), and assays for lupus anticoagulant. Warfarin decreases the levels of proteins C and S. The nutritional status of the patient is important because lack of vitamin K will not only prolong the prothrombin time but also decrease proteins C and S. Low levels of vitamin K occur in patients who have poor food intake, have been vomiting, or are receiving antibiotics.

MANAGEMENT OF ANTICOAGULATION IN THE PERIOPERATIVE PERIOD

Patients with the just-described disorders may be on long-term anticoagulant therapy. Should operative procedures become necessary, the anticoagulant regimen must be modified. In patients receiving warfarin, an INR of 1.5 or less indicates that surgery can be safely performed.[54] Stopping the warfarin 4–5 days before operation will permit the INR to decline to this level. The warfarin may then be resumed the evening of operation, with the anticipation that the INR will be in the therapeutic range (2–3) in approximately 3 days. Therefore, for about 6 days (3 days before and 3 days after surgery) the INR will be less than optimal, but it will be below 1.5 for probably less than 2 days. Thus, the actual risk period for recurrence of thrombosis is brief, but the degree of risk depends on a variety of factors, including whether thrombi have been in the arteries or veins, how recently they have occurred, and whether atrial fibrillation or a mechanical heart valve is present.

Kearon and Hirsh[54] recommend that patients with a history of recent venous thrombosis (within the previous 2 to 3 months) receive intravenous heparin postoperatively; for those with thrombosis before the previous 2 to 3 months, the usual postoperative prophylaxis with subcutaneous heparin is advised. Postoperative subcutaneous heparin is also given to patients with atrial fibrillation or mechanical heart valves. If at all possible, surgery should be avoided within the first month after an acute arterial or venous thrombosis. However, if an operation must be performed, intravenous heparin should be started when the warfarin is stopped, discontinued 6 hours preoperatively, and resumed 12 hours postoperatively as a continuous infusion without a bolus, provided that there is no bleeding. When a patient requires emergency surgery within 2 weeks of having a thrombotic event, a vena caval filter is placed. In addition, intravenous heparin is given preoperatively and resumed 12 hours postoperatively unless the patient has an unusual bleeding risk.

References

1. Saito H: Normal hemostatic mechanisms. In Ratnoff OD, Forbes CD (eds): Disorders of Hemostasis, 3rd ed. Philadelphia, WB Saunders, 1996, pp 23–52.
2. Demers C, Ginsberg JS, Hirsh J, et al: Thrombosis in antithrombin III deficient persons. Report of a large kindred and literature review. Ann Intern Med 1992; 116:754–761.
3. Thaler E, Lechner K: Antithrombin III deficiency and thromboembolism. In Prentice CRM (ed): Clinics in Hematology, Vol 10. London, WB Saunders, 1981, p 369.
4. Schulman S, Tengborn L: Treatment of venous thromboembolism in patients with congenital deficiency of antithrombin III. Thromb Haemost 1992; 68:634–636.
5. Teepe RG, Broekmans AW, Wermeer BJ, et al: Recurrent coumarin-induced skin necrosis in a patient with an acquired functional protein C deficiency. Arch Dermatol 1986; 122:1408–1412.
6. Green D, Otoya J, Oriba H, Rovner R: Protein S deficiency in middle-aged women with stroke. Neurology 1992; 42:1029–1033.
7. Dahlback B, Carlsson M, Svensson PJ: Familial thrombophilia due to a previously unrecognized mechanism characterized by poor anticoagulant response to activated protein C. Prediction of a cofactor to activated protein C. Proc Natl Acad Sci USA 1993; 90:1004–1008.
8. Zoller B, Dahlback B: Linkage between inherited resistance to activated protein C and factor V gene mutation in venous thrombosis. Lancet 1994; 343:1536–1538.
9. Rosendaal FR, Koster T, Vanderbroucke IP, Reitsma PH: High risk of thrombosis in patients homozygous for factor V Leiden (activated protein C resistance). Blood 1995; 85:1504–1508.
10. Ridker PM, Hennekens CH, Lindpainter K, et al: Mutation in the gene coding for coagulation factor V and the risk of myocardial infarction, stroke and venous thrombosis in apparently healthy men. N Engl J Med 1995; 332:912–917.
11. Ganesan V, Kelsey H, Cookson J, et al: Activated protein C resistance in childhood stroke. Lancet 1996; 347:260.
12. van der Bom JG, Bots ML, Haverkate F, et al: Reduced response to activated protein C is associated with increased risk for cerebrovascular disease. Ann Intern Med 1996; 125:265–269.
13. Simoni P, Prandoni P, Lensing AWA, et al: The risk of recurrent venous thromboembolism in patients with an Arg506 to Gln mutation in the gene for factor V (factor V Leiden). N Engl J Med 1997; 336:399–403.
14. Poort SR, Rosendaal FR, Reitsma PH, Bertina RM: A common genetic variation in the 3'-untranslated region of the prothrombin gene is associated with elevated plasma prothrombin levels and an increase in venous thrombosis. Blood 1996; 88:3698–3703.
15. van der Meer FJM, Koster T, Vandenbroucke JP, et al: The Leiden Thrombophilia Study. Thromb Haemost 1997; 78:631–635.
16. Rozen R: Genetic predisposition to hyperhomocysteinemia: Deficiency of methylenetetrahydrofolate reductase. Thromb Haemost 1997; 78:523–526.
17. Rodgers GM, Conn MT: Homocysteine, an atherogenic stimulus, reduces protein C activation by arterial and venous endothelial cells. Blood 1990; 75:895–901.
18. Harpel PC, Chang VT, Borth W: Homocysteine and other sulfhydryl compounds enhance the binding of lipoprotein (a) to fibrin: A potential biochemical link between thrombosis, atherogenesis, and sulfhydryl compound metabolism. Proc Natl Acad Sci 1992; 89:10193–10197.
19. den Heijer M, Koster T, Blom HJ, et al: Hyperhomocysteinemia as a risk factor for deep-vein thrombosis. N Engl J Med 1996; 334:759–762.
20. Perry IJ, Refsum H, Morris RW, et al: Prospective study of serum total homocysteine concentrations and risk of stroke in middle-aged British men. Lancet 1995; 346:1395–1398.
21. Clarke R, Daly L, Robinson K, et al: Hyperhomocysteinemia: An independent risk factor for vascular disease. N Engl J Med 1991; 324:1149–1155.
22. Malinow MR, Kang SS, Taylor LM, et al: Prevalence of hyperhomocyst(e)inemia in patients with peripheral arterial occlusive disease. Circulation 1989; 79:1180–1188.
23. Franken DG, Boers GHJ, Blom HJ, et al: Treatment of mild hyperhomocysteinemia in vascular disease patients. Arterioscler Thromb 1994; 14:465–470.
24. Stampfer MJ, Malinow MR: Can lowering homocysteine levels reduce cardiovascular risk? N Engl J Med 1995; 332:328–329.
25. Carter CJ, Anderson FA, Wheeler AB: Epidemiology and pathophysiology of venous thromboembolism. In Hull RD, Raskob GE, Pineo GF (eds): Venous Thromboembolism: An Evidence-Based Atlas. Armonk, NY, Futura Publishing, 1996, p 8.

26. Donati MB: Cancer and thrombosis: From phlegmasia alba dolens to transgenic mice. Thromb Haemost 1995; 74:278–281.
27. Scanu AM, Lawn RM, Berg K: Lipoprotein (a) and atherosclerosis. Ann Intern Med 1991; 115:209–218.
28. Triplett DA: Antiphospholipid antibody syndrome. In Seghatchian MJ, Samana MM, Hecker SP (eds): Hypercoagulable States. Boca Raton, FL, CRC Press, 1996, pp 223–232.
29. Arnout J: The pathogenesis of the antiphospholipid syndrome: A hypothesis based on parallelisms with heparin-induced thrombocytopenia. Thromb Haemost 1996; 75:536–541.
30. Marciniak E, Romond EH: Impaired catalytic function of activated protein C: A new in vitro manifestation of lupus anticoagulant. Blood 1989; 74:2426–2432.
31. Potzsch B, Kawamura H, Preissner KT, et al: Acquired protein C dysfunction but not decreased activity of thrombomodulin is a possible marker of thrombophilia in patients with lupus anticoagulant. J Lab Clin Med 1995; 125:56–65.
32. Carreras LO, Defreyn G, Machin SJ, et al: Arterial thrombosis, intrauterine death, and "lupus" anticoagulant; detection of immunoglobulin interfering with prostacyclin formation. Lancet 1981; i:244–246.
33. Chediak J: Lupus anticoagulants. In Green D (ed): Anticoagulants: Physiologic, Pathologic, and Pharmacologic. Boca Raton, FL, CRC Press, 1994, pp 143–156.
34. Ginsburg JS, Wells PS, Brill-Edwards P, et al: Antiphospholipid antibodies and venous thromboembolism. Blood 1995; 86:3685–3691.
35. Asherson RA, Khamashta MA, Gill A, et al: Cerebrovascular disease and antiphospholipid antibodies in systemic lupus erythematosus, lupus-like disease, and the primary antiphospholipid syndrome. Am J Med 1989; 86:391–412.
36. Triplett DA, Brandt JT, Kaczor D, et al: Laboratory diagnosis of lupus inhibitors: A comparison of the tissue thromboplastin inhibition procedure with a new platelet neutralization procedure. Am J Clin Pathol 1983; 79:678–682.
37. Thiagarajan P, Pengo V, Shapiro SS: The use of the dilute Russell viper venom time for the diagnosis of lupus anticoagulants. Blood 1986; 68:869–874.
38. Love PE, Santoro SA: Antiphospholipid antibodies: Anticardiolipin and lupus anticoagulant in systemic lupus erythematosus (SLE) and in non-SLE disorders. Ann Intern Med 1990; 112:682–698.
39. Ginsburg JS, Liang MH, Newcomer L, et al: Anticardiolipin antibodies and the risk for ischemic stroke and venous thrombosis. Ann Intern Med 1992; 117:997–1002.
40. Ginsberg JS, Wells PS, Brill-Edwards P, et al: Antiphospholipid antibodies and venous thromboembolism. Blood 1995; 86:3685–3691.
41. Stahl CP, Wideman CS, Spira TJ, et al: Protein S deficiency in men with long-term human immunodeficiency virus infection. Blood 1993; 81:1801–1807.
42. Khamashta MA, Cuadrado MJ, Mujic F, et al: The management of thrombosis in the antiphospholipid antibody syndrome. N Engl J Med 1995; 332:993–997.
43. Lubbe WF, Butler WS, Palmer SJ, Liggins GC: Fetal survival after prednisone suppression of maternal lupus-anticoagulant. Lancet 1983; i:1361–1363.
44. Boumpas DT, Fessler BJ, Austin HA, et al: Systemic lupus erythematosus: Emerging concepts. Ann Intern Med 1995; 123:42–53.
45. Danilenko-Dixon DR, van Winter JT, Homburger HA: Clinical implications of antiphospholipid antibodies in obstetrics. Mayo Clin Proc 1996; 71:1118–1120.
46. Selhub J, D'Angelo A: Hyperhomocysteinemia and thrombosis: Acquired conditions. Thromb Haemost 1997; 78:527–531.
47. Warkentin TE, Kelton JG: A 14-year study of heparin-induced thrombocytopenia. Am J Med 1996; 101:502–507.
48. Warkentin TE, Hayward CPM, Boshkow LK, et al: Sera from patients with heparin-induced thrombocytopenia generate platelet-derived microparticles with procoagulant activity: An explanation for the thrombotic complications of heparin-induced thrombocytopenia. Blood 1994; 84:3691–3699.
49. Warkentin TE, Levine MN, Hirsh J, et al: Heparin-induced thrombocytopenia in patients treated with low-molecular weight heparin or unfractionated heparin. N Engl J Med 1995; 332:1330–1335.
50. Greinacher A, Michels I, Mueller-Eckardt C: Heparin-associated thrombocytopenia: The antibody is not heparin specific. Thromb Haemost 1992; 67:545–549.
51. Refludan prescribing information.
52. British Society of Hematology, quoted by Alving BM: The hypercoagulable states. Hosp Practice 1993; 28:109–114, 119–121.
53. Lane DA, Mannucci PM, Bauer KA, et al: Inherited thrombophilia: Part 2. Thromb Haemost 1996; 76:824–834.
54. Kearon C, Hirsh J: Management of anticoagulation before and after elective surgery. N Engl J Med 1997; 336:1506–1511.

PART THREE

ARTERIAL DISEASES

10

Vascular Medicine and Vascular Rehabilitation

Mitzi A. Ekers, RN, MS, ARNP, and Alan T. Hirsch, MD

⥲ · ⥲

Peripheral arterial disease (PAD) is a prevalent, chronic atherosclerotic disease that limits the functional capacity of affected individuals, adversely affects their quality of life, and is associated with a 3- to 10-fold increased risk of myocardial ischemic events or death.[1–3] Progression of PAD to its most severe stages, in which refractory claudication, ischemic rest pain, or nonhealing wounds mandate surgical or percutaneous revascularization, is relatively rare, occurring in less than 5–8 percent of those with PAD.[4] When required, vascular surgical or percutaneous revascularization techniques can serve as effective interventions to alleviate disabling limb ischemic symptoms and may be essential to avoid the morbidity of amputation. However, the long-term benefits of successful limb revascularization may be limited if these interventions serve as the sole core of vascular care for this population. Successful palliative surgical interventions may actually contribute to the development of short-term, iatrogenic deconditioning from the bed rest required in the postoperative state. In the long term, limb revascularization does nothing to modify the underlying atherosclerotic disease process and might rarely provoke coronary ischemic symptoms in the postoperative state. *The successful long-term treatment of atherosclerotic PAD requires the creation of a medical management program that may delay PAD progression and prolong life.* The consistent, lifelong application of such medical therapeutic programs can be augmented by the development of a partnership between the patient with PAD, his or her family, and a devoted vascular health care team. Vascular rehabilitation can serve as an ideal environment for the creation of this partnership.

Although creation of such a vascular care partnership may be desirable, it is important for this generation of vascular clinicians to recognize the existence of potent barriers to the delivery of effective medical interventions for PAD. First, many primary care and vascular clinicians alike continue to believe that "conservative care" is an adequate care strategy for those who suffer from PAD. In the last decade, it has become clear that all individuals with PAD, whether symptomatic or asymptomatic, suffer high rates of stroke, myocardial infarction, and death. These outcomes can all be decreased by medical therapies but are generally left "unmanaged" by "conservative care." If global vascular health is our goal, then it is no longer acceptable for vascular clinicians to be unfamiliar with

TABLE 10–1. **The Effects of Selected Medical Interventions on PAD Outcomes**

INTERVENTION	IMPROVE CLAUDICATION SYMPTOMS	DECREASE CHD AND STROKE EVENT RATES	DECREASE MORTALITY
Tobacco cessation strategies	Minimal improvement	Yes	Yes
Antiplatelet therapies	Trend toward benefit	20–30%	Yes*
Lipid-lowering therapies	Unknown	Probable (as assessed in CAD)	Probable (as assessed in CAD)
Antihypertensive therapies	Unknown	20–35%	Yes

*The effect of aspirin, ticlopidine, and clopidogrel on mortality has not yet been directly compared to placebo in a single clinical trial powered to detect such an effect. However, the data for each of these drugs on event-free survival strongly suggest that each agent is likely to be effective in achieving this critical end-point.
PAD = peripheral artery disease; CHD = coronary heart disease; CAD = coronary artery disease.
Modified from Hirsch AT, Treat-Jacobson D, Lando HA, Hatsukam DK: The role of tobacco cessation, antiplatelet and lipid-lowering therapies in the treatment of peripheral arterial disease. Vasc Med 1997; 2:243–251.

those medical therapies that are effective in blunting the adverse ischemic events that frequently occur in PAD patients.

A second obstacle to the creation of a long-term medical intervention is the achievement of adequate patient compliance. The success of all medical therapies (e.g., smoking cessation, antiplatelet, lipid-lowering, antihypertensive, and diabetic therapies) requires a trusting, long-term therapeutic relationship. This relationship may encompass the physician, vascular nurse, rehabilitation staff, and many other vascular care professionals. Long-term compliance with medical interventions often requires patients to initiate selected, but potentially major, behavioral and lifestyle modifications that may affect their vocation, relationships, and life goals. Patients with PAD are often among the most motivated to undertake such efforts, as long as they can rely on their vascular clinicians to provide guidance, rationale for change, and specific tools for success. This chapter describes components of a comprehensive pharmacologic and behavioral approach to the treatment of PAD that can be utilized by all members of the vascular care team (Table 10–1). PAD is a chronic disease. Medical therapeutic interventions and vascular rehabilitation can serve together as the fulcrum of vascular health for most individuals with PAD.

A COMPREHENSIVE VASCULAR MEDICAL THERAPEUTIC APPROACH

Smoking and Peripheral Arterial Disease

Tobacco use in all forms is known to damage the vascular endothelium, promote intravascular coagulation, and accelerate the rate of progression of atherosclerosis. Tobacco use is the single most important cause of PAD. As delineated in Table 10–2, smoking is known to: (1) be the strongest risk factor for the development of de novo PAD, (2) foster progression of PAD from stable claudication to rest pain, (3) promote the failure of all surgical and percutaneous revascularization procedures, (4) increase rates of amputation, and (5) profoundly decrease patient survival.[5–8] The members of the vascular care team are, however, ideally positioned to provide therapeutic efforts to improve rates of long-term tobacco abstinence in patients with PAD. Central to the patients' long-term success

TABLE 10–2. **The Effects of Tobacco on PAD Disease Progression**

- Progression from asymptomatic PAD to stable claudication
- Conversion of stable claudication to rest pain—*such progression inevitably requires revascularization*
- Increased failure rate of limb bypass grafts and limb angioplasty
- Increased amputation rate
- Accelerated rates of cardiovascular ischemic events—*fatal and nonfatal MI, stroke*
- Decreased survival

PAD = peripheral arterial disease; MI = myocardial infarction.
Modified from Hirsch AT, Treat-Jacobsen D, Lando HA, Hatsukam DK: The role of tobacco cessation, anti-platelet and lipid-lowering therapies in the treatment of peripheral arterial disease. Vasc Med 1997; 2:243–251.

in quitting smoking is their access to a health care professional who can provide the educational links between tobacco use and their disease. Each day's use of tobacco can appropriately be linked, as a negative reinforcer, to the manifestations of PAD that cause pain or disability or mandate vascular surgery or amputation. Tobacco use in individuals with established PAD may so quickly shorten life as to prevent the completion of crucial life goals (e.g., watching children grow, enjoyment of retirement, or mere maintenance of a meaningfully independent, ambulatory lifestyle). Specific reasons to quit must be provided to the patient.

The attitudes of health care professionals have been demonstrated to be central to the success of those individuals who might quit smoking. It is important that all those who intend to aid the patient to quit smoking consider the principles outlined in Table 10–3. There is a prevalent myth that individuals with PAD may be particularly reluctant to quit smoking, although there are no data to support this supposition. Furthermore, the presumption of failure begets continued failure. In contrast, current data confirm that a high percentage of PAD patients successfully quit smoking. For example, approximately only 20–40 percent of elderly individuals with stable claudication are current smokers, although most of this patient group had smoked previously.[8, 9] Patients who present for surgical or percutaneous revascularization due to severe limb symptoms (e.g., severe claudication, ischemic rest pain, or gangrene) do represent a self-selected PAD population characterized by a high (80–90 percent) rate of current smoking. This is not surprising inasmuch as continued tobacco use is known to accelerate the atherosclerotic and pro-thrombotic processes that convert stable PAD to limb-threatening ischemia. Health care providers who are devoted to decreasing the suffering and societal costs of PAD can aid

TABLE 10–3. **Attitudes to Consider in Facilitating Successful Smoking Cessation**

- Do not blame the smoker. Recognize the patient as the victim of an addictive drug.
- Clarify the many specific links between the disease and smoking.
- Involve the whole family and children.
- Set realistic expectations for the patient and yourself.
- Be a partner: Help create an individualized smoking cessation plan.
- Invoke action: The patient must set a quit date.
- Utilize both behavioral and pharmacologic adjunctive measures.
- Maintain a reassessment schedule and utilize follow-up appointments.
- Approve and praise each passing success.
- Patients with PAD can successfully quit smoking.

PAD = peripheral arterial disease.

those individuals with mild-to-moderate (even asymptomatic) PAD to quit smoking in order to blunt their disease progression to more serious disability or critical limb ischemia.[10, 11]

Smoking cessation in patients with PAD has been proven to prolong life. The five-year mortality rate for patients with claudication who continue to smoke is approximately 40–50 percent. This high mortality of individuals with PAD is predominantly due to myocardial infarction because PAD is a marker of significant concomitant coronary artery disease. Successful abstinence from smoking in this population is associated with markedly decreased rates of myocardial infarction and stroke, resulting in an impressive improvement in survival.[6, 7] This accelerated mortality in PAD patients who smoke suggests that therapeutic interventions must be invoked immediately because delay by the patient ("I'm not ready to quit this year") or the health care system ("We hope to offer a smoking cessation program next year") may permit death to supervene before the first effective quit attempt is initiated.

Acknowledging the benefits of quitting smoking provides a first step toward success, but it remains challenging for patient and clinician alike to foster abstinence from tobacco use because tobacco products are unquestionably addictive substances. Smokers who attempt to quit without medical intervention generally encounter an abysmal 7–10 percent 1-year success rate, demonstrating the addictive potential of tobacco products, and providing a realistic baseline from which to judge the efficacy of programmatic efforts to help the patient quit smoking. Ideal tobacco intervention programs combine both behavioral and pharmacotherapeutic approaches. Long-term success rates from behavioral treatment alone are low. Only about 15–30 percent of smokers remain abstinent 1 year after treatment.[12, 13] More important, the vast majority of smokers with PAD are either not offered the opportunity or do not currently take the time to enroll in effective individual or group behavioral therapy. Special efforts to elicit the participation of smoking PAD patients into counseling interventions have rarely been attempted, and such behavioral interventions applied in isolation have not been proven to be very successful.[14]

Pharmacologic treatment of tobacco addiction has historically relied on nicotine replacement strategies. Nicotine replacement therapy is designed to relieve withdrawal symptoms by providing a substitute for the desired effects of nicotine while attenuating the reinforcing effects of continued nicotine self-administration.[15] Use of the nicotine patch in the general population of smokers has elicited smoking cessation success rates of 23–27 percent at 6–12 months, which is superior to rates achieved with use of placebo.[13] Nicotine patch therapy in patients with medical illnesses, such as smokers with cardiovascular disease, has been proven to be safe, and does not increase angina, palpitations, or heart attacks.[16] Patients and families also need to be informed that nicotine replacement therapies do *not* accelerate any adverse limb events (e.g., worsened limb ischemia) in patients with PAD. This is not surprising because nicotine replacement therapies do not cause comparable elevations in plasma nicotine levels to those that occur with smoking. Thus, nicotine replacement therapies are useful and safe. Although nicotine replacement is helpful, clinical experience suggests that additional adjunctive measures should be required to achieve tobacco abstinence in the PAD population.

Recent clinical trials have also demonstrated the efficacy of antidepressant therapy as an adjunct for smoking cessation. The use of these agents is based on the observation that nicotine may act as an antidepressant in some smokers.[17] Additionally, the development of a depressed affect or depression during smoking cessation may lead to a relapse.[18, 19] In this context, bupropion has now been shown to be an effective pharmacologic adjunct to improve rates of smoking cessation. Hurt and associates have demonstrated that bupropion promoted a 44.2 percent tobacco abstinence rate at 7 weeks and a 23.1 percent abstinence rate at one year in smokers in a well-designed, placebo-controlled trial.[20] Bupropion (Zyban) is also safe, although it should not be used in patients with a history of seizures, in those who actively abuse alcohol, or in whom bupropion would be contraindicated owing to the use of other psychotropic medications.

All vascular clinicians should inform their patients with PAD that tobacco is the single most important factor that has caused their disease and its associated claudication, rest pain, ischemic ulcers, a higher risk of amputation, and heart attack, stroke, or death. It is never too late to quit smoking. The entire family, spouses and children, should be encouraged to participate in the smoking cessation intervention. Patients with PAD are not intrinsically self-destructive tobacco users; in contrast, they are victims of a destructive, addictive drug (nicotine) as well as of PAD itself. We should seek to amplify the intrinsic motivation to quit tobacco use that accompanies the pain of claudication, rest pain and wounds, or revascularization procedures. The potential clinical implications of effective smoking cessation interventions in this cohort of patients are decreased cardiovascular event rates, blunted amputation rates, improved survival, and decreased health care costs.

Antiplatelet and Antithrombotic Strategies

PAD is but one overt manifestation of systemic atherosclerosis. Atherosclerosis is a disease that is characterized by disruption of the normal arterial architecture, by endothelial dysfunction, and by a propensity for thrombosis. Platelet aggregation plays a central role in the progression of peripheral atherosclerosis as hemodynamically stable disease progresses to thrombotic occlusion. Such progression can be clinically recognized in patients with PAD when stable claudication worsens suddenly, or when thromboembolism causes acute arterial occlusion, or when a nonhealing wound forms on a poorly perfused foot due to the formation of thrombus in the subdermal microcirculation. PAD progression can also be marked by the occurrence of thrombotic events in *other* circulations, as the patient with PAD suffers an adverse coronary or cerebrovascular ischemic event. The occurrence of such thrombotic events in any circulation heralds a marked deterioration in the quality of life of the patient with PAD. Thrombosis is the mechanism by which PAD can be interpreted as a lethal disease.

The natural history of PAD can thus be improved by antiplatelet therapies, which can potentially decrease the rate of progression of limb symptoms and blunt cardiovascular event rates. The potential beneficial effects of aspirin and an aspirin/dipyridamole combination on rates of femoral arterial atherosclerosis progression were reported by Hess and colleagues in a small cohort of patients followed over 2 years.[21] Over this short period of observation, femoral atherosclerosis progression was diminished by antiplatelet therapies. The effects of long-term administration of aspirin on the natural history of atherosclerotic arterial disease have also been reported from the Physicians Health Study.[22] This randomized, double-blind, placebo-controlled trial evaluated the effects of low-dose aspirin (325 mg every other day) in 22,071 male physicians over an average of 60 months of treatment. Those individuals who used aspirin required only half as many surgical limb revascularization procedures as in those in the placebo cohort. Aspirin use did not alter the incidence of claudication in the two treatment groups. These data suggest that aspirin decreased the frequency of those thrombotic events that convert stable claudication to critical limb ischemia, although the antiplatelet therapy most likely did *not* alter the primary atherosclerotic disease process. This is a remarkable result for a very inexpensive and safe pharmacologic intervention.

Although the benefits of aspirin use in the prevention of myocardial infarction and stroke are clearly defined—preventing as many as 20–30 percent of these ischemic events—many patients with atherosclerotic diseases still suffer such adverse outcomes. As well, there are individuals in whom aspirin use is not well tolerated, due to gastrointestinal irritation or rarely allergy. This has provided an impetus to evaluate potentially more potent or safer antiplatelet therapies. Ticlopidine has been evaluated extensively in patients with peripheral arterial occlusive disease and been shown to blunt ischemic event rates, to perhaps improve claudication symptoms, and to improve patient survival, as documented in the Swedish Ticlopidine Multicentre Study (STIMS) and smaller trials.[23-25] Picotamide, an investigational drug that is known to inhibit platelet thromboxane A2 (TxA2) synthase and to antagonize TxA2 receptors, has also been shown to reduce cardiovascular ischemic events and to improve symptoms in patients with PAD.[26] A randomized, prospective clinical investigation of 2304 patients treated with picotamide or placebo for 18 months has demonstrated that event-free survival was improved in those individuals who were assigned to picotamide therapy. Preliminary evidence has also suggested a beneficial effect of this antiplatelet drug on pain-free walking in patients with claudication.[27]

The relative benefits of aspirin and clopidogrel (a newer ticlopidine-like antiplatelet drug) on rates of myocardial infarction, stroke, and death have recently been reported from the prospective international Clopidogrel vs. Aspirin in Patients at Risk of Ischemic Events (CAPRIE) investigation.[28] CAPRIE recruited individuals with various manifestations of arterial atherosclerosis by including patients who had suffered a recent myocardial infarction, ischemic stroke, or who suffered from established PAD. The hypothesis of CAPRIE was that individuals who present with stroke, myocardial infarction, or PAD all suffer comparably high rates of subsequent heart attack, stroke, and vascular death. The CAPRIE investigators recruited 19,185 patients from these three eligible cohorts. The inclusion of 6452 individuals with PAD in the CAPRIE study marks this investigation as the largest prospective trial ever performed to evaluate any medical therapy for PAD. In CAPRIE, PAD was defined as either (1) self-reported claudication with an ankle-brachial index (ABI) less than 0.85, or (2) a history of prior lower-extremity arterial revascularization procedures (either angioplasty or vascular surgery) or amputation. Clopidogrel treatment was more effective than standard aspirin, eliciting an overall relative risk reduction of 8.7 percent in preventing subsequent ischemic stroke, myocardial infarction, or vascular death in the total study population in this well-controlled trial. Post hoc analysis demonstrated that patients with PAD, in particular, benefited from clopidogrel therapy inasmuch as this new antiplatelet agent effected a 23.8 percent risk reduction for these morbid events compared with aspirin treatment alone. The CAPRIE results suggest that PAD patients may constitute a population of individuals in which the atherosclerotic process can be effectively modulated by antiplatelet therapies.

Current clinical data therefore suggest that *all* patients with documented limb arterial occlusive disease should receive antiplatelet therapy unless otherwise contraindicated. These benefits of antiplatelet therapies for PAD have achieved broad acceptance by vascular clinicians. Nevertheless, as for many available and effective therapies, antiplatelet therapies remain underutilized in the "at risk" PAD population, inasmuch as many PAD patients remain untreated. In the Minnesota Regional Peripheral Arterial Disease Screening Study, as many as 40 percent of patients with PAD were receiving no antiplatelet therapies.[9] Thus, the potential benefits of antiplatelet therapies with aspirin, ticlopidine, and clopidogrel in preventing heart attack, stroke, and death in those with PAD will undoubtedly depend not only on the availability of these drugs at low cost but also on the commitment of both nurses and physicians to promote their long-term use by their patients with PAD.

Lipid-Lowering Strategies

Atherosclerosis is a complex, polygenic disorder that is modulated by serum lipids, in concert with a multitude of other factors that may damage the fragile endothelial lining of both large and medium-sized arteries and arterioles. The penetration of lipoproteins across the endothelium permits the initial development of a fatty streak, especially at sites of altered shear stress, such as at arterial bifurcations. Oxidation of these lipoproteins within the arterial wall may serve as a central mechanism that promotes the subsequent release of chemoattractant proteins, causing monocytes to bind to the arterial wall, to undergo conversion to macrophages, and to continue the oxidation of low-density lipoproteins (LDL). The early atherosclerotic plaque continues to accumulate cholesterol and macrophages, and to initiate a true inflammatory process that further promotes smooth muscle cell proliferation and inhibits endothelial healing of plaque ulcerations. Such complex atheromatous arterial lesions, regardless of the severity of the associated arterial stenosis, serve as the substrate upon which subsequent plaque fissuring can suddenly begin to attract platelets and initiate an aggressive thrombotic event.

Plasma lipids are transported in the blood attached to lipoproteins, which serve crucial functions in modulating the efficient transfer of cholesterol and triglycerides from the gut, to the liver, and to peripheral tissues. Lipoproteins include easily measured components, such as LDL, high-density lipoproteins (HDL), and very low-density lipoproteins (VLDL), as well as a number of other intermediate particles. Elevated plasma levels of LDL and VLDL are associated with an increased risk of atheroma development and of ischemic events. In contrast, high HDL levels subserve a protective role in transporting cholesterol from peripheral cells to the liver for processing and biliary excretion. Epidemiologic data confirm that elevations in LDL cholesterol are associated with an increased risk of cardiovascular disease, both in the general population as well as in individuals with PAD.[29] Patients with PAD may also demonstrate a pattern of lipid abnormalities that includes a low HDL–high triglyceride profile, which also confers cardiovascular risk.[30]

Effective lipid management should also be considered a mandatory component of the medical therapy of patients with objective evidence of lower-extremity arterial occlusive disease. This strategy has been sanctioned by the recent National Cholesterol Education Panel (NCEP) guidelines, which recommend that patients with objective evidence of atherosclerotic vascular disease be treated by diet and pharmacologic therapy to achieve an LDL cholesterol level of less than 100 mg/dl.[31] Such efforts should achieve a decreased rate of cardiovascular ischemic events in this fragile population. For individuals with PAD, these guidelines apply whether the patient is symptomatic or asymptomatic. The implication is that any objective evidence of PAD, such as the ankle-brachial index (ABI), defines a population at risk of coronary ischemic events. This is logical inasmuch as some individuals with moderately severe PAD may not present with classic claudication symptoms. For example, some elderly individuals who at one time were limited by claudication may so limit their activities of daily living that claudication is no longer induced. Other individuals with PAD may have concomitant illnesses (e.g., degenerative joint disease, and neuropathy) that can also limit functional status to levels below those required to unmask claudication. Finally, patients in whom limb revascularization strategies have been completely successful may have their claudication relieved while remaining at risk of the coronary and cerebrovascular events that occur in patients with a systemic atherosclerotic disease.

Lipid-lowering strategies have been demonstrated to have beneficial, though small, effects on the progression of femoral atherosclerotic arterial disease. The Cholesterol Lowering Atherosclerosis Study (CLAS) of Blankenhorn and colleagues assessed the rates of both coronary and femoral atherosclerosis disease progression in a cohort of 162 middle-aged, nonsmoking men in a double-blind, placebo-controlled study of dietary vs. aggressive lipid-lowering drug treatment.[32] Patients were either treated by combined dietary modification and colestipol and niacin therapy or by dietary management alone over a relatively brief 2-year study period. These data demonstrated that the rate of femoral arterial atherosclerosis progression, as assessed angiographically, was blunted and femoral arterial disease regression was greater in those subjects who achieved optimal effective lipid lowering. These relatively short-term angiographic observations have been extended in the Program on the Surgical Control of the Hyperlipidemias (POSCH) study.[33] In these patients, lipid lowering achieved by ileal bypass surgery extended the benefits of treatment throughout 10 years of follow-up. As in the CLAS trial, the rate of femoral arterial atherosclerosis disease progression was diminished; more impressively, the rate of development of symptomatic claudication was also reduced by 27 percent. During the past few years, data from coronary intervention trials suggest that life prolongation for individuals with PAD is likely if diet and drug intervention achieve an LDL cholesterol of 100 mg/dl or lower (the Scandinavian Simvastatin Survival Study [4S], West of Scotland, PLAC I and II, and CARE trials).[34, 35] Such lipid intervention trials have not yet been prospectively performed in cohorts of individuals with PAD. Unfortunately, despite the potential benefit of such intervention (and perhaps because of the absence of these prospective trials), data also suggest that less than 8–15 percent of individuals with PAD in the United States in 1996 were receiving lipid-lowering drug therapies.[9, 36]

Hypertension, Diabetes, and Estrogen Replacement Therapies

The progression of atherosclerosis is accelerated by the synergistic adverse effects of hypertension and diabetes. For women, epidemiologic data suggest that the manifestations of atherosclerosis are delayed by approximately a decade but accelerate in the postmenopausal state. Individuals with hypertension face approximately a twofold increased risk of developing claudication, and the risk of stroke, heart attack, and death from hypertension is magnified in individuals with PAD.[37] It is particularly important for all clinicians to be aware of the increased risk posed by isolated systolic hypertension, as well as diastolic hypertension. Treatment of elevated blood pressure, whether by lifestyle or pharmacologic means, should normalize both values in all hypertensive individuals.[38] Successful long-term treatment of high blood pressure should include the discussion of the goal blood pressure with the patient and an evaluation of the contribution of lifestyle factors (e.g., diet, weight, exercise, alcohol intake, stress) to high blood pressure, as well as education regarding the use of both lifestyle changes and medication. Although successful treatment of hypertension is known to reduce the risks of ischemic coronary and cerebrovascular events, the effect of treatment on the symptomatic progression of PAD has not yet been evaluated.

All vascular clinicians recognize the increased risk of atherosclerosis in the coronary, cerebrovascular, and limb circulations in individuals with diabetes. Diabetes is associated with more premature and rapid progression of PAD and involvement of more distal limb arterial sites. The neuropathy of diabetes increases the risk of development of foot ulcers and can either mask or mimic ischemic rest pain. The diagnostic sensitivity of the office-based ABI measurement can be decreased by the medial arterial calcification that can artifactually raise the ankle systolic blood pressure due to the noncompressibility of these arteries. Optimal achievement of tight glucose control in diabetics is associated with an improved natural history of microvascular disease (e.g., retinopathy and microalbuminuria). However, the effects of diabetic management on large-vessel arterial occlusive disease in this population have not yet been evaluated in a controlled, prospective clinical trial. The potential beneficial impact of ideal glucose management in the diabetic population should, nevertheless, not be discounted. Optimal diabetic management is presumed to improve the rate of lower-extremity disease progression, incidence of myocardial ischemic events, and incidence of wound infection, gangrene, and amputation. Estrogen replacement therapy in postmenopausal women with overt atherosclerosis is associated with a beneficial effect on cardiovascular ischemic event rates.[39, 40] Although the decision to initiate estrogens must always include an individualized discussion of the relative benefits and risks, postmenopausal women with PAD should be considered candidates by their vascular care clinician as well as their primary care physician.

The Crucial Role of Exercise in Management of Peripheral Arterial Disease

Symptomatic individuals with PAD, whether presenting with claudication, rest pain, or ischemic ulceration, have usually restricted their activities of daily living prior to their seeking medical help. The discomfort of intermittent or persistent limb pain contributes to a profound deconditioning that can be detected even in community-based (nonreferred) individuals with PAD.[9] Deconditioning may also be unavoidably induced iatrogenically by the postoperative bed rest required after successful surgical revascularization. Independent ambulation and freedom of mobility are the major end-organ functions of the lower extremities. This decreased mobility in patients with PAD represents a measurable factor that diminishes the quality of life of those with this disease.[41–44] Therefore, subjective patient-derived indices of improved ambulation, whether assessed by treadmill distances or questionnaire (vs. angiographic patency rates), serve as the optimal patient-focused treatment goal for individuals with claudication. In this light, exercise training and rehabilitation can serve as vitally important treatment modalities, and as a mainstay of treatment, for patients with claudication.

The efficacy of claudication exercise training has been established by numerous investigations over the past decade.[45–51] Essentially all studies of the efficacy of exercise training have demonstrated an improvement in both the pain-free walking time (the intermittent claudication distance or ICD) and the maximal walking time (the absolute claudication distance or ACD). Using a constant-load treadmill protocol, these investigations have demonstrated improvements that range from 50 to 300 percent. Similarly, exercise training may elicit improvements in maximal walking distance of 25 to 200 percent. The compliant patient in a supervised therapeutic program can reasonably expect to double the ICD and ACD. Although many clinicians continue to speculate that exercise training might improve performance in patients with claudication by augmentation of collateral blood flow, current data do not support this hypothesis. Alternative explanations remain plausible, such as exercise-induced decreases in blood viscosity, patients' learning to modify their walking techniques to involve more biomechanically efficient (and perhaps less ischemic) muscles, and alteration of the ischemic pain threshold. It has been speculated that abnormal skeletal muscle oxidative metabolism, with accumulation of acylcarnitines, denervation of muscle bundles (as documented by both electrophysiologic and histopathologic studies), and/or a selective loss of type II myofibers in ischemic limbs, could also underlie the disability of claudication and the mechanism of exercise-associated improvement.[52, 53] However, while the contribution of any (or of all) of these mechanisms in response to exercise training remains uncertain, clinical data unambiguously support the conclusion that impressive improvements in ambulation can be consistently gained for patients in such programs.

Many clinicians and patients may derive a sense of wonder that such functional improvements can be obtained from supervised exercise programs in the absence of a readily explicable and documented physiologic mechanism. Nevertheless, there are many effective medical interventions that yield beneficial results and that have achieved "market acceptance" with minimal question (e.g., physical therapy for low back and knee injuries in lieu of surgical approaches). Therefore, vascular clinicians might reserve greater wonder, perhaps, that the clinical database supporting a role for exercise rehabilitation has not yet led to the widespread promulgation of the technique. Dissemination of effective medical interventions has historically first required widespread education of clinicians, who can then create such programs, as well as acceptance of the intervention by health care payers. Integrated medical approaches to common vascular diseases always seek to utilize the most effective and the most cost-effective therapeutic interventions that can safely improve patient-focused outcomes. Rehabilitation techniques can serve this role for individuals with PAD.

VASCULAR REHABILITATION

Goals and Objectives

The ultimate goal of a vascular rehabilitation program (VRP) is to help patients gain control over their disease so that debilitating consequences may be avoided and improved physical function restored. This secondary prevention program uses a biopsychosocial approach to provide the crucial link between palliative and "curative" interventions to achieve this goal.

Improving functional capacity and controlling the progression of atherosclerosis demand major changes in behavior and lifestyle that patients often find difficult to make on their own. Through a structured VRP, the vascular clinician can empower patients to make these changes by focusing on two objectives: (1) to provide a sound knowledge base of vascular disease and its treatment and (2) to help patients discover their personal motivation to take action. Knowledge alone is not enough. Action provides the catalyst that results in the power to make effective change.[54] Whether in a center-based rehabilitation program or an office-based program, clinicians should devote considerable effort to helping patients develop and implement a personalized action plan that will work for them.

A Vascular Rehabilitation Model

Modeled after cardiac rehabilitation, most VRPs are offered in a formal rehabilitation center. However, primarily due to reimbursement constraints, very few of these programs have been established. In order to meet the needs of vascular patients who do not have access to a formal VRP, a home or office-based program could be developed through slight modification of the center-based model. Although not as effective as the center-based VRPs, these alternative programs are better than the expectation that patients will successfully modify their risks without any supervision or assistance.[55] In this home- or office-based program, a vascular nurse from the physician's office would perform the role and activities as described here for the rehabilitation staff nurse. Either program would consist of three phases of instruction (Table 10–4). Each phase is independent of the others and is designed to meet the needs of patients at different stages of their disease process.

Phase I

Patients hospitalized for a revascularization procedure may be particularly receptive to advice about vascular disease and how to avoid further invasive treatment. In Phase I of vascular rehabilitation, the rehabilitation nurse assists hospital staff nurses in initiating the educational process through one-on-one or group instruction. The objective of Phase I is not to teach patients everything they need to know about vascular disease but merely to increase their level of awareness of several key points.

First, patients need to be aware of what caused the disease that necessitated their

TABLE 10–4. **The Vascular Rehabilitation Model**

Phase I	Phase II	Phase III
• Inpatient education	• Outpatient physical reconditioning	• Maintenance program
• Introduction to Phase II	• In-depth patient education	• Minimal supervision
	• Home exercise program	

hospitalization. The disease process and the symptoms it causes, the risk factors, and the revascularization procedure performed to alleviate those symptoms are discussed. Excellent patient education booklets available from the Society for Vascular Nursing[56] will facilitate this part of the instruction.[57]

Second, patients need to become more acutely aware of their circulatory system. What improvements have they noticed since the surgery? Perhaps rest pain has been alleviated, or a walk down the entire length of the hallway no longer produces calf pain. On returning home, they need to constantly evaluate their improved walking ability. Any decrease in this level of functioning or a return of previous symptoms must be reported immediately. Instruction should be given on how to safely care for themselves at home during their recuperation. Precautions include careful inspection and meticulous care of feet and incisions.

Third, patients must understand that the procedure has not cured their vascular disease. They should accept the necessity of making significant lifestyle changes to control the disease and to enhance the long-term success of the revascularization. In many cases, patients know *what* they need to do but not *how* to do it. Providing a few initial actions such as a simple walking regimen, basic dietary instruction, and tips on smoking cessation reinforces the importance of immediately starting to make changes.

An active Phase I program provides an unprecedented opportunity for hospital staff nurses and rehabilitation staff to participate in secondary prevention teaching. It is at this stage when patients can be moved beyond merely contemplating behavior change to the action stage of "choosing a healthier lifestyle."[58] It is also an excellent method of identifying and initiating further discussions with potential candidates for Phase II of the VRP. While doing so, the rehabilitation nurse conveys an understanding of the difficulty in making lifestyle changes and informs patients that expert help is available through the Phase II component. Careful follow-up of these initial patient contacts will ensure timely referral into Phase II.

Phase II

Phase II of the VRP provides a thorough assessment, regular physical reconditioning sessions, and in-depth education on an outpatient basis. The success of this phase depends on integration of the classroom information and techniques into the patient's daily home routine. Frequent evaluation, continuous encouragement, and consistent reinforcement of information taught facilitate this process.

Candidates for Phase II must be referred by a physician and have a diagnosis of PAD that meets at least one of the following criteria:

- asymptomatic PAD (including asymptomatic carotid disease)
- a diagnosis of intermittent claudication
- a previous revascularization procedure
- severe arterial disease without possibility of revascularization

This diagnosis should be based on a history and physical assessment and an objective hemodynamic evaluation such as measurement of carotid duplex or Doppler pressures with a calculated ABI.

Assessment. Hemodynamic tests can document the presence and severity of the arterial disease, but they do not always correlate well with functional status or exercise capacity. Conversely, participation in a VRP may improve both functional status and exercise capacity without noticeable improvement in hemodynamic measurements. Therefore, patients must undergo a comprehensive assessment using appropriate tests and evaluation tools to determine their entry-level status. These baseline values will be used to determine the effectiveness of the VRP in achieving the desired outcomes. Areas to be assessed include

- evaluation of coronary artery disease
- evaluation of exercise capacity
- evaluation of functional status
- impact on quality of life
- presence and severity of atherosclerotic risk factors

Coronary Disease. Because PAD is a marker for cardiovascular disease, prospective Phase II patients must complete a graded exercise test, sometimes called a cardiac stress test. This test is necessary to determine the clinical significance of any cardiac disease, to evaluate the relative risk of entering the program, and to assist in documenting the patient's exercise capacity. Information obtained is also used in calculating the individual exercise prescription.

It is beyond the scope of this chapter to discuss all the different methods of graded exercise testing, the various protocols, and the clinical indications. The presence and severity of the patient's symptoms will determine the most appropriate method to use. Patients with asymptomatic PAD may be able to complete a treadmill evaluation using a standard Bruce protocol, but the patient with significant claudication will be severely limited, resulting in a submaximal effort. In this case, a bicycle test, or dipyridamole or thallium testing, will afford a more accurate evaluation of cardiac status. Detection of significant myocardial ischemia obviously warrants further evaluation and perhaps referral into a cardiac rehabilitation program.

Exercise Capacity. Historically, the treadmill has been used to evaluate the severity of claudication and effectiveness of various interventions, such as exercise therapy, revascularization procedures, and pharmacologic therapies. Traditionally, a constant-load treadmill test was performed, using a fixed speed (1.5–2.0 mph) and an unchanging, predefined grade (0–12 percent). The objective assessment of functional capacity was defined by the time to onset of claudication (the ICD) as well as the maximum claudication distance (or ACD). Several limitations to constant-load testing for PAD patients have recently been identified and the usefulness of the treadmill technique amplified by simple modifications.[59]

The objective functional assessment of patients with PAD may ideally be performed via application of treadmill protocols that can simultaneously assess both *exercise capacity* and *cardiac status*. Such simultaneous assessments often rely on the use of *graded* treadmill protocols. There are two graded protocols in common use that offer practical alternatives to the traditional constant-load (fixed) protocol. For each protocol, the treadmill speed is held constant at 2.0 mph and patients are asked to walk at an initial 0 percent grade. The Hiatt protocol is characterized by sequential 3.5 percent increases in grade every 3 minutes, whereas the Gardner-Skinner protocol increases the grade by 2.0 percent every 2 minutes.[60, 61] During these studies, patients are asked to indicate the location and time of onset of their claudication, and the maximum claudication distance is recorded. Any concomitant coronary ischemic symptoms are also recorded, and in many centers, simultaneous 12-lead cardiac monitoring may be performed in recognition of the coronary ischemic burden of the PAD population. These graded protocols have been validated in the PAD population, and initial data suggest that they demonstrate improved reproducibility as well as an ability to accommodate the patients of widely varied PAD functional limitations. In addition, patients accept them. The Vascular Clinical Trialists have proposed that one of these graded protocols be considered as an objective index of the effectiveness of any treatment for claudication, including exercise training.[59] Results of these objective exercise tests should be considered for inclusion as baseline and outcome measures for patients being considered for enrollment in a Phase II rehabilitation program.

In addition to providing the rehabilitation program with objective efficacy data, such testing may provide patients with a clear index of their current functional status and make it easier to set specific therapeutic goals to be reached by the completion of the VRP. As well, inasmuch as successful vascular rehabilitation can provoke major improvements in exercise capacity, graded stress testing performed initially with cardiac monitoring can demonstrate the safety of the exercise intervention if inducible coronary ischemia is not unmasked. In our experience, this added measure of safety can provide patient and rehabilitation therapist alike a "green light" for a vigorous exercise program. Confidence in such a program by patient and therapist may well increase the likelihood of long-term success.

Functional Status. The treadmill provides information about claudication distance in a "clinical" setting but does not determine the impact of claudication on the patient's ability to perform daily activities. Improved physical function is one of the goals of a VRP; therefore, baseline functional status must be documented and used as the standard against which the patient's improvement will be measured. Use of appropriate questionnaires, such as the Walking Improvement Questionnaire and the Peripheral Arterial Disease Physical Activity Recall Questionnaire, provide documentation of functional status before and after participation in the VRP.[59, 62]

Quality of Life. Determining the impact of disease on quality of life may provide some of the most useful information from the entire assessment process. Resumption of those important activities that patients no longer enjoy because of claudication becomes their motivation to make changes and stick with the program. At present there is no quality-of-life questionnaire specific to PAD. However, the Medical Outcomes Study (MOS SF-36) is one questionnaire that has been used to evaluate the impact of disease on general health perceptions in terms of mental health, social function, and vitality.[63, 64] Regardless of which questionnaire is used, it must be administered before starting Phase II and repeated at the completion of the program.

Atherosclerosis Risk Factors. During the assessment interview, document all existing risk factors for atherosclerosis (as outlined at the beginning of this chapter) and any treatment currently being provided. Obtain copies of the most recent lipid profiles from the referring physician. Too often cardiac and vascular rehabilitation programs focus solely on the exercise component of the program, with minimal attention to modification of risk factors. Physical reconditioning is only one intervention in the treatment regimen. Each contact with patients during the rehabilitation program must be fully utilized to reinforce teaching and monitor compliance with all aspects of treatment.

Once these physical parameters have been assessed, the assessment interview should focus on determining patients' goals and expectations of the program. They need a clear understanding of what the program does and does not offer. Some common misconceptions are that participation in the program will ensure that surgery can be avoided, that the disease or symptoms will not worsen, and that a 12- or 24-week program of exercise is all that is necessary to "cure" the problem.

Goals must be realistic, safe, practical, and mutually acceptable to the patient and rehabilitation staff. Long-term goals (3–6 months) are important, but realistic short-term goals (1–3 weeks) appear more achievable, encourage patients to start immediately, and serve as early determinants of progress. Early goal attainment is also its own reward, providing the positive motivation patients need to continue with the program.

Allocating sufficient time (perhaps up to 2 hours) for this initial assessment interview cannot be overemphasized. Davis encourages us to convey a "healing attitude" for patients and refers to this interaction as the "helping interview."[65] She cautions practitioners that first impressions do count and that obtaining the patient's trust as early as possible is crucial to the rehabilitation process. She says that this initial interview

. . . is the cornerstone for the structure of care we give. Patients come to us worried and often in pain. They feel vulnerable and in need of our help and understanding. . . . As health professionals, the burden is on us to recognize that the patient feels at a distinct disadvantage and to reassure and support. . . . At this initial meeting, interest, genuineness, acceptance and positive regard are critical to establishing a healing relationship.

By the end of the assessment, the interviewer should have some insight into the patient's level of commitment to the program. This should be discussed candidly. At this time, patients may be unsure of the depth of their commitment, but a willingness to *try* is essential. Without it, a successful rehabilitation course is dubious.

Physical Reconditioning

At the Rehabilitation Center. The cornerstone of Phase II of a VRP is the physical reconditioning instruction. The duration of the Phase II sessions varies, ranging from 12 to 24 weeks, although analysis of the literature shows optimal results achieved with a minimum of 24 weeks of therapy.[54] The results of the patient's graded exercise test and the guidelines established by the American College of Sports Medicine are used to calculate an individualized exercise prescription (Table 10–5).[66] The prescription includes the recommended time and intensity of exercise with a variety of equipment, as well as a target heart range to guide the patient's exercise. Proper use of the equipment as well as recording of the physical response to the exercise prescription is usually demonstrated before the first day of class, perhaps at the close of the initial assessment interview.

The actual format or degree of structure of the exercise sessions is not as important as making certain that the key elements of physical reconditioning—gradual warm-up, aerobic conditioning, and sufficient cool-down—are guided by safety and effectiveness. To reduce the risk of injury in this older group of patients, the importance of a gradual warm-up before more strenuous exercise cannot be overemphasized.[67, 68] Patients may warm up on the equipment, starting very slowly for 5 to 10 minutes. Another method that may also add interest and variety is to lead the entire group in a warm-up activity. This method makes it possible for proper techniques to be taught and observed and also provides a time of group interaction and support.

After sufficient warm-up, patients move to the various equipment stations. Walking provides the best exercise for improving claudication.[51] Patients with claudication should walk on the treadmill to the point of near-maximal pain (Fig. 10–1). Then while claudication subsides, patients can continue exercising on other equipment that is less strenuous on the calf muscle, such as stationary bicycles, Airdyne bikes (Fig. 10–2), arm ergometers, stairs (Fig. 10–3), and rowing machines. Use of a variety of equipment has the added advantage of improving total body fitness and preventing boredom. Patients should alternate back and forth from treadmill to other equipment so that several treadmill walks occur at each session.

The patient's tolerance of the prescribed exercise is recorded after each piece of equipment is used. This record includes the maximum heart rate achieved during exercise, the time to onset of claudication or other symptoms, the total exercise time on each piece of equipment, and the patient's rate of perceived exertion according to the Borg scale.[66, 69]

TABLE 10–5. **Exercise Prescription for Vascular Rehabilitation**

- Determined from the graded exercise test using the resting heart rate, maximum heart rate, and the maximum metabolic equivalent (MET) rate
- Calculations based on the American College of Sports Medicine Guidelines
- Entry training level set at 50% functional capacity
- Activity selected according to known energy expenditure at desired levels
- Subjective difficulty assessed with Borg's rate of perceived exertion

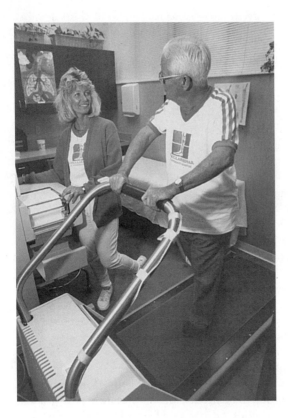

Figure 10–1. Treadmills are an excellent mode of conditioning to improve claudication.

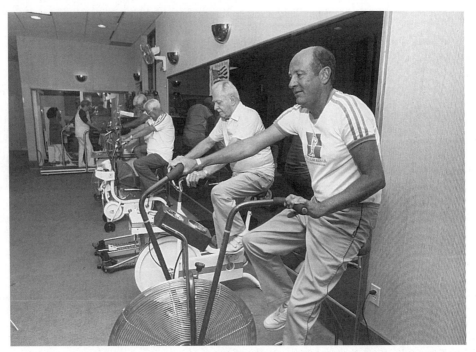

Figure 10–2. Stationary bicycles are more sparing of the calf muscle and may allow patients to continue exercise while claudication subsides.

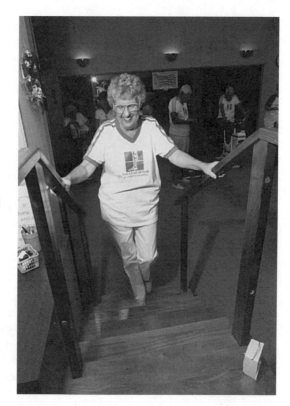

Figure 10–3. Stair-climbing improves overall fitness and stamina.

Adjustments to the exercise prescription are made at appropriate intervals throughout the program until the patient reaches a minimum of 35–40 minutes of discontinuous aerobic exercise per session.

Improving exercise tolerance in patients who are experiencing pain is a constant challenge to the staff. Patients need to learn the specific parameters of their symptoms. With claudication, does their discomfort get worse as they walk, forcing them to stop? Does it remain at a tolerable level or actually diminish, enabling them to walk through their pain?[70, 71] Once patients understand that claudication does not injure their legs, they may be able to push themselves to walk longer. Then significant progress can be made.

Each exercise session should end with several minutes of activity that allows the body to cool down gradually.[67, 68] This allows the heart rate and blood pressure to return to pre-exercise levels. Proper stretching at this time will improve flexibility and help prevent muscle soreness. As patients cool down and begin to relax, it may be helpful to incorporate stress-management techniques, such as guided imagery and total body relaxation.[72]

Even though a VRP can easily be incorporated into an existing cardiac program, it may be advisable to keep vascular patients separate from the cardiac group during the exercise sessions. Patients tend to identify and build supportive peer relationships more readily with others who have a similar diagnosis and symptoms. It is also easier for staff to manage a more homogeneous group. The exercise goals for vascular patients focus less on reaching target heart rates and more on walking beyond the initial onset of symptoms. This is not the goal with cardiac patients.

Supervised classes at a rehabilitation center are important in that they train patients in safe and effective guidelines for exercise to improve their stamina and fitness. These benefits continue only as long as the patient maintains a regular exercise program. Even during these exercise sessions at the center, the focus should be on developing a home exercise routine that the patient will continue after the supervised portion of the program.

Exercise Training at Home. Patients in supervised rehabilitation must understand the necessity of developing a pattern of daily exercise that can become an integral component of daily life. The development of a practical home exercise program during Phase II is essential for the establishment of long-term success. Such home-based programs are also essential inasmuch as many individuals with PAD may not be able or willing to participate in a structured center-based VRP. Barriers to participation in a center-based program include the following:

- The VRP may be too far from the patient's home.
- Adequate (available and inexpensive) transportation to the center may not exist.
- Program times may conflict with their daily schedule.
- There may be financial barriers to center-based participation.
- The patient may prefer exercising alone, instead of participating in group exercise.
- No center-based program may exist within the patient's health care system.

In order for these patients to benefit from a secondary prevention program, a home exercise program can be developed by a rehabilitation staff member in consultation with any primary care or vascular specialty clinician.

The clinician and patient must work together to plan the first stages of the home exercise plan, delineating specific steps for incorporating a regular exercise routine into the patient's day. Patients in Phase II of a VRP may particularly benefit from the overt creation of a home-based program, as they begin the transition from a supervised environment to including daily exercise in the activities of their home environment. The exercise therapist should discuss with each patient his or her current levels of exercise and activity in an effort to create a practical home program that is uniquely tailored to that patient. Many patients with PAD who are referred to a vascular rehabilitation program have never performed any regular, daily exercise and may doubt their ability to successfully initiate such a program at this stage of their lives. These patients may benefit from suggestions of various types of exercise, along with an exploration of different times and places in which such exercise might be most comfortable. Patients must develop their own practical regimen. Some patients find that exercising with a companion helps them follow their home program, whereas others prefer the introspection and relaxation that can be provided from such time alone. Patients should also be introduced to walking programs at local shopping malls and to various walking routes in their community, so as to lend variety and interest to the home program (Fig. 10–4). The home program should be considered a sign of a newly crafted independence, or as a "walk toward health."

Practitioners must plan home exercise individually. Prescribing too much could discourage the sedentary patient who has never exercised. Prescribing too little for a more active patient may cause him or her to lose interest. Regardless of the duration or intensity of exercise prescribed, the prescribed frequency should be the same for every patient, that is, to strive to exercise every day. If they follow this advice, patients can be sure of an adequate amount of exercise each week, even if they miss a day or two because of bad weather or unavoidable schedule conflicts. They also stand a better chance of developing a lifelong exercise habit.

A home exercise log is a useful tool for each patient to record the home exercise experience. Weekly review of this record by the staff allows appropriate changes in the program to be made and evaluated in a timely manner.[73]

Home exercise programs assist patients in making exercise a part of their daily routine. However, the key to developing the exercise habit is helping patients identify their exercise motivation. Gavin states that there are three types of exercise motives: body motives (look better, healthier body); psychologic motives (feel better, increased self-esteem); and social motives (exercise partners, social event). He believes that everyone has the motivation to exercise, although he admits that "it may be covered over by decades of suppression or accumulated fears about physical activity."[74] If vascular practitioners can encourage and

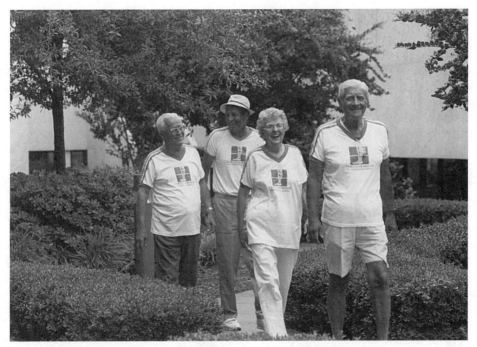

Figure 10–4. Walking clubs may improve compliance with a home exercise program.

assist patients in discovering exercise motives of all three types, there is a greater chance of long-term success.

Patient Education. Providing a sound knowledge base to patients means that clinicians must look for every opportunity to interact with patients, assess learning needs, and choose the best way to fill them. Increased understanding of the disease process and prognosis as well as the benefits of controlling risk factors may provide additional motivation for patients to modify behavior.

The rehabilitation program can offer a combination of formal and informal settings to enhance learning. A formal lecture series presented by the rehabilitation staff, vascular specialists, and allied health professionals is an excellent forum for delivering information on a selected topic to a large group of patients and their families. It also affords excellent visibility of the rehabilitation program and the hospital to the community if free lectures are offered and the public is invited to attend. The disadvantage of large-group instruction may be the varying levels of learning ability in the audience. Many people feel uncomfortable asking questions in front of a large group, so it may be difficult for the presenter to determine how well the information is understood. Follow-up time with each patient is needed to evaluate comprehension.

The physical reconditioning classes (usually a minimum of 24 sessions in a center-based program) provide follow-up time to reinforce classroom information. Informal discussions held with individual patients during these sessions enhance the patient-practitioner relationship and may serve two additional purposes. First, it is a good time to answer individual questions, personalizing and clarifying information. Second, it gives the patients something else to think about while exercising, keeping their eyes off the clock and perhaps allowing them to exercise longer.

Other informal teaching methods that reinforce classroom information include appropriate handouts, use of bulletin boards at the rehabilitation facility, video or audio tapes, a list of suggested reading material, and individual counseling sessions. Special presentations such as walking events, cooking classes, and restaurant expeditions provide practical "hands on" learning experiences where patients and families can put classroom information to use in real life.

Whether provided through formal classes at a rehabilitation center or one-on-one instruction in an office setting, educational content of VRPs should be the same. Patients need to hear basic information on the anatomy and physiology of the cardiovascular system, simple explanations of the pathophysiology of atherosclerosis and its associated symptoms, and the risk factors that contribute to the disease. Key points concerning each risk factor and how it contributes to the development of atherosclerosis, as discussed earlier in this chapter, should be incorporated into the patient education program. The importance of smoking cessation and stress management can be introduced during the risk factor lectures; however, the actual techniques are more effectively taught through separate, in-depth courses or individual counseling.

Although it is recommended that cardiac and vascular patients attend separate exercise sessions, it is entirely appropriate and perhaps even beneficial to include both groups of patients in the same education classes. They are facing the same disease with the same risk factors and need to realize the systemic nature of atherosclerosis. Cardiac patients need to know that they could experience leg symptoms, and vascular patients must realize that they may also have cardiac disease. Both groups need to know that they are at increased risk of having a stroke. Knowledge of these disease manifestations is essential for optimal management of this systemic disease.

Perhaps the one technique that has the greatest effect on behavior modification is that of role modeling. The more seasoned or "graduate" vascular rehabilitation patient serves as a role model for the novice, providing hope, empathy, and practical advice. Equally influential as role models are the members of the rehabilitation staff and the entire vascular team. They must be certain that the influence they exert on their patients is positive. Being a positive role model for health and fitness does not mean being "perfect." It does mean making a commitment to taking control and being responsible for one's own health. It also means being open, honest, and willing to share personal triumphs, defeats, strengths, and weaknesses.

Progress Evaluation. Progress is routinely discussed with patients during each exercise session, with more thorough evaluations scheduled halfway through the program. How much is accomplished in the final half of the program hinges heavily on this midpoint evaluation.

A graded treadmill walking test should be performed following the same protocol that was used during the initial assessment. Doppler studies need not be repeated unless there has been deterioration in symptoms and/or walking ability. If lipid-lowering agents are being used, updated laboratory values may be available from the physician and can be reviewed again with the patient. Particular attention is devoted to reviewing the home exercise records and planning the next stages of home exercise. Diet modifications are reviewed, and dietary consultations are arranged as needed. Progress with smoking cessation may be the most important aspect to evaluate, providing encouragement and adjusting interventions to help assure success.

The staff member conducting this evaluation should candidly discuss the patient's performance in terms of attendance, commitment, attitude, physical improvement, and knowledge attained. This is the time to acknowledge every measure of improvement or success, no matter how small, and to be generous with praise where deserved. If the patient has not shown improvement, staff and patient should try to determine why. Has the patient been making a serious effort? If so, he or she may need to be reminded that arteries do not occlude overnight and that improvement takes time. If the patient's attendance has been erratic, and no attempt has been made to exercise at home or to modify risk behaviors, this is the time for a frank discussion with the patient. There may be something in particular about the program that is upsetting and keeping the patient from participating. If no specific cause can be identified and the patient sincerely wants to continue, new goals and clear expectations should be identified for the remaining weeks of the program.

Phase III

On completion of the Phase II program, patients usually are afforded two options regarding a maintenance program: continue with a home exercise program or continue in the third phase of vascular rehabilitation. Ideally, most patients are well into their home exercise programs and are motivated enough to carry on without coming to the center for weekly supervised sessions. After these patients have been on their own for about 3 months, they return for a repeat evaluation. At that time, if they continue to show satisfactory improvement and adherence to their home routine, evaluations can be scheduled at 6-month intervals.

Occasionally, there are patients who know they are not sufficiently disciplined to continue on a program by themselves. These patients are likely candidates for a Phase III maintenance program offered at the rehabilitation center. These classes are usually offered three times a week with minimal supervision, and evaluations are scheduled every 3 months. To participate in this phase of the program, patients must be able to function fairly independently, continue to show improvement, and maintain regular attendance.

Results

The benefits of a structured VRP are significant for the vascular patient. A meta-analysis by Gardner and Poehlman of 21 programs in the country revealed a delayed onset of claudication and an increased maximal walking distance of 120–180 percent after exercise training.[51] This analysis also determined that the components most likely responsible for the improvement were using intermittent walking as the preferred exercise, exercising to the point of near-maximal pain, and continuing the program for at least 6 months. Another study by Carter and associates also demonstrated that improved treadmill walking distances may translate to even greater improvement during daily routine activities at home.[75]

Williams and colleagues reported a positive effect on other risk factors.[69] This included a significant reduction in serum triglyceride levels and a corresponding reduction in cholesterol levels after 1 year (Fig. 10–5). The VRP's in-depth education directed at risk

Figure 10–5. Reduction in serum triglyceride and cholesterol levels after 12 weeks, 1 year, and 2 years.

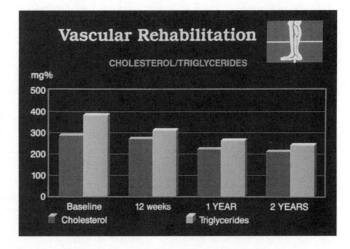

factor modification may account for this success, but equally important are peer pressure and support among the program participants.

Reimbursement Issues

A lack of consistent reimbursement policies has greatly hindered the proliferation of VRPs. There are currently no reimbursement codes for Medicare reimbursement of vascular rehabilitation. A few enlightened private insurance companies have seen the advantages of these programs and reimbursed accordingly. Several national concerns continue to address this issue with both the government and managed care administrators.

CONCLUSION

The ideal management of patients with PAD encompasses the skills of a multidisciplinary team of vascular nurses, vascular internists, vascular surgeons, interventional radiologists,

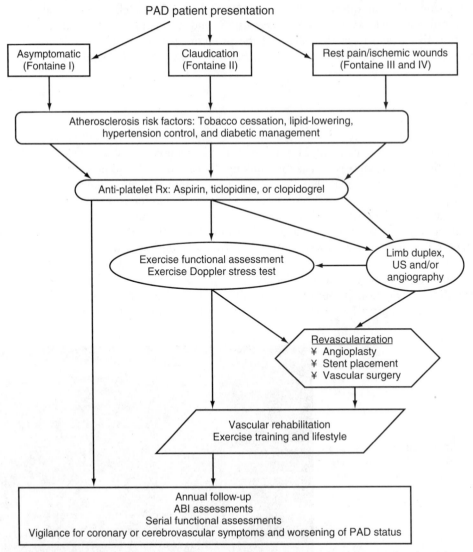

Figure 10–6. An integrated vascular medical/rehabilitation approach for community-based peripheral artery disease (PAD) care. US = ultrasonography; ABI = ankle-brachial index.

vascular technologists, and rehabilitation professionals. During the past decade, new data have demonstrated that patients with PAD benefit from preventive, palliative, and therapeutic medical interventions that can improve the natural history of PAD (limb arterial disease progression, and rates of myocardial infarction, stroke, and death), as well as functional outcomes (improved pain-free walking). Pharmacologic PAD interventions can now promote successful smoking cessation, normalize serum lipid levels, blunt the adverse effects of hypertension and diabetes, and prevent thrombotic events. Exercise training can markedly improve pain-free and total walking distances. However, the promise of these approaches, which are integral to both vascular medicine and vascular rehabilitation, must now become part of care management pathways for all patients with PAD (Fig. 10–6). The proposed integration of vascular medicine and rehabilitation can benefit patients with asymptomatic PAD, as well as those with claudication and severe limb ischemic symptoms, both prior to and after effective palliative revascularization procedures. All members of the health care team must see every encounter with patients with PAD as an opportunity to provide integrated vascular medical care. This opportunity is more than just a challenge, but defines our global responsibility as vascular clinicians for the long-term health of our patients.

References

1. Criqui MH, Langer RD, Fronek A, et al: Mortality over a period of 10 years in patients with peripheral arterial disease. N Engl J Med 1992; 326(6):381–386.
2. McKenna M, Wolfson S, Kuller L: The ratio of ankle and arm blood pressure as an independent risk factor of mortality. Atherosclerosis 1991; 87:119.
3. Newman AB, Siscovick DS, Manolio TA, et al for the Cardiovascular Health Study (CHS) Collaborative Research Group: Ankle-arm index as a marker of atherosclerosis in the Cardiovascular Health Study. Circulation 1993; 88:837.
4. Weitz, JI, Byrne J, Clagett P, et al: Diagnosis and treatment of chronic arterial insufficiency of the lower extremities: A critical review. Circulation 1996; 94:3026–3049.
5. Jonason T, Bergstrom R: Cessation of smoking in patients with intermittent claudication. Effects on the risk of peripheral vascular complications, myocardial infarction and mortality. Acta Med Scand 1987; 221:253–260.
6. Faulkner KW, House AK, Castleden WM: The effect of cessation of smoking on the accumulative survival rates of patients with symptomatic peripheral vascular disease. Med J Aust 1983; 1:217–219.
7. Lassila R, Lepantalo M: Cigarette smoking and the outcome after lower limb arterial surgery. Acta Chir Scand 1988; 154:635–640.
8. Hirsch AT, Treat-Jacobson D, Lando HA, Hatsukam DK: The role of tobacco cessation, anti-platelet and lipid-lowering therapies in the treatment of peripheral arterial disease. Vasc Med 1997; 2:243–251.
9. Hirsch AT, Baker S, Treat-Jacobson D, et al: The Minnesota regional peripheral arterial disease screening program: Toward a definition of community standards of care. Submitted to Circulation.
10. Quick C, Cotton L: The measured effect of stopping smoking on intermittent claudication. Br J Surg 1982; 69S:S24–26.
11. Gardner AW: The effect of cigarette smoking on exercise capacity in patients with intermittent claudication. Vasc Med 1996; 1:181–186.
12. Lando HA: Toward a comprehensive strategy for reducing the health burden of tobacco. In West R, Grunberg NE (eds): British Journal of Addiction, Vol 86. London, Carfax Publishing Company, 1991, pp 649–652.
13. Fiore MC, Bailey WC, Cohen SJ, et al: Smoking cessation. Clinical Practice Guideline No. 18. Rockville, MD: U.S. Department of Health and Human Services, Public Health Service, Agency for Health Care Policy and Research. AHCPR Publication No. 96-0692. April 1996.
14. Power L, Brown NS, Makin GS: Unsuccessful outpatient counseling to help patients with peripheral vascular disease to stop smoking. Ann R Coll Surg Engl 1992; 74:31–34.
15. Jasinski DR, Henningfield JE: Conceptual basis of replacement therapies for chemical dependence. In Pomerleau OF, Pomerleau CS (eds): Nicotine Replacement: A Critical Evaluation. New York, Alan R. Liss, 1988, pp 13–34.
16. Transdermal Nicotine Working Group: Nicotine replacement therapy for patients with coronary artery disease. Arch Intern Med 1994; 154:989–995.

17. Hughes, JR: Dependence potential and abuse liability of nicotine replacement therapies. In Pomerleau OF, Pomerleau CS (eds): Progress in Clinical Evaluation. New York, Alan R. Liss, 1988, pp 261–277.
18. Covey LS, Glassman AH, Stetner F: Depression and depressive symptoms in smoking cessation. Compr Psychiatry 1990; 31:350–354.
19. Ginsberg D, Hall SM, Reus VI, Munoz RF: Mood and depression diagnosis in smoking cessation. Exp Clin Psychopharmacol 1995; 3(4):389–395.
20. Hurt RD, Sachs DP, Glover ED, et al: A comparison of sustained-release bupropion and placebo for smoking cessation. N Engl J Med 1997; 337(17):1195–1202.
21. Hess H, Miewtaschik A, Deischel G: Drug-induced inhibition of platelet function delays progression of peripheral occlusive arterial disease: A prospective, double-blind arteriographically controlled trial. Lancet 1985; I:415–419.
22. Goldhaber SZ, Manson JE, Stampfer MJ, et al: Low-dose aspirin and subsequent peripheral arterial surgery in the Physicians Health Study. Lancet 1992; 340:143–145.
23. Janzon L, Bergquist D, Boberg J, et al: Prevention of myocardial infarction and stroke in patients with intermittent claudication; effects of ticlopidine. Results from STIMS, the Swedish Ticlopidine Multicentre Study. J Intern Med 1991; 27:301–308.
24. Arcan JC, Blanchard J, Boissel J, et al: Multicenter double-blind study of ticlopidine in the treatment of intermittent claudication and the prevention of its complications. Angiology 1988; 39:802–811.
25. Balsano F, Cocherri S, Libretti A, et al: Ticlopidine in the treatment of intermittent claudication: A 21-month double-blind trial. J Lab Clin Med 1989; 114:84–91.
26. Balsano F, Violi F: Effect of picotamide on the clinical progression of peripheral vascular disease. A double-blind placebo-controlled study. The ADEP Group. Circulation 1993; 87(5):1563–1569.
27. Coto V, Cocozza M, Oliviero U, et al: Clinical efficacy of picotamide in long-term treatment of intermittent claudication. Angiology 1989; 40(10):880–885.
28. CAPRIE Steering Committee: A randomized, blinded trial of Clopidogrel vs. Aspirin in Patients at Risk of Ischaemic Events (CAPRIE). Lancet 1996; 348(9038):1329–1339.
29. Stamler J, Wentworth D, Neatone JD: Is there a relationship between serum cholesterol and risk of premature death from coronary heart disease continuous and graded? Findings in 356,222 primary screenees of the Multiple Risk Factor Intervention Trial (MRFIT). JAMA 1986; 256:2823–2828.
30. Criqui MH, Wallace RB, Heiss G, et al: Cigarette smoking and plasma high density lipoprotein cholesterol. The Lipid Research Clinics Program Prevalence Study. Circulation 1980; 62(suppl IV):70–76.
31. Summary of the second report of the National Cholesterol Education Program (NCEP) expert panel on detection, evaluation, and treatment of high blood cholesterol in adults (Adult Treatment Panel II). JAMA 1993; 269:3015–3023.
32. Blankenhorn DH, Azen SP, Crawford DW, et al: Effects of colestipol-niacin therapy on human femoral atherosclerosis. Circulation 1991; 83:438–447.
33. Buchwald H, Varco RL, Matts JP, et al: Effect of partial ileal bypass surgery on mortality and morbidity from coronary heart disease in patients with hypercholesterolemia. Report of the Program on the Surgical Control of the Hyperlipidemias (POSCH). N Engl J Med 1990; 323:946–955.
34. Sacks FM, Pfeffer MA, Moye LA, et al, for the Cholesterol and Recurrent Events Trial Investigators: The effect of pravastatin on coronary events after myocardial infarction in patients with average cholesterol levels. N Engl J Med 1996; 335:1001–1019.
35. Scandinavian Simvastatin Survival Study Group: Randomized trial of cholesterol lowering in 444 patients with coronary heart disease: The Scandinavian Simvastatin Survival Study (4S). Lancet 1994; 344:1383–1389.
36. Hirsch AT, Garg R, Elam J, et al: Quality of life and walking impairment in peripheral arterial disease in the Arterial Disease Multiple Intervention Trial. Circulation 1996; 94:I-174.
37. Kannel WB, McGee DL: Update on some epidemiologic features of intermittent claudication. Lancet 1966; II:1093.
38. The Sixth Report of the Joint National Committee on Prevention, Detection, Evaluation and Treatment of High Blood Pressure. Arch Intern Med 1997; 137:2413–2446.
39. Grodstein F, Stampfer MJ, Colditz GA, et al: Postmenopausal hormone therapy and mortality. N Engl J Med 1997; 336(25):1769–1775.
40. Stampfer MJ, Colditz GA, Willett WC, et al: Postmenopausal estrogen therapy and cardiovascular disease. Ten year follow-up in the Nurses' Health Study. N Engl J Med 1991; 325(11):756–762.
41. Patterson RB, Pinto B, Marcus B, et al: Value of a supervised exercise program for the therapy of arterial claudication. J Vasc Surg 1997; 25:312–319.
42. Ponte E, Cattinelli S: Quality of life in a group of patients with intermittent claudication. Angiology 1996; 47:247–251.
43. Regensteiner JG, Steiner JF, Hiatt WR: Exercise training improves functional status in patients with peripheral arterial disease. J Vasc Surg 1996; 23:104–115.
44. Khaira HS, Hanger R, Shearman CP: Quality of life in patients with intermittent claudication. Eur J Vasc Endovasc Surg 1996; 11:65–69.
45. Larsen O, Lassen N: Effect of daily muscular exercise in patients with intermittent claudication. Lancet 1966; II:1093.

46. Dahloff A, Bjorntorp P, Holm J, Schersten T: Metabolic activity of skeletal muscle in patients with peripheral arterial insufficiency: Effect of physical training. Eur J Clin Invest 1974; 4:9.
47. Dahloff A, Holm J, Schersten T, Sivertsson R: Peripheral arterial insufficiency: Effect of physical training on walking tolerance, calf blood flow and blood flow resistance. Scand J Rehab Med 1976; 8:18.
48. Hiatt WR, Nawaz D, Regensteiner JG, et al: The evaluation of exercise performance in patients with peripheral arterial disease. J Cardpulm Rehabil 1988; 12:525–532.
49. Hiatt WR: Benefit of exercise conditioning for patients with peripheral arterial disease. Circulation 1990; 81:602.
50. Hiatt WR, Regensteiner JG: Exercise rehabilitation in the treatment of patients with peripheral arterial disease. J Vasc Med Biol 1990; 2:163.
51. Gardner AW, Poehlman ET: Exercise rehabilitation programs for the treatment of claudication pain: A meta-analysis. JAMA 1995; 274(12):975–980.
52. England JD, Regensteiner JG, Ringel SP, et al: Muscle denervation in peripheral arterial disease. Neurology 1992; 42:994.
53. Regensteiner JG, Wolfel EE, Brass EP, et al: Chronic changes in skeletal muscle histology and function in peripheral arterial disease. Circulation 1993; 87:413.
54. Robbins A: Unlimited Power. New York, Ballentine Books, 1986.
55. Patterson RB, Pinto B, Marcus B, et al: Value of a supervised exercise program for the therapy of arterial claudication. J Vasc Surg 1997; 25(2):312–318.
56. Barnes M: Vascular rehabilitation update: Components of a Phase I program. J Vasc Nurs 1992; 10(4):31.
57. Society for Vascular Nursing. 7794 Grow Drive, Pensacola, FL 32514.
58. Landis BJ, Brykczynski KA: Employing prevention in practice. AJN 1997; 97(8):40–46.
59. Hiatt WR, Hirsch AT, Regensteiner JG, et al: Clinical trials for claudication: Assessment of exercise performance, functional status, and clinical end points. Circulation 1995; 92:614–621.
60. Hiatt WR, Nawaz D, Regensteiner JG, et al: The evaluation of exercise performance in patients with peripheral vascular disease. J Cardpulm Rehabil 1988; 12:525–532.
61. Gardner AW, Skinner JS, Cantwell BW, et al: Progressive vs single-stage treadmill tests for evaluation of claudication. Med Sci Sports Exerc 1991; 23:402–408.
62. Regensteiner JG, Steiner JF, Panzer RJ, et al: Evaluation of walking impairment by questionnaire in patients with peripheral arterial disease. J Vasc Med Biol 1990; 2:142–152.
63. Ware JE, Sherbourne CD: The MOS 36-item short-form health survey (SF-36), I: Conceptual framework and item selection. Med Care 1992; 30:473–483.
64. McHorney CA, Ware JE, Raczek AE: The MOS 36-item short-form health survey (SF-36), II: Psychometric and clinical tests of validity in measuring physical and mental health constructs. Med Care 1993; 31:247–263.
65. Davis CM: Patient Practitioner Interaction: An Experiential Manual for Developing the Art of Health Care. Thorofare, NJ, Slack, 1989.
66. American College of Sports Medicine: Guidelines for Graded Exercise Testing and Exercise Prescription, 5th ed. Philadelphia, Williams and Wilkins, 1995.
67. Pollock ML, Wilmore JH: Exercise in Health and Disease: Evaluation and Prescription for Prevention and Rehabilitation, 2nd ed. Philadelphia, WB Saunders, 1990.
68. Cooper KH: The Aerobics Program for Total Well-Being. New York, Bantam Books, 1982.
69. Williams LR, Ekers, MA, Collins PS, et al: Vascular rehabilitation: Benefits of a structured exercise/risk factor modification program. J Vasc Surg 1991; 12:1636–1639.
70. Hubner C: Exercise therapy and smoking cessation for intermittent claudication. J Cardiovasc Nurs 1987; 1:50–58.
71. Taylor LM, Porter JM: Natural history and nonoperative treatment of chronic lower extremity ischemia. In Rutherford R (ed): Vascular Surgery, 3rd ed. Philadelphia, WB Saunders, 1989, pp 653–667.
72. Squires R, Gau GT, Miller TF, et al: Cardiovascular rehabilitation: Status 1990. Mayo Clin Proc 1990; 65:731–755.
73. Ekers MA: Vascular rehabilitation update. J Vasc Nurs 1992; 10(2):34.
74. Ekroth R, Dahlof AG, Gundevall B, et al: Physical training of patients with intermittent claudication: Indications, methods, and results. Surgery 1978; 84:640–643.
75. Carter SA, Hamel ER, Paterson JM, et al: Walking ability and ankle systolic pressures. J Vasc Surg 1989; 10:642–649.

11

Surgery of the Aorta

Jon S. Matsumura, MD

∽ · ∾

During the latter half of this century, reconstructive surgery of the aorta has become a relatively safe and effective treatment of aortic aneurysms, aortoiliac occlusive disease, and aortic dissection. Previously, these diseases were incurable and often led to serious morbidity and the patient's rapid demise. Currently, approximately 60,000 patients per year in the United States benefit from what has developed from experimental surgery into routine operations carried out in community hospitals. Perioperative mortality has fallen to single-digit levels in elective cases, and late complications are uncommon.[1, 2] These great strides in the care of these patients have been possible because of advances in surgical and anesthetic techniques, graft materials, and perioperative care.

Nursing management of patients undergoing aortic surgery encompasses a broad spectrum, ranging from preoperative teaching, intraoperative and intensive care, postoperative support, to recognition of complications. Knowledge of anatomy is key to understanding the manifestations of aortic diseases and the complications of aortic procedures. This chapter first reviews aortic anatomy, then discusses the three major diseases affecting the aorta with detailed discussion of presentation, diagnosis, and therapeutic options, and finishes with a description of short- and long-term complications. New findings and new endovascular treatments are emphasized.

ANATOMY AND FUNCTION

The aorta begins at the aortic valve, ascends in the anterior mediastinum, arches posteriorly, descends in the posterior mediastinum, and traverses the retroperitoneum to end at the bifurcation into the common iliac arteries (Fig. 11–1). The first branches are the left and right coronary arteries, which feed the myocardium. The arch vessels include the innominate artery, which branches into the right subclavian and right common carotid arteries, and also the left common carotid artery and the left subclavian artery. The descending aorta gives off intercostal branches, some of which (usually in the T9 to L1 region) anastomose with the crucial artery of Adamkiewicz, which feeds the spinal cord. Abdominal branches include the celiac artery, superior mesenteric artery, renal arteries, and inferior mesenteric artery.

Aortic diseases or surgical complications that impair the flow of blood to these branches affect the diverse functions of the corresponding organs. For instance, arch vessel embolism may manifest as transient ischemic attacks or hand ischemia, intercostal branch

Supported in part by the Baldwin Research Fund.

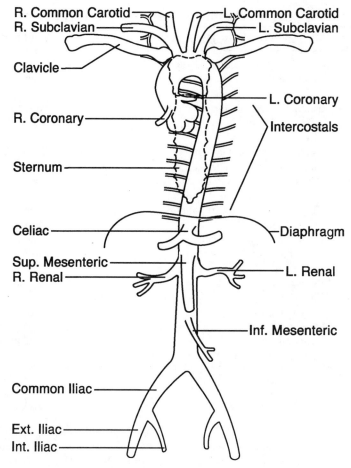

Figure 11-1. Anatomy of the aorta and its major branches.

occlusion may precipitate paraplegia, and renal artery thrombosis may lead to hypertension or renal failure. Onset of clinical symptoms usually correlates with the pace of blood flow reduction. For example, in the Leriche syndrome there is slow onset of decreased femoral pulses, buttock claudication, and erectile dysfunction as a result of gradual distal aorta and common iliac artery occlusion. In contrast, with acute thrombosis of the infrarenal aorta or saddle embolization of the aortic bifurcation, aortic occlusion occurs without sufficient time for collateral development, and hence there is acute bilateral leg ischemia with myonecrosis and symptoms of pelvic arterial insufficiency such as rectal ischemia.

AORTIC ANEURYSM

Aneurysms are diseased areas of artery that become dilated and lined with intraluminal thrombus. They can (1) rupture, causing pain and internal hemorrhage, (2) thrombose, leading to acute ischemia of all downstream branches, or (3) embolize, causing selective branch vessel symptoms. Most commonly, aortic aneurysms affect the infrarenal aorta and present with rupture. Screening of unselected adults and men with peripheral vascular disease reveals a prevalence of 3.2–9.6 percent,[3] and about 15,000 Americans die from aortic aneurysms each year. Fortunately, many aneurysms are detected when they are asymptomatic, by physical examination or by serendipity on radiographic tests. Many theories of aneurysm pathogenesis, which are not mutually exclusive, are reviewed in Table 11–1.

TABLE 11–1. **Theories of Aneurysm Pathogenesis**

ETIOLOGY	CLINICAL EVIDENCE	THEORY
Familial	Male siblings have up to 25% lifetime risk of aneurysm.	Genetic predisposition and specific defects in collagen (Ehlers-Danlos syndrome).
Atherosclerotic	Risk factors are similar to occlusive disease, including smoking, hypertension, and aging.	Compensatory dilation of the artery becomes uncontrolled.
Immunologic	A variant called inflammatory aneurysm is characterized by gross inflammation and microscopic leukocyte infiltrates.	Antigen, possibly through molecular mimicry, precipitates autoimmune response.
Degenerative	Hernias are common in patients with aneurysms.	Elastin and collagen aberrantly formed or digested.
Hemodynamic	Aneurysms typically occur proximal to bifurcations or distal to stenoses.	Wall tension is increased dynamically in these areas.
Iatrogenic	Aneurysms occur at graft anastomosis, after endarterectomy or angioplasty.	Structural injury, end-to-side anastomosis.
Infectious	*Salmonella* may be associated with aneurysms.	Microorganisms, as identified by PCR, may stimulate inflammation or degradation.

PCR = polymerase chain reaction.

The presentation of abdominal aortic aneurysm can be dramatic when rupture occurs. Typically, the patient complains of sudden onset of abdominal and lower back pain with physical findings of shock and abdominal tenderness. Most patients do not survive the rupture long enough to get to a hospital. Hypovolemic shock and a pulsatile abdominal mass are diagnostic. In these circumstances, simultaneous resuscitation and immediate operation are indicated. At other times, symptoms can be quite varied and include scrotal pain referred from retroperitoneal irritation; fever; uremia with inflammatory aneurysms that entrap the ureters; blue toe syndrome when microembolization from proximal lesions occurs (Fig. 11–2A); and even disseminated intravascular coagulation in the case of very large aneurysms. Computed tomography (CT) scans (Fig. 11–3) and abdominal ultrasound may be helpful in less obvious cases of acute onset and in chronic cases for planning treatment by assessing precise aneurysm size and its location relative to branches and for ruling out multiple aneurysms.[4]

Risk of rupture is related primarily to the size of the aneurysm, and hence observation is recommended for most small (<4 cm) and asymptomatic aortic aneurysms. Although aneurysms expand at an average rate of 10 percent per year, many will remain stable for years. Treatment is generally recommended for symptomatic aneurysms, rapidly enlarging aneurysms, and infrarenal aneurysms over 5 cm because the risk of rupture becomes excessive, although individual risk assessment is practiced.[5] The conventional operation is endoaneurysmal repair, which may be performed safely through a midline or transverse anterior approach or a retroperitoneal approach.[6] In the standard operation the aorta is exposed and clamped above and below the aneurysm and a graft sutured inside of the aneurysm sac to restore continuity (Fig. 11–4). Mortality in large series at experienced centers is less than 4 percent, and was 1.4 percent in the 25-year series reported by Crawford.[2, 3]

Alternative strategies for repair of aortic aneurysms include retroperitoneal ligation of the aneurysm and bypass to restore distal perfusion,[7] laparoscopic ligation and axillobifem-

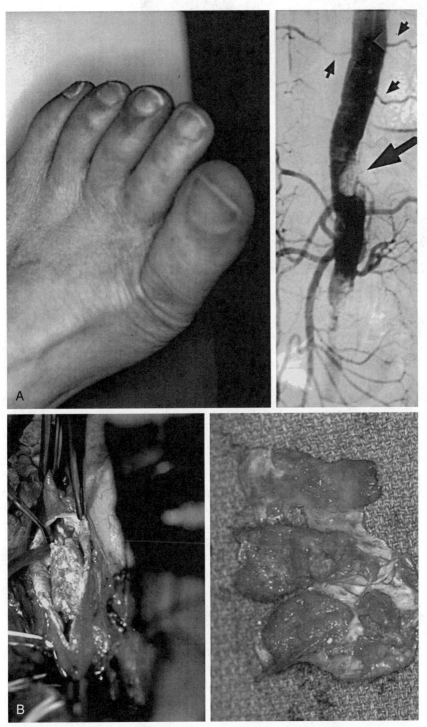

Figure 11–2. Blue toe syndrome. **A,** Upper left photograph shows mottling of distal aspects of toes. Upper right is a digital subtraction angiogram of the descending thoracic and abdominal segments of the aorta demonstrating plaque *(solid black arrow)*, with intercostal branches *(black arrowheads)*. **B,** Lower left is operative photograph of the aorta opened before endarterectomy, and lower right is a close-up view of the specimen of "coral reef"-like plaque, which is the source of the distal emboli.

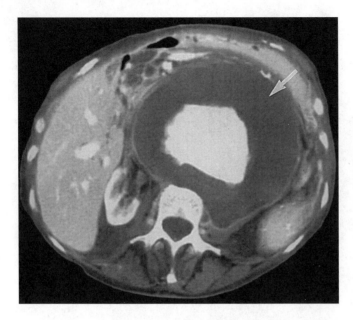

Figure 11–3. Computed tomography (CT) scan of an enormous aortic aneurysm with lumen enhanced by white appearing contrast and surrounded by thick intraluminal thrombus *(white arrow)*.

oral bypass,[8] and endovascular grafting. Endovascular treatment (Fig. 11–5) has received the greatest attention, with multiple clinical trials in progress worldwide. Preliminary results suggests that mortality and hospital stay may be reduced, although complete evaluation will require long-term follow-up.[9–11]

Aneurysms that extend above the renal arteries and into the thoracic aorta are more difficult to repair (Fig. 11–6). Their presentation is less distinct because high back pain and chest pain may be mistaken for angina and pulmonary diseases. These patients require more extensive incisions into the chest cavity and have greater blood loss and coagulopathy, and their reconstruction procedure must include additional attention to the important branches to the kidneys, bowel, and spinal cord. Often a larger cut-off size of 6 cm is utilized as an indication for repair of thoracic and thoracoabdominal aneurysms. Specialized intraoperative techniques to prevent complications include cold renal artery perfusion, atrial-to-femoral artery cardiopulmonary bypass, spinal fluid drainage, and regional epidural hypothermia. These techniques minimize organ metabolism and maximize collateral perfusion during the ischemic interval of aortic repair. Thoracoabdominal aneurysms are often treated in tertiary care institutions because of the higher risk of paraplegia, renal failure, and death.

AORTIC OCCLUSIVE DISEASE

Occlusive disease of the aorta is predominantly caused by atherosclerosis, with rare cases due to congenital coarctation, radiation injury, giant cell arteritis, or Takayasu's disease. Most symptomatic disease involves the infrarenal aorta and iliac arteries, and it is estimated that 1.8 percent, 3.7 percent, and 5.2 percent of adults less than 60 years old, 60–70 years old, and greater than 70 years old, respectively, experience claudication or intermittent leg pain with exercise.[12] Many of these patients' claudication symptoms are caused by aortoiliac disease. Aortic atherosclerosis can "spill over" into branch lesions, causing stenosis of the orifice of the main coronary, arch vessels, mesenteric, and renal arteries. These latter lesions and their treatment are covered in other chapters, although they are often treated with operations of the aorta that have similar complications.

Diagnosis of aortoiliac occlusive disease is by history and physical examination. Patients complain of lower-extremity muscle fatigue or cramping that occurs with a reproducible

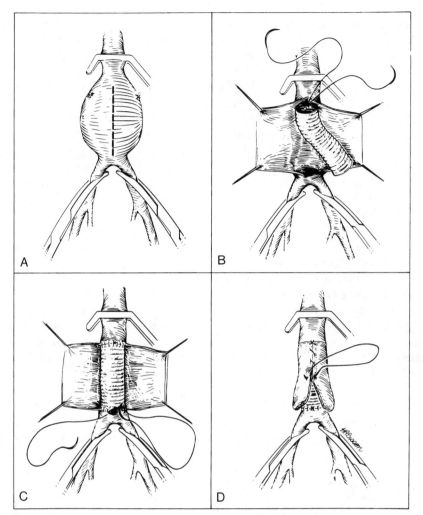

Figure 11–4. Classic endoaneurysmal repair of an abdominal aortic aneurysm. The aorta is controlled with vascular clamps **(A)**, and opened. The prosthetic graft is sutured from within the aneurysm attaching to the proximal **(B)** and distal **(C)** aorta. **D,** The aneurysm wall is closed over the graft to assist in hemostasis and prevent contact with the overlying bowel. (From Yao JST, Flinn WR, Bergan JJ: Technique for repairing infrarenal abdominal aortic aneurysm. In Nyhus LM, Baker RJ [eds]: Mastery of Surgery. Boston, Little, Brown & Co, pp 1361–1365. © 1984.)

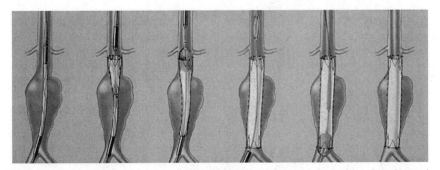

Figure 11–5. Ancure device for treatment of abdominal aortic aneurysm through endovascular approach. *Panel from left to right:* graft is sequentially implanted by a catheter inserted in the femoral artery; the proximal attachment system is released; balloon inflated below the renal arteries; distal graft deployed; balloon inflated above aortic bifurcation; and delivery catheter removed. This device is investigational at the time of writing. (Reproduced with permission: Endovascular Grafting System. Endo Vascular Technologies, Inc., 1996.)

walking distance and is relieved by standing. This contrasts with similar pain of neuro-spinal etiology, which occurs at variable exercise levels, requires positional change for relief, and has an electrical or shooting quality. In men, erectile dysfunction may occur due to arterial insufficiency to the pelvis through the internal iliac arteries. With advanced occlusive disease, often at multiple levels, critical ischemia develops with rest pain or gangrene. Physical findings include abdominal bruits and diminished or absent femoral pulses. Occasionally, normal pulses are present at rest but "disappear" when the patient walks, with consequent vasodilation of the distal vascular bed.

Initial treatment of patients with symptomatic aortoiliac disease begins with counseling on smoking cessation and an exercise program. Patients with persistent disabling symptoms and those with critical ischemia should be considered for revascularization. Aortobifemoral bypass is the gold standard and is performed through a combination of abdominal and femoral incisions (Fig. 11–7). Aortobifemoral bypass has a mortality of less than 3 percent and a remarkable 68 percent patency at 20 years according to the classic study by Szilagyi and confirmed in over 20 other series.[13, 14] Many alternative procedures exist, each with purported specific benefits, including endarterectomy (see Fig. 11–2B), which precludes the need for a prosthetic graft, axillobifemoral bypass (Fig. 11–8), which avoids aortic cross-clamping and major cavity invasion, and thoracofemoral bypass (Fig. 11–9), with possible improved long-term patency.[15] In the patient illustrated in Figure 11–2, not only did coral reef–appearing plaque impede blood flow, but also the irregular, ulcerated surfaces shed atheromatous debris, leading to the blue toe syndrome. Lately, laparoscopic aortobifemoral bypass has been explored and offers reduced recovery time while maintaining an anatomic revascularization.[16–18]

Endovascular approaches have revolutionized the treatment of these patients and are covered in detail in Chapter 6. Minimally invasive aortoiliac angioplasty has displaced bypass and endarterectomy as the primary procedure because of low complication rates and greatly reduced hospital stay and patient discomfort. Longer follow-up of randomized

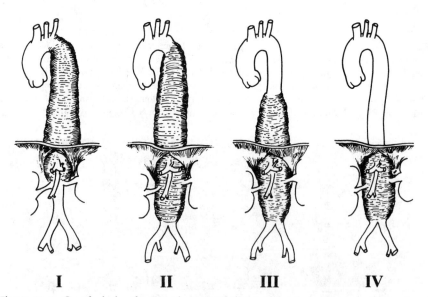

| I | II | III | IV |

Figure 11–6. Crawford classification of extent of thoracoabdominal aneurysms. Extent I and extent II aneurysms are associated with higher risks for paraplegia. (From Hamilton JN, Hollier LH: Thoracoabdominal aortic aneurysms. In Moore, W [ed]: Vascular Surgery: A Comprehensive Review, 5th ed. Philadelphia, W. B. Saunders, 1988, p 417.)

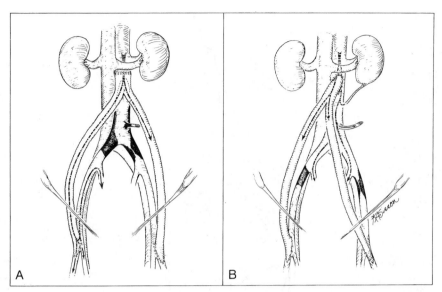

Figure 11–7. Aortobifemoral bypass. **A** illustrates an end-to-end configuration for the aortic anastomosis. **B** shows an end-to-side configuration, which preserves native flow to the pelvis, inferior mesenteric artery, and inferior pole renal artery. (From Schuler JJ, Flanigan DP: Aortobifemoral artery bypass. In Nyhus LM, Baker RJ [eds]: Mastery of Surgery. Boston, Little, Brown & Co, 1984, pp 1419–1427. © 1984.)

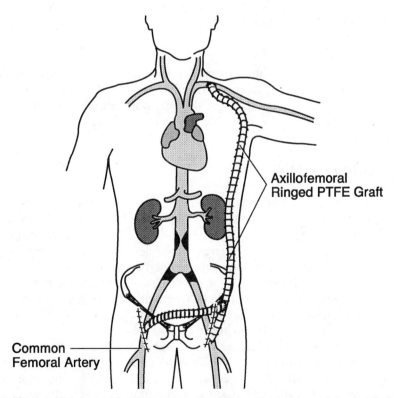

Figure 11–8. Axillobifemoral bypass connects the axillary artery just beyond the clavicle to the femoral arteries along the side of the torso, avoiding invasion of major body cavities. This bypass can even be performed under local and regional anesthesia. The externally supported grafts are usually palpable in the subcutaneous tunnels. PTFE = polytetrafluoroethylene.

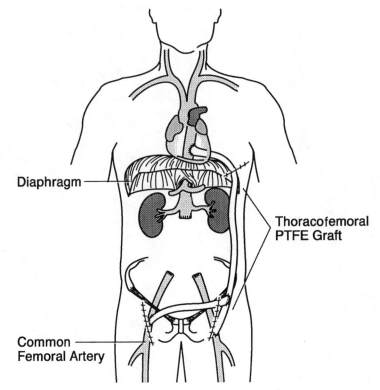

Figure 11–9. Thoracofemoral bypass uses the descending thoracic aorta for inflow source. This bypass is also useful when there has been previous infection in the abdomen and the iliac arteries are ligated. PTFE = polytetrafluoroethylene.

trials comparing angioplasty with conservative treatment has demonstrated improved arterial patency but equivalent patient satisfaction at 2 years.[19] Recent introduction of endovascular stenting and perhaps stent-grafting may provide improved long-term patency while maintaining the benefits of minimally invasive procedures.[20]

AORTIC DISSECTION

Dissection of the aorta is a condition in which the layers of the aortic wall have separated, creating a tear or opening into the lumen. Blood flows between the layers of the wall, "dissects" this space farther along the vessel, and creates a second blood-filled tube or "false lumen." In a dynamic process, different blood flow rates and pressures occur in the true and false lumen resulting in sudden impaired perfusion to any of the aortic branches. In some hospitals, aortic dissection is a much more common emergency than ruptured aneurysm. Risk factors for dissection include hypertension, male gender, trauma (particularly deceleration injuries), cystic medial necrosis (Marfan's syndrome), and iatrogenic injury from catheter interventions and aortic clamping.

Aortic dissection typically presents as acute onset of "tearing" chest or back pain, and can easily be mistaken for heart attack. Occasionally, patients will be pain-free and present only with symptoms of branch artery occlusion, mimicking arterial embolism. Rupture of a dissection can cause internal hemorrhage akin to ruptured aortic aneurysm (Fig. 11–10). Because of the variety of presenting symptoms (Table 11–2), aortic dissection may be considered a great masquerader and is often misdiagnosed on admission. Physical examination of carotid, brachial, and femoral pulses with measurement of limb pressures must be

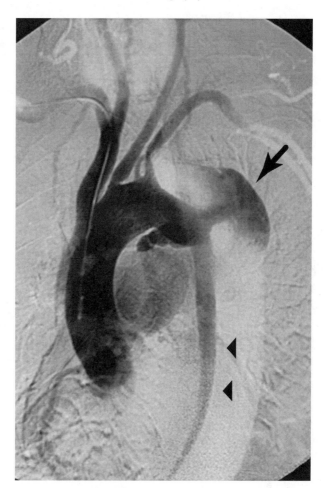

Figure 11–10. Arteriogram demonstrating dissection flap *(black arrowheads)* and impending rupture of false lumen *(black arrow).*

performed and documented carefully, and continued surveillance for symptoms or change in pulse examination is a vital component to the care of these patients. A new cardiac murmur may be the earliest sign of aortic valve involvement.

Classification of aortic dissection is crucial to predicting outcome and prescribing therapy. Acute dissection involving the ascending aorta may cause sudden death at a rate of 1–2 percent per hour because of the proximity to the coronary arteries, aortic valve involvement, or pericardial tamponade. These dissections are classified as Stanford type A (involves ascending) and DeBakey type I (ascending and descending) or type II (ascending only) and require immediate surgical treatment. Dissections limited to the descending aorta are classified as Stanford type B or DeBakey type III, and are often initially treated with medical therapy (Fig. 11–11).[21]

Several tests are available to confirm the diagnosis of aortic dissection and classify its location. Spiral CT scanning is widely available and with proper timing of the contrast bolus is a useful noninvasive screening test (Fig. 11–12). Transesophageal echocardiography has become our preferred test because it allows continued intensive care surveillance, is exceedingly accurate, and can provide additional information on ventricular function, aortic valve competency, and left main coronary patency.[22] Magnetic resonance imaging can be similarly helpful in an appropriate hospital setting.[23] Chest radiographs and electrocardiograms are nonspecific and helpful mainly to exclude other diagnoses. Angiography, formerly the standard diagnostic study, is rarely performed because of the risk of worsening the dissection.

TABLE 11–2. **Clinical Manifestations and
Pathogenesis of Aortic Dissection**

SIGN/SYMPTOM	FREQUENCY	STRUCTURE OR ARTERY	MECHANISM
Congestive heart failure	13–30%	Aortic valve	Ascending aortic tear results in deformation of aortic valve, with acute valvular insufficiency and left heart failure.
Hypotension	8–17%	Pericardium	False lumen ruptures through adventitia into pericardial space, causing pericardial tamponade. Also may rupture into pleura or mediastinum with internal hemorrhage and shock.
Myocardial ischemia	2%	Coronary	Dissection extends to coronary ostia, causing poor coronary perfusion and heart attack.
Neurologic deficit	2–6%	Arch vessels Intercostal vessels	Impaired perfusion to arch vessels causes stroke or to intercostal vessels causes paraplegia.
Visceral ischemia	5%	Mesenteric	Branch occlusion causes ischemic liver and bowel.
Hypertension, renal failure	5–10%	Renal	Decreased renal artery perfusion results in renin overproduction and renovascular hypertension. Complete occlusion results in tubular necrosis and renal failure.
Cold limb	17%	Iliac ubclavian	Dissection continues down entire length of aorta into iliac vessels, and the cold foot is the most common peripheral ischemic complication.
Aneurysm	20–50%	Aorta	Thinned aortic wall dilates, resulting in aneurysmal area. Persistent patent tear and large initial diameter predict enlargement.
Pain	90%	Aorta	Related to wall separation and often correlates with location and progression of dissection.

All patients with dissection require aggressive control of high blood pressure, usually in an intensive care unit with an arterial line. Beta-blockers have a theoretical advantage in reducing dp/dt (ratio of change of ventricular pressure to change in time) and wall stress, but several intravenous agents are available. As mentioned previously, constant surveillance for progression of dissection and branch vessel occlusion is necessary to detect peripheral ischemic complications rapidly.

Surgical treatment is indicated in several circumstances: (1) location of dissection in ascending aorta; (2) development of ischemic complication; (3) poor response to medical

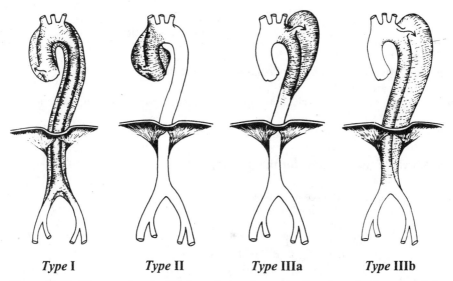

Type I   **Type** II   **Type** IIIa   **Type** IIIb

Figure 11–11. Two popular classification schemes for aortic dissections. Involvement of the ascending aorta has important prognostic and therapeutic implications. DeBakey type I and type II are called type A in the Stanford classification; DeBakey type III lesions are equivalent to Stanford type B. (From Hamilton JN, Hollier LH: Thoracoabdominal aortic aneurysms. *In* Moore W [ed]: Vascular Surgery: A Comprehensive Review, 5th ed. Philadelphia, W. B. Saunders, 1998, p 419.)

management with continued pain; (4) aneurysmal degeneration; and (5) in selected Stanford type B patients as dictated by local medical center experience.[24, 25] Operations may include complete aortic replacement, fenestration, interposition grafting, aortic valve resuspension, or extra-anatomic bypass. These patients have very high complication and death rates and are often referred to centers specializing in complex aortic operations. Endovascular interventions have also made a debut in this disease process with balloon fenestration and endovascular stenting, and offer hope of reduced morbidity and mortality in combination with standard surgical techniques.[26]

PERIOPERATIVE CARE

The preoperative evaluation of patients undergoing aortic operations includes a complete history and physical examination with attention to optimizing organ function in prepara-

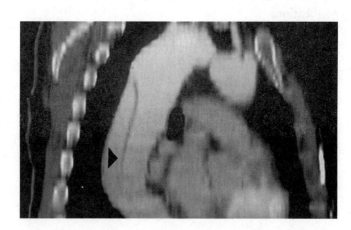

Figure 11–12. Helical CT scan in sagittal plane demonstrating a Stanford type B dissection flap *(black arrowhead)* limited to the descending thoracic aorta.

TABLE 11–3. **Teaching Plan***
(may vary from institution to institution)

PREOPERATIVE
Knowledge Deficit About Disease Process and Treatment
- Develop trusting relationship.
- Explain disease process and surgical procedure, using diagrams and written instructions when available.
- Teach and discuss with patient pre- and post-op routines: Assess level of understanding and reinforce teaching.

POSTOPERATIVE (Instructions for the patient)
Activity
- Ambulate as tolerated and increase activity gradually.
- Climbing stairs is acceptable in moderation.
- Going outdoors is acceptable.
- Regular exercise is important.
- No heavy lifting (more than 10 pounds) for 1 month after surgery.
- Sexual activity may be resumed in 3 to 4 weeks after discharge; discuss with physician if concerned.
- If leg swelling occurs, wear a 4-inch elastic bandage or elastic stockings when out of bed and elevate legs when sitting.

Bathing
- Bathing or showering is acceptable on the fifth day post-op. Clean the incision with mild soap and water, and dry it well.

Driving
- Driving is usually permissible after the first check-up with the doctor and you can move your legs normally. Do not drive if using narcotics or sleeping pills.

Wound Care
- No special care of wound is required unless otherwise indicated.

Avoiding Injury/Foot Care (see Table 12–6 for additional information)
- Inspect body daily and be aware of how incisions, feet, and legs look and feel post-op. This can help in recognition of early evidence of significant change.
- Wash feet regularly and dry well; have a podiatrist care for corns, calluses, or ingrown toenails.
- Protect limb from excessive heat or cold by avoiding heating pads, heat lamps, and hot water bottles on feet and legs.
- Avoid cream hair removers or any chemicals on legs. Use lanolin creams to prevent skin cracking.
- Avoid clothes such as tight socks, garters, or pantyhose that are constricting to the legs or feet.
- Wear shoes that fit well to avoid skin breakdown at pressure points. Wear socks or stockings with shoes at all times to prevent blistering, avoid walking barefoot, and inform physician if skin breakdown does occur.

Medications
- Explain medication, purpose of medication, dosage, and side effects.

Diet
- Inform patient that loss of appetite and changes in bowel habits may occur after surgery. Appetite will slowly return to normal.
- Instruct patient to maintain a diet that prevents extra pounds. If patient requires special diet, obtain a dietitian consult.

Risk Factor Modification
- To control progression of atherosclerosis, it is important to make the following lifestyle changes:
  - Control hypertension and diabetes.
  - Stop smoking.
  - Eat a low-fat, low-cholesterol diet.
  - Reduce stress in your life.
  - Exercise regularly.

TABLE 11–3. **Teaching Plan** *Continued*

POSTOPERATIVE
Abdominal Aortic Aneurysms
- There is evidence that the risk of abdominal aortic aneurysm (AAA) is greater in first-degree relatives of patients with AAA. Both brothers and sisters may be at increased risk of developing AAA. Please inform your siblings so they can discuss this with their doctor.

Medical Regimen/Indications for Physician Notification
- Emphasize the importance of follow-up visits with physician.
- Have the patient notify the doctor of any changes in incision, new or unusual drainage, change in color or amount of drainage, increase in temperature, swelling at the incision site, inflammation or tenderness around incision, any unusual or severe increase in pain in back or legs, sudden weight gain or swelling of feet or legs, loss of sensation or movement, unusual tingling/coldness/discoloration of the legs, or any skin breakdown on the foot.
- Inform patients to notify their physicians and/or dentist if they are undergoing any invasive procedure. Prophylactic antibiotics may be recommended during the first 6 months to 1 year after graft placement.

*By Victora A. Fahey, RN, MSN, CVN

tion for a major physiologic stress. Cardiac risk stratification is essential, as cardiac complications are the most frequent cause of early and late death, and aortic procedures are considered "high-risk" according to the American Heart Association guidelines.[2, 27, 28] Equally important is preparing the patient mentally for the operation. This includes a thorough discussion of the indications and conduct of the operation, alternative treatments, discussion of risks of the operation and alternatives, setting reasonable expectations of recovery, providing preoperative teaching, and initiating discharge planning (Table 11–3). This counseling needs to be performed in an informative but also reassuring manner that integrates patients actively into their care.

Patients having elective surgery without the need for preoperative hospitalization are routinely admitted on the morning of the operation without apparent increased morbidity. Reduction in intensive care use can be implemented by establishing a designated vascular unit with concentration of nursing skills.[29] However, in most hospitals, patients undergoing aortic surgery are admitted to the intensive care unit for invasive monitoring after operation. This includes arterial pressure measurement, arterial blood gas analysis, electrocardiography, bladder catheterization, pulse oximetry, and physical examination including monitoring of neurologic status, central organ perfusion and function, and ankle-brachial indices. Most patients require oxygen therapy and active topical warming. The necessity and benefits of routine pulmonary artery catheters are being questioned, and often only a central line is maintained for dependable intravenous access and infusion of vasoactive drugs.

Clinical pathways have become standard fare in medical centers. Clinical pathways with standardized order sheets may reduce unnecessary testing and with intermittent data analysis may identify areas of needed quality improvement.[30] Shifting care to the ambulatory setting during the preoperative and postoperative stages reduces hospital charges but has an unknown effect on total costs.[29] A clinical pathway for open surgical repair of an abdominal aortic aneurysm is given in Table 11–4.

SHORT-TERM COMPLICATIONS AND NURSING INTERVENTIONS

Early complications and nursing interventions after aortic surgery are summarized in Table 11–5. Many complications such as embolization occur intraoperatively, and patient

TABLE 11–4. **Clinical Pathway of Patient Undergoing Repair of Abdominal Aortic Aneurysm***

	POSTOP OR DAY DATE	ICU POD #1 DATE	FLOOR POD #1 DATE	POD #2 DATE	POD #3 DATE	POD #4 DATE	POD #5 DATE	POD #6 DATE
Vital Signs/ Parameters	VS q 1 hr I/O q 1 hr	VS q 1 hr I/O q 1 hr Weight	VS q 4 hr I/O q 4 hr Weight	VS q 4 hr I/O q 4 hr Weight	VS q 4 hr I/O q 4 hr Weight	VS q 8 hr I/O q 8 hr Weight	VS q 8 hr I/O q 8 hr Weight	VS q 8 hr I/O q 8 hr Weight
Pulse/Doppler Assessment	Doppler tones/ ABI q 2 hr	Doppler tones/ ABI q 2 hr	Pulse/Doppler tones q 4 hr	Pulse/Doppler tones q 4 hr	Pulse/Doppler tones q 4 hr	Pulse/Doppler tones q 8 hr	Pulse/Doppler tones q 8 hr	Pulse/Doppler tones q 8 hr
Tests	SMA-8, CBC, PT/PTT Chest x-ray ECG ABG prn Isoenzymes prn	SMA-8, CBC, PT/PTT prn ECG ABG prn Isoenzymes prn			CBC, SMA-8	Arterial blood flow study (selectively)		
Consult/ Discharge Planning		PCA prn Transfer to floor	Physical therapy prn	Discharge planner/social work prn Physical therapy prn	Discharge planner/social work prn	Discharge planner/social work prn	Rx and DC instruction sheet completed by MD May be discharged	Discharge Skilled nursing unit prn
IV and Oral Drugs	IV and A-line Antibiotic Pain medication prn Vasopressors prn	D/C A-line prn Pain medication prn Vasopressors prn	IV Pain medication prn	IV Pain medication prn	IV Pain medication prn	IV Pain medication prn	IV; DC prn Pain medication prn	Pain medication prn

226

Activity	Bed rest	OOB × 1 with assistance	OOB × 1 with assistance	Ambulate BID with assistance	Ambulate TID	Ambulate TID	Ambulate TID May shower	Ambulate TID May shower
Diet	NPO	NPO	NPO	NPO	Clear liquid diet after NG tube discontinued	Advance diet as tolerated	Low fat, low chol	Low fat, low chol
Treatment	NG tube Incentive spirometer TCDB q 2 hr O₂ prn Mouth care Incisional care Foley care	MD changes first dressing in AM NG tube prn Incentive spirometer TCDB q 2 hr Mouth care D/C Foley prn	NG tube prn Incentive spirometer TCDB q 2 hr Incisional care qd	NG tube prn Incentive spirometer TCDB q 2 hr Mouth care	Assess NG tube status prn Incisional care qd Mouth care	Assess NG tube status prn Incisional care qd Mouth care	Incisional care qd	Incisional care qd
Psychosocial	Provide support	Assess pt needs	Intervene w/ patient/family re psychosocial needs prn	Intervene w/patient/family re psychosocial needs prn	Intervene w/patient/family re psychosocial needs prn	Intervene w/patient/family re psychosocial needs prn	Intervene w/patient/family re psychosocial needs prn	Intervene w/patient/family re psychosocial needs prn
Patient Education	Assess patient's/family's level of understanding Discuss postoperative course with family	Assess patient's/family's level of understanding Discuss postoperative course with family			Review patient education material including risk reduction	Discharge teaching	Discharge teaching	Discharge teaching

*By Victora A. Fahey, RN, MSN, CVN.

OR = operating room; ICU = intensive care unit; POD = postoperative day; VS = vital signs; I/O = intake and output; ABI = ankle-brachial index; SMA = Sequential Multiple Analysis; CBC = complete blood count; PT/PTT = prothrombin time/partial thromboplastin time; ECG = electrocardiogram; ABG = arterial blood gas; PCA = patient-controlled analgesia; prn = as needed; Rx = prescription (drugs and other medicaments); DC = discharge; D/C = discontinue; A-line = arterial line; IV = intravenous; PO = orally; OOB = out of bed; BID = twice a day; TID = three times a day; NPO = nothing by mouth; NG = nasogastric; TCDB = turn, cough, deep breathe; qd = every day; pt = patient; q = every.

227

TABLE 11–5. **Potential Postoperative Complications, Causes, and Nursing Interventions**

COMPLICATION	PATHOGENESIS	NURSING INTERVENTIONS
Myocardial ischemia or infarction	Supply: coronary thrombosis, hypoperfusion, anemia, hypoxemia Demand: hypertension, tachycardia, hypothermia	Monitor oximetry, vital signs; implement adequate analgesic regimen; monitor electrocardiogram; restart appropriate cardiac medications; actively rewarm
Renal failure	Embolization, renal artery damage, renal vein ligation, ureteral injury, dehydration	Monitor blood pressure, urine output, creatinine, and fluid balance; check for hematuria
Congestive heart failure	Fluid overload, myocardial ischemia	Monitor fluid balance; anticipate "mobilization" of third-space fluids; initiate appropriate diuretic prescription
Atelectasis	Decreased lung function, incisional pain	Implement analgesic regimen; encourage incentive spirometry/deep breathing; assist early mobilization
Nosocomial infection	Invasive monitoring/tubes, aseptic technique break	Check dressings and observe quality of drainage; observe strict aseptic technique; monitor for fever
Hemorrhage	Technical error, coagulopathy, hypothermia, hypertension	Monitor vital signs and for abdominal or back pain or increase in abdominal girth; check laboratory values and notify physician if abnormal; check dressings and incisions for hematoma and bleeding, and transfuse as necessary; actively rewarm and maintain euthermia
Leg ischemia	Embolization, graft occlusion, hypoperfusion	Monitor limb pulses, color, temperature, motor and sensory functions and Doppler pressures; with axillofemoral and femoral-femoral grafts, also monitor donor limb pulses
Paraplegia	Spinal cord ischemia, hypotension, cord swelling	Monitor neurologic function; maintain spinal drainage as indicated
Ischemic colitis	Inferior mesenteric and hypogastric artery ligation, embolization, hypoperfusion	Maintain adequate hydration; monitor vital signs; monitor for abdominal distention or pain, excessive third spacing, elevated white blood count, and diarrhea
Dysrhythmia	Hypoxemia, myocardial ischemia, electrolyte imbalance, pulmonary artery catheter	Monitor oximetry, vital signs, and electrocardiogram; review chest radiography and lab values
Prolonged ileus	Extensive operation, other postoperative complications	Maintain nasogastric drainage; monitor for abdominal tenderness and distention; institute necessary nutritional support
Graft occlusion	Technical error, hypotension	Monitor limb perfusion and ankle pressures
Erectile dysfunction	Disruption of periaortic sympathetic plexus	Document baseline status, preoperative patient counseling, referral to urologist if necessary

morbidity can be minimized with good postoperative support. Some problems such as bleeding and graft occlusion mandate immediate recognition and treatment to avoid a fatality. Others require delicate management of fluid and electrolyte balance inasmuch as many of the patients have compromised cardiac, pulmonary, and renal function that limits their reserve. Foremost in the care of these patients is a familiarity with the normal postoperative track so that departure from this course is sensed early. Extensive team experience is an important component of the postoperative care of patients after aortic operations.

LATE OUTCOME

Segmental aortic graft replacement does not influence the natural history of either more proximal aortic or distal iliac arterial disease. Typical late complications are graft infection, limb occlusion, pseudoaneurysms, and development of secondary aneurysms.[2, 31–36] These complications are uncommon but often require reoperative aortic surgery several years after the first operation.

Subsequent Aneurysm

Rupture of a second aneurysm is a leading cause of death after abdominal aortic aneurysm repair.[2] In a recent survey of 10 years of reoperative aortic surgery at Northwestern, we identified 67 secondary aneurysms in 50 patients (Fig. 11–13). Presenting symptoms included rupture, limb ischemia, abdominal pain or mass, and hydronephrosis. One-third of subsequent aneurysms were not palpable and were asymptomatic. Reoperations occurred an average of 9 years after the first operation, and elective repair was safe compared with emergency operation. Similarly, of 26 patients presenting to the Mayo Clinic with

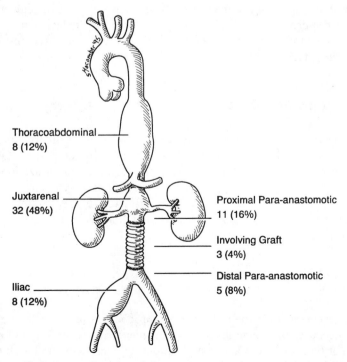

Figure 11–13. Location of 67 consecutive aneurysms in 50 patients.

rupture of a recurrent aneurysm, only one survived (4 percent).[37] This striking mortality after rupture requires that any patient fit to undergo an operation have a secondary aneurysm repaired. Finally, routine radiographic imaging is advisable at least every 5 years after aortic operations because these second aneurysms are often not palpable.[27, 38]

Subsequent Occlusion

Graft occlusion presents as recurrent claudication or limb ischemia, and these patients usually had occlusive disease as the indication for their primary surgery. Progression of disease below the aortobifemoral bypass is the most common cause of late graft occlusion. Several options, including observation, extra-anatomic bypass, and thrombectomy with outflow revision are available as alternatives to reoperative aortic surgery for graft occlusion.[39] Whether widespread use of angioplasty and primary stenting for occlusive disease will reduce the need for reoperative aortic surgery or increase the use of aortic surgery for management of failure of endovascular treatment is unknown. Nevertheless, mortality is 5 percent in elective reoperation similar to primary surgery.[40]

Subsequent Infection

Fortunately, graft infections occur in less than 1 percent of patients after aortic operation. Antibiotic prophylaxis is recommended for dental procedures and other interventions likely to result in bacteremia for the first 6 months after aortic graft placement. The interval between primary procedure and subsequent infection is shorter than with other late complications after aortic operation. Presenting symptoms include fever, abdominal or groin mass, groin wound infection, and the dramatic aortoenteric fistula. The last problem may manifest as exsanguinating gastrointestinal hemorrhage that requires emergent operation in an unstable patient. Graft infections often require total graft removal with extra-anatomic bypass and remain a challenging problem with high morbidity and mortality.[41] Other approaches in selected patients are in situ replacement with prosthetic grafts, cadaveric allografts, or autogenous femoral vein, and improved results have been described with these techniques.[42-44]

Long-Term Mortality

Patient longevity after aortic surgery is reduced in some studies, primarily due to increased heart-related mortality,[45] although in others it was found to be comparable to age-matched controls.[46, 47] These differences may be dependent on different utilization of coronary revascularization.[48] Overall survival is about 90 percent at 1 year and 65 percent at 5 years. Intensive study in this area is needed to evaluate whether strategies of coronary artery revascularization at the time of presentation with aortic disease will have significant benefits in long-term patient survival.

SUMMARY

Significant improvements over the past hemi-century have resulted in the development of safe surgical procedures for aortic disease. Aortic aneurysm, occlusion, and dissection are now treatable entities. Early and late complications are well defined. The future management of these disorders lies in the emerging endovascular and other minimally invasive therapies. Perioperative nursing care will remain an important component of high-quality patient care well into the next century.

References

1. Brewster DC, Darling RC: Optimal methods of aortoiliac reconstruction. Surgery 1978; 84:739–748.
2. Crawford ES, Saleh SA, Babb JW, et al: Infrarenal abdominal aortic aneurysm: Factors influencing survival after operation performed over a 25-year period. Ann Surg 1981; 193:699–709.
3. Taylor LM Jr, Porter JM: Abdominal aortic aneurysms. In Porter JM, Taylor LM Jr (eds): Basic Data Underlying Clinical Decision Making in Vascular Surgery. St. Louis, Quality Medical Publishing, 1994, pp 98–100.
4. Crawford ES, Cohen ES: Aortic aneurysm: A multifocal disease. Arch Surg 1982; 117:1393–1400.
5. Cronenwett JL: Abdominal aortic aneurysms: Predicting the natural history. In Yao JST, Pearce WH (eds): Progress in Vascular Surgery. Stamford, CT, Appleton & Lange, 1997, pp 127–138.
6. Sicard GA, Reilly JM, Rubin BG, et al: Transabdominal versus retroperitoneal incision for abdominal aortic surgery: Report of a prospective randomized trial. J Vasc Surg 1995; 21:174–83.
7. Paty PSK, Darling RC III, Chang BB, et al: A prospective randomized study comparing exclusion technique and endoaneurysmorrhaphy for treatment of infrarenal aortic aneurysm. J Vasc Surg 1997; 25:442–445.
8. Murayama KM, Grune MT, Baxter BT: Minimally invasive approaches to aneurysmal and occlusive disease of the aorta. In Yao JST, Pearce WH (eds): Techniques in Vascular and Endovascular Surgery. Stamford, CT, Appleton & Lange, 1998, pp 109–119.
9. Moore WS, Rutherford RB, for the EVT investigators: Transfemoral endovascular repair of abdominal aortic aneurysm: Results of the North American EVT phase I trial. J Vasc Surg 1996; 23:543–553.
10. Matsumura JS, Pearce WH, McCarthy WJ III, et al: Reduction in aortic aneurysm size; early results after endovascular graft placement. J Vasc Surg 1997; 25:113–123.
11. Ivancev K, Malina M, Lindblad B, et al: Abdominal aortic aneurysms: Experience with the Ivancev-Malmo endovascular system for aortomonoiliac stent-grafts. J Endovasc Surg 1997; 4:242–251.
12. McDaniel MD, Cronenwett JL: Basic data related to the natural history of intermittent claudication. Ann Vasc Surg 1989; 3:273–277.
13. Szilagyi DE, Elliott JP Jr, Smith RF, et al: A thirty-year survey of the reconstructive surgical treatment of aortoiliac occlusive disease. J Vasc Surg 1986; 3:421–436.
14. de Vries SO, Hunink MGM: Results of aortic bifurcation grafts for aortoiliac occlusive disease: A meta-analysis. J Vasc Surg 1997; 26:558–569.
15. McCarthy WJ, Mesh CL, Mcmillan WD, et al: Descending thoracic aorta-to-femoral artery bypass: Ten years' experience with a durable procedure. J Vasc Surg 1993; 17:336–438.
16. Ahn SS, Clem MF, Braithwaite BD, et al: Laparoscopic aortofemoral bypass. Ann Surg 1995; 222:677–683.
17. Dion YM, Katkhouda N, Rouleau C, Aucoin A: Laparoscopy-assisted aortobifemoral bypass. Surg Lap Endosc 1993; 3:425–429.
18. Fabiani J-N, Mercier F, Carpentier A, et al: Video-assisted aortofemoral bypass: Results in seven cases. Ann Vasc Surg 1997; 11:273–277.
19. Whyman MR, Fowkes FGR, Kerracher EMG, et al: Is intermittent claudication improved by percutaneous transluminal angioplasty? A randomized controlled trial. J Vasc Surg 1997; 26:551–557.
20. Marin ML, Veith FJ, Sanchez LA, et al: Endovascular aortoiliac grafts in combination with standard infrainguinal arterial bypasses in the management of limb-threatening ischemia: Preliminary report. J Vasc Surg 1995; 22:316–325.
21. Glower DD, Wolfe WG: Management of dissecting aortic aneurysms. In Yao JST, Pearce WH (eds): Aneurysms: New Findings and Treatments. East Norwalk, CT, Appleton & Lange, 1994.
22. Blanchard DG, Kimura BJ, Dittrich HC, DeMaria AN: Transesophageal echocardiography of the aorta. JAMA 1994; 272:546–51.
23. Nienaber CA, von Kodolitsch Y, Nicolas V, et al: The diagnosis of thoracic aortic dissection by noninvasive imaging procedures. N Engl J Med 1993; 328:1–8.
24. Glower DD, Speier RH, White WD, et al: Management and long-term outcome of aortic dissection. Ann Surg 1991; 214:31.
25. Fann JI, Smith JA, Miller DC, et al: Surgical management of aortic dissection during a 30-year period. Circulation 1995; 92[suppl II]:II-113.
26. Slonim SM, Nyman U, Semba CP, et al: Aortic dissection: Percutaneous management of ischemic complications with endovascular stents and balloon fenestration. J Vasc Surg 1996; 23:241.
27. Edwards JM, Teefey SA, Zierler RE, Kohler TR: Intraabdominal paraanastomotic aneurysms after aortic bypass grafting. J Vasc Surg 1992; 15:344–353.
28. Eagle KA, Brundage BH, Chaitman BR, et al: Guidelines for perioperative cardiovascular evaluation for noncardiac surgery: Report of the American College of Cardiology/American Heart Association Task Force

on Practice Guidelines (Committee on Perioperative Cardiovascular Evaluation for Noncardiac Surgery). Circulation 1996; 93:1278–1317.

29. Calligaro KD, Dandura R, Dougherty MJ, et al: Same-day admissions and other cost-saving strategies for elective aortoiliac surgery. J Vasc Surg 1997; 25:141–144.

30. Muluk SC, Painter L, Sile S, et al: Utility of clinical pathway and prospective case management to achieve cost and hospital stay reduction for aortic aneurysm surgery at a tertiary care hospital. J Vasc Surg 1997; 25:84–93.

31. Stoney RJ, Albo RJ, Wylie EJ: False aneurysms occurring after arterial grafting operations. Am J Surg 1965; 110:153–161.

32. Mikati A, Marache P, Watel A, et al: End-to-side aortoprosthetic anastomoses: Long-term computed tomography assessment. Ann Vasc Surg 1990; 4:584–591.

33. den Hoed PT, Veen HF: The late complications of aorto-ilio-femoral Dacron prostheses: Dilatation and anastomotic aneurysm formation. Eur J Vasc Surg 1992; 6:282–287.

34. Szilagyi DE, Smith RF, Elliott JP, et al: Anastomotic aneurysms after vascular reconstruction: Problems of incidence, etiology, and treatment. Surgery 1975; 78:800–816.

35. Crawford ES, Manning LG, Kelly TF: "Redo" surgery after operations for aneurysm and occlusion of the abdominal aorta. Surgery 1977; 81:41–52.

36. Coselli JS, LeMaire SA, Büket S, Berzin E: Subsequent proximal aortic operations in 123 patients with previous infrarenal abdominal aortic aneurysm surgery. J Vasc Surg 1995; 22:59–67.

37. Plate G, Hollier LA, O'Brien P, et al: Recurrent aneurysms and late vascular complications following repair of abdominal aortic aneurysms. Arch Surg 1985; 120:590–594.

38. Berman SS, Hunter GC, Smyth SH, et al: Application of computed tomography for surveillance of aortic grafts. Surgery 1995; 118:8–15.

39. Brewster DC, Meier GH, Darling RC, et al: Reoperation for aortofemoral graft limb occlusion: Optimal method and long-term results. J Vasc Surg 1987; 5:363–374.

40. Erdoes LS, Bernhard VM, Berman SS: Aortofemoral graft occlusion: Strategy and timing of reoperation. Cardiovasc Surg 1995; 3:277–283.

41. McCarthy WJ, McGee GS, Lin WW, et al: Axillary-popliteal artery bypass provides successful limb salvage after removal of infected aortofemoral grafts. Arch Surg 1992; 127:974–8.

42. Bandyk DF, Bergamini TM, Kinney EV, et al: In situ replacement of vascular prostheses infected by bacterial biofilms. J Vasc Surg 1991; 13:575–583.

43. Kieffer E, Bahnini A, Koskas F, et al: In situ allograft replacement of infected infrarenal aortic prosthetic grafts: Results in forty-three patients. J Vasc Surg 1993; 17:349–356.

44. Clagett GP, Valentine RJ, Hagino RT: Autogenous aortoiliac/femoral reconstruction from superficial femoral-popliteal veins: Feasibility and durability. J Vasc Surg 1997; 25:255–270.

45. Johnston KW and the Canadian Society for Vascular Surgery Aneurysm Study Group: Nonruptured abdominal aortic aneurysm: Six-year follow-up results from the multicenter prospective Canadian aneurysm study. J Vasc Surg 1994; 20:163–170.

46. Feinglass J, Cowper D, Dunlop D, et al: Late survival risk factors for abdominal aortic aneurysm repair: Experience from fourteen Department of Veterans Affairs hospitals. Surgery 1995; 118:16–24.

47. Stonebridge PA, Cullam MJ, Bradbury AW, et al: Comparison of long term survival after successful repair of ruptured and nonruptured abdominal aortic aneurysms. Br J Surg 1993; 80:585–586.

48. O'Hara PJ, Hertzer NH, Krajewski LP, et al: Ten year experience with abdominal aortic aneurysm repair in octogenarians: Early results and late complications. J Vasc Surg 1995; 21:830–8.

12

Arterial Reconstruction of the Lower Extremity

Victora A. Fahey, RN, MSN, CVN, and Walter J. McCarthy, MD

Innovations in surgical technique and perioperative management during the last three decades have made femoral artery reconstruction a standard in modern medicine. Patients who once faced primary amputation because of leg ischemia are now candidates for endovascular or bypass surgery. Although this field is continuously evolving, many basic principles are well established. Selection of patients for these procedures has been standardized, and the expected patency rates for the different operations and interventions are generally predictable.

Lower-extremity arterial occlusive disease is often a chronic process and when it becomes symptomatic, it can alter a person's lifestyle in many ways. Although it seldom causes death, it may result in limb loss and devastating disability. In contrast, acute arterial occlusion can be limb- as well as life-threatening. In both cases, the patients are usually elderly and often have many complicated medical problems. Because of these factors and the multisystem involvement of atherosclerosis, these patients are at high risk and present many challenging problems to nursing.

ANATOMY

The abdominal aorta bifurcates into the common iliac arteries, each of which divides into an internal iliac artery to supply the pelvis, and an external iliac artery. Anatomically the aortic bifurcation is at the level of the umbilicus. The external iliac artery becomes the common femoral artery when it passes under the inguinal ligament into the upper leg. The common femoral artery gives rise to the superficial femoral artery and the profunda femoris artery, which supplies the muscles of the thigh.

The superficial femoral artery becomes the popliteal artery as it passes through the adductor hiatus in the distal thigh. The popliteal artery gives rise to the anterior tibial artery. Several centimeters below the origin of the anterior tibial artery are the origins of the posterior tibial and peroneal arteries. The posterior tibial artery continues down the medial aspect of the leg, passing behind the medial malleolus into the foot. The anterior tibial artery lies in the anterior compartment of the leg and continues onto the dorsum of the foot as the dorsalis pedis artery. The peroneal artery courses through the center of the leg and terminates in the distal leg, giving rise to two major branches capable of serving as collateral circulation to the pedal arch. A figure illustrating lower-extremity arterial anatomy is found in Chapter 1 (Fig. 1–3).

DIAGNOSTIC EVALUATION

The history and physical examination of the patient with lower-extremity arterial disease are discussed in Chapter 4. In addition to eliciting a description of the patient's chief complaint, a complete evaluation includes assessment of risk factors for atherosclerosis, and a history of arterial occlusion in other systems (e.g., cerebrovascular disease, cardiac disorders, renal failure), an occupational profile, and medication history should be included. The physical examination can often determine the proximal site of involvement by pulse deficits and the presence of bruits.

The noninvasive laboratory plays an important role in the evaluation of patients with lower-extremity arterial disease. Segmental arterial pressures and/or pulse volume recordings provide an objective assessment of lower-extremity circulation by localizing the occlusive lesion and determining the degree of ischemia. They also provide a baseline against which future changes can be measured. Noninvasive testing is also helpful in predicting the possibility of healing following a toe amputation or other surgical procedures involving the foot.[1]

Yao determined the ankle-to-brachial blood pressure index (ABI) in normal individuals to be slightly greater than 1.0; in patients with intermittent claudication, the ABI averaged 0.6; and in patients with rest pain or gangrene, the ABI was less than 0.3.[2] It is important to obtain bilateral brachial pressures, because in order to determine the correct ratio, the ankle pressure must be divided by the highest brachial pressure. If a difference between the right and left arm pressures is greater than 20 mmHg, a subclavian stenosis may be present.

Occasionally, the need arises to perform segmental arterial blood flow measurements after the patient has exercised. This is because patients with claudication may have ankle pressures near normal at rest but develop a significant blood pressure drop following exercise. This decrease occurs as the lower-extremity muscular demand for blood outstrips the ability of the proximal diseased arterial segment to supply it. Routine exercise arterial blood flow studies are conducted by measuring ankle pressures before and after a standard walk on a motorized treadmill.

Ultrasonic duplex scanning is used in establishing the presence of an adequate saphenous or upper-extremity vein for bypass grafting and it also assists in planning the incision. The course of the veins may be mapped on the skin to guide the surgeon in the operating room. The aforementioned tests are discussed in greater detail in Chapter 5.

Other diagnostic tests may be required for patients with pain in the lower extremities that does not appear to be arterial occlusive disease. For example, electromyography, measurements of nerve conduction velocity, and lumbar spine x-rays may be useful in patients with diabetic neuropathy or neurogenic claudication caused by spinal stenosis. Laboratory testing for coagulopathies should be analyzed in patients with atypical arterial thrombosis (see Chapter 9). In the case of acute arterial occlusion, echocardiography, transesophageal echocardiography, Holter monitoring, and computed tomography (CT) scanning may be performed to identify a proximal source of emboli.[3]

Once the diagnosis of arterial insufficiency has been demonstrated by noninvasive testing and therapeutic intervention is contemplated, angiography or magnetic resonance angiography (MRA) may be performed. Angiography, which demonstrates the location and extent of arterial disease, is the most precise diagnostic tool for the assessment of arterial anatomy in the lower extremity and is used to depict the aorta, iliac, femoral, popliteal, and tibial arterial segments. MRA is an evolving technology (see Chapter 6 for further details).

Because the etiology, clinical manifestations, and treatment vary between chronic and acute arterial ischemia, further discussion will be divided into chronic and acute problems.

CHRONIC ARTERIAL ISCHEMIA

Etiology

Atherosclerosis is the most common cause of chronic arterial occlusive disease of the lower extremity. The risk factors for atherosclerosis of the lower extremity are the same as for the other vascular beds: advanced age, male sex, diabetes mellitus, cigarette smoking, hypertension, and increased lipid levels.[4] Rare conditions including popliteal artery entrapment and adventitial cystic disease of the popliteal artery also can result in arterial occlusion. Other causes of chronic arterial occlusion are discussed in Chapter 1. The superficial femoral and the proximal popliteal arteries are the most susceptible to atherosclerosis; however, the aortoiliac segment and the tibial and peroneal arteries are also commonly affected. The arterial stenosis or occlusion that occurs reduces the blood flow to the lower limb during exercise or at rest.

Clinical Manifestations and Natural History

Patients with chronic arterial occlusive disease most often complain of cramping pain in the muscles of the lower extremity during exercise that disappears after rest. This condition is known as *intermittent claudication*. The distance a patient can walk before the onset of pain is usually consistent for that patient. The occluded arterial segment is the one just proximal to the symptomatic muscle group; thus, superficial femoral artery occlusion causes calf pain, external iliac artery disease produces thigh pain, and aortic disease is heralded by cramping of the buttock muscles (see Fig. 4–5). Most patients with claudication will remain stable throughout their lifetime, with approximately 20 percent of patients deteriorating to the extent that incapacitating symptoms require surgical intervention,[5] and ultimate limb loss limited to 1 percent per year.[6]

As arterial occlusive disease progresses to involve multiple arterial segments, patients complain of continuous pain even at rest. *Rest pain* is a specific term referring to discomfort in the forefoot, often across the metatarsal heads, that is aggravated by elevation and diminished by hanging the foot in a dependent position. It usually begins as an isolated nocturnal event reflecting a patient's decreased cardiac output while asleep and the effect of the relative elevation of the extremity in the supine position. It occurs when resting blood flow is insufficient to meet the maintenance metabolic requirements for nonexercising tissue.[7]

Tissue necrosis and *gangrene* may also be present with severe disease. Areas of an ischemic foot subject to local pressure that may develop skin necrosis include the medial and lateral metatarsal heads and the tip of the heel. Skin ulcerations heal slowly, if at all, in the ischemic limb. Areas of tissue necrosis may degenerate to wet or dry gangrene. Dry gangrene is a mummification of tissue, which, if left untreated, may progress slowly to involve the entire foot or leg. Wet gangrene manifested by blebs, bullae, and violaceous discoloration implies significant underlying tissue infection and is often complicated by a rapid progression. Critical ischemia, as evidenced by rest pain or tissue necrosis, is associated with inevitable amputation for most patients unless surgical correction is undertaken.

One of the hallmarks of chronic arterial insufficiency is the dusky, purplish discoloration of the foot and leg when the foot is placed in a dependent position. This "dependent rubor" changes to a characteristic chalky white "pallor on elevation" of the extremity. Changes in the skin related to insufficient delivery of nutrients by the inadequate blood flow result in atrophy and dryness, with thin, shiny skin and diminished or absent hair growth. The toenails become brittle and opaque, and the affected extremity is often cooler to touch than the opposite foot (see Chapter 4).

Medical Treatment

The treatment of lower-extremity ischemia is based on the severity of the patient's symptoms and the overall medical condition of the individual. Full evaluation is necessary prior to arterial surgery. Some patients may require carotid endarterectomy or coronary artery bypass grafting before femoral reconstruction is undertaken.

The majority of patients with claudication are managed conservatively with an exercise program and modification of associated risk factors, especially smoking cessation. However, some patients who are younger or severely disabled by their claudication may undergo an endovascular or a bypass procedure (see Chapter 10).

Exercise Therapy

Exercise therapy designed to increase exercise tolerance has been found to be the most consistently effective medical treatment for claudication.[8] Studies report an increase in treadmill exercise performance and decreased claudication during exercise.[9] Patients are advised to walk to the limit of their discomfort on a daily basis to develop collaterals in the affected leg. The precise mechanism accounting for the improvement in pain-free walking capacity remains unknown but probably involves adaptation of skeletal muscle to hypoxic conditions.[4]

Exercise therapy may also be used in conjunction with bypass surgery. Additive beneficial effects of bypass surgery and subsequent exercise training when compared with operation or exercise training alone have been reported. Exercise therapy may be part of a vascular rehabilitation program (see Chapter 10).

Risk Factor Modification

The risk factors for atherosclerosis of the lower-extremity arteries are the same as those for other vascular beds and include advanced age, male sex, diabetes mellitus, cigarette smoking, hypertension, and increased lipid levels.[4] Chapter 10 discusses risk factor modification in more detail.

Pharmacologic Therapy

The role of pharmacologic therapy in the treatment of chronic lower-extremity arterial occlusive disease is yet to be defined. In the last few years, there has been increased development of some new pharmacologic agents potentially useful in the treatment of lower-extremity ischemia. These include antithrombotic agents (anticoagulants, antiplatelet agents, thrombolytic agents, and dextran), rheologic agents, prostaglandins, calcium channel blockers, lipid-lowering agents, and others.[7, 10] Chapters 8 and 10 discuss some of these drugs in more detail.

Thrombolytic therapy has been used selectively for the treatment of lower-extremity arterial occlusion. The Surgery versus Thrombolysis for Ischemia of the Lower Extremity (STILE) trial was designed to investigate the results of traditional surgical revascularization compared with those of thrombolytic therapy. This trial concluded that surgical revascularization for lower-extremity native artery occlusions is more effective and durable than thrombolytic therapy. Thrombolysis used initially provides a reduction in the extent of the surgical procedure for a majority of patients; however, long-term outcome is inferior, particularly for patients who have a femoropopliteal occlusion, diabetes, or critical ischemia.[11]

Chapters 8 and 10 discuss pharmacologic therapy in the treatment of arterial occlusive disease in detail.

Radiologic Interventional Procedures

Percutaneous transluminal balloon angioplasty (PTLA) and stenting have become an accepted therapy for certain iliac artery stenoses and are selectively used in more distal arteries.[12, 13] Results of arterial dilation/stenting below the inguinal ligament are not as promising as those at the iliac level, but some success has been reported. The long-term role of endovascular intervention in the treatment of arterial disease is yet to be determined. Angioplasty may be used in conjunction with surgery, such as with the stenting of a proximal iliac lesion prior to a femoral-to-popliteal artery bypass.[14] Refer to Chapter 6 for additional information.

Surgical Treatment

Patients with claudication may be candidates for bypass surgery if the disability severely limits their lifestyle or occupational activity. In the presence of rest pain, a nonhealing ulceration, gangrene of the toes or foot, or embolization from a peripheral aneurysm, surgical revascularization is usually necessary to restore and/or maintain limb viability. After bypass surgery, rest pain is relieved, ulcerations heal with standard attention, and gangrenous tissue can usually be amputated with prompt healing. An arterial reconstruction may thus allow substitution of a minor toe or forefoot amputation for an inevitable below-the-knee or above-the-knee amputation. Patients with limb-threatening ischemia with no potential for rehabilitation or who are bedridden with limited life expectancy may be treated conservatively.

Because arterial disease is often present in several areas, it is essential to determine the arterial segment with the hemodynamically significant stenosis responsible for the patient's problems. For example, the stenosis may be at the aortoiliac level, affecting arterial inflow to the legs. It is a fundamental principle that the inflow should be corrected before the outflow to the foot is repaired. This prevents a newly placed bypass graft from thrombosing because of inadequate blood flow through the graft.

If the aortoiliac segment is diseased as well as the femoral/popliteal/tibial arteries, an aorta–femoral artery graft (see Fig. 11–7) or angioplasty may be necessary to provide inflow prior to femoral bypass surgery. Patients who cannot tolerate an abdominal operation may undergo an axillofemoral reconstruction (see Fig. 11–8). This operation supplies the legs with blood flow using one of the axillary arteries placed through a graft tunneled in the subcutaneous tissue. If iliac blood flow to the noninvolved leg is adequate, a femoro-femoral bypass graft is sometimes used.

After it is ascertained that the inflow to the femoral system is adequate, femoral reconstruction can be undertaken. The two traditional approaches for correcting arterial occlusion are (1) to position a bypass around the obstruction and (2) to open the artery and remove the obstruction by performing an endarterectomy. Thirty years of experience has established bypass of an arterial occlusion as the dominant technique, but endarterectomy is occasionally used in the correction of lower-extremity ischemia.

The choice of surgical procedure depends on the level of arterial disease. Selecting the proper bypass involves determining the best proximal site for inflow and the best distal site for outflow (Fig. 12–1). Generally, the proximal anastomosis is anastomosed to the common femoral artery. Under unusual circumstances, the graft may be attached to the limb of an aortobifemoral graft, the superficial femoral artery, the popliteal artery, or the deep femoral artery. The distal graft is anastomosed to the most cephalic portion of the leg that allows unobstructed blood flow to the foot.

Bypass Procedures

Femoropopliteal Bypass

The most common point of arterial occlusion in the leg is at the lower portion of the superficial femoral artery as it passes through the medial adductor muscles just above the knee. Therefore, a femoral–to–above-knee popliteal graft is frequently performed. If the upper popliteal artery is diseased, the graft may be sewn to the below-knee popliteal

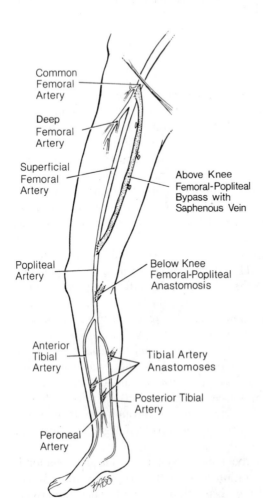

Figure 12–1. Femoral artery bypass grafts may be anastomosed to the popliteal or any one of the 3 tibial arteries. (From McCarthy WJ, Williams LR: Femoral artery reconstruction. Critical Care Quarterly 1985; 8:43. Reprinted with permission of Aspen Publishers, Inc., © 1985.)

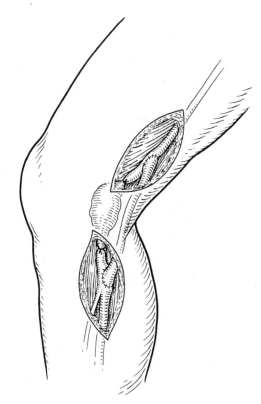

Figure 12–2. Popliteal artery aneurysm repair. (From Clyne CA: Aneurysm of the popliteal artery. In Bell PR, Jamieson CW, Ruckley CV [eds]: Surgical Management of Vascular Disease. Philadelphia, WB Saunders, 1992, p 880.)

artery. A popliteal aneurysm is ligated above and below the aneurysm with the bypass placed around the ligatures to eliminate it from the circulation (Fig. 12–2).

Infrapopliteal Bypass

In the event that there are no tibial branches remaining in continuity with the popliteal artery, the graft may be sewn directly to one of the three tibial/peroneal arteries. The tibial vessel of largest diameter with the least disease and the best outflow to the foot should be selected for the distal anastomosis. Arterial reconstructions to the small arteries of the distal leg and foot, most frequently the dorsalis pedis artery, have also been performed.[15]

If the tibial vessels are poorly visualized on the preoperative arteriogram, an arteriogram may be performed in the operating room at the time of surgery. After completion of the bypass, an arteriogram is usually performed in the operating room to identify technical problems or an arteriovenous fistula that may be present after an in situ bypass. A duplex scan may also be used in assessing the bypass at this time. If a technical flaw is discovered, it can be corrected while the bypass is still exposed.

Axillopopliteal Bypass

An axillopopliteal bypass (Fig. 12–3) is used when amputation is otherwise imminent and a more standard arterial reconstruction is not feasible because of groin infection, previous scarring, or very rarely because of extensive bilateral atherosclerosis of the femoral arteries, when the femoral vessels would not provide sufficient outflow to support a graft limb.[16]

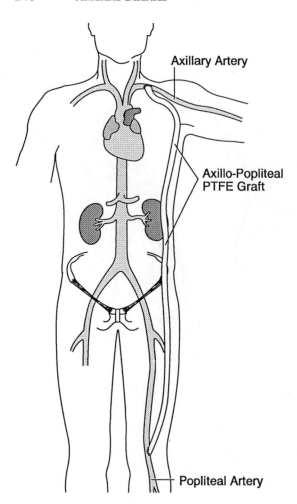

Axillary Artery

Axillo-Popliteal PTFE Graft

Popliteal Artery

Figure 12–3. Axillopopliteal bypass. PTFE = polytetrafluoroethylene.

Polytetrafluoroethylene (PTFE) is usually used for these grafts and there may be an advantage to using a ringed (externally supported) graft.

Obdurator Foramen Bypass

The obdurator foramen bypass (Fig. 12–4) is used to revascularize an extremity in which the femoral area is infected or inappropriate for dissection because of previous surgery or previous irradiation. The graft originates in the retroperitoneum at a point proximal to the infection and is sewn to the iliac artery. It is then brought through the obturator foramen in a clean field and anastomosed to a distal uninvolved artery.[17]

Endarterectomy/Profundaplasty

Endarterectomy may be useful as an adjunct to bypass grafting or alone in the repair of a stenotic profunda femoris artery (the deep femoral artery). The profunda femoris artery is the main component of an important collateral system that provides arterial flow when there is occlusive disease of inflow arteries and also provides alternative flow to the foot in presence of superficial artery occlusion. A patch angioplasty using vein or prosthetic

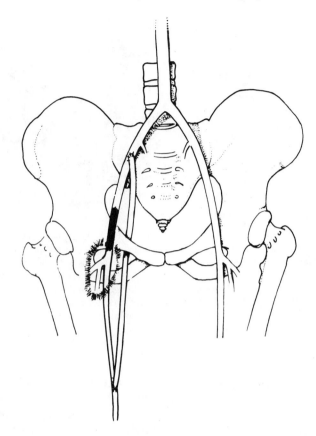

Figure 12–4. Obturator foramen bypass. (From Brief DK, Brener BJ: Extraanatomic bypass. In Wilson SE, Veith FJ, Hobson RW II, Williams RA [eds]: Vascular Surgery Principles and Practice. New York, McGraw-Hill, 1987, p 422.)

material may also be used to widen the lumen of the profunda after endarterectomy; this is called a profundaplasty.[18]

Graft Material

A variety of conduits are available for bypass grafting to the lower-extremity arteries. Two types of conduits are used: autogenous (vein) and synthetic (artificial) grafts.

Reversed Greater Saphenous Vein

The saphenous vein has a series of valves permitting blood flow only in the direction of the heart. The traditional way of using autologous saphenous vein tissue as an arterial bypass is to reverse the vein, which allows blood to flow unobstructed through the vein valves. This reversal necessitates attaching the small end of the saphenous vein to the common femoral artery and the large end of the saphenous vein to a smaller-diameter popliteal or tibial artery at the distal anastomosis.

In Situ Saphenous Vein

The inevitable size mismatch of the reversed vein graft prompted the development of a technique using the vein in its natural position without reversal; this is known as the *in situ technique*. Besides the obvious advantage of anastomotic size match, the in situ

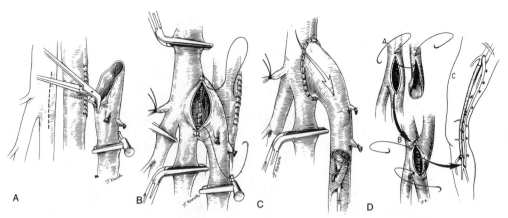

Figure 12–5. A, In the in situ method, the saphenofemoral junction is transected in the groin, the venotomy in the femoral vein oversewn, and the proximal end of the saphenous vein prepared for anastomosis. **B,** After the first venous valve is excised under direct vision, the graft is anastomosed end to side to the femoral artery. **C,** Flow is then restored through the vein graft and the valvulotome inserted through side branches at appropriate intervals to lyse residual valve cusps. **D,** The distal anastomosis is completed, in this case at the level of the distal tibioperoneal trunk. (From Whittemore AD: Infrainguinal bypass. In Rutherford RB: Vascular Surgery, 4th ed. Philadelphia, WB Saunders, 1995, p 800.)

technique provides physiologic preservation of venous endothelium. This is because the long saphenous vein is not entirely removed from its bed in the subcutaneous position, and therefore it retains its adventitial blood supply. Deprivation of a vein's blood supply for longer than 30–40 minutes creates a flow surface that is conducive to thrombus deposition, particularly in low-flow states. In addition, this technique allows more frequent use of small veins and thus a higher vein utilization rate.[19] Disadvantages of the in situ technique include problems with rendering valves incompetent (retained valve cusps), the learning curve of the surgeon, and difficulty in locating and controlling arteriovenous (AV) fistulae.

In situ surgery entails mobilization of the vein's ends for construction of the proximal and distal arterial anastomoses, removal of the valvular obstructions to arterial flow by rendering the valves incompetent, and interruption of the venous branches to prevent AV fistulae (Fig. 12–5).[20] The vein may be exposed through multiple interrupted (closed) or continuous (open) incisions (Fig. 12–6). Angioscopic guidance providing direct visualization for valve interruption and localization of AV fistulae has increased the use of the

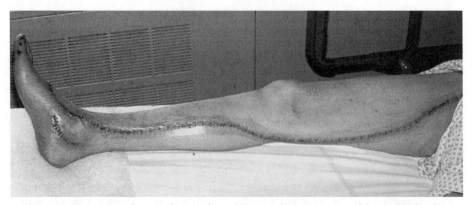

Figure 12–6. Incision of in situ bypass along the entire leg to expose and ligate arteriovenous (AV) fistulae.

closed technique.[21] The use of such minimally invasive techniques has resulted in fewer wound complications, diminished pain, and possibly decreased length of hospital stay. However, the superiority of any one in situ technique over another has not yet been clarified.

Nonreversed Greater Saphenous Vein

The use of a nonreversed greater saphenous vein graft provides optimal size match between the artery and vein at each anastomosis. The most common indication for use of this graft is when a contralateral greater saphenous vein is required for a long bypass graft. One study produced results equivalent to those achieved in a series of in situ bypass procedures.[22]

Lesser Saphenous Vein

Although the lesser saphenous vein may be used, it has limitations because it extends only from the ankle to the knee.[23]

Arm Vein

Cephalic and basilic veins (Fig. 12–7) from the upper extremity constitute viable alternatives for use as infrapopliteal bypass grafts when other sources of autogenous vein are

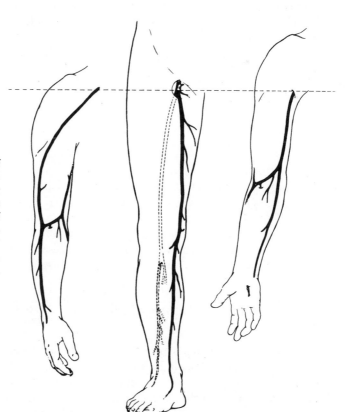

Figure 12–7. Relative lengths of the cephalic and basilic veins as potential bypass grafts in the lower extremity. (From Andros G, Harris RW, Dulawa LB, et al: The use of arm veins as lower extremity arterial conduits. In Kempczinski RF [ed]: The Ischemic Leg. Chicago, Year Book Medical Publishers, 1985, p 427.)

unavailable (utilized for coronary artery or peripheral bypass surgery, a vein stripping, or the vein is inadequate, e.g., with phlebitis, variations in venous anatomy, chronic venous insufficiency, or a small saphenous vein).[23] The preferred arm vein for grafting is the forearm cephalic vein. When a single arm vein is not long enough to span blocked segments, two or three veins can be spliced to create a composite arm vein graft. Disadvantages of arm veins are that they tend to be thin walled, thus requiring careful dissection; their use is associated with an increased incidence of aneurysmal change; they may be too small; and they are prone to intimal fibrosis.[1, 24]

There are several recommendations for successful use of arm veins as conduits. These include protocols to preserve arm veins, the education of patients and health care professionals, and the training of surgical nurses related to the maneuvers for arm vein implantation. Use of physician orders, periodic in-service training programs, posting of signs in patient rooms, and wrapping the patient's arm with gauze can be helpful. The protection of arm veins from venipuncture or intravenous therapy is essential to prevent phlebitis.[25]

Synthetic Prosthetic

The choice of conduit in the absence of adequate vein is made of expanded PTFE.[26] Dacron may also be used. Prosthetic grafts can also be used for extended conduits such as axillary-to-femoral (see Fig. 11–8) or axillary-to-popliteal artery bypasses (see Fig. 12–3). Potential advantages of a prosthetic bypass are decreased dissection in an ischemic limb and decreased time of operation.

Because results achieved with distal PTFE grafts have proved to be less than optimal, several modifications of the standard approach have been attempted. A collar of vein may be interposed between the distal arteriotomy and the distal PTFE graft (Miller cuff) or a vein patch across the distal anastomosis (Taylor patch) to decrease the chance of smooth muscle AV fistula constructed in conjunction with the distal anastomosis or at a more remote site in an effort to augment flow through the prosthetic graft and enhance patency.[1]

Umbilical Vein

Grafts constructed from human umbilical cord vein may be used for arterial bypass surgery. Umbilical veins are treated with glutaraldehyde, which acts as a tanning agent, increasing strength and also preventing antigenic recognition and rejection by the graft recipient. They are wrapped with a Dacron mesh to help prevent aneurysm formation. Although the patency rate compares favorably to that of PTFE grafts, there remains a high incidence of aneurysmal degeneration with these grafts.[27]

Composite Sequential Bypass Graft

A composite-sequential bypass graft is made up of prosthetic material and autogenous vein. A prosthetic graft, usually PTFE, is used from the femoral to the popliteal level and a vein graft is then placed directly onto the PTFE material and brought down through an anastomotic tunnel to the selected site for tibial outflow (Fig. 12–8). These grafts may be necessary because of the lack of available vein length.[28]

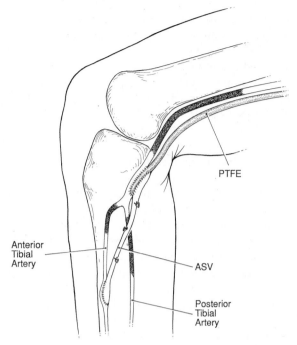

Figure 12–8. Composite-sequential bypass graft. PTFE = polytetrafluoroethylene; ASV = autogenous saphenous vein. (From Mc-Carthy WJ, Pearce WH, Flinn WR, et al: Long-term evaluation of composite sequential bypass for limb threatening ischemia. J Vasc Surg 1992; 15(5):765.)

Results

Technical advances in the last decade have contributed to improved success with several studies documenting the ability of surgical revascularization to provide durable salvage of ischemic limbs in 85–90 percent of cases.[29–31] The long-term patency and success of these grafts are influenced by a variety of factors, including the indications for surgery, the bypass conduit, the anatomic and hemodynamic characteristics of the inflow artery, the site of the distal anastomosis and associated outflow, distal arterial anatomy, diabetes, smoking, the use of anticoagulation, primary or secondary procedure, the progression of atherosclerosis, and the development of fibromuscular hyperplasia. Unless patients have been stratified for these factors, it is difficult to draw meaningful conclusions from the results of numerous studies of lower-extremity bypass surgery.[4]

Intact greater saphenous vein is the conduit of choice for an infrainguinal bypass.[4] The superior patency of vein grafts over PTFE prosthetic conduit is well documented by a multicenter randomized trial. At 5 years, the primary patency rate for autogenous vein grafts to the popliteal artery was 68 percent.[32] In grafts to the infrapopliteal artery, the 5-year patency rate for vein was 49 percent compared to 12 percent patency rate for PTFE.[32]

PTFE has been shown to provide patency nearly equal to that of saphenous vein when placed in the femoral–to–above-knee popliteal position. However, PTFE is considerably inferior to saphenous vein when placed below the popliteal artery.[32–34] Results of a multicenter randomized prospective trial demonstrated there was no statistically significant difference in observed primary or secondary patency rates between PTFE and Dacron grafts used in the above-knee position.[35]

The question of which vein graft is the best conduit remains an unanswered question requiring further study.[1] In several studies, long-term outcome of femoropopliteal bypass was satisfactory using both in situ and reversed vein grafts.[36, 37] The results achieved with alternate autogenous vein grafts (arm veins, lesser saphenous veins) are generally inferior to those achieved with intact ipsilateral greater saphenous vein. One study demonstrated that the patency results of the alternate vein bypass graft to infrapopliteal arteries are superior to those achieved with prosthetic grafting.[38] However, the results of alternate autogenous vein bypass are not clearly superior to those achieved with prosthetic grafting, especially in view of recently reported improved results of prosthetic grafting using modified anastomoic techniques and long-term anticoagulation with warfarin.[39]

Composite sequential bypass grafts have better patency than an all-prosthetic bypass to the tibial level, providing a 40 percent patency rate at 4 years.[28] Benefits are compounded if the venous graft crosses the knee joint.

Bypass and Free Tissue Transfer

Some patients present with such extensive tissue loss that primary wound healing is not expected even after successful arterial reconstruction. This situation, most often seen in diabetic patients with severe peripheral neuropathy, occurs on the weight-bearing plantar surface of the foot. The performance of distal arterial reconstruction and microvascular tissue transfer provides an opportunity for limb salvage in these patients who would normally be candidates for amputation. Advantages to free tissue transfer include: (1) adequate debridement of infected tissue is possible; (2) adequate bulk is restored to weight-bearing surface; (3) local infection is better controlled; and (4) neovascularization from the free flap may improve local tissue perfusion. Close collaboration between the plastic and vascular surgeons is necessary.[40]

Amputation

In some neglected cases, extensive gangrene with major foot destruction, infection, or osteomyelitis is best handled by a primary leg amputation. This approach also is used if no distal arteries remain for a bypass. All effort is made to preserve as much of the extremity as possible so that the potential for rehabilitation is optimal.

Adjunctive Medical Management

The variable patency of all lower-extremity arterial bypasses, regardless of the type of conduit, suggests the need for adjunctive postoperative thrombotic therapy. There is no consensus as to the optimal form of pharmacotherapy that should be used to prevent graft failure. A number of agents are used, including aspirin, dipyridamole, dextran, low-dose heparin, intravenous heparin, low-molecular-weight heparin (Lovenox), and warfarin.[10]

Antiplatelet drugs are believed to inhibit platelet aggregation, preventing their deposition on the surface of thrombogenic grafts, and may help prevent perianastomotic fibrous hyperplasia. Aspirin, 325 mg/day, may be useful in patients undergoing prosthetic femoro-popliteal grafts. In patients with vein grafts, aspirin is recommended to reduce the incidence of myocardial infarction and stroke.[10]

Warfarin has been used in patients undergoing infrainguinal bypass surgery in an attempt to decrease the incidence of graft failure. The effectiveness of warfarin varies among studies and its exact role remains unanswered.[41] It may be recommended for patients undergoing prosthetic bypasses, long bypasses to small arteries, composite bypasses or complex procedures, or redo of a failed bypass graft, and after a compromised operation, i.e., with poor distal runoff or a very small diameter vein graft.[10, 42] It may also have a role in patients with hypercoagulable states and grafts.[42] Warfarin may be used in conjunction with aspirin. Hemorrhagic complications remain and risk needs to be addressed. There is an important need for clinical trials evaluating warfarin and aspirin in the treatment of these patients.

The principal difference between thrombotic occlusion of vein and prosthetic bypassses has to do with surface thrombogenicity. Because vein grafts are lined with endothelium, they are inherently less thrombogenic than prosthetic grafts. Vein grafts may lose variable amounts of their endothelial lining during harvesting and implantation, which may contribute to early occlusion. This suggests the rationale for early thrombotic therapy that could be discontinued after healing at anastomotic sites and repavement of graft with endothelium. Prosthetic grafts, however, remain highly thrombogenic.[10]

When perioperative anticoagulation is recommended, low-molecular-weight heparin (LMWH) provides a safe and effective alternative to intravenous heparin for infrageniculate PTFE bypass graft procedures.[43] LMWH may reduce the number of postoperative hospital days and coagulation studies by allowing discharge before therapeutic anticoagulation with warfarin.[44]

Dextran 40 may also be beneficial in preventing postoperative thrombosis following lower-extremity bypass. It should not be used routinely because of its side effects and cost and should be reserved for complex cases.[10]

Refer to Chapter 8 for additional information.

ACUTE ARTERIAL ISCHEMIA

Acute arterial occlusion (AAO) of the lower extremity refers to the sudden interruption of arterial blood supply. Regardless of etiology, AAO differs from chronic occlusion in that good collateral circulation is lacking. With chronic occlusion, symptoms develop slowly because as the artery narrows, collateral vessels develop around the blockage. With abrupt occlusion, critical ischemia of the extremity results within hours. AAO represents a vascular emergency that may result in both limb loss and life.

Etiology

Embolism, thrombosis, and trauma are the primary causes of acute arterial occlusion in the lower extremity. Venous outflow obstruction, including phlegmasia cerulea dolens and compartment syndrome, and low-flow states may also result in acute occlusion (Table 12–1).

Embolism

Emboli are fragments of thrombus, atheromatous debris, tumor, or other material that has migrated from another source. Causes of embolism are included in Table 12–1. Many patients with embolization of cardiac origin are in atrial fibrillation or recently converted from fibrillation to a sinus rhythm (Fig. 12–9). Mitral stenosis produces a high left atrial pressure, and stasis predisposes the affected person to thrombus formation. Following myocardial infarction, thrombotic debris forms on the surface of the injured endocardium. Thrombus may embolize from the sewing rings of a prosthetic valve or from deposits on the valve leaflets. With appropriate anticoagulation and the introduction of tissue valves, there has been a reduced incidence of embolization from these sources.[45]

Noncardiac (artery to artery) emboli originate from proximal aortic plaque, such as an ulcerated aortic atheroma or an aneurysm usually occluding smaller distal vessels (see Fig. 12–9).[46] Paradoxical emboli, in which venous thrombus embolizes into the arterial circulation, can occur in the presence of an intracardiac right-to-left shunt such as a patent foramen ovale. The source of embolism remains unknown in approximately 5–20 percent of cases of acute ischemia.

TABLE 12–1. **Etiology of Acute Arterial Ischemia**

Embolic	Traumatic
Heart	Penetrating trauma
Atherosclerotic heart disease	Direct vessel injury
Coronary heart disease	Indirect injury
Acute myocardial infarction	Missile emboli
Dysrhythmia	Proximity
Valvular heart disease	Blunt trauma
Rheumatic	Intimal flap
Degenerative	Spasm
Congenital	Iatrogenic
Bacterial	Intimal flap
Prosthetic	Dissection
Artery-to-artery	Presence of medical device
Aneurysm	Space-occupying thrombosis
Atherosclerotic plaque	Clot propagation
Idiopathic	External compression
Paradoxical embolus	Drug abuse
Thrombosis	Intra-arterial administration leading to
Atherosclerosis	mycotic aneurysm
Aneurysm of popliteal artery	Drug toxicity
Arterial dissection	Contaminant
Low-flow states	Microembolization
Congestive heart failure	**Outflow Venous Occlusion**
Hypovolemia	Compartment syndrome
Hypotension	Phlegmasia cerulea dolens
Hypercoagulable states	**Low-Flow States**
Disseminated intravascular coagulation	Cardiogenic shock
Antithrombin III, protein C, or protein S	Hypovolemic shock
deficiency	Drug effect
Malignancy-related heparin-induced	Mesenteric
thrombocytopenia and thrombosis	Digoxin
syndrome (HITTS)	H_2 blockers
Polycythemia vera	
Collagen vascular disease	
Vascular grafts	
Progression of disease	
Intimal hyperplasia	
Mechanical failure	

Adapted from Quinones-Baldrich WJ: Acute arterial and graft occlusion. In Moore W (ed): Vascular Surgery: A Comprehensive Review. Philadelphia, WB Saunders, 1998, p 670.

Most emboli lodge where the vessel suddenly tapers or branches and consequently are located most often in the lower extremities (Fig. 12–10). An embolus that lodges at the bifurcation of the aorta is known as a saddle embolus.[47]

Thrombosis

Acute arterial thombosis may be the result of local arterial factors or a consequence of systemic diseases (see Table 12–1). Local factors include thrombosis of a previously narrowed atherosclerotic artery and a popliteal aneurysm. Popliteal aneurysms, which account for 70 percent of all peripheral aneurysms, contain intraluminal clot, which may

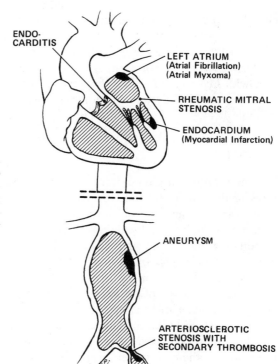

Figure 12–9. Sources of emboli. Most emboli originate in the diseased heart, but they may also represent debris from aneurysm or atherosclerotic arteries. (From Zimmerman JJ, Fogarty TJ: Acute arterial occlusion. In Moore WS [ed]: Vascular Surgery: A Comprehensive Review. New York, Grune & Stratton, 1983, p 694.)

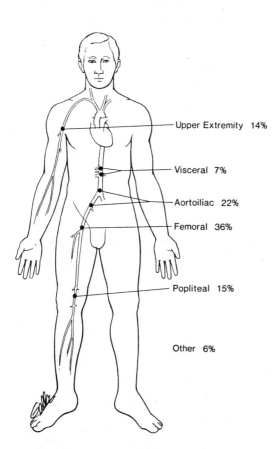

Figure 12–10. Incidence of embolic occlusion at different sites. (From Brewster DC, Chin AK, Hermann GD, Fogarty TJ: Arterial thromboembolism. In Rutherford RB [ed]: Vascular Surgery, 4th ed. Philadelphia, WB Saunders, 1995, p 650.)

embolize to the tibial circulation.[48] Patients with a popliteal aneurysm have a 43 percent chance of popliteal aneurysm in the contralateral leg.[49] Popliteal artery entrapment or adventitial cystic disease of the popliteal artery may also result in popliteal artery thrombosis. Dissection of the aorta can also result in acute lower-extremity ischemia. Severe back pain with hypertension and differential or loss of extremity pulses suggest the diagnosis (see Chapter 11).[47] Systemic conditions predisposing to arterial thrombosis are included in Table 12–1.

Trauma

Trauma resulting in arterial injury may be responsible for acute arterial occlusion. Fractures of the femur and tibial plateau, dislocations (knee), and crushing and penetrating injuries are all common problems that can lead to arterial occlusion from direct transection or secondary to intimal disruption with subsequent thrombosis of the artery (Fig. 12–11).[50] Although laceration and transection of the artery are most frequent, mural contusion and isolated intimal injury of an intact artery also are encountered, sometimes leading to a delayed arterial occlusion.

With increased use of percutaneous catheters for diagnostic and therapeutic procedures, iatrogenic trauma from arterial catheterization has become a more frequent source of acute arterial occlusion.[51] Many such patients have underlying arterial disease. Clinical manifestations may appear during a procedure while indwelling arterial catheters are in place or after the catheter has been removed.

Outflow Venous Occlusion

Compartment syndrome causes a rise in intracompartmental pressure, which may exceed capillary filling pressure. This leads to impedance of venous outflow. If this process goes

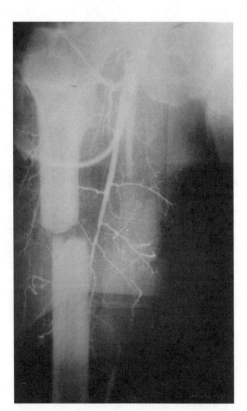

Figure 12–11. Fracture of femur resulting in acute arterial occlusion of the superficial femoral artery.

unchecked, arterial inflow is eventually restricted, leading to nerve and muscle ischemia. Compartment syndrome is seen most frequently after limb trauma or after revascularization of an acutely ischemic limb (see Chapter 21).[47] Phlegmasia cerulea dolens, the most severe form of iliofemoral venous thrombosis, can lead to acute arterial occlusion and limb ischemia.[50]

Low-Flow States

Low-flow states can potentiate ischemia, especially when superimposed on pre-existing atheroslerotic disease. Cardiogenic or hypovolemic shock, sepsis, congestive heart failure, myocardial infarction, dehydration, and pulmonary embolism may all be associated with significant reduction in cardiac output.[47] This occurs because of peripheral vasoconstriction with resultant decrease in blood flow through collateral circulation.[3]

Pathophysiology

The impact of sudden arterial occlusion is related to several factors including the site of obstruction, extent of thrombus propagation, adequacy of collateral circulation, and the hemodynamic state of the patient. Because of differences in tissue tolerance to ischemia, severe and sometimes irreversible anoxic injury occurs in skeletal muscle or peripheral nerves about 4–6 hours after the onset of ischemia; skin and subcutaneous tissue remain viable for longer.[3, 50]

In cases of massive ischemic myopathy, systemic metabolic abnormalities can occur during the acute phase of occlusion or after revascularization in the reperfusion stage.[3] These include metabolic acidosis, hyperkalemia, elevated muscle enzymes, and myoglobinuria. The venous effluent from the revascularized limb may contain high concentrations of lactic acid, potassium, creatine phosphokinase (CPK), and lactate dehydrogenase (LDH), resulting in an abrupt and rapid metabolic acidosis. Severe hyperkalemia and acidosis are most dangerous because they can result in cardiac depression and dysrhythmia. Myoglobin and metabolic products released from ischemic muscle may have nephrotoxic effects (renal failure) when myoglobin is deposited in the renal tubules.[52]

Clinical Manifestations

Clinical manifestations of AAO, which occur distal to the site of arterial occlusion, will vary depending on the level and severity of obstruction and the adequacy of collateral circulation.[3] The patient may exhibit signs of pain, pallor, pulselessness, and poikilothermy (coolness) in the affected extremity. The extent of paresthesia and paralysis is a good index of the degree of ischemic injury to nerves and muscle and correlates well with the ultimate prognosis. Preservation of sensitivity to light touch is often the best guide to viability. Its absence and paralysis are grave signs with potential irreversibility.[45]

Irreversible nerve damage manifested as a foot drop may also occur.[3] An ischemic blue toe, known as blue toe syndrome, may result from distal embolization from a proximal source such as an aneurysm, heart, or any proximal atherosclerotic lesion. Phlegmasia cerulea dolens is characterized by pain, massive swelling, tenderness, and cyanosis of the lower extremity.

Diagnosis

An accurate diagnosis of an arterial occlusion as embolic or thrombotic in origin is necessary in order to initiate appropriate treatment (Table 12–2). When arterial thrombosis occurs in a nonatherosclerotic artery, signs and symptoms are similar to those of embolism.

Evaluation of the consistency of skeletal muscle is an important part of the physical exam to determine the severity of ischemia. With increased ischemia, cellular swelling occurs and the muscle no longer feels soft but becomes thick and inelastic. As this worsens, the extremity becomes stiff and firm. This rigidity, which may occur many hours before clinical and laboratory abnormalities become apparent, is an ominous sign.[50, 52]

Treatment

Initial Treatment

The approach to acute leg ischemia varies significantly from treatment used in the chronic situation, because immediate intervention is usually required. Because a delay in or inadequate treatment may result in limb loss, damage to vital organs, or death, prompt treatment of the patient is crucial to successful management. The severity of ischemia, the amount of ischemic tissue, and the underlying cardiopulmonary status of the patient play a significant role in determining the patient's outcome.[47]

After the diagnosis of acute leg ischemia has been confirmed, if there are no immediate life-threatening contraindications, systemic anticoagulation with heparin is initiated with a 10,000 unit bolus followed by a continuous drip of 1000 units each hour. This helps to prevent thrombus propagation and thrombosis of arteries distal to the occlusion as well as prevent proliferation of new emboli.[10, 50]

Thrombolytic Therapy

Thrombolytic therapy may be used to treat recently formed arterial and bypass graft occlusions, addressing the unmasked lesions with an operative or endovascular approach. The key to prolonging patency is identification and correction of the underlying lesion. Research is ongoing to define the exact role of thrombolytic therapy in the treatment of acute arterial occlusion. The risk/benefit relation of thrombolytic therapy remains unclear

TABLE 12–2. **Acute Arterial Occlusion (AAO): Embolism Versus Thrombosis**

Embolism
Sudden onset of pain in an extremity without prior symptoms of arterial insufficiency
Loss of pulses in one leg with normal pulses in contralateral extremity
Presence of likely source of emboli, e.g., with atrial fibrillation, valvular heart disease, recent myocardial infarction, ventricular aneurysm

Thrombosis
Gradual onset of symptoms in an extremity with antecedent symptoms of arterial insufficiency, e.g., claudication
Contralateral disease
No proximal source of emboli

in most clinical settings. Recent data suggest that bypass graft occlusions may be associated with a better thrombolytic response than native arterial occlusions. Only in rare cases of embolic events or prosthetic graft occlusion will thrombolysis be sufficient as the sole intervention.[53]

A multicenter trial of thrombolysis or peripheral arterial surgery (TOPAS) was organized to compare the use of recombinant urokinase (rUK) with surgery for the initial treatment of acute lower-extremity ischemia. The preliminary results suggested that an initial rUK dose of 4000 IU/min is safe and efficacious in the treatment of acute limb-threatening ischemia in native arterial or bypass graft. Therapy with rUK is associated with limb salvage and patient survival rates similar to those achieved with surgery, concurrent with a reduced requirement for complex surgery after thrombolytic intervention.[54] For patients without diabetes who have older vein grafts, thrombolysis may provide significant improvement in patency rates. However, in diabetics, thrombolytic therapy is unlikely to result in durable patency or limb salvage even if newly discovered disease is corrected.[55]

Selective intra-arterial delivery of a thrombolytic agent has been used with the advantage of local thrombolysis and minimizes risk of systemic effects. Thrombolytic therapy may require 8–72 hours to be successful and can only be used in patients who do not require immediate restoration of blood flow. For patients with severe ischemia, surgical exploration may afford a more expeditious restoration of blood flow. Thrombolytic therapy may be used alone or in conjunction with surgical intervention (refer to Chapter 6).

Surgical Intervention

Embolism

Arterial embolism can often be corrected by an embolectomy, the extraction of the embolus using a Fogarty embolectomy catheter with a small balloon at one end (Fig. 12–12).[3] Through an opening in the artery, the catheter is passed down the affected arterial segment with the balloon deflated. When the tip is beyond the obstruction, the balloon is inflated and the catheter and embolus are withdrawn. This procedure can be performed using local anesthesia. If an embolus is present in a badly diseased artery, an embolectomy may fail and a bypass graft may be required. Most patients are maintained on heparin and warfarin postoperatively.

Thrombosis

Arterial thrombosis is treated in much the same way as is chronic ischemia, with a bypass procedure to the appropriate nonoccluded arterial segment. Depending on the location of thrombosis, aortofemoral, femoral-femoral, or femoral-to-popliteal or distal artery bypass may be performed. Ligation of a popliteal aneurysm may also be necessary. With an arterial graft thrombosis, thrombectomy of the graft may be adequate or a new bypass graft may be necessary. However, the surgical management of a failed graft depends on the cause of the failure.

Trauma (see Chapter 21)

After the evaluation of an injured patient, if there is any suggestion of arterial injury, an ABI must be obtained in the affected leg. In blunt trauma, following crush injury, fracture,

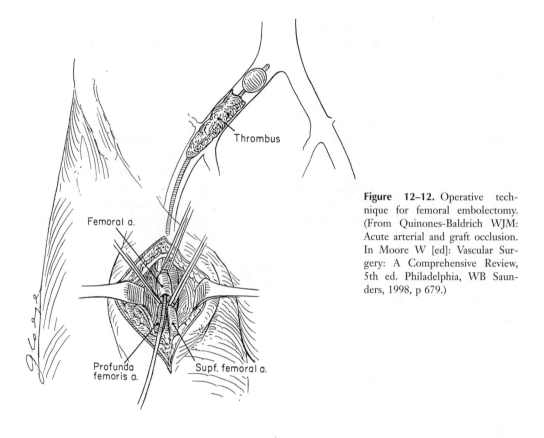

Figure 12–12. Operative technique for femoral embolectomy. (From Quinones-Baldrich WJM: Acute arterial and graft occlusion. In Moore W [ed]: Vascular Surgery: A Comprehensive Review, 5th ed. Philadelphia, WB Saunders, 1998, p 679.)

or major dislocation, an arteriogram should be obtained when the Doppler examination suggests a blood pressure drop in the affected extremity. Certain types of blunt trauma are so likely to produce arterial injury that an arteriogram is recommended even without any Doppler evidence of arterial injury. These injuries include dislocation of the knee, which causes popliteal artery injury in about one-third of all cases. Patients with an associated fracture and arterial obstruction may need external fracture stabilization or reduction at the time of arterial repair.[50]

Blunt arterial injury sometimes precipitates leg ischemia chronologically remote from the initial accident. An arterial stretch injury may produce intimal tearing that slowly progresses and occludes the vessel. This produces severe leg pain hours or even days after the initial injury, at a time when the extremity may be surrounded by a well-fitted plaster cast. These painful complaints demand rapid Doppler assessment of ankle pressure and must not be attributed to inadequate analgesia or benign swelling beneath the plaster. Delays under these circumstances often result in leg amputation.

Penetrating leg wounds may produce severe leg ischemia similar to that seen in blunt trauma from arterial contusion, or the patient may present with massive external bleeding from the wound. Injured patients should always be examined with a stethoscope to detect an arteriovenous fistula between the injured artery and adjacent vein.

Leg injuries caused by bullet wounds or stabbing require liberal evaluation with arteriography if occult vascular injuries are to be avoided. Arterial injuries of the thigh and leg require an attempt at direct vascular reconstruction because arterial ligation frequently leads to amputation. Information from World War II, before arterial repair was commonly used, reminds us that leg amputation is necessary following simple ligation in 81 percent of common femoral arteries and in 55 percent of popliteal arteries.[56]

Arterial reconstruction in blunt or penetrating arterial trauma is usually undertaken

TABLE 12–3. **Signs and Symptoms of Compartment Syndrome**

Pain disproportional to injury
Tenseness and fullness of compartment
Pain on passive muscle stretching
Decreased muscle strength within the compartment
Decreased simple touch perception
Decreased sensation or anesthesia of nerves in the compartment
Pulses: normal or diminished or absent in late stage

using a saphenous vein graft from the uninjured leg. Experience has shown that if the adjacent vein is also injured, it should be repaired at the time of initial reconstruction.

Compartment Syndrome

The compartment of the leg contains bone, muscle, nerve tissue, and blood vessels all wrapped in a fascia membrane. After an episode of prolonged ischemia or after revascularization, there may be considerable swelling of skeletal muscle. This muscle swelling may eventually produce a destructively high pressure within the leg compartments, giving rise to a compartment syndrome. This increased pressure will first cause nerve injury, then muscle cell necrosis, and, finally, occlusion of the tibial vessels or a bypass graft.[3] Signs and symptoms of compartment syndrome are included in Table 12–3.

If a compartment syndrome is present, a fasciotomy is performed, which allows expansion of the edematous muscle, resulting in decompression of the compartment and relief of pressure. Incisions are made over the leg compartments, and the underlying fascia is opened from the knee to the ankle (Fig. 12–13). Immediate identification of compartment syndrome and prompt fasciotomy can reduce the sequelae of muscle necrosis, nerve damage, and possible limb amputation.

Muscle debridement may be necessary until healthy granulation tissue is present. A fasciotomy wound can either be closed once swelling resolves or may be covered with a skin graft.[45] Complications after fasciotomy result from infection, bleeding from anticoag-

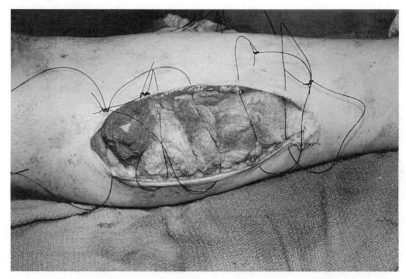

Figure 12–13. Fasciotomy performed for compartment syndrome.

ulation, or peroneal nerve injury. Vigorous physical therapy and a splint to prevent foot drop may be necessary. (Refer to Table 12–4 and Chapter 21.)

Amputation

Amputation may be an acceptable alternative under certain circumstances. Attempted revascularization can be inappropriate and potentially dangerous due to metabolic complications. Primary amputation may be urgent if advanced tissue ischemia has led to systemic toxicity or the leg is irreversibly anesthetic or paralytic.

Metabolic Complications

As discussed previously, serious systemic complications, acidosis, hyperkalemia, and renal failure secondary to myoglobinuria can follow revascularization of a severely ischemic limb. Treatment is directed at maintaining normal physiologic functions and ameliorating systemic effects caused by metabolic derangements. Aggressive fluid resuscitation and careful attention to cardiac and renal function is needed. Metabolic acidosis should be anticipated and can be treated with sodium bicarbonate during the early stages of reperfusion. Leakage of potassium during cell death leads to hyperkalemia. Administration of glucose and insulin drives potassium into cells, thus controlling hyperkalemia. Oral or rectal administration of exchange resins or even hemodialysis may be necessary. This may be aggravated by acute renal failure secondary to myoglobin precipitation in the collecting tubules. Maintaining a high urine output with an alkaline urine is the best way to control the myoglobinuria and potential renal failure. This can be achieved by the systemic adminstration of mannitol to promote osmotic diuresis and bicarbonate to maintain an alkaline urine.[3]

Treatment of Underlying Conditions

In addition to restoring blood supply to an extremity, underlying medical conditions leading to emboli or thrombosis also require treatment. If the patient is at risk for further embolization from a proximal source, the source must be treated. Warfarin may be prescribed in the case of atrial fibrillation and cardiac surgery may be indicated to replace diseased valves. An abdominal aortic aneurysm or popliteal aneurysm should be repaired if it is the cause of embolism. If heparin-induced thrombocytopenia occurs, heparin must be stopped promptly.

Because renal or mesenteric infarction can also occur, the patient should be monitored for abdominal, flank, or back pain; hematuria and gut emptying; and an elevated white blood count. These may be indicative of acute renal or visceral ischemia.

POTENTIAL COMPLICATIONS/MEDICAL AND NURSING MANAGEMENT

Cardiac

Patients with lower-extremity ischemia have significantly higher mortality because atherosclerotic disease is multifocal, in most instances including the coronary or cerebral vessels. The clinically silent or apparently stable coronary disease is unmasked by the stress of

TABLE 12–4. **Postoperative Care (may vary from institution to institution)**

Hematoma and/or Hemorrhage
- Observe for signs of shock including increase in pulse, decrease in blood pressure, anxiety, restlessness, pallor, cyanosis, thirst, oliguria, clammy skin, venous collapse, and level of consciousness.
- Check incision and dressing for excessive drainage, the presence of a hematoma; a pulsatile mass at the incision site is indicative of a false aneurysm.
- Assess pulmonary artery pressures and/or cardiac output if parameters are available.
- Check daily weights; monitor intake and output closely.
- Check lab values, e.g., hematocrit, hemoglobin, and notify doctor if abnormal.
- Check creatinine level after angiography.

Lower-Extremity Ischemia
- Check pedal pulses and ankle-brachial indices every hour for 24 hours, then every shift or as ordered.
- Monitor pain status of leg.
- Check sensory and motor function of extremities.
- Avoid raising knee gatch and placing pillows under the knees because pressure may increase possibility of thrombosis.
- Monitor for abdominal, flank, or back pain, decreased urine output, hematuria, or gut emptying (vomiting or diarrhea), which could indicate renal or mesenteric infarction from additional arterial occlusion.

Compartment Syndrome/Myoglobinuria/Metabolic Complications
- Assess foot and leg for motor and sensory function, the presence of foot drop, and for pain out of proportion to the situation.
- Assess the patient's leg for hematoma, severe swelling and/or a tense calf, and consistency of muscle (doughy gastrocnemius muscle indicative of compartment syndrome). Severe swelling may impede blood flow through the graft. Remove dressing when necessary to provide complete examination.
- Observe for change in color (reddish brown) and presence of red blood cells in urine secondary to release of myoglobin, secondary to ischemia of muscle. Monitor urine output and creatinine level and maintain urine output at 100 ml/hr.
- Watch for hyperkalemia and acidosis because of increased concentration of lactic acid and potassium. Monitor creatine phosphokinase (CPK) levels.
- Use sterile technique for dressing changes of fasciotomy.
- The extremity with a compartment syndrome should be positioned at a level no higher than the heart.

Prevention of Tissue Damage
- Separate toes that press on each other with lambswool or dry gauze.
- Use sheepskin to reduce friction under the heels as the patient moves in bed.
- Elevate the heels off the bed.
- Remove pressure on the toes from bed linen.
- If bed cradle is used, position it properly.

Impaired Physical Mobility
- Assess for the presence of neurologic deficits or foot drop.
- Assess causative factors for immobility, the patient's range of motion, and ability to ambulate.
- Encourage progressive ambulation and range of motion while in bed.
- Request physical therapy consult when appropriate.
- Encourage independence in activities of daily living.

Pain
- Assess patient's level of pain, type, duration, and location.
- Avoid elevation of limb.
- Provide comfort measures and means of distraction.
- Medicate with prescribed analgesics as needed (prn).
- Evaluate effectiveness of pain medication after each administration.

Disturbance in Self-Concept/Change in Body Image
- Establish a trusting relationship with patient.
- Encourage patient to verbalize feelings.
- Promote social interaction.
- Make appropriate referrals if indicated.

surgery. Myocardial ischemia in this patient population occurs more often postoperatively than during surgery.

Graft Thrombosis

Failure of a graft will result in an acutely ischemic limb or a return to its preoperative status. The causes of graft thrombosis are multifactorial (Table 12–5). Early recognition and aggressive treatment of failed bypass grafts may result in successful restoration of graft patency in most patients. The appropriate treatment of graft failure depends on several variables including the timing of the occlusion, the cause of occlusion, type of graft material, limb viability, the patient's ability to tolerate reoperation, continued validity of original indications for operation or new indication, the condition of the proximal and distal arteries, and likelihood of success of reoperation.

If graft failure is secondary to a problem with anticoagulation, graft thrombectomy or thrombolytic therapy may be adequate to restore blood flow. Neointimal hyperplasia usually requires a new bypass or revision of the distal anastomosis with a patch angioplasty. Progression of distal disease may require a completely new or an extended graft with a new distal anastomotic site.

Following femoral artery bypass, the dorsalis pedis and posterior tibial artery pulses

TABLE 12–5. **Causes of Graft Failure**

Immediate to Early (within 30 days of surgery)
Technical defects
Anastomosis
Sewing vein shut with suture
Intimal flap
Retained valve cusp
Compression/twisting of graft
Hypercoagulability/clotting disorder
Inadequate anticoagulation
Hypercoagulable state
Decreased antithrombin III
Heparin-induced thrombocytopenia
Decreased cardiac output (i.e., hypotension/myocardial infarction)
Poor runoff
Poor patient selection
Unexplained
Intermediate (30 days to 2 years)
Graft stenosis
Myointimal hyperplasia
Embolization
Inadequate/failure of anticoagulation
Unexplained
Late (greater than 2 years)
Progression of disease (inflow/outflow)
Thrombosis of proximal reconstruction
Embolization from proximal source
False aneurysm
Inadequate/failure of anticoagulation
Graft infection
Valvular fibrosis

should be assessed frequently to assess graft patency. However, Doppler-derived blood pressure measurements at the ankle level provide the best means for monitoring the patency of femoral artery bypasses. These pressures vary postoperatively depending on the type of graft, the location of the distal anastomosis, and the degree of arterial disease beyond the bypass graft. Because PTFE is relatively noncompressible, ankle pressure with the blood pressure cuff over a PTFE graft is usually greater than 200 mmHg, which represents a false elevation.

Patients with normal arteries distal to the bypass, or with bypasses extending to near the ankle, should have ABIs of approximately 1.0. Arterial occlusive disease distal to the bypass will not permit an elevation in ankle-level blood pressure to a systemic level. A reduction in the ABI of greater than 0.15 may be indicative of a graft occlusion and warrants prompt physician notification. Ankle pressure measurements are not recommended when a bypass to the dorsalis pedis or posterior tibial artery has been performed.

Although discomfort is expected after a femoral artery bypass, this must be differentiated from the extreme pain of lower-extremity ischemia or compartment compression. Severe pain in the foot across the metatarsal leads may be the first sign of graft occlusion. Sudden motor weakness or limb anesthesia may also reflect graft occlusion.

Noninvasive segmental arterial pressures of infrainguinal bypass grafts should be determined on a regular basis.[57] Sustained graft patency is enhanced with graft surveillance and intervention before graft thormbosis occurs.[35] Tests are usually recommended 6 months after surgery, and yearly thereafter. Any significant change in pressure, or new symptoms, warrants further evaluation. More frequent evaluation is sometimes recommended for certain types of bypasses. Duplex scanning may also be performed in certain vein bypass grafts.

Bleeding/Hematoma

Any bleeding from the wounds following surgery is cause for concern. Suture line disruption, pseudoaneurysm formation, or failed ligature must be corrected in the operating room. A tense hematoma can present as a compartment syndrome and compromise arterial blood flow and nerve function. Hematomas related to femoral grafts should be evacuated promptly in the operating room to prevent skin damage and graft infection.

Renal Failure

A complication of compartment syndrome is the release of myoglobin by the damaged muscle cells. The first evidence of this is usually a reddish-brown discoloration of the urine. Patients with preoperative muscle paralysis or rigor should have urine checked for the presence of myoglobin. If myoglobinuria is anticipated, alkalinization of the urine with sodium bicarbonate, as well as osmotic diuresis using mannitol, is employed (see Chapter 21).[52]

Edema

Leg edema following femoral revascularization is common. The exact etiology is not clear but is believed to be a result of interstitial fluid accumulation, dissection around perivascular lymphatics, lymphatic obstruction, and a loss of subcutaneous venous channels.[58] Edema can inhibit wound healing and a mild diuretic may sometimes be necessary. An elastic bandage applied below the knee when the patient is out of bed can help to control edema; however, elastic bandages may not be recommended if an in situ vein bypass has

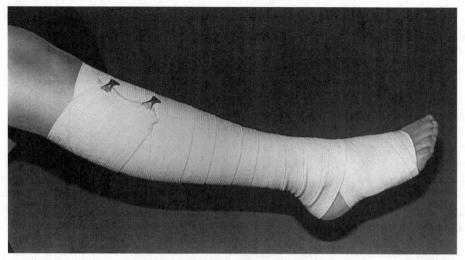

Figure 12–14. Elastic bandage wrapped from toe to below the knee.

been performed because of the graft's location (Fig. 12–14). Patients should understand that edema usually resolves within the first 8–12 postoperative weeks but can last many months after surgery. If swelling continues, the patient may be fitted for an elastic stocking. Leg elevation is also beneficial to control the edema.

Wound Care

Observe strict aseptic technique during dressing changes. Leg incisions may be covered with dry dressings held in place with a light, rolled gauze wrap. Tape should be avoided on the sensitive skin of the distal lower extremity to prevent skin damage or loss when the tape is removed. The foot and leg must be handled with extreme care, because a severe reduction in blood flow may render the leg more vulnerable to external forces.

Wounds that develop evidence of infection should be cultured and appropriate antibiotics ordered. Wound dehiscence or exposure of the graft necessitates immediate readmission of the patient to the hospital. Minor amputation wounds may not be completely healed at the time of discharge but should be clean and granulating well. Monitor for any signs of infection—low-grade fever, elevated white blood cell count, drainage from wound, cellulitis, and delayed healing and graft exposure—during each shift.

Perigraft Seroma

Vascular surgical wounds, expecially in the groin, may develop lymphatic collections between the arterial dissection and the skin. Lymphoceles often appear between the fifth and seventh postoperative days. The discharge of clear, pale yellow fluid begins a few days later. The lymphatic fistula usually heals after treatment with bed rest, antibiotics, and dressing changes. Direct operative exploration with lymphatic suture and the use of a suction drain may be necessary. In rare cases, a lymphocele may develop after the patient is home when the wound is well healed. A perigraft seroma may be seen along the length of a subcutaneous synthetic graft; this usually is benign and resolves over time. Owing to increased risk of infection, these collections of fluid usually should not be aspirated. The late appearance of a fluid collection may also indicate graft infection.

TABLE 12–6. **Postoperative/Discharge Teaching Plan (may vary from hospital to hospital)**

Graft Patency
- Review disease process and surgical procedure with patient and family. Use diagram and written information when available.
- Teach the patient/family how to palpate pulses in the foot.
- Teach the patient signs and symptoms of graft failure that need to be reported to the physician.

Activity
- Regular exercise is important, and climbing stairs, going out of doors, and bending knee are acceptable. There is no danger of disrupting an anastomosis by normal convalescent activity.
- Avoid heavy lifting.
- Sexual activity may be resumed in 2 weeks; discuss with physician if concerned.

Bathing
- Bathing or showering is acceptable on the fifth day after surgery or on an individual basis if there are open wounds or skin lesions.
- Clean incision gently with mild soap and water; dry it well.

Presence of Prosthetic Graft
- Inform patient if a prosthetic graft is used; patient should notify other physicians and dentist if undergoing any invasive test or procedure or extensive dental work.
- Inform patient that prosthetic graft is not rejectable.

Wound Care
- Instruct patient that no special care of wound is required unless otherwise indicated. If oozing from the incision is present, the area should be covered with dry gauze. If sutures are subcuticular, the patient should be informed that sutures do not require removal.
- Avoid tape on the skin below the knee. Use gauze such as Kling or Kerlix and tape the gauze. Physicians' opinions on dressing material for open wounds or ulcers vary widely. Saline, Betadine ointment, Silvadene, Garamycin ointment, Neosporin, Polysporin, and Betadine solution are some of the choices. The first six keep the wound moist while exerting a bacteriostatic action on the wound. Betadine solution has a drying effect unless kept constantly wet as a wet dressing. It exerts a debriding effect each time the gauze is changed.

Foot Care
- Inspect body on a daily basis and be aware of how incisions, feet, and legs look and feel after surgery. This can help in the recognition of early evidence of significant change. Use a mirror if necessary.
- Wash feet and clean between toes regularly and dry well. Mild soap and warm water should be used. Check the water temperature with the hand or a thermometer each time the feet are bathed. A warm, moist washcloth will remove dry, scaly skin.
- Apply a lubricating cream to the feet, except between the toes and near open ulcers. The lubricant should be used sparingly and rubbed into the skin. Avoid perfumed preparations.
- If the feet perspire excessively, a hypoallergenic, nonmedicated talcum powder should be lightly dusted on the feet twice a day. Avoid powder in the presence of cracked skin or ulcerations.
- Nail care should be performed under good lighting while the nails are softened from the bath. If nail care cannot be performed then, soak the feet for 5–10 minutes before to soften the nails. Do not trim nails if they are hypertrophic, badly ingrown, infected, or painful. Toenails are to be cut straight across. The corners are filed slightly to rid the edges of sharp points, but they should not be cut back. See a podiatrist for assistance especially with corns, calluses, or ingrown toenails. Make sure the podiatrist is aware of the vascular status of the patient.
- Corns and calluses should not be trimmed or cut. A pumice-impregnated soap bar used regularly on the heels and the bony prominences during bathing can help impede callus formation.
- Lambswool (Fig. 12–15), cotton, or gauze pads may be placed between the toes to prevent pressure. The bony prominences of each toe put pressure on the adjoining toe, which can result in a pressure ulcer. Change the padding daily or when it becomes wet.
- Report skin breakdown to the physician.

Table continued on following page

TABLE 12–6. **Postoperative/Discharge Teaching Plan** *Continued*

Footwear/Avoiding Injury

- Wear properly fitting shoes to avoid skin breakdown at pressure points. It is best to buy shoes midday to take into account some edema that may develop.
- Shoes should be soft, flexible leather. Manmade materials such as patent leather and plastic should be avoided because they prevent evaporation and may contribute to fungal infections. Since athletic shoes have become more popular, more styles with proper support are available. Avoid sandals.
- Break new shoes in gradually.
- Wear socks or stockings with shoes at all times to prevent blistering.
- Socks should be clean, preferably cotton or wool, nonmended, and without seams, to prevent skin breakdown.
- Stockings should not be held up with garters or by twisting at the knee. Men's socks should not constrict the ankle or the leg below the knee.
- Inspect shoes for foreign objects, holes, or nail points in the soles. Decreased sensory perception in the diabetic foot makes it possible for patients to be unaware of sharp objects, stones, or other debris for extended periods of time. Any potential area of damage should be eliminated because pressure may result in skin breakdown with subsequent infection and potential limb loss.[64]
- Avoid clothes such as tight socks, garters, or pantyhose that constrict the legs or feet.
- Wear protective shoes or slippers when out of bed. Avoid walking barefoot. Simple debris or splinters on the floor or in the carpet can go unnoticed in a foot that lacks sensory perception or be noticed only after the injury is inflicted.
- Protect feet/legs from excessive heat or cold by avoiding heating pads/cold packs, heat lamps, or hot water bottles, and cream hair removers, adhesive corn pads, or any harsh chemicals.

Elastic Support

- Inform patient that leg swelling is normal after surgery. Because of decreased postoperative activity and immobilization during the surgical procedure, fluid accumulates in lower leg.
- If ordered, instruct patient how to wrap 4-inch elastic bandage snugly from the toe to just below the knee (see Fig. 12–14), to apply bandage before ambulation, to remove at night, to wear bandage for 2 weeks or until swelling disappears. Elastic bandages can be washed with mild soap and water and can be reused. They can be purchased at most drug stores. Elastic bandages are usually not recommended with in situ bypass grafts.

Medications

- Instruct patient regarding medications with which he or she will be discharged, their purposes, dosages, and side effects. Document teaching (see Chapter 8).

Driving

- Driving may be possible after returning to first office visit or possible when patient has returned to baseline in terms of mobility.

Risk Factor Modification (refer to Chapter 10)

Medical Follow-Up/Indications for Doctor Notification

- Instruct patient regarding importance of follow-up visits with doctor and arterial blood flow studies on regular basis.
- Inform patient to notify doctor of any changes in incision; new or unusual drainage; change in color or amount of drainage; increase in temperature; swelling or pulsatile mass at the incision site; inflammation or tenderness around incision; any unusual or severe increase in pain in leg, especially when it is severe enough to prevent sleep; sudden weight gain or swelling of feet or legs; fever; loss of sensation or movement of legs; unusual tingling, coldness, or discoloration of the feet or legs; and any skin breakdown on the foot.

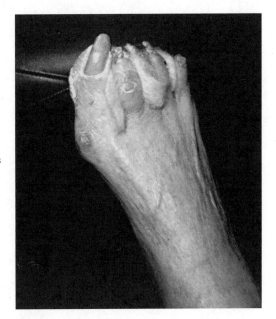

Figure 12–15. Lambswool to separate the toes. It is woven in and out, not wrapped around the toes.

Graft Infection

Infection is one of the most serious complications of bypass surgery and threatens both limb and life. If a prosthetic graft becomes infected, it usually must be removed. Causes of graft infection include contamination of the graft during insertion, penetrating injury from an angiography catheter, or blood-borne inoculation. Broad-spectrum antibiotic coverage should be started preoperatively and continued for at least the first postoperative day. Patients are carefully monitored for low-grade fever, an elevated white blood count, septic emboli, or hemorrhage, which are all suggestive of infection.

Poorly nourished patients appear to be most prone to wound disruption, graft infection, and possible graft thrombosis.[59] These patients may be identified preoperatively by their low serum albumin levels. Dietary supplementation by enteral or parenteral routes is beneficial in patients with delayed wound healing. Because of the severe consequences of graft infection, patients require appropriate antibiotic prophylaxis during any subsequent invasive procedures, including dental procedures.

Nerve Damage

Following bypass grafting, a saphenous neuropathy may occur. The patient may complain of pain along the medial aspect in the lower part of the thigh and medial aspect of the leg. The severity of the pain varies from patient to patient.[60] This pain is related to an operative injury to the nerve or may result from nerve entrapment in the scar tissue in the lower thigh. It may appear as a mild transient discomfort or may assume a burning character or more rarely may be persistent and disabling.

Pharmacologic Management

Depending on the type of anticoagulation therapy used postoperatively, patients may require frequent monitoring of their partial thromboplastin time/prothrombin time (PTT/PT) or International Normalized Ratio (INR). With heparin therapy, the platelet count

TABLE 12–7. **Clinical Pathway of Patient Undergoing Lower-Extremity Bypass Surgery (may vary from institution to institution)**

	POSTOP OR DAY DATE	ICU POD #1 DATE	FLOOR POD #1 DATE	POD #2 DATE	POD #3 DATE	POD #4 DATE	POD #5 DATE
Vital Signs/ Parameters	VS q 1 hr I/O q 1 hr	VS q 1 hr I/O q 1 hr	VS q 4 hr I/O q 4 hr	VS q 4 hr I/O q 8 hr	VS q 4 hr I/O q 8 hr	VS q 4 hr I/O q 8 hr	VS q 8 hr
Pulse/Doppler Assessment	ABI q 1 hr	ABI q 1 hr	Pulse/Doppler tones q 4 hr	Pulse/Doppler tones q 4 hr	Pulse/Doppler tones q 4 hr	Pulse/Doppler tones q 4 hr ABI prior to d/c	Pulse/Doppler tones q 4 hr
Activity	Bed rest	OOB in chair with assistance	Ambulate with assistance 1–2×	Ambulate BID	Ambulate TID	Ambulate TID	Ambulate TID May shower
Medication	IV; A-line prn ASA or anti-coagulation Pain meds prn Platelet count if on heparin ECG prn	IV; D/C A-line prn ASA or anti-coagulation Pain meds prn	IV Antibiotic (if ulcer) ASA or anti-coagulation Pain meds prn	IV: D/C prn Antibiotic (if ulcer) ASA or anti-coagulation Pain meds prn	Assess IV status ASA or anti-coagulation Pain meds prn	Assess IV status ASA or anti-coagulation Pain meds prn	Assess IV status ASA or anti-coagulation Pain meds prn
Tests	SMA-8, CBC, PTT/PT Platelet count if on heparin prn	SMA-8, CBC, PTT/PT Platelet count if on heparin	PTT/PT Platelet count if on heparin	PTT/PT Platelet count if on heparin	PTT/PT Platelet count if on heparin	PTT/PT Platelet count if on heparin Arterial blood flow study	PTT/PT Platelet count if on heparin
Consult/ Discharge Planning		Transfer to floor	Discharge planner/social worker prn Physical therapy prn Skilled unit prn	Discharge planner/ social worker Physical therapy prn	Discharge planner/ social worker Physical therapy prn May be discharged to skilled unit	Rx & d/c instruction sheet completed by MD Pt may be discharged to home/skilled unit	Patient discharged

264

Diet	NPO	Clear liquid diet	Clear liquid diet advance as tolerated to low-fat/low-choles diet (step 2)	Low-fat/low-choles	Low-fat/low-choles	Low-fat/low-choles	Low-fat/low-choles
Treatment	Observe for bleeding, hematoma, q 1 hr TCDB q 2 hr	D/C Foley Incentive spirometer prn TCDB q 2 hr Observe for bleeding, hematoma, q 1 hr 4" elastic bandage below knee (not in situ grafts)	Incentive spirometer prn Observe for bleeding, hematoma, q 4 hr 4" bandages below knee (not in situ grafts)—rewrap q 8 hr	Incisional care qd Elastic bandages—rewrap q 8 hr	Incisional care qd Elastic bandages q 8 hr	Incisional care qd Elastic bandages—rewrap q 8 hr	Incisional care qd Elastic bandages—rewrap q 8 hr
Psychosocial	Provide support	Assess pt/family needs	Assess pt/family needs	Intervene with pt/family psychosocial needs prn	Intervene with pt/family psychosocial needs prn	Intervene with pt/family psychosocial needs prn	Intervene with pt/family psychosocial needs prn
Patient Education	Assess family's level of understanding Discuss postop course with family	Assess family's level of understanding Discuss postop course with family		Discuss pt progress w/ pt and family Begin anticoagulation therapy instruction prn	Discharge teaching including risk reduction Anticoagulation Rx teaching prn	Discharge teaching including risk reduction Anticoagulation Rx teaching prn	Discharge teaching Teach pt and family elastic bandage application prn Anticoagulation Rx teaching prn

OR = operating room; ICU = intensive care unit; POD = postoperative day; VS = vital signs; I/O = intake & output; ABI = ankle-brachial index; d/c = discharge; OOB = out of bed; BID = twice a day; TID = three times a day; IV = intravenous; D/C = discontinue; ASA = acetylsalicylic acid (aspirin); prn = as needed; A-line = arterial line; SMA = Sequential Multiple Analysis; CBC = complete blood count; PTT/PT = partial thromboplastin time/prothrombin time; ECG = electrocardiogram; SW = social worker; Rx = drug; NPO = nothing by mouth; TCDB = turn, cough, deep breathe.

should be checked before any heparin is administered and every day starting on day 5 to monitor for heparin-induced thrombocytopenia. A drop in platelet count to less than 100,000/mm³ can be indicative of this problem. Observe patients for skin breakdown or necrosis, called Coumadin necrosis, which can result from warfarin therapy. Patients who are anticoagulated should be assessed for signs of bleeding, including local as well as systemic problems, including mental status changes. Patients receiving thrombolytic therapy must have fibrinogen levels and coagulation parameters monitored regularly (see Chapter 8).

Foot Care

Because of the importance of skin integrity in vascular patients, particularly those with diabetes, it is imperative to establish a detailed plan for foot maintenance. The patient must be educated about specific maintenance steps and their significance, so that foot problems can be avoided. Foot care, footwear, and steps to avoiding injury are included in Table 12–6.

The nurse should inform the patient of the hazard of cutting skin during nail care and should assess the patient's visual acuity to perform this task. A tiny break in the skin can allow a host of organisms to penetrate it. With impaired arterial flow, the potential for infection is high and the results can be limb-threatening.

Psychosocial

Delivery of comprehensive care to a person with vascular disease is based on an understanding of disease pathophysiology, associated risk factors, and an awareness of the patient's response to the disease. Vascular patients and their families vary greatly in their responses to the diagnosis and chronicity of arterial insufficiency. Although some patients may express a positive outlook, others express anger, anxiety, depression, guilt, uncertainty, or helplessness. Psychologic variables can affect the patient's ability to adapt to altered function and comply with the prescribed medical regimen.[61] Nursing interventions can be enhanced by an understanding of how the disease affects feelings, coping capabilities, self-esteem, and psychosocial resources of the person, all of which are reflected in general well-being.[62]

Little research has been completed on how vascular patients adapt to chronic illness. One study that examined the psychologic variable of uncertainty after vascular surgery implied that patients need accurate information about their disease process, clear cues regarding their recovery from surgery, and an explanation of the meaning of residual symptoms. Congruence between expected outcomes and experienced events will aid in the patient's physiologic and psychosocial adaptation.[63]

Nursing intervention should focus on the patient's perceived needs. It is important to explore social, financial, and safety issues as well as to help the patient retain a comfortable level of control while attaining self-care skills.

Patient Education

Additional nursing care of the patient undergoing lower-extremity surgery is discussed in Table 12–4. Nurses play a significant role in the care and education of the patient and the family. Table 12–6 outlines a postoperative/discharge teaching plan. A clinical pathway of the patient undergoing lower-extremity bypass surgery is outlined in Table 12–7.

SUMMARY

Nurses play a significant role in the care of patients with lower-extremity arterial disease. High-quality patient care includes the identification of potential problems and appropriate nursing action as well as provision for patient education. Nurses must also take an active role in educating patients about risk factor modification.

References

1. Sanchez LA, Veith FJ: Femoral-popliteal-tibial occlusive disease. In Moore WS (ed): Vascular Surgery: A Comprehensive Review, 5th ed. Philadelphia, WB Saunders, 1998, pp 497–520.
2. Yao JST, Hobbs JT, Irvine WT: Ankle systolic pressure measurements in arterial disease affecting the extremities. Br J Surg 1969; 56:677–683.
3. Quinones-Baldrich WJ: Acute arterial and graft occlusion. In Moore W (ed): Vascular Surgery: A Comprehensive Review. Philadelphia, WB Saunders, 1998, pp 667–689.
4. Weitz JI, Byrne J, Clagett P, et al: Diagnosis and treatment of chronic arterial insufficiency of the lower extremities: A critical review. Circulation 1996; 94(11):3026–3049.
5. Whittemore AD: Infrainguinal bypass. In Rutherford RB (ed): Vascular Surgery, 4th ed. Philadelphia, WB Saunders, 1995, pp 794–814.
6. Walsh DB, Gilbertson JJ, Swolak RM, et al: The natural history of superficial femoral artery stenoses. J Vasc Surg 1991; 14:299–304.
7. Taylor LM, Porter JM: Natural history and nonoperative treatment of chronic lower extremtiy ischemia. In Rutherford RB (ed): Vascular Surgery, 4th ed. Philadelphia, WB Saunders, 1995, pp 751–766.
8. Ernst E, Fialka V: A review of the clinical effectiveness of exercise therapy for intermittent claudication. Arch Intern Med 1993; 153:2357–2360.
9. Regensteiner JG, Hiatt WR: Exercise rehabiliation for patients with peripheral arterial disease. In Holloszy JO (ed): Exercise and Sports Sciences Reviews. Baltimore, Williams and Wilkins, 1995, pp 1–24.
10. Clagett GP, Krupski WC: Antithrombotic therapy in peripheral arterial occlusive disease. Chest 1995; 108(4)431S–443S.
11. Weaver FA, Comerota AJ, Youngblood M, et al, and the STILE Investigators: Surgical revascularization versus thrombolysis for nonembolic lower extremity native artery occlusions: Results of a prospective randomized trial. J Vasc Surg 1996; 24:513–523.
12. Dalsing MC, Harris VJ: Intravascular stents. In White RA, Fogarty TJ (eds): Peripheral Endovascular Interventions. St. Louis, Mosby, 1996, pp 315–339.
13. Zarge JI, Duke DN, White JV: Balloon angioplasty. In White RA, Fogarty TJ (eds): Peripheral Endovascular Interventions. St. Louis, Mosby, 1996, pp 258–275.
14. Brewster DC: Staged inflow angioplasty and femoral bypass. In Yao JST, Pearce WH (eds): Techniques in Vascular and Endovascular Surgery. Stamford, CT, Appleton & Lange, 1998, pp 361–366.
15. Akbari CM, LoGerfo FW: Saphenous vein bypass to pedal arteries in diabetic patients. In Yao JST, Pearce WH (eds): Techniques in Vascular and Endovascular Surgery. Stamford, CT, Appleton & Lange, 1998, pp 227–232.
16. McCarthy WJ, McGee GS, Lin WW, et al: Axillary popliteal artery bypass provides successful limb salvage after removal of infected aortofemoral grafts. Arch Surg 1992; 127:974–978.
17. Rutherford RB, Baue A: Extra-anatomic bypass. In Rutherford RB (ed): Vascular Surgery, 4th ed. Philadelphia, WB Saunders, 1995, pp 705–716.
18. Deaton DH, Quinones-Baldrich WJ: Infrainguinal revascularization to the popliteal and proximal tibial arteries. In Callow AD, Ernst CB (eds): Vascular Surgery: Theory and Practice. Stamford, CT, Appleton & Lange, 1995, pp 689–705.
19. Leather RP, Veith FJ: In situ vein bypass. In Haimovici H, Ascer E, Hollier LH, et al (eds): Vascular Surgery, 4th ed. London, Blackwell Science, 1996, pp 632–641.
20. Mannick JA, Whittemore AD, Donaldson MC: In situ saphenous vein graft for lower extremity occlusive disease. In Ernst CB, Stanley JC (eds): Current Therapy in Vascular Surgery. St. Louis, Mosby, 1995, pp 469–472.
21. Rosenthal D, Piano G, Martin JD, et al: Angioscopic-assisted in situ vein graft. In Yao JST, Pearce WH (eds): Techniques in Vascular and Endovascular Surgery. Stamford, CT, Appleton & Lange, 1998, pp 259–264.
22. Belkin M, Magruder DC, Whittemore AD: Nonreversed saphenous bypass graft for infrainguinal arterial reconstruction. In Yao JST, Pearce WH (eds): Techniques in Vascular and Endovascular Surgery. Stamford, CT, Appleton & Lange, 1998, pp 233–242.

23. Londrew GL, Bosher LP, Brown PW, et al: Infrainguinal reconstruction with arm vein, lesser saphenous vein, and remnants of greater saphenous vein: A report of 257 cases. J Vasc Surg 1994; 20:451–457.
24. Hertzer NR, Sesto ME: Arm veins for lower extremity revascularization. In Ernst CB, Stanley JC (eds): Current Therapy in Vascular Surgery, 3rd ed. St. Louis, Mosby, 1995, pp 476–480.
25. Lovell MB, Harris KA, DeRose G, Jamieson WG: The use of arm vein as an alternative conduit for lower-extremity bypass. J Vasc Nurs 1996; 14:98–101.
26. Suggs WD, Veith FJ: Expanded polytetrafluoroethylene graft for atherosclerotic lower extremity occlusive disease. In Ernst CB, Stanley JC (eds): Current Therapy in Vascular Surgery, 3rd ed. St. Louis, Mosby, 1995, pp 480–484.
27. Karkow WS, Cranley JJ, et al: Extended study of aneurysm formation in umbilical grafts. J Vasc Surg 1986; 4:486–492.
28. McCarthy WJ, Shireman PK: Composite prosthetic-vein grafts. In Whittemore AD (ed): Advances in Vascular Surgery, Vol 2. St. Louis, Mosby, 1994, pp 121–131.
29. Mannick JA: Infrainguinal arterial reconstruction. Historical perspective. In Whittemore AD (ed): Advances in Vascular Surgery. St. Louis, Mosby, 1994, pp 3–8.
30. Taylor LM, Hamre D, Dalman RL, et al: Limb salvage vs amputation for critical ischemia: The role of vascular surgery. Arch Surg 1991; 126:1251–1258.
31. Veith FJ, Gupta SK, Wengerter KR, et al: Changing arteriosclerotic disease patterns and management strategies in lower-limb threatening ischemia. Ann Surg 1990; 212:402–414.
32. Veith FJ, Gupta SK, Ascer E, et al: Six-year prospective multicenter randomized comparison of autologous saphenous vein and expanded polytetrafluoroethylene grafts in infrainguinal arterial reconstructions. J Vasc Surg 1986; 3(1):104–114.
33. Veteran Administration Cooperative Study Group 141: Comparative evolution of the prosthetic, reversed, and in situ vein grafts in distal popliteal and tibial peroneal revascularization. Arch Surg 1988; 123:434–438.
34. Quinones-Baldrich WJ, Prego AA, Ucelay-Gomez R, et al: Long-term results of infrainguinal revascularization with polytetrafluoroethylene: A ten year experience. J Vasc Surg 1992; 16:209–217.
35. Abbott WM, Green RM, Matsumoto, et al: Prosthetic above-knee femoropopliteal bypass grafting: Results of a multicenter randomized prospective trial. J Vasc Surg 1997; 25:19–28.
36. Leather RP, Veith FJ: In situ vein bypass. In Haimovici H (ed): Vascular Surgery, 4th ed. London, Blackwell Science, 1996, pp 632–641.
37. Watelet J, Soury P, Menard J, et al: Femoropopliteal bypass: In situ or reversed vein grafts? Ten-year results of a randomized prospective study. Ann Vasc Surg 1997; 11:510–519.
38. Calligaro KD, Syrek JR, Dougherty MJ, et al: Use of arm and lesser saphenous vein compared with prosthetic grafts for infrapopliteal arterial bypass: Are they worth the effort? J Vasc Surg 1997; 26:919–927
39. Taylor RS, Loh A, McFarlan RJ, et al. Improved techniques for polytetrafluoroethylene bypass grafting long term results using anastomotic vein patches. Br J Surg 1992; 79:348–354.
40. Matsumura JS, Cabellon A, Fine N: Extended limb salvage: Combined distal vein bypass and free tissue transfer. In Yao JST, Pearce WH (eds): Techniques in Vascular and Endovascular Surgery. Stamford, CT, Appleton & Lange, pp 265–274.
41. Kretschner GJ, Holzenbein: The role of anticoagulation in infrainguinal bypass surgery. In Yao JST, Pearce WH (eds): The Ischemic Extremity: Advances in Treatment. Norwalk, CT, Appleton & Lange, 1995, pp 447–454.
42. Liem TK, Silver D: Options for anticoagulation. In Whittemore AD, Bandyk DF, Cronenwett JL, et al (eds): Advances in Vascular Surgery. St. Louis, Mosby, 1997, pp 201–221.
43. Edmundson RA, Cohen AT, Das SK, et al: LMWH vs aspirin and dipyridamole after femoro-popliteal bypass grafting. Lancet 1994; 344:914–918.
44. McMillan WD, McCarthy WJ, Lin SJ, et al: Perioperative low molecular weight heparin for infrageniculate bypass. J Vasc Surg 1997; 25:796–802.
45. Brewster DC, Chin AK, Hermann GD, et al: Arterial thromboembolism. In Rutherford RB (ed): Vascular Surgery, 4th ed. Philadelphia, WB Saunders, 1995, pp 647–668.
46. Tunick PA, Perez JL, Kronzon I: Protruding atheromas in the thoracic aorta and systematic embolization. Ann Intern Med 1991; 115(6):423–27.
47. Ascer E, Gennaro M, Mohan C, et al: Management of acute lower extremity ischemia. In Callow AD, Ernst CB (eds): Vascular Surgery: Theory and Practice. Stamford, CT, Appleton & Lange, 1995, pp 715–734.
48. DeWeese JA, Shortell C, Green R, et al: Operative repair of popliteal aneurysms. In Yao JST, Pearce WH (eds): Long Term Results in Vascular Surgery. Norwalk, CT, Appleton & Lange, 1993, pp 287–293.
49. Shortell CK, DeWeese JA, Ouriel K, et al: Popliteal artery aneurysm: A 25 year surgical experience. J Vasc Surg 1991; 14:771–79.
50. Perry MO: Acute limb ischemia. In Rutherford RB (ed): Vascular Surgery, 4th ed. Philadelphia, WB Saunders, 1995, pp 641–647.
51. Ettles DE, Earnshaw JJ: Complications in interventional radiology and thrombolysis. In Campbell B (ed): Complications in arterial surgery: A practical approach to management. Oxford, England: Butterworth/Heinemann, 1996, pp 159–170.
52. Haimovici H: Metabolic complications of acute arterial occlusions and skeletal muscle ischemia: Myonephro-

pathic-metabolic syndrome. In Haimovici H, Ascer E, Hollier LH, et al (eds): Vascular Surgery, 4th ed. London, Blackwell Science, 1996, pp 509–530.

53. Ouriel K: Current status of thrombolytic therapy in occlusion of native arteries and bypass grafts. In Yao JST, Pearce WH (eds): Progress in Vascular Surgery. Stamford, CT, Appleton & Lange, 1997, pp 277–285.

54. Ouriel K, Veith FJ, Sasahara AA for the TOPAS Investigators: Thrombolysis or peripheral arterial surgery: Phase I results. J Vasc Surg 1996; 23:64–75.

55. Nackman GB, Walsh DB, Fillinger MF, et al: Thrombolysis of occluded infrainguinal vein grafts: Predictors of outcome. J Vasc Surg 1997; 25:1023–32.

56. DeBakey ME, Simeone FA: Battle injuries of the arteries in World War II. Ann Surg 1946; 123:534–579.

57. Sumner DS, Mattos MA: Influence of surveillance programs on femoral-distal bypass graft patency. In Pearce WH, Yao JST (eds): The Ischemic Extremity. Stamford, CT, Appleton and Lange, 1995, pp 455–474.

58. Smith SRG, Wolf JHN: Convalescent problems in arterial surgery. BMJ 1991; 303:1388–1391.

59. Casey J, Flinn WR, Yao JST, et al: Correlations of immune and nutritional status with wound complications in patients undergoing vascular operations. Surgery 1983; 93:822–827.

60. Veith FJ, Haimovici H: Femoropopliteal arteriosclerotic occlusive disease. In Haimovici H (ed): Vascular Surgery, 4th ed. London, Blackwell Science, 1996, pp 605–631.

61. Pollock SE, Christian BJ, Sands D: Responses to chronic illness: Analysis of psychological and physiological adaptation. Nurs Res 1990; 39:300–304.

62. Crosby FE, Ventura MR, Frainier MA, et al: Well-being and concerns of patients with peripheral arterial occlusive disease. J Vasc Nurs 1993; 11(1):5–11.

63. Ronayne R: Uncertainty in peripheral vascular disease. Can J Cardiovasc Nurs 1989; 1:26–30.

64. Helt J: Foot wear and foot care to prevent amputation. J Vasc Nurs 1992; 9(4):2–8.

13

Extracranial Cerebrovascular Disease

Mimi Bradley, RN, BSN, and William H. Pearce, MD

❦ · ❦

Stroke is the leading cause of disability in the United States and the third leading cause of death, behind heart disease and cancer. Each year it is estimated that 500,000 Americans will suffer a stroke. The mortality rate following a stroke ranges from 26 to 52 percent. According to the most recent American Heart Association statistics, it is estimated that stroke accounts for half of all hospital admissions for acute neurologic disease. In addition, 28 percent of annual stroke victims are under the age of 65.[1] Although stroke may be caused by a variety of diseases, atherosclerosis is the most common contributing factor. The focus of this chapter will be the anatomy, pathophysiology, diagnosis, treatment, and nursing management of patients with extracranial cerebrovascular disease.

ANATOMY OF THE EXTRACRANIAL VASCULAR SYSTEM

Blood is supplied to the brain through paired carotid and vertebral arteries. These arteries are present in nearly constant configuration across the population. The unique anatomy and collateral blood supply to the brain is such that loss of a single or several vessels is tolerated. However, stroke is unavoidable with embolization.

Carotid Arteries

The blood supply to the anterior brain is provided by the carotid arteries (Fig. 13–1). The territory of the brain supplied by the internal carotid artery includes the frontal and temporal lobes. The right common carotid artery takes its origin from the innominate artery (brachiocephalic trunk), which is the first major branch of the aortic arch. The left common carotid artery originates directly from the arch. At the angle of the jaw and the superior border of the thyroid cartilage, the common carotid artery bifurcates into the internal and external carotid arteries. The external carotid artery lies anterior to the

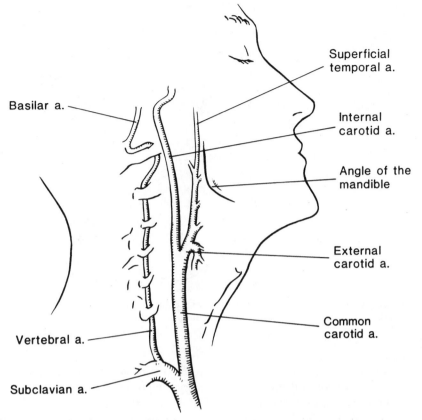

Figure 13–1. Arterial anatomy of the neck. (Reprinted from *Critical Care Nursing Quarterly*, Vol. 8, No. 2, p. 12, with permission of Aspen Publishers, Inc., © 1985.)

internal carotid artery and gives off numerous branches, which supply the face. The first section of the internal carotid artery is enlarged and is known as the carotid bulb or sinus. The carotid body is both a baroreceptor for blood pressure and a chemoreceptor for CO_2. The internal carotid artery has no major branch until the ophthalmic artery, which gives rise to the superficial and deep circulations of the eye. Since the ophthalmic artery is the first branch of the internal carotid artery, atherosclerotic emboli of this branch give rise to amaurosis fugax (transient monocular blindness).

Vertebral Arteries

The vertebral arteries originate from the subclavian arteries bilaterally and provide blood to the posterior circulation (main stem, cerebellum, and occipital lobes). They are surgically accessible for a short distance in the neck before entering the bony canal at the C6 vertebra and again at the base of the skull (C2). The vertebral arteries enter the skull and fuse in the midline to form the basilar artery. The basilar artery is the major blood supply to the anterior spinal artery, and provides posterior circulation to the main spinal artery. This posterior circulation communicates with the carotid circulation via the posterior communicating arteries.

Circle of Willis

The four extracranial vessels—two vertebral and two carotid arteries—join at the base of the brain and form the anastomotic network known as the circle of Willis. The anterior,

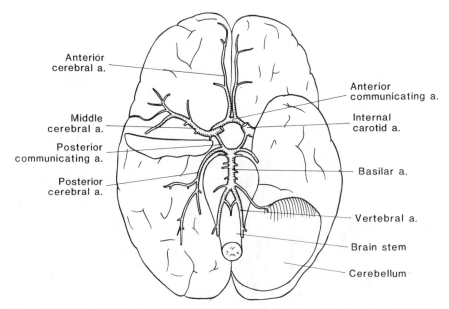

Figure 13–2. Cerebral blood supply. (Reprinted from Critical Care Nursing Quarterly, Vol. 8, No. 2, p. 13, with permission of Aspen Publishers, Inc., © 1985.)

middle, and posterior cerebral arteries arise from this network (Fig. 13–2). The circle provides the potential for collateral flow anteriorly or posteriorly to compensate for the loss of a carotid or vertebral artery, respectively. There is also the potential for "cross-over flow" from side to side through the anterior communicating arteries. Unfortunately, the circle of Willis may be incomplete, either congenitally or because of atherosclerotic occlusion, in as much as 50 percent of the population.[2]

PATHOPHYSIOLOGY OF THE EXTRACRANIAL VASCULAR SYSTEM

The most common cause of cerebrovascular disease in the United States is atherosclerosis, which accounts for 90 percent of all cases.[2, 3] The causes of the remaining 10 percent of cases of cerebrovascular disease include fibromuscular dysplasia, irradiation, carotid dissection, and arteritis. In any case, symptoms occur whenever arterial flow to an area is insufficient to support neuronal function.[2]

Atherosclerosis

The pathologic characteristics of atherosclerosis are described in Chapter 1 of this text. As in other areas of the body, most extracranial lesions occur at branch points and areas in which the artery is either fixed by the surrounding structures or curved. In arteriographic studies of patients with cerebrovascular insufficiency, Hass and associates[4] found that 75 percent of patients with symptoms had extracranial, surgically correctable lesions. Nearly 34 percent of all the extracranial lesions were at the common carotid bifurcation. Lesions of the vertebral arteries were most common at the origin and proximal one-third of the arteries. The same study population demonstrated a 40 percent rate of intracranial lesions. These were most common at the carotid siphon, the basilar artery, and the terminal portion of the vertebral artery. This is significant because it can be difficult to

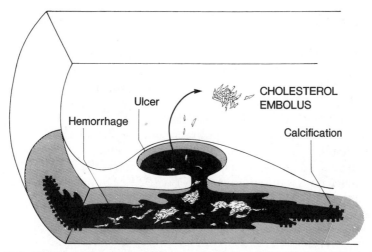

Figure 13–3. Cholesterol embolization. (From Lugsby RJ, Farrell LD, Wylie EJ: The significance of intraplaque hemorrhage in the pathogenesis of carotid atherosclerosis. In Bergan JJ, Yao JST [eds]: Cerebrovascular Insufficiency. New York, Grune & Stratton, 1983, p 450.)

determine whether symptoms are due to the intracranial or extracranial lesions when both are present.

The major mechanisms by which atherosclerosis causes ischemic symptoms are embolization and thrombosis.[5] Ulcerated lesions occur when the lining of the artery (endothelium and fibrous cap) ruptures, exposing cholesterol deposits, which may become emboli to the brain (Fig. 13–3). At Northwestern Memorial Hospital in Chicago, the carotid plaques from 44 patients undergoing carotid endarterectomy were studied. Plaque rupture occurred in 74 percent of symptomatic patients as compared with 32 percent of asymptomatic patients. With plaque rupture and high-grade stenosis with greater than 90 percent occlusion of the internal carotid artery, thrombosis may occur because of sluggish flow across the lesion (Fig. 13–4). In patients with an incomplete circle of Willis, thrombosis of a carotid artery will produce a significant stroke.

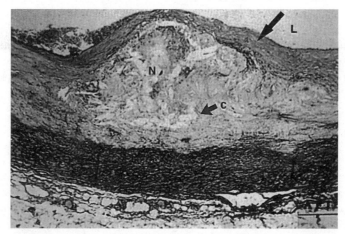

Figure 13–4. Histologic section of diagram in Figure 13–3. Mature atherosclerotic plaque with an intact fibrous cap *(arrow* near L*)* covering the necrotic core (N). The shoulder of the fibrous cap contains many inflammatory cells and is thought to represent a weak point in the plaque. L = lumen, C = cholesterol in plaque, which can become an embolus. (From Carr SC, Cheanvechai V, Virmani R, Pearce WH: Histology and clinical significance of the carotid atherosclerotic plaque: Implications for endovascular treatment. J Endovasc Surg 1997; 4:322.)

Fibromuscular Dysplasia

Fibromuscular dysplasia (FMD) occurs primarily in white females and involves larger arteries (renals, iliac, internal carotid arteries). The disease is usually bilateral, and is characterized by fibromedial or internal hyperplasia, which leads to focal stenosis and dilation of the artery. Of the extracranial vessels, the internal carotid artery is most often affected, although the vertebral arteries may demonstrate the disease as well.

Most patients have no symptoms; however, cerebral embolization may occur. Since fibromuscular dysplasia is well above the carotid bifurcation, arteriography is needed to make the diagnosis. In these cases, first-line therapy involves the use of antiplatelet agents. In general, percutaneous transluminal angioplasty (PTLA) of the carotid artery or surgery is needed to correct the problem.[6] Anticoagulation is required for those few persons who continue to have ischemic symptoms.

Cervical Irradiation

External irradiation for malignant cervical lesions damages the entire vessel wall and may accelerate atherosclerosis. Endarterectomy in these vessels is possible, although the lesions are longer. Wound problems may occur as a result of prior scarring and fibrosis of neck tissue. An increased probability of postoperative airway compromise in this population has been reported.[7]

Carotid Artery Dissection

Blunt trauma, sudden extension of the neck, or even paroxysms of coughing or vomiting may cause intimal tearing with subsequent carotid artery dissection. This entity is more common in persons under the age of 50 years, those with hypertension, and those with fibromuscular dysplasia.[8] Arteriographically, the result is a tapered stenosis in the shape of a bird's beak.

Most commonly, these patients present with ipsilateral headaches, ocular or cerebral ischemic events, and Horner's syndrome. Less frequent symptoms include a variety of cranial nerve disturbances such as slurred speech, facial nerve palsy, and dysphagia.[6] Commonly, the arterial dissection passes into the bony canal, making surgery impossible. Observation and anticoagulation constitute the treatment of choice. If surgery is required, a bypass from the carotid to the intracranial circulation (extracranial-intracranial [ECIC] bypass) is performed by a neurosurgeon. However, in the majority of the patients, the dissection will heal without consequence.[9]

Arteritis

Takayasu's arteritis is a vasculitis of the giant-cell type, often involving the aortic arch and its branches. Young women, especially those of Asian descent, are most commonly affected. Symptoms of carotid artery involvement can include transient ischemic attacks (TIAs), stroke, and cranial neuropathies. Corticosteroids are usually given for acute disease. Some patients with aggressive disease have been reported to benefit from the addition of the cytotoxic agent cyclophosphamide (Cytoxan).[10] However, there are no controlled studies to confirm this combined approach. For upper-extremity or cerebral ischemia that has not responded to medical therapy, arterial bypass may be required. Surgery is not usually performed during the active phase of the disease.[11]

CLINICAL MANIFESTATIONS

The symptoms related to carotid artery disease may be divided into several broad categories (Table 13–1). The first group is patients without symptoms. Atherosclerotic occlusion of the carotid artery may build up slowly without symptoms. The remaining three blood vessels increase blood flow to accommodate the decrease in blood flow in the diseased artery. When followed over long periods of time, patients with asymptomatic stenosis may develop symptoms (3 to 5 percent per year). The natural history of these lesions is often erratic, and a minor stenosis may rapidly progress to plaque hemorrhage and rupture.

However, the majority of patients present with symptoms, which can be divided into focal, global, and vertebrobasilar. Focal symptoms are any that produce discrete, unilateral findings. Embolic debris from the proximal carotid artery may lodge in the retinal artery, producing visual field deficits and visual loss. Ocular examination may detect the Hollenhorst plaque or cholesterol emboli within the retinal vessels. Emboli to the retinal artery may also result in total occlusion, producing monocular blindness with or without retinal vein occlusion. If the embolic debris passes into the brain and lodges within one of the terminal branches of the middle cerebral artery, the patient may experience hemiparesis, hemiplegia, or aphasia.

If the neurologic deficit lasts less than 24 hours, it is termed a transient ischemic attack (TIA). If the event lasts greater then 24 hours but resolves over a period of weeks, it is called a reversible ischemic neurologic deficit (RIND). Any event that lasts greater than 24 hours and does not resolve is termed cerebrovascular accident or stroke. These terms are arbitrary and do not reflect the exact nature of the insult to the brain. Ischemic

TABLE 13–1. **Summary of Ischemic Neurologic Events**

CATEGORY	DURATION OF SYMPTOMS (hr)	SYMPTOMS	DEGREE OF RECOVERY
ASYMPTOMATIC			
SYMPTOMATIC			
Focal			
TIA	<24	Hemiparesis, monoparesis, aphasia	Complete
RIND	>24 but <72	Any of the above	Complete
CVA		Hemiparesis, monoparesis, aphasia	Permanent deficit
Amaurosis fugax	<24	Monocular blindness: at times described as a shade over a portion of the eye	Complete. Rarely, blindness may be permanent
Global			
Stroke	>24	Any of the above	Permanent deficit; some improvement may occur with time
Dizziness, syncope	Nonspecific	Nonspecific	Usually not permanent
Vertebrobasilar	<24	Dysarthria, global aphasia, diplopia, vertigo, syncope, dizziness, confusion, drop attacks	Complete

TIA = transient ischemic attack; RIND = reversible ischemic neurologic deficit; CVA = cerebrovascular accident.

damage can be detected by magnetic resonance arteriography (MRA) or computed tomography (CT) in patients suffering a simple TIA. Patients with diffuse extracranial vascular disease may also present with focal symptoms when the responsible ("watershed") area of the brain becomes more ischemic than others. Watershed infarcts are usually in the terminal branches of the cortex, and are best detected by CT scans. Finally, there are a few patients who have multiple-vessel occlusions leading to ocular ischemia of the eye, producing the "red-eye syndrome." The red-eye syndrome is extremely rare but should not be missed because of the potential for eventual blindness.

Patients may also present with global symptoms reflecting decreased perfusion to all areas of the brain. These patients most often have multiple-vessel occlusions and present with dizziness, syncope, and occasional ocular manifestations. These patients may be difficult to separate from patients with vertebrobasilar symptoms (vertebrobasilar infarcts [VBIs]). Patients with vertebrobasilar symptoms have decreased perfusion to the brain stem and as a result may complain of dizziness, syncope, ocular symptoms, and neurologic deficits of the arms and legs. The patients with global and vertebrobasilar symptoms are most difficult to separate from those with nonspecific neurologic diseases. Such patients often require neurologic evaluation in addition to assessment of the cerebral circulation.

PATIENT EVALUATION

History

Evaluation of the patient with known or suspected extracranial cerebrovascular disease includes a thorough history and physical examination along with noninvasive vascular testing. For the patient with symptoms, the goals of history taking are to characterize the neurologic event and identify any coexisting medical problems. The ischemic event should be described in detail, including symptoms and findings noted by others at the time of the incident. Family members may provide details that the patient is unable to recall. The assessment should include questions about speech difficulties, visual disturbances, motor weakness or paralysis, vertigo, syncope, and confusion and memory loss. Timing of the incident would include time of day, activity the patient was involved in at the time, the duration of symptoms, and the frequency of episodes.

Because atherosclerosis accounts for the majority of ischemic episodes, the patient should be evaluated for risk factors that may be modified. Risk factors include tobacco use, hypertension, diabetes mellitus, hyperlipidemia, and family history of disease. Other evidence of the systemic nature of the disease includes intermittent claudication, angina, congestive heart failure, myocardial infarction, prior cardiac or vascular surgery, or known aneurysms.

Any indication of cardiac disease should be carefully evaluated. Hertzer and colleagues[12] found that more than half of all persons with peripheral arterial disease had clinically suspected coronary artery disease. This included 57 percent of those evaluated for cerebrovascular disease. Severe coronary artery disease was demonstrated by angiography in 35 percent of the cerebrovascular patients. Detection is essential for proper management of the cardiac disease as well as for determining whether the patient may be a candidate for surgery. Some patients may require either staged or combined repair of both the coronary and extracranial cerebrovascular disease.

Physical Examination

Extracranial artery disease can be assessed through careful evaluation of the head and neck. Bilateral pulse examination should include the superficial temporal artery, which can be palpated just anterior to the ear. The carotid artery should be palpated low in the neck to avoid dislodging plaque from the bifurcation. Massage of the carotid sinus may also lead to bradycardia or asystole. The neck should be evaluated for the presence of bruits, which are best heard with the bell of the stethoscope. The location of the bruit should be described as being at the angle of the jaw, in the midportion of the neck, or low in the neck. Particular attention should be paid to carotid bruits heard in both systole and diastole, as they indicate severe stenosis. However, severe stenosis may not be associated with a bruit. Vertebral artery bruits may be heard posterior to the sternocleidomastoid muscle.[13] A variety of clues to vascular disease may be found during the fundoscopic examination. Signs of hypertension, diabetic retinopathy, Hollenhorst plaque (atheromatous debris), and retinal ischemia can be seen on the funduscopic exam.

Sometimes a bruit will be detected during a routine examination or during the evaluation of another problem. These asymptomatic patients should receive the same careful attention as those with symptomatic disease. Although there are a variety of opinions concerning the natural history of asymptomatic carotid artery disease,[14] one study demonstrated a significantly increased stroke rate among those persons with more than 60 percent stenosis of the internal carotid artery.[15]

In addition to the vascular exam, a complete neurologic examination should be performed. This includes an evaluation of sensory and motor function, visual acuity, speech, memory, level of consciousness, and comprehension. In some cases, deficits may help to identify the areas of the brain affected and indicate the location of the diseased arterial segment. The initial neurologic examination will also serve as a baseline to detect postoperative complications.

The remainder of the evaluation should focus on the degree of arterial insufficiency in other areas of the body. Bilateral upper-extremity blood pressures are measured to detect hypertension and occlusion of either the innominate or subclavian arteries. Cardiac evaluation should include auscultation for rhythm, murmurs, and the presence of abnormal heart sounds. Peripheral edema, shortness of breath, and jugular vein distention may also point to cardiac dysfunction. Finally, the extremities should be observed for the presence of ulcers, ischemic skin changes, and peripheral pulses.

Noninvasive Testing

Further evaluation of the patient is based on the findings from the history and physical examination. The primary tool for the evaluation of the neck arteries is duplex ultrasonography. The duplex scan is accurate in quantifying carotid artery stenosis and is described in detail in Chapter 5. Because of the high accuracy of the duplex scan and the risk of arteriography, many surgeons are performing surgery based solely upon the duplex scan itself. Noninvasive testing is used for routine follow-up of the patient to detect recurrent stenosis after carotid endarterectomy.

CT scanning may be performed to identify those patients whose symptoms are due to tumors, hemangiomas, intracranial vascular disease, or subdural hematomas. The scan is also used to detect stroke and is used postoperatively for any neurologic complication. However, a recent study found that CT results did not influence the operative decisions in 496 consecutive patients over a 5-year period.[16] Also, the CT results did not correlate with any of the postoperative neurologic events.

Invasive Diagnostic Studies

Invasive testing is usually reserved for patients in whom the cause of the neurologic event is questioned or when the duplex study is inadequate.[2] Arteriography of the aortic arch,

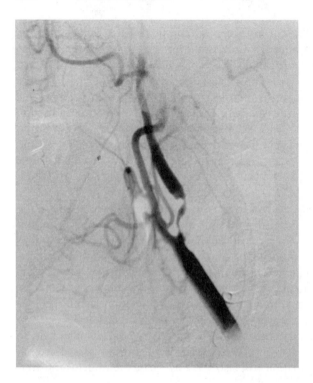

Figure 13–5. Carotid angiogram demonstrating stenotic lesion of the internal carotid artery.

neck vessels, and cerebral circulation identifies the exact location and extent of disease (Fig. 13–5). Arteriography is particularly helpful in the identification of lesions of the distal cerebral circulation, which are not surgically accessible. Angiography is more fully described in Chapter 6.

Conventional arteriography has been enhanced by the addition of digital subtraction techniques. Digital subtraction angiography (DSA) is a computerized fluoroscopic method that subtracts the bone and soft-tissue structures from a stored summation of all of the contrast that has circulated in the arterial tree. The information is displayed on a screen and can be printed as other arteriograms are. Although DSA can be performed intravenously, the images are usually inferior to those obtained with an intra-arterial injection. Also, the arterial route allows for the use of less contrast material.

Magnetic resonance angiography (MRA) is available in most areas. This technology is developing and the degree of resolution improving. The recent use of intravenous gadolinium has improved image quality. In many areas MRA has replaced angiography[17] (Fig. 13–6) for severe carotid stenosis. MRA requires only a peripheral injection of gadolinium and does not require an arterial puncture.

MEDICAL AND SURGICAL MANAGEMENT

Carotid endarterectomy (CEA) is currently the most frequently performed vascular surgical procedure in the United States.[18] The goal of this surgery is to prevent stroke from occurring. In the mid 1980s the efficacy of CEA in preventing stroke was questioned. As a result, a number of randomized prospective studies were performed comparing surgery with best medical management in both symptomatic and asymptomatic patients. The two most significant symptomatic trials are the North American Symptomatic Carotid Endarterectomy Trial (NASCET)[18] and the European Carotid Surgery Trial (ECST).[19] Both studies demonstrated a significant benefit of carotid endarterectomy for patients with symptoms in whom there was more than 70 percent stenosis of the internal carotid

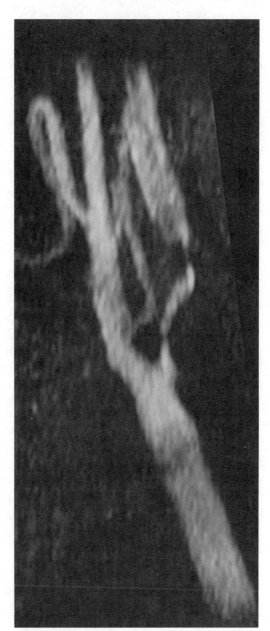

Figure 13–6. Magnetic resonance arteriography (MRA) demonstrating stenosis of the internal carotid artery in the same patient as Figure 13–5.

artery. Endarterectomy in patients with symptomatic moderate carotid stenosis of 50 to 69 percent yielded only a moderate reduction in the risk of stroke.[20] For patients with less than 30 percent stenosis, surgery was not beneficial.

Asymptomatic carotid disease, as mentioned earlier, does not always remain asymptomatic. In a large Veterans Affairs Cooperative Study, carotid endarterectomy reduced the incidence of an ipsilateral neurologic event in men without symptoms and a greater than 50 percent stenosis. The incidence of ipsilateral neurologic event was 8 percent in the surgical group as compared with 20.6 percent in the medical group ($p < 0.001$).[14] In the more recent Asymptomatic Carotid Atherosclerosis Study (ACAS), asymptomatic patients with a stenosis of 60 percent or greater had a reduced 5-year risk of ipsilateral stroke with carotid endarterectomy, provided they were good surgical candidates and aggressively managed modifiable risk factors.[15]

The natural history of disease must be weighed against the risks of mortality and morbidity associated with surgery.[21] Carotid endarterectomy is now recommended for patients with more than 70 percent stenosis if the operation can be done with little risk.[22-24] Others who may benefit from surgery include those patients with bilateral stenosis of more than 50 percent, unilateral stenosis of more than 60 percent with a contralateral occlusion, and a rapidly progressing stenosis of more than 50 percent.[24]

Medical Management

Aspirin, other antiplatelet agents, and anticoagulants have been studied for their effectiveness in preventing stroke in cases of carotid and vertebral atherosclerosis. Recent research indicates that daily doses of aspirin after TIA result in a 15–30 percent reduction in stroke rate.[15] Research doses have ranged from 40–1300 mg daily. Doses of 325 mg daily have been shown to be as effective as higher doses and to have fewer side effects.[23] The role of aspirin has yet to be clarified in the treatment of women, patients with ulcerative carotid artery lesions, and persons with asymptomatic disease.[15] It is important to remember that aspirin does not change the progression of the arterial plaque. Also, it is not likely to prevent thrombosis of highly stenotic lesions.[2]

Ticlopidine is another antiplatelet agent that has recently received attention. Patients who received ticlopidine after a stroke demonstrated a 30.2 percent lower risk of subsequent stroke, myocardial infarction, and vascular death than in similar patients who received a placebo. This effect was the same for both men and women.[25] However, ticlopidine has significant side effects, including white blood cell abnormalities and thrombotic thrombocytopenic purpura (TTP). Other antiplatelet agents given with aspirin, such as sulfinpyrazone and dipyridamole, have shown little additional benefit over aspirin alone.[2, 23]

Anticoagulation with heparin or warfarin has been studied with varying results. Although some studies would advocate this treatment for certain patients, others indicate that anticoagulation may actually be harmful.

Surgical Management

Indications for CEA are in Table 13–2. When surgery is being considered, the risk of stroke must be weighed against the risk of mortality and morbidity associated with the operation in the specific institution.

Perioperative Care

Each patient should have an intra-arterial catheter to monitor blood pressure during carotid endarterectomy so that cerebral perfusion can be maximized. Wide fluctuations in the patient's blood pressure are common and excessive hypertension or hypotension may produce stroke. The operation may be performed with local, regional, or general inhalation anesthesia. The risk of stroke during surgery is related not to the type of anesthesia but rather to the surgeon's qualifications and experience. Because the benefit of this surgery is based on a low perioperative stroke rate, the surgeon performing this procedure must be very experienced, with an operative stroke rate of less than 3 percent in asymptomatic patients and less than 6 percent in the symptomatic patient.

The skin incision is made either along the anterior border of the sternocleidomastoid muscle or transversely in a skin crease. All of the dissection is performed gently to avoid atheroembolization. Once the bleeding vessels are controlled, the patient is given heparin

TABLE 13–2. **Indications for Carotid Endarterectomy (CEA)**

Symptomatic
- **Proven**
  - Surgical morbidity and mortality < 6%
  - Transient ischemic attack (TIA) or mild stroke with ≥ 70% stenosis
- **Acceptable**
  - TIA or mild stroke with 50–69% stenosis
  - Progressive stroke ≥ 70%
  - CEA ipsilateral to TIA or stenosis ≥ 70% and associated coronary artery surgery

Asymptomatic
- Surgical morbidity and mortality < 3%
- 60% or greater stenosis (primarily men)

Data from Moore WS, Barnett HJM, Beebe HG, et al: Guidelines for carotid endarterectomy: A multidisciplinary consensus statement from the ad hoc committee, American Heart Association. Circulation 1995; 91:566–579.

to prevent thrombosis. A longitudinal arteriotomy is performed. The plaque and arterial intima, along with portions of the media of the artery, are then removed. A patch of autogenous vein or prosthetic material may be used if primary closure of the carotid artery will cause narrowing of the artery or when the endarterectomy is being repeated. The use of routine patching is debated, with literature support for either selective or routine patching.[26]

During CEA, cerebral perfusion is a primary concern. Theoretically, this should occur via collaterals and the circle of Willis. However, collateral flow is not always adequate and an intraluminal shunt is placed (Fig. 13–7). Some surgeons use shunting routinely, whereas others use it selectively. Other methods of monitoring cerebral perfusion during clamping

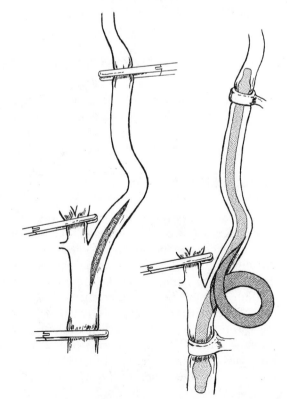

Figure 13–7. Intraluminal shunt placement during carotid endarectomy. (Reprinted from Critical Care Nursing Quarterly, Vol. 8, No. 2, p. 18, with permission of Aspen Publishers, Inc., © 1985.)

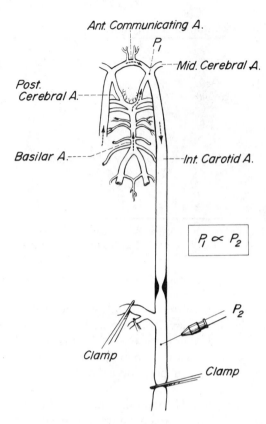

Figure 13–8. Stump pressure measurement. (From Moore WS, Hall CD: Carotid artery back pressure. Arch Surg 1969; 99:705. © 1969, American Medical Association.)

include electroencephalography (EEG) monitoring and the use of the stump pressure (Fig. 13–8). A stump pressure of greater than 50 mmHg is considered safe to proceed with clamping alone.

POSTOPERATIVE COMPLICATIONS

Postoperative problems include perioperative stroke, cranial nerve injuries, and wound complications. Cardiac events are the major cause of the few deaths that occur following surgery.

Perioperative Stroke

Because of improvements in anesthesia, operative procedure, and shunting, the incidence of perioperative stroke has decreased to 2 percent in some institutions. Immediate postoperative deficits may be due to embolization of the atheromatous debris during dissection, low flow while the carotid artery is clamped, or technical complications such as a raised intimal flap, resulting in carotid artery thrombosis.

With an acute stroke, the patency of the carotid artery must be promptly determined either by obtaining a noninvasive study or taking the patient directly back to surgery. If the carotid artery is patent, heparinization is suggested. If the artery is not patent, thrombectomy is urgently performed. The artery is explored to locate any luminal irregularities that may have led to occlusion. On closure, patch angioplasty is sometimes used to widen the lumen of the artery if that was not done previously. Heparin may be added after the second operation. Deficits due to acute occlusion will often resolve when flow is restored. Deficits due to atheromatous embolization may or may not resolve.

Cranial Nerve Injuries

Some patients will experience sensory or motor deficits involving the cranial nerves or the greater auricular nerve, which may be misinterpreted as a stroke. The most frequent injures are summarized in Table 13–3. These result from traction or inadvertent transection during the operation. The neuroanatomy of the neck is demonstrated in Figures 13–9 and 13–10. Although most of these injuries resolve in time, patients undergoing staged bilateral endarterectomies may require laryngoscopy between the operations to identify any vocal cord paralysis.

Wound Complications/Respiratory Distress

Wound complications are infrequent after carotid endarterectomy. Bleeding and wound hematomas should be aggressively managed because the airway may be compromised by tracheal compression. Cervical hematomas are usually the result of coughing or straining during extubation. Reoperation is performed to identify and correct a suture line bleed and to drain the hematoma. A small closed drain is used in these situations.

SPECIAL CONSIDERATIONS

Currently, a few issues remain in the surgical management of extracranial cerebrovascular disease. These include surgery for treatment of vertebrobasilar insufficiency, treatment of recurrent carotid disease, and carotid stenting.

Vertebrobasilar symptoms may be due to brain tumors, cervical spine injuries, or diseases of the vertebral or basilar arteries. Therefore, careful evaluation is required before surgery is considered. Arterial symptoms may be transient, resolving with no treatment.

TABLE 13–3. **Summary of Nerve Injuries After Carotid Endarterectomy**

CRANIAL NERVE	POSTOPERATIVE INJURY
Hypoglossal (XII)	Affects the ipsilateral tongue, difficulties with speech and mastication; patient will be hoarse and have difficulty attaining high-pitched phonation
Superior laryngeal vagus (X) branch	Minor swallowing problems and easily fatigued voice
Recurrent laryngeal-anterior vagus (X)	Vocal cord paralysis, hoarseness present, and inadequate gag reflex
Glossopharyngeal (IX)	Difficulty swallowing with ipsilateral Horner's syndrome (ptosis, exophthalmos, reduced sweating); a rare injury
Facial (VII)	Drooping of the corner of the lip on the ipsilateral side and inability to smile symmetrically
Spinal accessory (XI)	Limitations in neck, shoulder movement in terms of alignment and horizontal motion
Greater auricular	(A branch of brachial plexus rather than a cranial nerve) Paresthesias of the face and ear

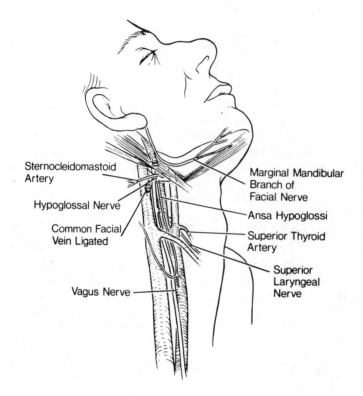

Sternocleidomastoid Artery

Hypoglossal Nerve

Common Facial Vein Ligated

Vagus Nerve

Marginal Mandibular Branch of Facial Nerve

Ansa Hypoglossi

Superior Thyroid Artery

Superior Laryngeal Nerve

Figure 13–9. Cranial nerves in relation to the carotid artery. (From Bergan JJ, Flinn WR, Yao JST: Cranial nerve injury in carotid surgery. In Bergan JJ, Yao JST [eds]: Cerebrovascular Insufficiency. New York, Grune & Stratton, 1983, p 454.)

Figure 13–10. Greater auricular and facial nerves in relation to the carotid artery. (From Bergan JJ, Flinn WR, Yao JST: Cranial nerve injury in carotid surgery. In Bergan JJ, Yao JST [eds]: Cerebrovascular Insufficiency. New York, Grune & Stratton, 1983, p 452.)

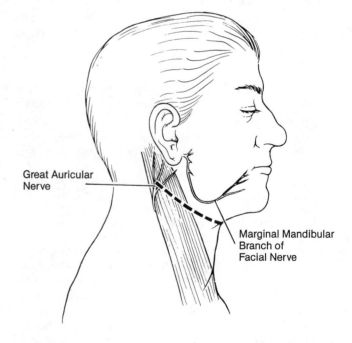

Great Auricular Nerve

Marginal Mandibular Branch of Facial Nerve

Medical therapy is much the same as for carotid artery disease. However, some patients with severe symptoms have been treated with bypass procedures.[27] Carotid endarterectomy has also been used to treat this problem. Increasing the anterior circulation reaching the circle of Willis allows for sufficient collateral perfusion of the posterior portions of the brain.[28]

Patients and health care providers alike are often frustrated by recurrent carotid artery disease. Exact rates of recurrence vary among reports in the literature. One study demonstrated early restenosis (in less than 24 months) to be due most often to myointimal hyperplasia.[29] Stenoses occurring after 24 months were usually due to atherosclerotic lesions. The only significant variable in late restenosis was continued smoking. Of the patients with recurrent disease, 64 percent continued to smoke, whereas only 26 percent of those without recurrent disease were smokers. All patients should be counseled to refrain from smoking. Management of recurrent disease requires an annual examination and ultrasonographic scanning. If the restenosis exceeds 50 percent or if the patient has symptoms, reoperation may be required.

Recently, angioplasty with stenting has been used for the treatment of carotid artery stenosis. This technique is highly controversial and early results are poor. The combined stroke and death rate for carotid stenting is between 5.9 and 11 percent.[30, 31] It is no surprise that the stroke rate is so high given the friable nature of the carotid lesion. Until the results are dramatically improved, carotid stenting should be performed only as a part of a national study and only by highly qualified individuals.

POSTOPERATIVE NURSING CARE

Following carotid endarterectomy, the patient may recover on a surgical unit or may require an intensive care unit (ICU) bed. A patient requiring close monitoring can remain

TABLE 13–4. **Potential Postoperative Complications and Nursing Management**

Blood Pressure Deviation

Monitor for hypotension and hypertension. Administer appropriate medication as ordered.

Neurologic Problems

Monitor patient for increased blood pressure, decreased heart rate, and Cheyne-Stokes respiration (increased intracranial pressure secondary to hemorrhage); decreased blood pressure, increased heart rate and respirations (due to cerebral ischemia); symptomatic bradycardia (due to vagal nerve stimulation).

Assess level of consciousness. Is patient oriented to time, date, place, and person? Does patient respond appropriately to command and/or pain? Check response to auditory and tactile stimuli.

Assess pupils. Are they equal in size? Do they respond to light equally and briskly? Is the resting position of the eyes at midline?

Assess motor function. Can patient move all extremities in response to command (flexion and extension)? Are hand grips equal in strength?

Cranial Nerve Injury

See Table 13–3 for summary of nerve injuries and presenting symptoms.

Hematoma/Respiratory Distress

Monitor for excessive bleeding, swelling at incisional site, or sudden increase in neck circumference. Observe for signs of respiratory distress, shortness of breath, changes in vital signs, anxiety, restlessness, pallor, cyanosis, or changes in level of consciousness.

TABLE 13–5. **Patient Education**

PREOPERATIVE TEACHING

Explain to patient that carotid artery disease is usually the result of atherosclerosis. Carotid endarterectomy is the surgical removal of atherosclerotic plaque from the artery. Surgery is performed to prevent symptoms from occurring and to decrease the incidence of stroke. The surgeon will discuss potential neurologic deficits and cranial nerve injuries preoperatively with the patient and the family.

Teach and discuss preoperative and postoperative routines with patient. Assess level of understanding and reinforce teaching.

Provide written material if available.

POSTOPERATIVE TEACHING

Activity

Recovery from surgery varies from person to person. Return to normal activity at a gradual but regular pace using common sense. Move the neck as you would normally. No heavy lifting (greater than 10 lbs) is allowed for 1 month after surgery.

Restriction on sexual activity depends on the philosophy of the physician.

Bathing

Instruct the patient that: bathing or showering is acceptable on the third day after surgery if subcuticular sutures are used: Clean the incision with mild soap and water and dry well; and no special wound care is required unless otherwise indicated.

Risk Factor Reduction (see Chapter 10)

Risk factors are habits, traits or conditions that may increase a person's likelihood of developing atherosclerosis. Review pertinent risk factors with the patient and family.

* **Diet**—Instruct patient on a low-fat, low-cholesterol diet unless specified. When appropriate, diet for modification of hyperlipidemia, hypertension, or diabetes should also be reviewed. American Heart Association guidelines specify that a total cholesterol level should be less than 200 mg/dl with low-density lipoprotein (LDL) of less than 130.
* **Smoking**—Explain to the patient that smoking accelerates atherosclerosis, increases blood pressure, and decreases heart rate. Encourage the patient to quit smoking.
* **Hypertension**—Instruct patient to resume preoperative antihypertensive medication and emphasize importance of future blood pressure management.

Driving

Inform patients that they may resume driving when they can move the neck as freely as they did before surgery. Instruct patients not to drive after taking narcotic pain medicine or sleeping pills. They should check with their physician.

Wound Care

Inform patient that bruising, discoloration, and swelling are not uncommon and will disappear. Inform patient that sutures are internal and do not need to be removed.

Men may shave around the incision using an electric razor. Use of a bladed razor should be avoided until the swelling around the incision is gone.

Cranial Nerve Deficits

Instruct patient regarding any postoperative cranial nerve deficits. Instruct patient that problems with swallowing and tongue coordination are the most common and will resolve in time.

Medical Follow-up/Indications for Physician Notification

Instruct patient/significant other to inform physician of recurrent or new symptoms:

* Transient ischemic attack (TIA) or permanent (stroke)
  * Motor or sensory deficits in extremities
  * Speech impairments (difficulty expressing self or understanding spoken words)
* Visual deficits, especially loss of vision in one eye.
* Sudden onset of swelling around the incision, increase in the size of the neck, or difficulty breathing
* Sudden severe headache

Do not ignore any symptoms.

Attend scheduled follow-up visits. (Both duplex scan and office visit, time frame specified per physician's preference.)

up to 4 hours in the recovery room and in an ICU for 8–24 hours. Frequent neurologic and hemodynamic assessments will be required in either setting. New neurologic deficits require prompt attention and sometimes reoperation. Hypertension is a common problem, which can threaten the arterial anastomosis. Hypotension may also occur and predispose the patient to carotid artery thrombosis. Extremes in blood pressure may complicate any existing cardiac disease. Thorough assessment and timely treatment can aid in preventing undesirable outcomes. Standard nursing care after CEA is described in Table 13–4.

Because of the shortened length of stay, nurses are required to provide comprehensive teaching in a shorter period of time. Discharge teaching is directed toward a return to normal activities and modification of risk factors for atherosclerosis. Control of risk factors and behavioral modification is critical for optimal long-term outcome.[32] Specific instructions regarding driving, bathing, and other activities may vary with physician preference. In general, there are very few limitations in the uncomplicated postoperative course. Table 13–5 provides further teaching information. A duplex scan may be recommended 6 months to a year after surgery to assess any restenosis of the carotid arteries. The scan may then be performed on an annual basis. For the unfortunate person who has sustained a perioperative stroke, more extensive planning and placement may be required.

In this time of increased health care costs, cost containment, and increased utilization of ICU beds, nurses are striving to find methods for efficient utilization of resources without compromising the quality of patient care. Clinical pathways are one tool utilized to streamline the patient's hospital course.[33] Table 13–6 presents a clinical pathway for care of a patient undergoing carotid endarerectomy. One study demonstrated that the introduction of clinical pathways reduced cost without increasing risk in patients undergoing CEA.[34]

Other studies have attempted to determine a predictable postoperative course in patients undergoing CEAs. In the past 5 years, dramatic strides have been made in reducing both ICU bed need and decreasing hospital stay after carotid endarterectomy. Lipsett[35] found that patients with numerous preoperative risk factors had an increased need for an ICU bed. Hypertension is the risk factor that best correlates with ICU bed need.[36] Hirko and colleagues reduced the ICU stay from 94.8 percent in 1990 to 12.5 percent in 1993.[37] This study also revealed a significant decrease in length of stay. The total length of stay was reduced from an average of 6.18 days to 2.0 days. This study also confirmed that these changes have not adversely affected the safety of the operation.

CONCLUSION

Although a variety of diseases may produce cerebrovascular insufficiency, the most common cause is atherosclerosis. Careful evaluation of the patient by physical examination and noninvasive testing will define the extent of disease and direct planning for the appropriate treatment. Carotid endarterectomy is indicated for patients with greater than 70 percent stenosis, regardless of symptoms, and with no contraindications to surgery. The surgeon must have a combined mortality and morbidity of less than 3 percent for asymptomatic patients and less than 6 percent for symptomatic patients. The value of CEA in patients with symptoms who have lesser degrees of stenosis is uncertain. Carotid stenting at present cannot be recommended until the procedural stroke rate is comparable to surgery. Nurses are instrumental in providing education and support for lifestyle changes to reduce the risk of further disease.

TABLE 13–6. **Clinical Pathway for Same-Day Admission Carotid Endarterectomy**

	PREADMIT	OR DAY; ICU/FLOOR	POD #1; FLOOR	POD #2
Vital Signs/ Parameters		VS/neurochecks q 1 hr I/O q 1 hr	VS/neurochecks q 4 hr I/O q 8 hr	VS/neurochecks q 4
IV and PO Drugs	D/C aspirin	Aspirin (recovery room) Antibiotic, pain med prn IV vasopressors prn IV; A-line	Aspirin q day Pain med prn Discontinue A-line, IV line prn	Aspirin q day
Treatment		Observe for hematoma, respiratory distress q 1 hr Elevate HOB 30°	Observe for hematoma and respiratory distress Discontinue Foley catheter prn MD changes first dressing in AM	Observe for hematoma and respiratory distress
Consult/ Discharge Planning	Cardiology consult prn Evaluate discharge needs Anesthesia	Transfer when appropriate	Rx and discharge instruction sheet completed by MD May be discharged Discharge planner prn	Rx and discharge instruction sheet completed by MD Discharge home
Activity	Ad lib	Bed rest	OOB 2–3 × Ambulate as tolerated	OOB ad lib
Diet	Low fat, low cholesterol NPO after midnight	NPO	Advance diet as tolerated; low fat, low cholesterol	Low fat, low cholesterol
Tests	Bloodwork (SMA 20) CBC with diff coag profile, cardiac risk panel prn Carotid duplex scan Cardiac evaluation prn UA ECG, chest x-ray Angiogram/MRA CT head prn T & S	ECG prn Labs prn ABGs prn O_2 prn	EKG prn CBC, SMA-7, PTT/PT prn ABGs prn O_2 prn	

Psychosocial	Admission profile Assess patient/family psychosocial needs	Provide support	Intervene w/pt & family re psychosocial needs prn	Intervene w/pt & family re psychosocial needs prm
Patient Education	Preop teaching Provide patient with education material Review clinical path w/patient & family Review postop course Assess pt/family level of understanding	Assess family level of understanding Discuss postop course with family	Discuss progress w/patient & family Provide discharge teaching Offer risk reduction class and information	Provide discharge teaching
Expected Outcomes	Pt's lab values are within normal range Pt's neurologic exam is within normal limits or has not deteriorated from baseline exam Pt receives educational material Pt receives cardiac evaluation Pt verbalizes understanding of preadmission teaching Pt verbalizes understanding of diagnostic testing and preop teaching	Pt verbalizes satisfaction with pain relief Pt's cardiac parameters remain within normal limits Pt's neurologic exam is within normal limits or has not deteriorated from baseline exam Pt demonstrates no signs/symptoms of neck hematoma or respiratory distress	Pt's cardiac parameters remain within normal limits Pt verbalizes satisfaction with pain relief Pt's neurologic exam is within normal limits or has not deteriorated from baseline exam Pt demonstrates no signs/symptoms of neck hematoma	Pt verbalizes understanding of discharge instructions and warning signs of stroke Pt/family verbalizes risk factors and application of lifestyle modification

OR = operating room; ICU = intensive care unit; POD = postoperative day; VS = vital signs; I/O = intake & output; D/C = discontinue; prn = as needed; IV = intravenous; PO = by mouth (oral); A-line = arterial line; HOB = head of bed; Rx = prescription (for drugs and other medicaments); ad lib = freely; OOB = out of bed; NPO = nothing by mouth; SMA = Sequential Multiple Analysis; CBC = complete blood count; UA = urinalysis; ECG = electrocardiogram; MRA = magnetic resonance angiography; CT = computed tomography; T & S = type and screen; ABG = arterial blood gas; PTT/PT = partial thromboplastin time/prothrombin time.

References

1. A to Z Stroke Guide. http://www.americanheart.org/Heart_and_Stroke_A_Z_Guide.
2. Sullivan ED, Herzter NR: Extracranial cerebrovascular arterial disease. In Young JR, Graor RA, Olin JW, et al: (eds): Peripheral Vascular Disease, 2nd ed. St. Louis, Mosby–Year Book, 1996, pp 288–304.
3. Moore WS: Fundamental consideration in cerebrovascular disease. In Rutherford RB (ed): Vascular Surgery. Philadelphia, WB Saunders, 1995, pp 1456–1473.
4. Hass WK, Fields WS, North RR, et al: Joint study of extracranial arterial occlusion. II. Arteriography, techniques, sites and complications. JAMA 1968; 203:961–968.
5. Carr SC, Cheanvechai V, Virmani R, Pearce WH: Histology and clinical significance of the carotid atherosclerotic plaque: Implications for newer methods of treatment. J Endovasc Surg 1997; 4:321–325.
6. Lee NS, Jones HR: Extracranial cerebrovascular disease. Cardiol Clin 1991; 9:523–534.
7. Francfort JW, Smullens SN, Gallagher JF, et al: Airway compromise after carotid surgery in patients with cervical irradiation. J Cardiovasc Surg 1989; 30:877–881.
8. Spittell JA, Spittell PC: Dissection of the aorta and other arteries. In Young JR, et al (eds): Peripheral Vascular Diseases. St Louis, Mosby–Year Book, 1991, pp 321–329.
9. Green RM: Management of spontaneous dissection and fibromuscular dysplasia of the carotid artery. In Yao JST, Pearce WH (eds): Arterial Surgery: Management of Challenging Problems. Norwalk, CT, Appleton & Lange, 1996, pp 127–139.
10. Calabrese LH, Clough JD: Systemic vasculitis. In Young JR, Graor RA, Olin JW, et al (eds): Peripheral Vascular Diseases, 2nd ed. St Louis, Mosby–Year Book, 1996, pp 380–406.
11. Anderson CA: Takayasu's arteritis. J Vasc Nurs 1992; 10:17–19.
12. Hertzer NR, Beven EG, Young JR, et al: Coronary artery disease in peripheral vascular patients: A classification of 1000 coronary angiograms and results of surgical management. Ann Surg 1984; 199:223–233.
13. Young JR: Physical examination. In Young JR, Graor RA, Olin JW, et al (eds): Peripheral Vascular Diseases, 2nd ed. St Louis, Mosby–Year Book, 1996, pp 18–32.
14. Hobson RW, Weiss DG, Fields WS, et al: Efficacy of carotid endarterectomy for asymptomatic carotid stenosis. N Engl J Med 1993; 328:221–227.
15. Executive Committee for the Asymptomatic Carotid Atherosclerosis Study (ACAS). Endarterectomy for asymptomatic carotid artery stenosis. JAMA 1995; 273:1421–1428.
16. Martin ID, Valentine RI, Meyers SI, et al: Is routine CT scanning necessary in the preoperative evaluation of patients undergoing carotid endarterectomy? J Vasc Surg 1991; 14:267–270.
17. Currie IC, Lamont PM, Baird RN: Magnetic resonance imaging and duplex scanning for carotid artery disease. In Greenhalgh RM (ed): Vascular Imaging for Surgeons. London, WB Saunders, 1995, pp 95–106.
18. North American Symptomatic Carotid Endarterectomy Trial (NASCET) Steering Committee: North American Symptomatic Carotid Endarterectomy Trial: Methods, patient characteristics and progress. Stroke 1991; 22:711–720.
19. European Carotid Surgery Trialists' Collaborative Group: MRC European Carotid Surgery Trial: Interim results for symptomatic patients with severe (70–99%) or with mild (0–29%) carotid stenosis. Lancet 1991; 337:1235–1243.
20. Barnett, HJ, Taylor DW, Eliasziw M, et al: Benefit of carotid endarterectomy in patients with symptomatic moderate or severe stenosis. N Engl J Med 1998; 339:1415–1425.
21. Moneta GL, Taylor DC, Nicholls SC, et al: Operative versus nonoperative management of asymptomatic high-grade internal carotid artery stenosis: Improved results with endarterectomy. Stroke 1987; 18:1005–1010.
22. Grotta IC: Current medical and surgical therapy for cerebrovascular disease. N Engl J Med 1987; 317:1505–1516.
23. Gent M, Blakely TA, Easton ID, et al: The Canadian American Ticlopidine Study (CATS) in thromboembolic stroke. Lancet 1989; 1:1215–1220.
24. Callow AD: Carotid endarterectomy: Ten-year follow up. In Yao JST, Pearce WH (eds): Long-Term Results in Vascular Surgery. Norwalk, CT, Appleton & Lange, 1993, pp 61–68.
25. American College of Physicians: Indications for carotid endarterectomy. Ann Intern Med 1989; 111:675–677.
26. Rosenthal D, Archie JP, Garcia-Rinaldi R, et al: Carotid patch angioplasty: Immediate and long-term results. J Vasc Surg 1990; 12:326–333.
27. Humphries AW, Young JR, Beven EG, et al: Relief of vertebrobasilar symptoms by carotid endarterectomy. Surgery 1965; 57:48–52.
28. Moore DI, Miles RD, Gooley NA, et al: Noninvasive assessment of stroke risk in asymptomatic and nonhemispheric patients with suspected carotid disease. Ann Surg 1985; 212:491–504.
29. Sterpetti AV, Schults RD, Feldhaus RJ, et al: Natural history of recurrent carotid artery disease. Surg Gynecol Obstet 1989; 227–234.
30. Wholey MH, Wholey MH, Jarmolowski CR, et al: Endovascular stents for carotid artery occlusive disease. J Endovasc Surg 1997; 4:326–338.

31. Dietrich EB, Ndiaye M, Reid DB.: Stenting in the carotid artery: Initial experience in 110 patients. J Endovasc Surg 1996; 3:42–62.
32. Wilson PWF, Hoeg JM, D'Agostino RB, et al: Cumulative effects of high cholesterol levels, high blood pressure, and cigarette smoking on carotid stenosis. N Engl J Med 1997; 337:516–22.
33. Christensen CR: Carotid endarterectomy clinical pathway: nursing perspective. J Vasc Nurs 1997; 15:1–7.
34. Morasch MD, Hodgett D, Burke K, Baker WH: Selective use of the intensive care unit following carotid endarterectomy. Ann Vasc Surg 1995; 9:229–234.
35. Lipsett PA, Tierney S, Gordon TA, Perler BA: Carotid endarterectomy—Is intensive care unit necessary? J Vasc Surg 1994; 20:403–10.
36. Back MR, Harward TRS, Huber TS, et al: Improving the cost-effectiveness of carotid endarterectomy. J Vasc Surg 1997; 26:456–464.
37. Hirko MK, Morash MD, Burke K, et al: The changing face of carotid endarterectomy. J Vasc Surg 1996; 23:622–627.
38. Moore WS, Barnett HJM, Beebe HG, et al: Guidelines for carotid endarterectomy: A multidisciplinary consensus statement from the ad hoc committee, American Heart Association. Circulation 1995; 91:566–579.

14

Upper-Extremity Problems

Larry R. Williams, MD, John F. Lee, MD,
and Cynthia J. McNeave, RN

∽ · ∾

Upper-extremity ischemia is much less common than lower-extremity ischemia, due in part to the fact that arteries of the upper extremity are relatively spared from the atherosclerotic process. Extensive collateral pathways effectively compensate in most cases when major arterial obstruction threatens the upper extremities, making upper-extremity limb loss an unusual circumstance.

Gradual onset of physiologic dysfunction is unusual. However, acute vasospasm, or Raynaud's phenomenon, may be associated with collagen vascular disease and with a host of other underlying disease processes. The upper extremity is particularly prone to trauma, exposure to cold, and occupational injuries. Thoracic outlet syndrome, as well as upper-extremity sympathectomy, will be addressed in this chapter. In addition, increased use of upper-extremity arteries for invasive diagnostic procedures, for monitoring of critically ill patients, and for access to the circulatory system for chronic hemodialysis has brought a new generation of iatrogenic causes of upper-extremity arterial ischemia.

Although the upper extremities and hands are often taken for granted, humans depend tremendously on them to carry out the simple routines of life. For most persons, the prospect of amputation or disability of an upper extremity represents a considerably greater impairment than the loss of a lower extremity. For this reason, the diagnosis and treatment of upper-extremity problems presents a distinct challenge.

ANATOMY

Knowledge of upper-extremity anatomy is essential to an understanding of factors responsible for arm ischemias and their treatment (Fig. 14–1). The subclavian artery originates from the brachiocephalic trunk on the right side and from the distal transverse aortic arch on the left and exits from the chest over the first rib on each side. At its junction with the first rib, the subclavian artery passes just behind the anterior scalene muscle, giving off the vertebral, internal mammary, and thyrocervical branches. Just beyond the anterior scalene muscle, the subclavian artery becomes the axillary artery, at which point close approximation with the axillary vein and brachial plexus occurs. The axillary artery then becomes the brachial artery and courses through the medial upper arm to just below the

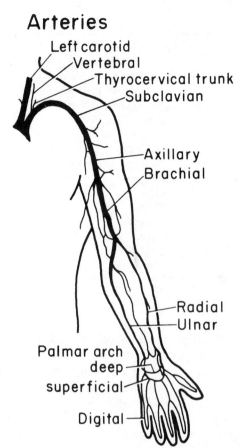

Arteries

Left carotid
Vertebral
Thyrocervical trunk
Subclavian

Axillary
Brachial

Radial
Ulnar

Palmar arch
deep
superficial

Digital

Figure 14–1. Anatomy of the major arteries of the upper extremity. (From Pearce WH, Ricco JB, Yao JST, et al: Upper extremity diagnosis. In Zweibel WJ [ed]: Introduction to Vascular Ultrasonography. Orlando, Grune & Stratton, 1982.)

antecubital fossa, where it divides into the ulnar, radial, and interosseous arteries. These branches course deep to the flexor muscles of the forearm.

The radial artery (lateral) and the ulnar artery (medial) supply most of the hand circulation. Intercommunications at the palmar level are multiple, with one dorsal and two palmar arches (superficial and deep) providing a variety of inflow pathways to the digits. In most persons the superficial palmar arch is the dominant arterial circulation to the fingers, supplying common digital arteries that then branch into proper digital arteries on either side of the fingers. The distal circulation of the hand tends to be much more variable than that of the larger, proximal arteries of the upper extremity.

ETIOLOGY

Unlike lower-extremity ischemia, in which the majority of patients suffer from atherosclerotic arterial occlusive disease, upper-extremity ischemia may have a wide variety of etiologic factors. An exhaustive listing is beyond the scope of this chapter. However, Table 14–1 summarizes the pathologic processes commonly responsible for upper-extremity arterial problems.

Atherosclerosis

Although unusual, upper-extremity atherosclerosis is well recognized; the proximal left subclavian artery is involved twice as often as the right subclavian artery, with innominate

TABLE 14–1. **Etiology of Upper-Extremity Problems**

Atherosclerosis	Posttraumatic pain syndrome
Generalized atherosclerosis	Ischemic monomelic neuropathy
Subclavian steal syndrome	Immune arteritis
Atherosclerotic embolization	Polyarteritis
Atherosclerotic aneurysms	Hypersensitivity
Emboli	Giant-cell
Cardiac source	Buerger's disease
Proximal arterial source	Thoracic outlet syndrome
Inadvertent drug injections	Hyperhidrosis
Iatrogenic	
Trauma	
Violent	
Iatrogenic	
Occupational	
Frostbite	
Irradiation	

artery involvement a distant third.[1, 2] As with atherosclerosis elsewhere, the disease process is one of advancing age, with most patients being more than 50 years old. For reasons that are not entirely clear, subclavian artery blockage usually occurs at the origin of these vessels, most often proximal to the vertebral arteries. Thus the development of collateral circulation often finds major contributions from the vertebral arteries.

In cases of left subclavian artery occlusion, for example, a significant amount of blood may flow to the arm because of reversal of blood flow in the left vertebral artery (Fig. 14–2). The source of this flow is the basilar artery in the brain, which has received its circulation from the right vertebral artery or the carotid arteries via the circle of Willis. This forms the basis of the *subclavian steal syndrome*. It has been suggested that patients who complain of vertigo, dizziness, drop attacks, or visual disturbances suffer because the arm "steals" blood from the circulation intended for the posterior aspect of the brain. In fact, very few patients actually have these symptoms, despite reversed flow in the vertebral arteries. The current theory is that patients who present with cerebral symptoms have associated or coincidental stenosis of the carotid arteries.[3] Treatment of the carotid artery lesions usually relieves these symptoms.

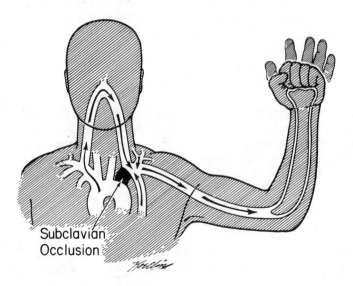

Figure 14–2. Demonstration of "subclavian steal syndrome" with reversal of vertebral artery flow due to proximal subclavian artery occlusion. (From Moore WS: Clinical manifestations of cerebrovascular insufficiency. In Rutherford RB [ed]: Vascular Surgery. Philadelphia, WB Saunders, 1977, p 1054.)

Subclavian
Occlusion

It is also because of rather extensive collateral circulation from the vertebral arteries and around the shoulder that patients seldom develop symptoms of arm ischemia from proximal subclavian artery occlusive disease alone. In some patients, however, these atherosclerotic lesions may be the source of distal embolization of atherosclerotic debris or small organized clots resulting in digital artery occlusion.[4] Small areas of tissue loss or even significant major ischemia may occur as a result.

Although atherosclerosis is commonly responsible for the development of aneurysms elsewhere in the body, aneurysms of the upper-extremity arteries are exceedingly uncommon. In addition to atherosclerosis, aneurysms may be associated with trauma, infections, or thoracic outlet syndrome.[5, 6]

Embolism

Embolization to the upper extremity is a relatively common cause of acute arm ischemia, but only 10 percent of all embolic episodes involve the upper extremities.[7, 8] These emboli may originate from proximal arterial lesions; however, most often they come from the heart (Table 14–2). In general, emboli that originate from the heart are larger than emboli from proximal arterial sources and contain mainly thrombus (thromboembolism). Cardiac emboli, therefore, lodge primarily in the larger vessels of the upper extremity, involving the subclavian (10 percent), axillary (22 percent), and brachial arteries (64 percent).[9] Emboli that originate from proximal arterial sources are usually the result of platelet deposition and thrombus formation at points of atherosclerotic arterial damage. Emboli formed by this thrombus and atherosclerotic debris (atheroembolism) lodge more distally in the palmar arches or digital vessels and at times in the ulnar or radial arteries.[9, 10] Mural thrombus that has developed in subclavian artery aneurysms may also embolize to the distal arm arteries. Inadvertent arterial injection of drugs of abuse, embolization during arterial catheterization procedures or arteriography, and embolization from indwelling arterial monitoring lines also may be seen.

Trauma

Traumatic injuries of the upper extremities stand out as a leading cause of upper-extremity ischemia. Penetrating injuries from knife wounds, lacerations, and gunshot wounds present a relatively straightforward mechanism for arterial injury. Blunt injuries to arterial structures may result from clavicular fractures, inferior shoulder dislocations, dislocations of the elbows, or humeral fractures. Prolonged use of crutches may result in continued trauma to the axillary artery and either arterial thrombosis or axillary aneurysm formation.

A wide variety of iatrogenic arterial injuries are likewise now being recognized. Diagnostic and therapeutic procedures that require arterial puncture may lead to arterial thrombosis, hemorrhage, or distal embolization. Cardiac catheterization, commonly performed through the brachial artery (Sones technique), is often performed in patients with generalized atherosclerosis. The brachial artery may be difficult to repair after

---

TABLE 14–2. **Emboli From the Heart**

Left atrial thrombi in patients with atrial fibrillation
Left ventricular mural thrombi after myocardial infarction
Cardiac tumors such as atrial myxoma
Debris from diseased cardiac valves
Thrombi that have developed on prosthetic valves

catheterization.[11] Puncture of the brachial or axillary arteries for arteriography likewise may be complicated by arterial thrombosis or hemorrhage. Bleeding into the axillary sheath may result in significant nerve compression and dysfunction without the loss of distal pulses. Radial arterial lines for blood pressure monitoring and blood specimen withdrawals in critically ill patients likewise may result in arterial thrombosis and hand ischemia.

Increasing use of upper-extremity arteries and veins as access sites for chronic hemodialysis has resulted in a proportionate increase in iatrogenic hand ischemia. Several mechanisms may be at fault, including arterial injury at operation, distal embolization, pseudoaneurysm formation, or infection and mycotic aneurysm formation at anastomotic sites.[12]

Although many occupations lend themselves to an inordinate risk of blunt or penetrating trauma of the upper extremities, one particular mechanism for arterial damage and hand ischemia stands out. The "hypothenar hammer syndrome" reported by Conn and associates[5] in 1970 describes the association of ulnar artery injury with use of the heel of the palm to hammer, push, or twist objects. Ulnar artery thrombosis or aneurysm formation with distal embolization then causes digital ischemia. Another mechanism recently described in association with digital ischemia has been the chronic use of vibratory tools. Unlike hypothenar hammer syndrome, in which intermittent severe blows are incurred, the vibratory tool syndrome results in arterial injury due to prolonged repetitive vibratory damage from pneumatic tools.[13]

Frostbite, of course, is the tissue injury that occurs as a result of overexposure to cold temperatures. The severity varies with the temperature and the duration of exposure, with most injuries occurring on exposure at temperatures between $0°$ C and $-7°$ C for more than 7 hours. Increased humidity and wind velocity accelerate the withdrawal of heat from the body and may shorten the exposure time necessary to result in significant tissue damage. Although some acclimatization may occur, extremities previously injured from frostbite remain permanently susceptible to future cold injury because of an intensified vasoconstrictor response. Although direct freezing with cell membrane disruption may play a significant role in extremely low temperature frostbite injuries, many authorities believe that the mechanisms of vasoconstriction, decreased blood flow, arterial thrombosis, and ischemic necrosis are responsible in the majority of frostbite cases.[14]

Radiation therapy for various malignant processes can result in arterial injury.[2] Intimal thickening, cellular infiltration, and scarring result in arterial lesions very similar in appearance to those of atherosclerosis. Small-artery occlusion and large-artery stenosis may occur soon after irradiation or may develop gradually over many years. Irradiation of various cancers of the head, neck, breast, and lung most commonly results in subclavian artery lesions, while irradiation of soft tissue tumors of the arm causes axillary or brachial artery damage. Another problem that may arise after irradiation is exposure of underlying arteries as a result of breakdown of overlying skin and subcutaneous tissue. Resultant arterial infection, desiccation, or disruption with blow-out are complications that may arise because of inadequate coverage of underlying vascular structures.

Posttraumatic Pain Syndrome

Posttraumatic pain syndromes (causalgia, reflex sympathetic dystrophy) are intensely painful symptom complexes that are poorly understood and difficult to diagnose accurately. Posttraumatic pain may develop after peripheral nerve injury or irritation. Frequently, ischemia may be the inciting event. However, at times, the cause may be so insignificant as not to be readily apparent.

Three clinical stages of posttraumatic pain syndrome have been recognized. The acute stage is reversible, and the patient experiences burning, redness, swelling, sweating, and extreme tenderness to light tactile stimuli. After 2 months, symptoms may resolve spontaneously or patients may exhibit patchy areas of osteoporosis. In the dystrophic stage, symptoms progress to coolness, cyanosis, brawny edema, continuous pain, and diffuse osteoporosis. The atrophic phase is characterized by increasingly severe pain, even beyond the injured area. This is accompanied by skin atrophy, muscle wasting, and trophic ulceration. Bones show advanced demineralization with joint contractures and ankylosis.

Patients who exhibit a majority of these symptoms are more likely to have an accurate diagnosis and are considered to have "major causalgia." Most patients, on the other hand, present with "minor" or "mimo" causalgia and complain of only certain of these symptoms.

The differential diagnosis may include nerve entrapments, Raynaud's syndrome, arterial ischemia, and thoracic outlet syndrome. Response to sympathetic nerve block may help make the diagnosis. Patients with posttraumatic pain syndromes experience dramatic relief of pain with sympathetic nerve block, and this may be a useful predictor of the result of surgical sympathectomy.

Ischemic Monomelic Neuropathy

Ischemic monomelic neuropathy is a rare pain syndrome with a predilection for the upper extremity. It was originally described as a consequence of acute arterial compromise and now is more often seen in diabetic renal failure patients following upper-extremity dialysis graft insertion. The pathologic feature of multiple axon-loss mononeuropathies distally in the limb without muscle necrosis is diagnostic.[15, 16]

The clinical presentation includes prominent sensory symptoms of numbness, dysesthesias, and burning causalgia-type pain with milder levels of motor weakness and coordination loss in conjunction with acute ischemia. The pain is continuous, may persist for months, and rarely disappears completely even in the face of correction of the inciting ischemic event. The syndrome has no clinical, arterial, or neurologic predictors, and delay in diagnosis is common.

Immune Arteritis

Immune arteritis is a complex topic with many different categories and classifications (see Chapter 1). The specific term *arteritis* implies inflammation of the arterial wall with cellular infiltrates and eventual necrosis. The term does not imply the arterial involvement that is inevitable in the multitude of inflammatory processes with perivascular round-cell infiltrates. Immune arteritis is associated with intimal damage, scarring, and stenosis leading to arterial occlusions.[17] Most commonly, the small and medium-sized arteries are involved, although Takayasu's arteritis involves only the large aortic branch arteries.

Although an in-depth discussion is beyond the scope of this chapter, features that serve to distinguish the types of arteritis will be briefly discussed.

The polyarteritis nodosa group of diseases most commonly affects older patients, with male/female ratio of 2:1. Focal, transmural inflammation of the small and medium-sized arteries results in necrosis, arterial thrombosis, and formation of small aneurysms. The hepatic, renal, and mesenteric circulations are frequently involved. Although significant upper-extremity involvement is not common, Raynaud's phenomenon and upper-extremity symptoms may be the first clue to the underlying disease.

Hypersensitivity angiitis encompasses a broad group of problems affecting the small arteries. Characteristic arterial thickening, connective tissue swelling, and vascular occlusion occur with relatively little inflammatory reaction. Except for scleroderma, most of these conditions result from exposure to some antigen, with the formation of antigen/

antibody immune complexes. At times, the inciting antigen is not known, but fragments of DNA, RNA, hepatitis B virus, or specific tumor antigens are commonly responsible.

Giant-cell arteritis is characterized by localized periarteritis with mononuclear and giant-cell infiltrates and disruption of elastic fibers of the arterial wall. Temporal arteritis or systemic giant-cell arteritis may involve any artery but most commonly involves the branches of the carotid arteries of older women. Takayasu's arteritis affects younger Oriental women, with typical involvement of the aortic arch and its branches and, less frequently, involvement of the pulmonary artery.

Buerger's disease (thromboangiitis obliterans) represents a controversial clinical condition that is believed to represent a severe form of distal atherosclerotic arterial occlusive disease. Significant evidence, however, supports the feeling that it does exist as a discrete pathologic entity.[4] The disease occurs predominantly in young men of Jewish familial descent who have a strong history of cigarette smoking. Transmural cellular infiltration of the small and medium-sized arteries results in fibrous obliteration of vascular lumen. Superficial thrombophlebitis and venous involvement are characteristic, involving the lower extremities more commonly than the upper extremities. Specific cellular immunity against antigens has been suggested as an etiologic factor.

Thoracic Outlet Syndrome

The thoracic outlet syndrome entails a complex of upper-extremity symptoms of the neurovascular bundle as it exits from the thoracic cage (Fig. 14–3). The disorder affects women more commonly than men and is usually seen in young and middle-aged adults. Neurologic symptoms due to brachial plexus compression predominate. Vascular compression, arterial or venous, is occasionally responsible for symptoms associated with thoracic outlet syndrome.

The peculiar anatomic relationships of the thoracic outlet are keys to an understanding of thoracic outlet syndrome. The first rib forms the floor of the thoracic outlet, with the clavicle and the subclavius muscle forming the superior portion. Laterally, the scalenus medius muscle inserts inferiorly on the first rib and is in close proximity to the posterior aspect of the brachial plexus. The subclavian artery lies just anterior to the brachial plexus, so that the neurovascular bundle (brachial plexus and subclavian artery) lies between the scalenus medius and scalenus anticus muscle bundles. The scalenus anticus muscle inserts on the first rib between the subclavian artery and the subclavian vein and, with the subclavius muscle tendons, forms the medial border of the thoracic outlet by inserting on the first rib at its junction with the costal cartilage. Therefore any affliction that impinges

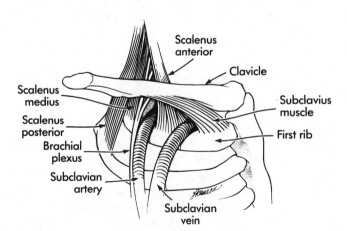

Figure 14–3. Diagram of the right thoracic outlet demonstrating the relationship of the vein and artery and brachial plexus to the clavicle, first rib, and scalenus muscles. (From Beven EG: Thoracic outlet syndrome. In Young JR, Olin JW, Barthlomew JR [eds]: Peripheral Vascular Diseases. Chicago, Mosby–Year Book, 1996.)

on this rather limited outlet may result in compression of the nerve, artery, or vein, and symptoms may be extremely variable, depending on the nature of the process involved.

Both congenital and acquired factors may upset this delicate balance of structures and result in thoracic outlet symptoms. A congenital cervical rib is a common mechanism. This may take the form of a complete bony rib or of multiple fibrous bands that stretch from an elongated cervical transverse process to the first rib. Because the nerve courses in close proximity to the posterior aspect of this brachial plexus, nerve irritation is caused by the scissor compression action of the cervical rib/fibrous band anomalies.

Trauma is frequently associated with the thoracic outlet syndrome. Callus formation due to a fractured clavicle or first rib may cause obvious outlet narrowing. Hyper-extension-flexion (whiplash) injuries may be followed acutely or even remotely by severe spasm of multiple cervical or upper back muscle groups. Involvement of the scalenus medius muscle may be responsible for the symptoms related to overdevelopment of the muscles of the neck and shoulder region that occurs in baseball pitchers, golfers, swimmers, and weight lifters.

In many patients, thoracic outlet syndrome has no obvious congenital or traumatic cause. Although it has been suggested that shoulder girdles that lie exceptionally low in the thorax may be associated with a narrow costoclavicular space, this is not always the case. In many patients no particular etiologic factor can be identified.

Pain is the most common complaint in patients with thoracic outlet syndrome. Although symptoms are quite subjective, patients commonly describe a dull, aching pain that radiates down the arm from the shoulder. At times patients may experience sharp pains limited to specific muscle groups. Pain may involve the neck, shoulder, forearm, or hand, may be constant or intermittent, and may be related to specific physical activities such as lifting or working with the arms overhead. Numbness and paresthesia may accompany the pain. The ulnar nerve distribution is most commonly affected, with or without median nerve involvement. Radial nerve symptoms are infrequently seen. Although sensory symptoms predominate in the early stages, longstanding neurovascular compression frequently results in weakness of upper-extremity muscle groups; with time, muscle wasting may be seen.

Arterial complications that may result from thoracic outlet syndrome include thickening and fibrosis with early atherosclerotic changes and plaque formation because of continued arterial trauma. Poststenotic dilation and actual aneurysm formation may result. Complications include arterial thrombosis and distal embolization of thrombotic and atherosclerotic debris, whereas rupture is rarely seen. At times hypertrophy of the anterior scalenus muscle in athletes may result in arterial compression during hyperabduction (Fig. 14–4). Subclavian venous compression may cause thrombosis with resultant swelling and pain, in addition to an increased risk of pulmonary embolization.

Hyperhidrosis

Hyperhidrosis is a peculiar condition in which sweating exceeds thermoregulatory needs. Sweat glands are anatomically normal but respond abnormally to certain stimuli such as emotion, chewing, or sudden temperature shifts. The cause is not known but may be related to hyperactivity of the sudomotor center of the brain. Symptoms range from occasional excessive sweating to constant wetness, social embarrassment, chronic dermatitis, and fungal infections. The diagnosis is relatively straightforward, and specific testing is usually not required.

CLINICAL PRESENTATION

The symptoms of upper-extremity arterial insufficiency vary considerably, depending on the level and acuteness of obstruction, the degree of collateral circulation, and the presence

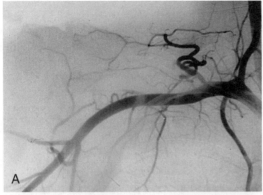

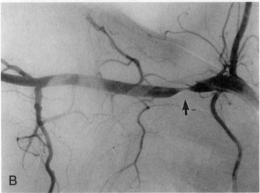

Figure 14–4. Arteriogram of a professional baseball pitcher demonstrating **(A)** neutral position of subclavian artery and **(B)** compression of the subclavian artery *(arrow)* in the pitching position (hyperabduction). (From Yao JST: Occupational vascular problems. In Rutherford RB [ed]: Vascular Surgery. Philadelphia, WB Saunders, 1989, p 1203.)

of vasospasm. In the majority of patients, the diagnosis is determined by careful history and physical examination.

History

The identification of acute hand ischemia temporally related to upper-extremity trauma, cardiac catheterization, or other arterial diagnostic or monitoring procedures is relatively straightforward. A history of renal failure requiring hemodialysis should include diagrams of previous arteriovenous fistulae or shunts. Previous infections, graft problems, and ischemic symptoms should be noted. When a history of previous cardiac valve prosthesis, cardiac arrhythmias (especially atrial fibrillation), or myocardial infarction is obtained, embolization is the likely cause. Intra-arterial injection of drugs of abuse can be determined by history as well.

An occupational history may be revealing because repetitive trauma to the hand by either blunt (hypothenar hammer syndrome) or vibratory mechanisms may result in acute or chronic hand ischemia. Specific questions regarding athletic endeavors, training methods, or repetitive strenuous motions may prove enlightening. Many cases of atherosclerotic upper-extremity arterial disease have a history of atherosclerotic problems elsewhere, most commonly coronary artery disease, cerebrovascular disease, or lower-extremity arterial occlusive disease. Documentation of tobacco use, sensitivity to cold, diabetes mellitus, familial diseases, medication history (especially vasoconstrictors, ergot alkaloids, dopamine), drug sensitivities, and previous operations or irradiation is of importance as well.

Physical Examination

Physical examination of the upper extremity should proceed in a logical fashion, beginning with inspection. The presence of gangrene, muscular atrophy, swelling or edema, and discoloration, such as blanching, erythema, or cyanosis, should be thoroughly documented. Microemboli from proximal atherosclerotic or cardiac sources produce characteristic punctate lesions on the fingertips that are associated with cyanosis (Fig. 14–5). Ischemic changes secondary to scleroderma can often be identified because of the tight, shiny, atrophic skin characteristic of this systemic disorder.

Exposure to the cold may prompt the characteristic color changes associated with Raynaud's phenomenon. Symmetric blanching of the digits due to spastic closure of the small arterioles is followed by cyanotic mottling as cutaneous flow resumes sluggishly. This is followed by a hyperemic phase, with purplish rubor that remains for several minutes after rewarming.

In cases of trauma, careful description with drawings of upper-extremity wounds, puncture sites, and arm circumferences is vital. In some patients with acute arterial ischemia, increases in the pressure within the muscular compartments of the forearm may result in a tense, swollen, painful arm. Recognition of this compartmental hypertension and prompt treatment are necessary to avoid further nerve and muscular damage with significant loss of function. Measurement of upper arm and forearm circumferences at initial assessment and at later examinations may be extremely valuable.

Auscultation may reveal bruits at areas of arterial stenosis and should be performed over the subclavian, axillary, and brachial arteries in both neutral and hyperabducted arm positions. Palpation for pulses in the carotid, axillary, brachial, radial, and ulnar arteries is of paramount importance. The examination should include a notation of the strength of the pulse, an estimation of the character of the underlying artery (compliant versus sclerotic), and a description of any aneurysm dilation or tortuosity. The disappearance of upper-extremity pulses during hyperabduction may provide a clue to the diagnosis of thoracic outlet syndrome.

Adson's maneuver is one method of demonstrating compression of the subclavian artery at the thoracic outlet. With the patient sitting erect, the radial pulse is located and continuously palpated while the patient inspires deeply and turns the head strongly to the affected side. The tension of the scalenus anticus muscle against the first rib results in compression of the subclavian artery in the narrow thoracic outlet. Although the Adson maneuver may be positive in a significant number of persons who have no evidence of upper-extremity ischemia, it may be of considerable importance in patients with no

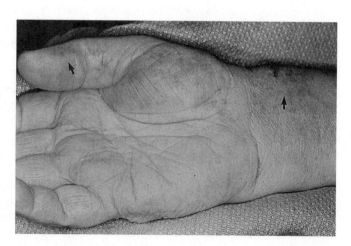

Figure 14–5. Pseudoaneurysm of the radial artery *(right arrow)* due to arterial line trauma. Note the punctate lesions on the thenar eminence *(left arrow)* from distal microembolization.

obvious source of upper-extremity ischemia and may lead to the diagnosis of potentially curable lesions.

The Allen test is another maneuver that should be performed routinely to assess patency of the palmar arch. In this maneuver, the radial and ulnar arteries are compressed while the patient makes a fist to evacuate the blood from the hand. When the hand is open, the palm appears pale and mottled. In a patient with a normally patent palmar arch, release of either the radial or the ulnar artery results in prompt, even reactive hyperemia of the entire palm, with disappearance of the pallor and mottling. In the presence of radial artery occlusion, however, release of radial artery compression while occlusion of the ulnar artery is maintained does not relieve the pallor and mottling. Only on release of the ulnar artery compression does perfusion return to the hand. Likewise, with ulnar artery occlusion, color returns to the hand only after release of the radial artery, which is supplying the majority of perfusion to the hand (see Fig. 4–3).

Upper-extremity examination should be supplemented by a complete physical examination. Specific areas of interest would include examination for signs of previous cerebrovascular accident, auscultation of the carotid arteries for bruits, complete cardiac evaluation, and a thorough investigation for abdominal or lower-extremity atherosclerotic processes. At times, systemic diseases responsible for upper-extremity ischemia result in signs or symptoms in the feet or lower extremities that are similar to those seen in the upper extremities.

DIAGNOSTIC EVALUATION

The diagnostic evaluation of patients with symptoms suggestive of upper-extremity arterial ischemia centers on establishment of the diagnosis and documentation of the location and degree of hemodynamically significant lesions. Noninvasive vascular testing (see Chapter 5) has become an important supplement to the clinical evaluation of patients with a variety of arterial and venous diseases but is especially applicable to upper-extremity arterial insufficiency. Although arteriography remains the definitive diagnostic tool, especially in patients who require operative intervention, it can now be used selectively on the basis of noninvasive hemodynamic test results.

Noninvasive Testing

The continuous-wave direction Doppler probe is the instrument most commonly used for upper-extremity arterial examinations. Flow velocity wave forms obtained by placement of the ultrasound probe over the subclavian, axillary, brachial, ulnar, radial, and digital arteries normally are triphasic. In the presence of significant proximal arterial stenosis, however, the arterial signal becomes damped and monophasic. Comparison with the opposite upper extremity is useful.

Patency of the palmar arterial arch can be determined by obtaining arterial wave forms at the midthenar and hypothenar regions in the hand. By alternately compressing the ulnar and radial arteries, the examiner can easily determine the vessel responsible for supplying the palmar arch and the one most responsible for the circulation of the hand. This is similar to the Allen test.

Arterial wave forms can also be obtained at the common digital vessel at the base of each finger and at the proper digital vessels along the shaft of each finger. Again, interpretation is dependent on comparison with more proximal wave forms and with the opposite extremity. The inability to detect any flow in an underlying artery with the directional Doppler probe is usually diagnostic of total occlusion of that particular artery.

In addition to the wave form analysis, the continuous-wave Doppler probe can be used to determine systolic blood pressures at different levels in the upper extremity. This is done by placing a regular blood pressure cuff on the upper arm and forearm and listening with the Doppler probe at the brachial, radial, and ulnar arteries, respectively. More distal blood pressure measurements are possible with the use of very small (2.5 cm) specialized blood pressure cuffs at the base of each finger. A reduction in the systolic blood pressure of more than 20 mmHg is significant. For example, a reduction in the upper arm blood pressure when compared with the opposite extremity signifies innominate, subclavian, axillary, or proximal brachial arterial stenosis. A normal upper arm blood pressure in conjunction with a reduction in the forearm blood pressure is diagnostic of distal brachial, radial, or ulnar arterial occlusive disease. Similarly, if the forearm blood pressure is normal, reduction in digital pressure implies occlusive disease distal to the major forearm arteries.

At times, in patients in whom arterial ischemia is suspected, various maneuvers may be extremely helpful in establishing the cause of upper-extremity symptoms. Patients with intermittent obstruction of the subclavian artery as a result of thoracic outlet syndrome may have an entirely normal upper-extremity arterial examination at rest. The exaggerated military position (with shoulders back and chest forward), hyperabduction of the arm, or the Adson maneuver (abduction and external rotation of the arm with the head turned first toward the arm, and then away) may result in damping of the brachial artery wave form and reduction in the upper arm systolic blood pressure.

In patients with no evidence of proximal or digital arterial occlusion, a useful means of documenting vasospastic disorders is the digital temperature recovery time. In normal persons, the finger temperature returns to normal within 10–15 minutes after a 20-second submersion in an ice water bath. In patients with an abnormal vasospastic response to cold (Raynaud's phenomenon), finger skin temperatures return to normal much more slowly (recovery times exceeding 20–25 minutes). Bilaterally symmetric responses to cold submersion are characteristic of vasospasm. In patients with an asymmetric response, or those in whom only selected digits are affected, digital artery occlusive disease should be suspected.

As with ultrasound techniques elsewhere in the body, B-mode scanning and color flow imaging are especially useful in the diagnosis of arterial aneurysms. Atherosclerotic subclavian aneurysms, poststenotic subclavian dilatation, mycotic aneurysms, traumatic pseudoaneurysms, and even arteriovenous fistulae can be documented noninvasively.[20] Detection of small aneurysms or pseudoaneurysms, even at the palmar arch level, is possible as well (Fig. 14–6). In addition, occlusive lesions due to emboli, atherosclerotic plaque, or traumatic thrombosis at the axillary, brachial, and more distal arteries can be diagnosed with ultrasound imaging.[21]

Diagnostic Imaging

Arteriography continues to be the definitive test for the diagnosis of most arterial problems and is essential if operative intervention is to be considered. With the increasing use of noninvasive Doppler testing, however, arteriography plays a less prominent role in the evaluation of vasospastic disorders, especially when the extremity is not in jeopardy.

The transfemoral route, in which the Seldinger technique and catheters are used to selectively inject upper-extremity arteries, is the preferred method. Visualization of the aortic arch and proximal arch arteries is essential, and proximal arterial occlusive lesions, including subclavian and axillary aneurysms and ulcerative plaque, are easily identified. In assessing for thoracic outlet compression, hyperabduction maneuvers are used during arteriography. Proximal subclavian occlusion with subclavian steal and retrograde flow in the vertebral artery is easily demonstrated arteriographically if delayed films are obtained. It is more difficult, however, to determine when angiographically detected "steal" is of clinical significance.

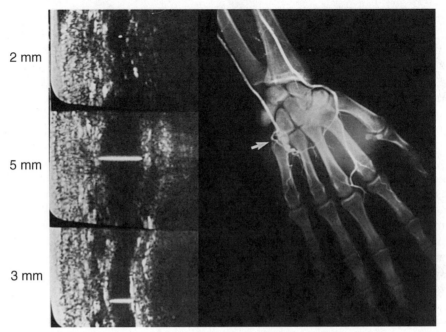

Figure 14–6. B-mode ultrasound image of a 5-mm ulnar artery aneurysm *(left)*. The corresponding angiogram *(right)* demonstrates the aneurysm *(arrow)*.

Arteritis of the aortic arch vessels usually causes solitary or multiple tapered stenosis without atherosclerotic plaques or ulcerations. Distinction between giant-cell arteritis and Takayasu's arteritis is difficult, however, on the basis of arteriography alone.

Atherosclerotic occlusions, embolic occlusions, traumatic lesions, and vasospasm usually are readily diagnosed by arteriography. In addition, variations in the normal arterial anatomy, which may be an important consideration at operation, and the degree of collateral circulation and distal runoff can be documented on arteriography.

Several techniques that have significantly improved the ability to visualize the small hand and digital arteries have been developed (Fig. 14–7). Warming of the hand and intra-arterial injection of vasodilators, such as tolazoline hydrochloride (Priscoline) or papaverine, prevent vasospasm, which is often induced by high-pressure injection of contrast. In this way, the more distal arterial tree can usually be visualized and the vasospastic hypersensitivity characteristic of Raynaud's disease can be differentiated from vasospasm (Raynaud's phenomenon) that implies underlying arterial disease. In patients with underlying collagen vascular disease, arteriographic findings include the bilateral occurrence of distal lesions with no evidence of atherosclerosis. Typical smooth, tapering, stringlike arteries or multiple segmental lesions may be seen. Collateral circulation is limited and often appears as winding "corkscrew" vessels. Routine and computerized digital subtraction techniques eliminate overlying bony shadows and significantly improve image quality as well.

Refinements in computed tomography (CT) and magnetic resonance techniques have added new dimensions to diagnostic imaging for upper-extremity maladies. Cross-sectional display of vascular structures with magnetic resonance angiography (MRA), now available in most medical centers, may supplement arteriography or may offer a less invasive alternative. Technologic advances have come so rapidly that equipment and institutional experience vary widely, making comparisons of applicability difficult.

Spiral CT, electron beam CT, spin echo, and two-dimensional time-of-flight MRA imaging are just a few examples of the emerging vocabulary necessary to keep pace in this rapidly advancing field.[22] Although most operative decisions and transcatheter treatment

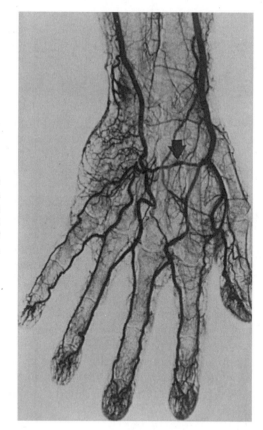

Figure 14–7. Excellent visualization of digital arteries demonstrating a patent palmar arch *(arrow)*. (From Janevsky BK: Arteriography of the upper extremity: Technique and essentials of interpretation. In Bergan JJ, Yao JST [eds]: Evaluation and Treatment of Upper and Lower Extremity Circulatory Disorders. Orlando, Grune & Stratton, 1984, p 223.)

options continue to be directed by conventional arteriography, the complicated anatomy of the thoracic outlet is displayed much more thoroughly by CT or magnetic resonance imaging (MRI). Fully three-dimensional vascular imaging is now possible, but the role of this exciting new information is yet to be determined.

Laboratory Evaluation

Routine hospital admission laboratory testing is usually not helpful in patients with upper-extremity arterial ischemia. In patients with atherosclerotic arterial occlusive disease, additional information is seldom provided by laboratory evaluation; however, appropriate testing for diabetes mellitus (fasting glucose, glucose tolerance test), hyperlipidemia (serum lipid profile), renal disease (creatinine, blood urea nitrogen, serum electrolytes, urinalysis), hypercalcemia (serum calcium, phosphorus, albumin, protein), or hypercoagulable states (see Chapter 9) may be extremely important.

Although careful inspection of the routine chest radiograph may identify a cervical rib that is causing thoracic outlet syndrome, cervical spine films may be necessary to adequately rule out this diagnosis. Electrocardiography may lead to the diagnosis of recent or remote myocardial infarction, atrial fibrillation, or other cardiac abnormalities, which might be responsible for upper-extremity embolization. More complete investigation would include 24-hour Holter monitoring, echocardiography, or transesophageal echocardiography.

Although a wide variety of serologic tests are available, they are not all useful in any individual patient. The sequence of workup for patients in whom a systemic cause of upper-extremity arterial insufficiency is suspected may vary depending on the clinical situation. Scleroderma (systemic sclerosis) and the CREST syndrome (calcinosis cutis, Raynaud's phenomenon, esophageal stricture, sclerodactyly, telangiectasis) may be suspected in patients with skin atrophy or calcinosis. Radiographs of the hands may reveal distal phalangeal tuft reabsorption or evidence of soft tissue atrophy, and barium swallow may be diagnostic of an esophageal motility disorder. The immunologic abnormalities are less specific and include hypergammaglobulinemia, elevated serum rheumatoid factor, and antinuclear antibodies in 40–70 percent of cases.

Systemic lupus erythematosus is characterized by elevated anti-DNA antibodies, low levels of serum complement, and the presence of acute-phase reactants such as C-reactive protein and elevated fibrinogen and erythrocyte sedimentation rates. Mixed connective tissue disease, a variant of systemic lupus erythematosus, is often associated with Raynaud's phenomenon in the upper extremity. Circulating antinuclear antibodies directed against acidic nuclear proteins is the distinguishing feature of this systemic abnormality. In patients with suspected immune arteritis, the erythrocyte sedimentation rate is usually elevated; however, this test is nonspecific. At times, skin or temporal artery biopsies may be necessary before the diagnosis can be made. In patients with suspected thromboangiitis obliterans (Buerger's disease), precise diagnosis is possible only on microscopic evaluation of the involved small arteries and veins.

The detection of the abnormal serum protein cryoglobulin, which precipitates on exposure to cold, may provide a clue to excessive upper-extremity sensitivity to cold temperatures. Cryoglobulinemia may occur in an essential form or may be associated with abnormal protein production caused by other collagen vascular disorders, myeloma, lymphosarcoma, or macroglobulin anemia. In some cases, cold agglutination of red blood cells occurs when exposed to extremely cold temperatures.

TREATMENT

Methods of treatment of upper-extremity ischemia depend on the severity of ischemia, the cause, and at times the potential for future problems.

Operative Treatment

The clinical history is the best means of identifying patients who may be candidates for operative intervention. Patients with chronic upper-extremity ischemia and potentially curable lesions, skin necrosis, gangrene, and severe pain at rest are considered for operation. Patients who have arm claudication or symptoms only after strenuous exercise are not usually considered candidates for operative treatment. At times, cerebrovascular symptoms in association with subclavian steal are indications for repair of a subclavian artery occlusion.

Patients who have acute arterial occlusions as a result of trauma or emboli are almost always considered for early operation. Traumatic lacerations or arterial intimal injuries, however trivial, should be promptly repaired, because these may take the form of chronic thrombosis, arteriovenous fistulae, or pseudoaneurysms.[23] The treatment of embolic lesions is dependent on the severity of ischemia and the overall condition of the patient. In seriously ill patients with complicated cardiac abnormalities, the decision concerning operation may be tempered by the patient's ability to withstand that operation.

Aneurysms of the subclavian artery are considered for operative treatment to prevent distal embolization and thrombosis. Distal aneurysms likewise have a tendency to embolize and are also most often considered for resection as opposed to alternate treatment. If there is any question of infection (mycotic aneurysm), or if the arterial wall is disrupted (pseudoaneurysm), operation is indicated because these aneurysms will rupture in addition to the problem of distal embolization.

Incisions commonly used for upper-extremity arterial operations are depicted in Figure 14–8. Arterial bypass is usually the recommended treatment for significant proximal arterial occlusive lesions, although endarterectomy of localized areas with vein patch angioplasty is an alternative. At the present time, bypass with prosthetic graft materials (usually expanded polytetrafluoroethylene) is optimal because of appropriate size match and proven long-term patencies.[20] For the most part, intrathoracic procedures (aortic-subclavian artery bypass) have been replaced by extra-anatomic bypasses (axillary-axillary bypass, carotid-subclavian bypass, carotid-axillary bypass) because hemodynamic improvement obtained is adequate and the complications of thoracotomy are avoided (Fig. 14–9).[24]

In patients with subclavian artery aneurysms or arterial injury secondary to thoracic outlet syndrome, resection of the diseased artery with interposition bypass grafting of prosthetic material is accompanied by resection of the first rib. In this way, the thoracic outlet compression is relieved in addition to removal of the arterial abnormality. The pros and cons of treatment in patients with symptomatic thoracic outlet syndrome without obvious arterial damage are quite variable and beyond the scope of this chapter. Division of hypertrophied scalenus anticus muscles (scalenotomy or scalenectomy) in highly developed athletes may provide relief of symptoms secondary to intermittent arterial entrapment.

In cases of chronic arterial occlusion more distal in the arm, arterial bypass has likewise been shown to be an effective treatment.[25, 26] Use of reversed autogenous saphenous vein as the bypass graft material is the procedure of choice.

In patients with aneurysm formation in the distal arteries of the forearm or hand from occupational trauma or atherosclerosis, resection with interposition grafting is indicated

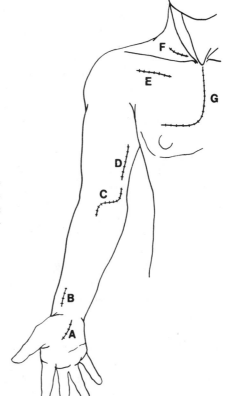

Figure 14–8. Standard incisions commonly used for upper-extremity arterial operations. (From Roos D: The management of neurovascular diseases involving the upper extremity: Overview. In Rutherford RB: Vascular Surgery, 2nd ed. Philadelphia, WB Saunders, 1977, p 686.)

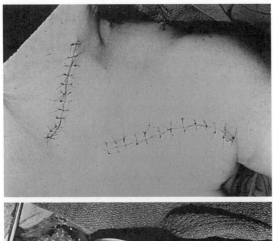

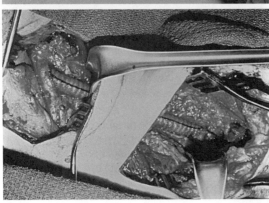

Figure 14–9. Left carotid-axillary artery bypass: Prosthetic bypass graft *(bottom)*. Sutured incisions over the left carotid and left axillary arteries *(top)*.

(Fig. 14–10). In patients with infected aneurysms or pseudoaneurysms, resection with ligation of the proximal and distal vessels is adequate, if collateral circulation maintains the viability of the distal extremity. At times, extra-anatomic bypass with reversed saphenous vein through uninvolved tissues is necessary (Fig. 14–11).

Treatment of traumatic injuries is relatively straightforward and depends to a great degree on the amount of tissue injury involved. With many iatrogenic or laceration injuries, minimal debridement with primary repair of the injured artery will suffice. At times vein-patch angioplasty is necessary to avoid narrowing of the arterial lumen. In patients with blunt injuries and contaminated penetrating injuries or gunshot wounds, excision of devitalized tissue is necessary; although end-to-end arterial anastomoses are at times possible, interposition grafts of reversed saphenous vein are often required. In cases of high-velocity gunshot wounds, injuries to the accompanying nerves are responsible for the majority of functional disability postoperatively.

Thromboembolectomy can at times be a fairly simple procedure in patients with acute occlusions of proximal large arteries with relatively little distal arterial thrombosis. A limited arteriotomy followed by removal of thrombotic debris with a balloon catheter suffices to restore distal circulation. More complicated situations, especially those that involve distal thrombotic debris, require systemic heparinization to discourage additional thrombosis of digital arteries in association with vasospasm.

Interventional Techniques

Thrombolytic therapy, percutaneous angioplasty, and intravascular stents and stented grafts are now emerging as alternative means of treatment for thrombotic and occlusive arterial lesions. Although reports of upper-extremity transcatheter treatment experiences

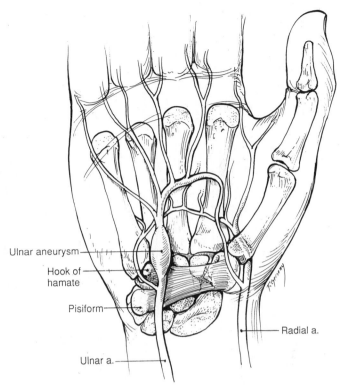

Figure 14–10. Posttraumatic ulnar artery aneurysm in the typical anatomic position adjacent to the hamate bone and distal to the deep palmar artery. (From Dalman RL: Upper extremity arterial bypass distal to the wrist. Ann Vasc Surg 1997; 11:551.)

are limited, the results are good and parallel the broader experience in lower-extremity disease.[27]

Thrombolysis may play a role as both primary treatment and as an adjunct to surgical treatment, such as bypass or thromboembolectomy. Transcatheter approaches allow access to the upper-extremity vessels through remote routes, thus limiting direct arterial trauma and providing a means of regional delivery of thrombolytic agents such as urokinase, streptokinase, or recombinant tissue–type plasminogen activator.

Lysis of even well-organized thrombus in larger arteries is routine, and recanalization of smaller peripheral vessels may restore flow when thromboembolectomy might not have been technically feasible. Alternatively, lysis of obscuring luminal thrombus may reveal underlying causative arterial lesions and help direct definitive treatment.[28]

Thrombolytic therapy is limited at times by the potential for serious hemorrhage either at the catheter insertion site or at remote areas. Other limitations include the relative inability of the forearm fascial compartments to expand, increasing the possibility of compartmental hypertension, and the tendency of the upper-extremity arteries to vasospasm.

Regardless, wider experience has shown that serious complications are actually rare and most often correctable. Moreover, should attempts at thrombolytic therapy fail to achieve acceptable distal perfusion, additional damage is usually not inflicted and the patient is no worse off than prior to its use.

Suboptimal results following arterial dilation can often be improved by the placement of an intra-arterial stent. Residual stenosis due to arterial recoil, subintimal dissection, and at times even arterial rupture can be treated successfully by stent placement.

Use of stents as primary treatment of arteriovenous fistulae or arterial lacerations secondary to subclavian trauma is inviting because direct operative repair in this area is technically challenging. Longer segments of arterial disease not amenable to dilation alone are now being treated with prosthetic grafts secured intramurally by stents. Early success

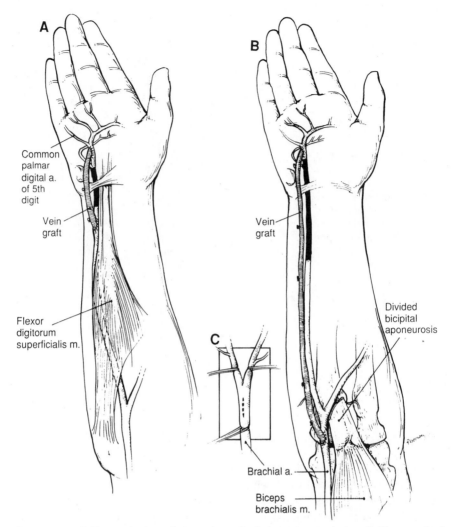

Figure 14–11. A, Reversed vein graft, bypassing a distal ulnar artery occlusion. **B,** More proximal ulnar artery disease requiring a graft from the brachial artery to the palmar ulnar artery. **C,** Brachial artery exposure may be facilitated by division of the bicipital aponeurosis. (From Dalman RL: Upper extremity arterial bypass distal to the wrist. Ann Vasc Surg 1997; 11:553.)

in patients with aorto-ilio-femoral disease suggests that stented grafts may be a popular option in the future but it is difficult to predict that this modality will fulfill a similar role in upper-extremity arterial disease.[29, 30]

Upper-Extremity Sympathectomy

In the past, removal of the sympathetic ganglia (sympathectomy) was a popular treatment for a variety of upper-extremity maladies, including severe ischemia, when direct arterial repair and bypass were not possible. The theoretic benefits of sympathectomy are based on the fact that the sympathetic chain innervates arterial vasoconstrictor fibers as well as eccrine (sweat) glands. Sympathectomy removes these potential vasoconstrictors and eliminates the stimulus for sweat production. Unfortunately, the diseased atherosclerotic peripheral arteries are minimally influenced by this fine sympathetic innervation, and lasting improved perfusion is not usually seen.

Experts disagree on the extent of nerve division necessary in all cases, but most agree that severing the sympathetic trunk below the third thoracic ganglion and cutting the rami communicantes of the second and third thoracic ganglia effectively denervate the upper extremity. Additional division below the fourth thoracic ganglion is necessary to denervate the axillary sweat glands completely.[31, 32]

Several surgical approaches, including supraclavicular, axillary, transthoracic, and cervical, are available. Sugical complications are included in Table 14–3. Inadvertent division of the long thoracic nerve during the axillary approach will result in the disfiguring complication of winging of the scapula.[33] Horner's syndrome (ptosis, miosis, and anhidrosis) should be avoidable. However, if the stellate ganglion is included in the resection, its occurrence is troublesome. Endoscopic and percutaneous sympathectomy are newly developed alternatives that may offer lower complication rates, but their benefit is not yet proven.[34]

Sympathectomy is seldom used now in the treatment of arterial ischemia in view of the disappointing and unpredictable results in patients with atherosclerosis and the uniform failure in patients with underlying connective tissue disease. Some practitioners continue to use it as a last resort in selected patients with ischemic ulceration or gangrene. Short-term relief of pain, decreased tissue loss, and improved wound healing may be seen. Patients with Raynaud's syndrome in the absence of digital arterial occlusion seldom benefit from this treatment.

Recent resurgence of the microsurgical technique of adventitial stripping of sympathetic fibers at the common digital and proper digital levels has met with limited success. Patients with chronic arterial ischemia are strictly selected based on arterial testing and response to cold stress testing after local anesthetic block in the distal palm. In spite of a time-consuming, extensive dissection, results are mixed, especially over the long term, with hand specialists hopeful and vascular specialists remaining skeptical.

Posttraumatic pain syndromes (causalgia or reflex sympathetic dystrophy) may respond favorably to sympathectomy in severe cases. Best results are achieved if sympathectomy is performed before the development of fixed pain patterns or atrophic skin changes.[37] Treatment may also include physical therapy, analgesia, and stellate ganglion nerve blocks prior to sympathectomy. Patients with mild cases of hyperhidrosis may be treated with topical antiperspirants or atropine-like medications.

Medical Treatment

The medical management of patients with upper-extremity ischemia is extremely variable and can be broken down into three main areas: (1) treatment of vasospasm; (2) protection from further injury; and (3) treatment of systemic diseases.

Because vasospasm is commonly a reaction to exogenous stimuli, simple removal of the stimulus is often effective. Keeping the upper extremity warm with gloves, cotton batting, or a warm water bath is an effective method of preventing cold-induced vasospasm.

Medical management of vasospasm is not uniformly effective; however, oral administration of guanethidine or calcium channel blockers such as nifedipine has shown some promise. Short-term relief may be provided in some cases by the intravenous or intra-

TABLE 14–3. **Complications of Surgical Sympathectomy**

Atelectasis	Pneumothorax
Horner's syndrome	Postsympathetic neuralgia
Pleural effusion	Winged scapula
Pneumonia	

arterial administration of arterial smooth muscle relaxants (vasodilatory agents: papaverine, reserpine, Priscoline).

Protection of the upper extremity from obvious or subtle injury includes the avoidance of continued occupational trauma. Avoidance of hyperabduction of the upper extremity is important to avoid compression of the subclavian artery at the thoracic outlet. Circumferential dressings, tourniquets, and tight casts should be avoided, and in patients with limited mobility or neurologic abnormalities, pressure on the upper extremity for prolonged periods of time should be avoided.

Although there are a variety of specific medical treatments for the multitude of underlying systemic conditions that may be associated with upper-extremity ischemia, their discussion is beyond the scope of this chapter. In general, anticoagulation, regional sympathetic blockade, and administration of vasodilators, both systemically and locally, have shown no convincing proof of efficacy.[6] In the treatment of giant-cell arteritis, early initiation of steroid therapy is of proven value and often results in the restoration of upper-extremity pulses. In Takayasu's arteritis, steroids are less beneficial.

Systemic anticoagulation with heparin is indicated in patients with acute upper-extremity ischemia caused by embolization. In most instances, chronic anticoagulation should be continued with warfarin (Coumadin) in an attempt to decrease the risk of re-embolization of thrombotic material from proximal sources. Low-molecular-weight heparin products are now available as an alternative method of long-term outpatient anticoagulation.

NURSING INTERVENTION

General Measures

Conscientious nursing care may have a significant impact on the outcome of treatment in patients with upper-extremity ischemia, who may have a variety of systemic disorders responsible for or in conjunction with their upper-extremity problem. An overall nursing plan is vital.

In general, an ischemic upper extremity should not be elevated or dependent but should be kept at the level of the heart. The arms should be protected from further injury by avoidance of areas of increased pressure for any prolonged period of time. Cold stimuli should be avoided, and soft cotton batting is an effective means of providing gentle warmth in addition to even pressure distribution. Constrictive circumferential dressings should be avoided, and any cast materials should be inspected for tightness on a regular basis. The forearm should be assessed for excessive swelling or tightness that might be a sign of compartmental hypertension. Hematomas which may compress the brachial plexus or axillary nerve are at times subtle and the resulting nerve damage may be permanent if decompression is not carried out promptly. Routine serial physical examinations with circulatory and neurologic assessments, including Doppler evaluation as outlined earlier in this chapter, are likewise of critical importance.

Postoperative Monitoring

Patients who have had arterial repairs, upper-extremity bypass, or diagnostic or therapeutic interventions require aggressive postoperative monitoring to assure early, and eventually long-term, success. Pulses should be assessed by palpation and by Doppler examination on an hourly basis for the first 24 hours postoperatively and at less frequent intervals throughout the patient's recovery. Forearm Doppler blood pressure measurements should be performed every 2–4 hours postoperatively for the first 24 hours and on a daily basis after that. Pain in the hand or fingers may be the first sign that ischemia has returned and that the arterial repair or bypass has stopped functioning. The distal extremity should be assessed from a neurologic standpoint by examination of motor and sensory function, and the hand should be checked regularly for warmth and capillary refill.

Although mild swelling in the upper extremity often accompanies revascularization in both acute and chronic ischemia, severe swelling is abnormal and may indicate hemorrhage and hematoma formation or compartmental hypertension. Hemorrhage may also take the form of frank bleeding from the wound, and in these instances prompt exploration is often indicated. Any evidence of acutely intensified postoperative pain, upper-extremity swelling, or hemorrhage should be brought to the immediate attention of the surgeon. Mild swelling may be relieved by elevation of the arm. Nonconstricting elastic bandages may prove useful, and a sling may provide added support during ambulation.

Revascularization of acutely ischemic muscular tissue may result in systemic elevations in serum creatine phosphokinase, potassium, and myoglobin levels. This may result in excretion of these byproducts in the urine, causing dark urine and at times renal dysfunction. The patient's potassium, urine output, and creatinine levels should be monitored closely in the postoperative period.

Wound Care

Operative incisions for upper-extremity arterial repairs or bypass operations can ordinarily be covered with dry gauze for 1–2 days postoperatively. Ischemic ulcerations or gangrenous areas on the hands or fingers are managed with gentle cleansing, conservative debridement, and light dressings. Tape on the skin should be avoided. At times wet-to-dry dressings will hasten debridement of slightly dirty wounds. Traumatic wounds of the upper extremity likewise need to be kept very clean. Dressing changes should be preformed with an aseptic technique. Sharp debridement frequently plays a role in the ultimate healing process. Excessive moisture between the fingers can be prevented by lightly bandaging the hand with gauze between the fingers. Any bandages on the upper extremity should allow easy access for frequent physical examination of the digits and access to the radial and ulnar pulses for examination. Bleeding from any wound requires accurate physical assessment of the cause and appropriate physician notification. Avoid reinforcing dressings with excessive bandaging. A variety of newly developed gel dressings and enzymatic debriding agents are useful adjuncts for lesser amounts of tissue necrosis.

Patient Education

The nursing staff caring for the patient with upper-extremity ischemia plays a vital role in the patient education process, with regard to both in-hospital care and posthospitalization management. Patients welcome additional information about the disease process responsible for their upper-extremity problems, as well as information regarding the operation performed. Diagrams of upper-extremity anatomy and the specific procedures performed on individual patients are extremely useful. Patients should be informed about their activity level postoperatively. Exercises of gradually increasing duration and intensity can be coordinated through the occupational and physical therapy departments. Information with regard to bathing is usually straightforward; however, it may require alteration, depending on upper-extremity wounds. Including the patient and the family in dressing changes and wound management allows them to acquire the skills necessary to perform dressing changes independently.

Patients usually need counseling concerning medications that will be required after their discharge from the hospital. In the case of anticoagulation (see Chapter 8) the patient should be advised of the dangers of discontinuing the medication without consulting the physician and should also be advised with regard to any bleeding complications that should be brought to the physician's attention.

Although uncommon, arterial ischemia and other upper-extremity problems may be the cause of significant morbidity and disability. Recognition of the multitude of causes requires a careful, systematic approach to achieve an accurate diagnosis and ultimately to provide the appropriate treatment.

References

1. Ehrenfeld WK, Rapp JH: Direct revascularization for occlusion of the trunks of the aortic arch. J Vasc Surg 1985; 2:228–230.
2. Machleder HI: Vascular disease of the upper extremity and the thoracic outlet syndrome. In Moore WS (ed): Vascular Surgery: A Comprehensive Review. Philadelphia, WB Saunders, 1998, pp 613–625.
3. Walker PM, Paley D, Harris KA, et al: What determines the symptoms associated with subclavian artery occlusive disease? J Vasc Surg 1985; 2:154–157.
4. Taylor LM, Bauer GM, Porter JM: Finger gangrene caused by small artery occlusive disease. Ann Surg 1981; 193:453–461.
5. Conn J, Bergan JJ, Bell JL: Hypothenar hammer syndrome: Post traumatic digital ischemia. Surgery 1970; 68:1122–1128.
6. Miller CM, Sanginiolo P, Schanyer H, et al: Infected false aneurysms of the subclavian artery: A complication in drug addicts. J Vasc Surg 1984; 1:684–688.
7. Banis JC, Rich N, Whelan TJ: Ischemia of the upper extremity due to noncardiac emboli. Am J Surg 1977; 134:131–139.
8. Ahmed AM, Eduards JM, Porter JM: Nonatherosclerotic vascular disease. In Moore WS (ed): Vascular Surgery: A Comprehensive Review. Philadelphia, WB Saunders, 1998, pp 111–145.
9. Gross WS, Flanigan DP, Kraft RD, et al: Chronic upper extremity arterial insufficiency: Etiology, manifestations and operative management. Arch Surg 1978; 113:419–422.
10. Dietrich EB, Koopot R, Kinard SA, et al: Treatment of microemboli of the upper extremity. Surg Gynecol Obstet 1979; 148:584–587.
11. Finkelmeier WR: Iatrogenic arterial injuries resulting from invasive procedures. J Vasc Nurs 1991; 9:12–17.
12. Valji K, Hye RJ, Roberts AC, et al: Hand ischemia in patients with hemodialysis access grafts; angiographic diagnosis and treatment. Radiology 1995; 196:696–701.
13. Bartel P, Blackburn D, Peterson L, et al: The value of noninvasive tests in occupational trauma of the hands and fingers. Bruit 1984; 8:15–18.
14. Porter JM, Snider RL, Bardana EJ, et al: The diagnosis and treatment of Raynaud's phenomenon. Surgery 1975; 88:11–23.
15. Wilbourn AJ, Furlan AJ, Hulley W, et al: Ischemic monomelic neuropathy. Neurology 1983; 33:447–51.
16. Hye RJ, Wolf YG: Ischemic monomelic neuropathy: An under-recognized complication of hemodialysis access. Ann Vasc Surg 1994; 8:578–582.
17. Fauci AS, Haynes BF, Katz P: The spectrum of vasculitis. Ann Intern Med 1978; 206:521–528.
18. Sanders RJ, Cooper MA: Thoracic outlet syndrome. In Dean RH, Yao JST, Brewster DC (eds): Current Diagnosis and Treatment in Vascular Surgery. Norwalk, CT, Appleton & Lange, 1995, pp 133–152.
19. Matsumara JS, Yao JST: Thoracic outlet arterial compression: Clinical features and surgical management. Semin Vasc Surg 1996; 9:125–133.
20. Brewster DC, Moncure AC, Darling RC, et al: Innominate artery lesions; problems encountered and lessons learned. J Vasc Surg 1985; 2:99–112.
21. Payne KM, Blackburn DR, Peterson LK, et al: B-mode imaging of the arteries of the hand and upper extremity. Bruit 1986; 10:168–174.
22. Esposito MD, Arrington JA, Blackshear MN, et al: Thoracic outlet syndrome in a throwing athlete diagnosed with MRI and MRA. J Magn Reson Imaging 1997; 7:598–599.
23. Hardin WD, O'Connell RC, Adinolfi MF, et al: Traumatic arterial injuries of the upper extremity: Determinants of disability. Am J Surg 1985; 150:266–270.
24. Moore WS; Extra-anatomic bypass for revascularization of occlusive lesions involving the branches of the aortic arch. J Vasc Surg 1985; 2:230–232.
25. McCarthy WJ, Flinn WR, Yao JST, et al: Result of bypass grafting for upper limb ischemia. J Vasc Surg 1986; 3:741–746.
26. Dalman RL: Upper extremity arterial bypass distal to the wrist. Annals Vasc Surg 1997; 11:550–557.
27. Bonn J, Soulen MC: Thrombolysis and angioplasty in upper extremity arterial disease. In Strandness DE, Van Breda A (eds): Vascular Diseases: Surgical and Interventional Therapy. New York, Churchill Livingstone, 1995, pp 539–555.

28. Wheatley MJ, Marx MV: The use of intraarterial urokinase in the management of hand ischemia secondary to palmar and digital artery occlusion. Ann Plast Surg 1996; 37:356–363.
29. Martinez R, Rodriguez-Lopez J, Torruella L, et al: Stenting for occlusion of the subclavian arteries: Technical aspects and followup results. Texas Heart Institute 1997; 24:23–27.
30. Kumar K, Dorros G, Bates MC, et al: Primary stent deployment in occlusive subclavian artery disease. Cathet Cardiovasc Diagn 1995; 34:281–285.
31. Welch E, Geary J: Current status of thoracic dorsal sympathectomy. J Vasc Surg 1984; 1:202–214.
32. Mattassi R, Miele F, D'Angelo F: Thoracic sympathectomy: Review of indications, results and surgical techniques. J Cardiovasc Surg 1981; 22:336–339.
33. May J, Harris JP, Upper extremity sympathectomy: A comparison of the supraclavicular and axillary approaches. In Bergan JJ, Yao JST (eds): Evaluation and Treatment of Upper and Lower Extremity Circulatory Disorders. Orlando, Grune & Stratton, 1985, pp 69–85.
34. Malone PS, Cameron AEP, Rennie JA: Endoscopic thoracic sympathectomy in the treatment of upper limb hyperhidrosis. Ann R Coll Surg Engl 1986; 69:93–94.

15

Renovascular Hypertension

Alyson J. Breisch, RN, MS, ANP

❧ · ❧

Renovascular hypertension (RVH) refers to blood pressure elevation that develops as a result of renal ischemia. Renal artery stenosis (RAS) may occur in patients with essential hypertension and may also be present in normotensive individuals.[1] The finding of renal arterial occlusive disease does not establish the diagnosis of renovascular hypertension. Renovascular hypertension is confirmed by improvement in, or cure of, hypertension following correction of the stenosis. Renovascular hypertension is ruled out when no RAS is found or RAS is present but no blood pressure improvement response occurs after angioplasty or surgical revascularization.

PATHOLOGY

The renin-angiotensin-aldosterone cascade is integral to renal regulation of blood pressure and intravascular volume (Fig. 15–1A). Continuing research on this mechanism has identified new concepts regarding its role in blood pressure regulation.[2] Specialized renal cells, the juxtaglomerular cells, produce renin. Renin interacts with circulating angiotensinogen, an alpha$_2$ globulin produced by the liver, to form the decapeptide angiotensin I. Angiotensin-converting enzyme (ACE), produced by lung tissue, converts angiotensin I to the octapeptide angiotensin II. Angiotensin II is a very potent vasoconstrictor. It also stimulates the adrenal gland production and release of aldosterone and increases the retention of sodium and water. Research has also identified angiotensin II–specific receptors that may be significantly involved in many cardiovascular reactions.[3]

Decreased renal perfusion pressure activates the renin-angiotensin-aldosterone cascade. The result is excess production of renin from the ischemic kidney, which results in a further decrease in renal blood flow secondary to arterial vasoconstriction. Glomerular filtration rate also decreases. The intravascular volume is increased secondary to the aldosterone production and sodium and water retention. The consequences of this mechanism vary in unilateral and bilateral RAS.

Unilateral RAS activates the renin-angiotensin-aldosterone mechanism in both kidneys (Fig. 15–1B). The kidney with normal renal artery lumen compensates by suppressing its production of renin, and diuresis occurs. The intravascular volume is restored toward normal. In the early stages of unilateral RAS, hypertension is dependent on angiotensin II and, therefore, responds to ACE inhibitors. Over time, the ACE inhibitors become less

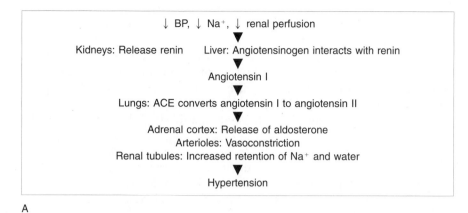

Figure 15-1. Renin-angiotensin-aldosterone cascade. **A,** Physiologic mechanisms. **B,** Unilateral renal artery stenosis. **C,** Bilateral renal artery stenosis. BP = blood pressure; Na⁺ = sodium; ACE = angiotensin-converting enzyme.

effective in regulating blood pressure, and chronic decreases in renal perfusion pressure may result in hypertension that is not relieved by revascularization procedures.

In bilateral RAS, both kidneys are influenced by the renin-angiotensin-aldosterone mechanism and there is no diuresis of sodium (Fig. 15–1C). The resulting intravascular volume overload that develops is the primary cause of hypertension. Use of ACE inhibitors, which reduce blood pressure and thus decrease renal perfusion, may actually worsen the renal insufficiency. The patient may present with acute pulmonary edema.[4]

ETIOLOGY

A variety of renal arterial lesions may cause RVH. Ninety percent of all lesions are either atherosclerosis or fibromuscular dysplasia. Other causes include Takayasu's arteritis, renal artery aneurysms, embolism, polyarteritis nodosa, arteriovenous fistulae, and RAS after renal transplantation.[5-7] Children may present with RVH secondary to developmental lesions of the renal arteries. These lesions are frequently bilateral and are often associated with congenital narrowing of the aorta.

Atherosclerosis accounts for two-thirds of all diagnosed cases of RVH. The incidence in men is double that in women. Clinical presentation often occurs between ages 50 and 55. The ostium and proximal third of the main renal artery are most commonly affected. The left renal artery is more often involved than the right renal artery. The lesions are often less than 1 cm in length. Approximately one-third of the patients have bilateral stenoses.

Fibromuscular dysplasia (FMD) is the leading underlying disorder in RVH in persons younger than 40 years of age. There are three subcategories to FMD: intimal dysplasia, medial hyperplasia, and perimedial (subadventitial) fibrodysplasia. The most common form is medial fibromuscular dysplasia or hyperplasia and occurs most often in young women. Fibromuscular dysplasia is 4–5 times more common in women. Most patients present in their third or fourth decade. The presentation is often bilateral, although the right side tends to be more severely involved. There are usually multiple lesions with the appearance of microaneuryms in a series of constricted lesions alternating with areas of greater diameter. This corrugated effect results in the angiographic appearance termed the *string of beads*, as illustrated in Figure 15–2.

The etiology of fibromuscular dysplasia is not certain. Immunologic factors and smoking have been implicated. The higher prevalence in women raises the possibility of hormonal influences. Many patients with FMD have a ptotic kidney (Fig. 15–3), which has led to the proposal that arterial stretching may be an etiologic factor.

INCIDENCE

The true incidence of RVH is not known. It has been reported to be as little as 1 percent and possibly as high as 10 percent of the 60 million persons with hypertension in America. This lack of certainty is partly due to the difficulty of accurately diagnosing RAS as the etiology in large screening endeavors without the use of angiography. The incidence of RVH increases in selected populations.

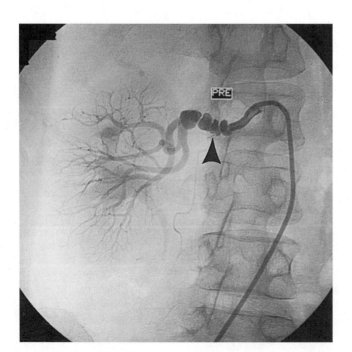

Figure 15–2. Arteriogram depicting characteristic "string of beads" appearance *(arrowhead)* of fibromuscular dysplasia of the renal artery.

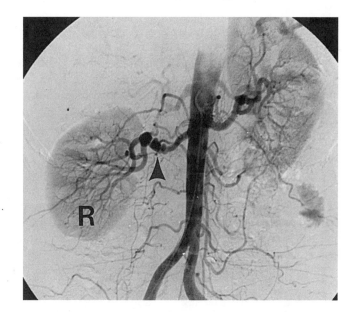

Figure 15–3. Arteriogram depicting right renal fibromuscular dysplasia. Note the "string of bead" appearance *(arrowhead)* and also note ptosis, or downward displacement, of the right kidney *(R)*.

The incidence of RAS rises in patients with evidence of atherosclerosis in other arterial segments. Louie et al[8] found that patients with RAS have a high prevalence of carotid and lower-extremity arterial disease. In another series of 100 patients with peripheral vascular disease (PVD), 31 percent were found to have RAS (14 percent with greater than 50 percent stenosis).[9] Table 15–1 illustrates the incidence of renal artery disease in patients with other patterns of atherosclerotic disease.[10, 11]

The overall prevalence of RAS in one series of patients over the age of 40 with myocardial infarction was reported as 12 percent.[12] The authors found the prevalence of RAS in patients with fatal myocardial infarction (MI) to be 19 percent of those with hypertension, 39 percent of those with proteinuria, and 39 percent of those with renal insufficiency. Other investigators have found that as the severity of coronary artery disease increased, the prevalence of RAS increased.[11]

RAS is more prevalent in Caucasian patients. It has frequently been stated that African Americans have a low incidence of RAS and RVH. However, studies in clinically selected populations suggest a 6–13 percent incidence of RAS. One series of 79 selected black hypertensive subjects found 18 percent with RAS.[12] Thus it is estimated that 582,000 American blacks have diastolic blood pressures greater than 115 mmHg, which is a criterion for RVH, and may benefit from further diagnostic evaluation.

NATURAL HISTORY

Limited available data suggest both fibromuscular dysplasia and atherosclerotic renal artery disease are progressive.[13] It has been estimated that renovascular disease may be

TABLE 15–1. **Incidence of Renal Artery Stenosis**

ASSOCIATED ATHEROSCLEROTIC DISEASE	INCIDENCE (%)
Abdominal aortic aneurysms	38
Aortoiliac occlusive disease	33
Lower-extremity occlusive disease	39
Significant coronary lesion (>75% stenosis)	15
≥2 vessel coronary artery disease	30

the etiology for as many as 15 percent of all patients who develop end-stage renal disease.[14] In another retrospective study,[15] patients with RAS underwent serial angiography. Approximately 50 percent of the subjects showed progression of stenosis over a mean follow-up time of 5 years. Nine percent of the subjects developed total renal artery occlusion. Patients with greater than 60 percent stenosis were at greatest risk for progression to total occlusion. In this series, at 1 year, 23 percent had progressed from less than 60 percent to greater than 60 percent. At 2 years, 42 percent underwent this progression.

Another group of 76 patients with RAS was followed by serial duplex scanning.[16] The incidence rates for progression from under 60 percent RAS to over 60 percent RAS were 30 percent at 1 year, 44 percent at 2 years, and 48 percent at 3 years. Of the patients who demonstrated greater than 60 percent at the initial visit, 4 percent progressed to total occlusion at 1 year, 4 percent at 2 years, and 7 percent at 3 years. The overall combined rate of progression of RAS was 7 percent per year for all degrees of baseline RAS. In another series, 54 patients underwent serial duplex studies at 6-month intervals. Only those patients with a 60 percent or greater degree of stenosis had more than 1-cm decrease in renal size. Loss of renal mass is an important consequence of high-grade RAS.[17] These findings suggest that patients with advanced degrees of RAS should be referred for revascularization.

DIAGNOSIS

Clinical Signs

Certain clinical findings are suggestive of RVH. RVH should be suspected when hypertension presents before the age of 30 (especially with diastolic pressures greater than 110 mmHg), or onset occurs after age 55. It should also be suspected when well-controlled hypertension becomes more difficult to control, changes to malignant or accelerated hypertension, or becomes resistant to pharmacologic agents.[1, 7] Deterioration of renal function after treatment of hypertension with ACE inhibitor medications strongly suggests bilateral renal artery disease or stenosis. Patients should have creatinine values monitored after initiating therapy with ACE inhibitors. Transient decline in renal function can also be seen in unilateral RAS.

Hypertensive patients with extensive clinical evidence of atherosclerosis should be evaluated for RAS. The presence of claudication is a strong indicator of significant coronary artery disease, which in turn increases the possibility of RAS. The presence of an abdominal bruit was found to be strongly associated ($p < 0.0005$) with RAS in a retrospective study that examined the ability of common clinical features to predict RAS.[18] In patients without an abdominal bruit, refractory hypertension only was found to be associated with radiographically documented RAS.

In more recent studies, a subset of patients with recurrent pulmonary edema as their presenting clinical sign of RVH has been identified.[4, 19] The authors describe episodes of recurrent pulmonary edema as a clinical marker for severe bilateral renal artery occlusive disease. In one series, 65 percent of patients with bilateral RAS developed pulmonary edema despite normal left ventricular function.[19] These patients may develop worsening renal insufficiency when ACE inhibitors are used to treat their hypertension. As absolute pressure is decreased, renal perfusion is decreased and thus there is an increased likelihood of volume overload. Aggressive management of these patients' hypertension may improve control of hypertension but worsen renal insufficiency. A rising creatinine level after the introduction of an ACE inhibitor should raise the question of bilateral RAS. Clinical criteria for RVH are summarized in Table 15–2.[12]

TABLE 15–2. **Clinical Criteria for Diagnosis
of Renovascular Hypertension**

Hypertension before age 25 or after age 45
Recent onset of hypertension
Systolic blood pressure (SBP) > 200 mmHg
Diastolic blood pressure (DBP) > 115 mmHg
Malignant hypertension or encephalopathy
Progressive hypertension (15% increase in SBP or DBP) unexplained by change
  in medication in last 6 months
Hypertension refractory to 3 antihypertensive medications
Grade III hypertensive retinopathy
Abdominal bruit
Previous urogram suggestive of renal artery stenosis

Blood Pressure Evaluation

Blood pressure is the primary clinical measurement used in diagnosis of RVH and also as a clinical marker to evaluate the outcome of renal revascularization. Although blood pressure measurement is a commonly performed clinical procedure, with serious implications associated with inaccuracy, studies have shown a lack of compliance with the basic techniques for use of sphygmomanometers.[20, 21] The major sources of error are faulty equipment, observer error, and failure to standardize the techniques of measurement.[22]

When systolic pressure is near normal or normal in a patient with clinical signs of severe hypertension, the blood pressure should be taken with careful attention to assessment for an auscultatory gap.[21] One cross-sectional study of 168 persons with hypertension revealed auscultatory gaps in 21 percent of the patients. Auscultatory gaps were associated with older age, increased arterial stiffness and atherosclerotic plaques, and a 67 percent incidence in women.[23] The presence of an auscultatory gap may result in underestimation of the systolic pressure or overestimation of the diastolic pressure. This can be avoided by palpating the pulse while inflating the cuff to ensure that the radial pulse has been obliterated by the inflation pressure. The systolic pressure is recorded as the first audible sound heard as the cuff is deflated. The diastolic sound is recorded as the pressure where the Korotkoff sounds disappear.[22]

A standardized technique for measuring blood pressure is crucial to monitoring patients over time. Two readings should be taken at each visit. There should be at least 1 minute between the two readings. If there is a significant difference between the readings, a third should be taken. The patient should sit in a chair with arm support. The forearm should be level with the junction of the fourth intercostal space and the lower left sternal border.[21, 22] Disparities have been documented between readings taken while the subject sits in a chair with legs supported and those taken with the subject on the examining table with legs dangling.[24] Studies describing outcomes after angioplasty or surgical revascularization should include descriptions of the techniques used for monitoring blood pressure.

Patient self-monitoring of blood pressure may be a component of care in patients with RVH. Demonstrations and supervised return demonstrations of patient technique for blood pressure measurement are recommended to ensure accuracy. Patients should be informed about the importance of position, accuracy of equipment calibration, as well as influences such as activity, meals, smoking, over-the-counter medications, and emotions. Because blood pressure normally fluctuates throughout the day, patients should measure blood pressure at two different specified times of day and keep a running record of the measurements.

Screening Tests

The ideal screening test should be simple, safe, inexpensive, sensitive, and specific. Currently none of the screening tests for RVH meet all of these criteria. Tests to detect renal physiologic abnormality include intravenous pyelography, renal scanning, plasma renin levels, and captopril renography. Diagnostic studies that can detect RAS include duplex ultrasonography, magnetic resonance angiography (MRA), and arteriography. Blood and urine analyses include blood urea nitrogen and creatinine, and 24-hour urine collections for creatinine clearance and protein.

Renal vein renin assays, which have been used to assess the functional significance of a renal artery lesion, have relatively low specificity and sensitivity in diagnosing RVH.[25] Many medications, including beta-adrenergic blocking agents, suppress renin output. Sodium intake, patient position, age, sex, race, timing of obtaining samples, as well as transit time to laboratory, may result in falsely nonlateralizing results. Many centers no longer use renal vein renin assays as a component for diagnosis. One clinical setting in which renal vein renin assay may be useful involves severe hypertension in the setting of angiographically identified unilateral total occlusion of a renal artery. Selective renal vein renin assays may assist in determining if the occluded kidney is secreting high levels of renin in comparison to the perfused kidney. High renal vein renin levels from the unperfused kidney may favor nephrectomy as a component to achieve blood pressure regulation in severely hypertensive patients with known total renal artery occlusions.

The more recent trend in diagnostic studies includes ACE inhibitor renal scintigraphy, Doppler sonography, MRA, and renal angiography. The limitations in sensitivity and specificity of these tests as well as costs influence current controversies related to their use as screening tools for RVH.

The physiologic response to ACE inhibitors is applied in diagnostic renal radionuclide scintigraphy studies. Administration of an ACE inhibitor results in decreased angiotensin II production and efferent arteriolar vasodilation. A kidney with RAS may exhibit decreased function when a converting enzyme inhibitor is administered. Because of the fixed stenosis, there is a decrease in glomerular filtration, and isotope clearance in the stenotic kidney is decreased. Renal scintigraphy with technetium Tc 99m MAG$_3$ before and after administration of captopril or enalaprilat are compared for levels of residual cortical activity (RCA). Significant changes in the time-activity curves indicate loss of excretory function.[26] A normal person or a patient with essential hypertension will not demonstrate a change in glomerular filtration rate after captopril administration.

ACE inhibition renal scanning is performed as an outpatient procedures. Patients who are taking ACE inhibitors must discontinue these medications for at least 48 hours prior to the study. Blood pressure is monitored before, during, and after the study. Patients may present with markedly elevated systolic and diastolic pressures because of withholding their antihypertensive medications. Depending on criteria for a positive result, captopril scintigraphy has a sensitivity of approximately 80 percent and specificity of 100 percent for detection of RVH. A marked decline in blood pressure after the administration of captopril may produce a false-positive bilateral disease pattern.[27] False-negative studies may occur in patients with poorly functioning kidneys. The test is usually followed by angiography for confirmation of RAS.

Doppler sonography is an inexpensive and noninvasive diagnostic tool for detecting RAS. Patients should fast prior to the study to enhance visualization of the renal arteries. There are numerous techniques using Doppler wave forms to show RAS. These include renal artery to aorta velocity ratio, acceleration time, acceleration index, and tardus-parvus wave form. The normal renal artery Doppler wave form has a rapid or steep upstroke and a small peak in early systole. In contrast, a tardus-parvus wave form distal to the stenosis lacks both of these features. The wave form has a slowed systolic acceleration (tardus) and low amplitude of the systolic peak (parvus).[27] The accuracy of the study is influenced by blood flow criteria used by the interpreter, patient preparation, and technique and skill of the sonographer in obtaining Doppler wave forms. Recent studies suggest that simple pattern recognition of the tardus-parvus wave form yields a sensitivity of 95 percent in detecting RAS in high-risk patients.[28]

MRA may be indicated in settings in which intravenous iodinated contrast is contraindicated. Images are usually obtained in two planes: axial and coronal. Following acquisition, the series is reconstructed for imaging. MRA is a reliable way of detecting single or dominant renal arteries but is not helpful for identification of accessory or small arterial branches. This diagnostic approach to detection of RAS continues to evolve. It is best suited for patients with atherosclerotic disease. It may serve a role in screening for RAS. If results of MRA are negative, some authors suggest no further evaluation is necessary. If a stenosis is identified, then conventional angiography should be performed to quantitate the stenosis.[29]

Digital subtraction angiography (DSA) is another advance in radiologic technique.[1] A baseline image is obtained without contrast—called the mask—and stored in a computer. A second image obtained using contrast is compared with the mask. Although the procedure is less expensive, more convenient, and carries less risk, there are several limitations to DSA. The technique is affected by motion artifacts. Patients must be able to remain still during the image acquisition. Fibromuscular dysplasia lesions may not be well visualized because of the decreased spatial resolution. The images may be uninterpretable in obese patients and those with cardiac decompensation.

Renal arteriography remains the gold standard for diagnosing RAS. This invasive study is indicated in patients who are being considered for balloon angioplasty or surgical revascularization. Percutaneous retrograde transfemoral technique is widely used to perform flush aortography and selective renal artery injections of contrast media. Arteriography defines the aorta and main renal artery, extent of poststenotic dilatation, presence of collateral circulation, and visualization of vessels that may be used for vascular repair or bypass. Renal arteriography can be performed as an outpatient procedure. If a significant stenosis is identified, it may be possible to perform balloon angioplasty at the same time.

TREATMENT

Comparison of percutaneous transluminal renal angioplasty (PTRA) and surgical interventions as treatment for RVH is limited by the lack of controlled trials and the differences in patient characteristics. Although there is still debate as to what is appropriate treatment for RVH, there is unequivocal evidence that a functionally significant lesion should be corrected. In the past several years, PTRA has become the preferred treatment for RAS causing RVH. Figure 15–4 illustrates percutaneous and surgical options for renal revascularization.

Angioplasty

Angioplasty of stenosis caused by fibromuscular dysplasia is effective in approximately 87–100 percent of patients.[6, 30] In contrast, the success rate of PTRA for atherosclerotic lesions ranges from as low as 30 percent to 90 percent. Some of this variation is influenced by the type of atherosclerotic lesion. Ostial lesions have a lower success rate than nonostial lesions. There is a higher initial technical failure rate and restenosis rate for ostial lesions. This may in part be due to the bulky aortic plaque impinging on the renal ostium and also arterial wall recoil at the ostium. In the last several years, stenting of renal ostial lesions has been performed with nearly 100 percent technical success rate.[31]

Renal angioplasty and stenting is performed in the vascular radiology suite or interven-

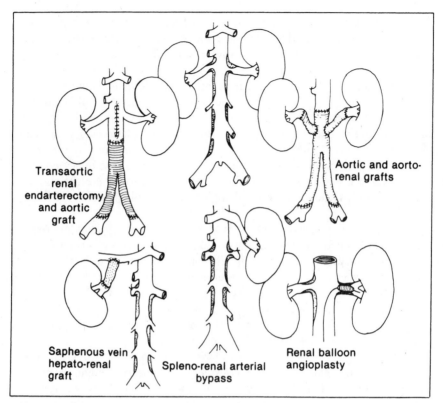

Figure 15–4. Options for renal revascularization for atherosclerotic disease. (From Hallet JW, Brewster DC, Darling RC: Patient Care in Vascular Surgery, 2nd ed. Boston, Little Brown & Co, © 1987.)

tional catheterization laboratory. The technique involves percutaneous insertion of a radiopaque guidewire, usually into the femoral artery, using local anesthesia. The guidewire is advanced retrograde fashion to the aorta. Arterial pressures are recorded proximal and distal to the stenotic lesion. The balloon-tipped catheter is advanced over the guidewire and positioned in the center of the renal artery lesion. The balloon is inflated, deflated, and pressures are remeasured. A significant decrease in the pressure differential indicates a successful dilation. A similar technique is employed for stent placement (Figs. 15–5 and 15–6). Following the procedure, the catheters and guidewires are removed and firm pressure is applied over the arterial access site for hemostasis and sealing of the arteriotomy.

The advantages of PTRA include lower morbidity and mortality than surgery, less expense, reduced hospital length of stay, and reduced loss of productive time. Subsequent surgery is usually not excluded by renal angioplasty. Elderly patients with multisystem disease or bilateral renal artery stenoses who would be at high risk for surgery may safely undergo PTRA.

In some hospitals, patients may be observed in the intensive care unit after PTRA, whereas in other institutions, patients may be placed in intermediate or step-down observational units. Patients should be carefully observed for precipitous decline in arterial blood pressure, changes in renal function as indicated by rising creatinine, and signs and symptoms of vascular access complications. Potential complications of PTRA are listed in Table 15–3. The patient remains on bed rest for several hours after the procedure and is often discharged from the hospital the next morning.

The local arterial trauma produced by the inflated balloon is thought to enhance platelet aggregation and thrombosis and even accelerate atherogenesis. Various anticoagu-

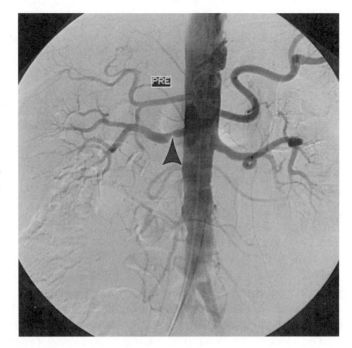

Figure 15–5. Arteriogram of atherosclerotic lesion of right artery with poststenotic dilatation *(arrowhead)* prior to renal angioplasty.

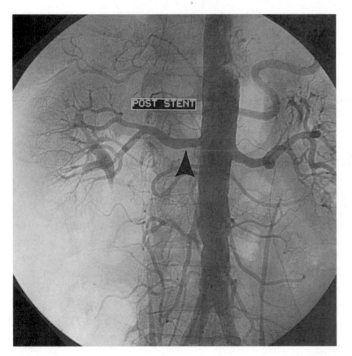

Figure 15–6. Arteriogram of same vessel *(arrowhead)* as in Figure 15–5 following angioplasty and placement of stent.

TABLE 15–3. **Potential Complications of PTRA**

PROCEDURAL COMPLICATIONS	VASCULAR ACCESS COMPLICATIONS
Arterial thrombosis	Retroperitoneal hemorrhage
Arterial rupture at time of balloon inflation	Distal embolization
Embolization of atherosclerotic plaque into kidney	Arteriovenous fistula, pseudoaneurysm, or hematoma

PTRA = percutaneous transluminal renal angioplasty.

lant or antiplatelet regimens may be used after PTRA including warfarin, ticlopidine, and aspirin. Intimal hyperplasia may develop, present as restenosis within the first 6 months after angioplasty, and require redilatation.

Surgical Revascularization

A variety of surgical techniques may be used to correct RAS or occlusion. The choice of technique is influenced by the nature and anatomic location of the obstructive lesion, presence and extent of aortic atherosclerotic disease, as well as experience and preference of the surgeon. The operative risk is influenced by these characteristics as well as by the patient's age, duration of hypertension, and comorbid disease states.[32]

The most common surgical approach, aortorenal bypass, uses an autogenous vessel, either artery or vein, to bypass from the aorta to beyond the renal artery lesion. Prosthetic materials such as polytetrafluoroethylene (PTFE) may also be used. The surgical approach is made through an oblique incision from the tip of the eleventh rib on the involved side to the lateral border of the opposite rectus muscle. The bypass conduit saphenous vein is obtained from either thigh. The bypass is usually accomplished with an end-to-end anastomosis between the saphenous vein and the renal artery beyond the stenotic lesion. The renal artery is clamped proximal and distal to the stenosis during the anastomosis of the bypass conduit. After the conduit is anastomosed to the renal artery, the aorta is cross-clamped proximally and distally. An arteriotomy is made and the bypass conduit vessel is anastomosed to the side of the aorta. Timing is essential because the kidney and lower extremities may suffer ischemic injury with prolonged clamping.

Other approaches to surgical revascularization include extra-anatomic bypass using splenic artery, mesenteric artery, or hepatic artery, and thromboendarterectomy. Figure 15–4 illustrates several surgical approaches to renal revascularization. A nephrectomy may be indicated when the involved kidney has nonreconstructible vessels and minimal to no excretory function.

After surgical renal revascularization, patients are routinely monitored in intensive care settings for 1–3 days. The nursing care during this period is similar to other aortic surgery (see Chapter 11). The goals of postoperative care include regulation of blood pressure, stabilization of cardiopulmonary function, prevention of or management of postoperative complications, and assessment of renal function.

OUTCOMES

The goals of renal revascularization are to preserve and stabilize renal function and control hypertension. Renal angioplasty with or without stent placement and surgical revascularization techniques offer patients with RVH the potential for improved control of hypertension and slowing of the progression of renal insufficiency.[33–35] Medical management of RVH should be limited to those patients unwilling to undergo or with contraindications to interventional procedures.

Patients with FMD have a higher chance for total cure than do those with atherosclerosis. Results are less favorable in bilateral renal artery stenoses and ostial lesions. Although the cure rate for RVH remains low, blood pressure improves in the majority of patients. There have also been improvements in total renal function as evidenced by increased glomerular filtration rate and decreased serum creatinine levels.

NURSING CARE

Nursing care of patients with RVH is both challenging and rewarding. Nurses provide care to patients at presentation and during the diagnostic, treatment, and follow-up periods. Patient evaluation in each of these phases should include physical examination, blood pressure monitoring, documentation of antihypertensive medications (number of medications and doses), and ongoing evaluation of renal patency and function through serial diagnostic testing. Patient education should provide explanations of renal anatomy and function; preparation for diagnostic studies; information on doses, actions, and side effects of medications; and preparation for treatment techniques. Patients with atherosclerotic etiology for RAS should be informed of strategies to reduce modifiable risk factors. Key points for nursing interventions are listed in Table 15–4.

SUMMARY

Fibromuscular dysplasia or atherosclerosis should be considered as the possible cause of poorly controlled hypertension, especially in the young and in the elderly. The possibility of RAS as the etiology of hypertension should be raised in patients presenting with

TABLE 15–4. **Nursing Care in Renovascular Hypertension**

Screening
- Identify high-risk patients.
- Perform physical assessment to identify clinical signs:
  Standardized blood pressure measurement, auscultate for abdominal bruit, eye exam for hypertensive retinopathy, survey patient for symptoms of coronary artery disease, carotid disease, peripheral vascular disease
- Evaluate presentation and course of hypertension:
  New onset, early or late stage, progressive, refractory to 3 medications, malignant

Diagnostic Phase
- Provide patient education and instructions for diagnostic studies.
- Observe patients for side effects and complications during periprocedural period.

Treatment
- Administer antihypertensive medications and document response.
- Provide patient education related to planned intervention and risk factor modification.
- Provide nursing care during periprocedural period.
- Observe and document blood pressure response and laboratory test results.

Maintenance/Monitoring
- Monitor blood pressure and renal function with serum creatinine, 24-hour urine samples.
- Assess for patency/restenosis:
  Abdominal physical examination for presence of bruit, observe trends in blood pressure levels, schedule serial diagnostic studies as indicated

coexisting evidence of coronary, cerebral, or peripheral vascular insufficiency. Appropriate diagnostic studies should be performed to screen for RAS as the basis for hypertension. Renovascular hypertension is amenable to percutaneous and surgical revascularization techniques. Elevated blood pressure is often adequately controlled, and, to a lesser degree, may even be cured, in patients who undergo revascularization techniques. Equally as important, revascularization may retard the progressive decline in renal tissue mass and function. Patients who undergo PTRA or surgical revascularization may develop restenosis or progression of disease. Serial monitoring of renal function and renal artery patency is vital. Recognition and management of a potentially curable form of hypertension require diligence during all phases of care.

References

1. Ram CV, Clagett G, Radford R: Renovascular hypertension. Semin Nephrol 1995; 15(2):152–174.
2. Goldfarb DA: The renin-angiotensin system: New concepts in regulation of blood pressure and renal function. Urol Clin North Am 1994; 21(2):187–194.
3. Edwards RM, Aiyar N: Angiotensin II receptor antagonists as a treatment for hypertension. J Am Soc Nephrol 1993; 3(10):1643–1652.
4. Pickering TG, Herman L, Devereux RB, et al: Recurrent pulmonary oedema in hypertension due to bilateral renal artery stenosis: Treatment by angioplasty or surgical revascularisation. Lancet 1988; 2(8610):551–552.
5. Olin JW, Novick AC: Renovascular disease. In Young JR, Graor RA, Olin JW, et al (eds): Peripheral Vascular Diseases. St. Louis, Mosby–Year Book, 1991, pp 267–284.
6. Nabel EG, Dzau VJ: Renal vascular hypertension. In Loscalzo J, Creager MM, Dzau M (eds): Vascular Medicine. Boston, Little, Brown & Co, 1992, pp 867–886.
7. Gunnells JC, McCann RL: Renovascular disease. In Sabiston DC Jr (ed): Textbook of Surgery: The Biological Basis of Modern Surgical Practice, 15th ed. Philadelphia, WB Saunders, 1996, pp 1759–1767.
8. Louie J, Isaacson JA, Zierler RE, et al: Prevalence of carotid and lower extremity arterial disease in patients with renal artery disease. Am J Hypertens 1994; 7(5):436–439.
9. Wachtell K, Ibsen H, Olsen M, et al: Prevalence of renal artery stenosis in patients with peripheral vascular disease and hypertension. J Hum Hypertens 1996; 10(2):83–85.
10. Olin JW, Melia M, Young JR, et al: Prevalence of atherosclerotic renal artery stenosis in patients with atherosclerosis elsewhere. Am J Med 1990; 88(1N):46N–51N.
11. Harding M, Smith L, Himmelstein S, et al: Renal artery stenosis: Prevalence and associated risk factors in patients undergoing routine cardiac catheterization. J Am Soc Nephrol 1992; 2(11):1608–1616.
12. Emovon OE, Klotman PE, Dunnick NR, et al: Renovascular hypertension in blacks. Am J Hypertens 1996; 9(1):18–23.
13. Schreiber MJ, Pohl M, Novick A: The natural history of atherosclerotic and fibrous renal artery disease. Urol Clin North Am 1984; 11(3):383–392.
14. Rimmer JM, Gennari FJ: Atherosclerotic renovascular disease and progressive renal failure. Ann Intern Med 1993; 118(9):712–719.
15. Tollefson D, Ernst C: Natural history of atherosclerotic renal artery stenosis associated with aortic disease. J Vasc Surg 1991; 14(3):327–331.
16. Zierler RE, Bergelin RO, Davidson RC, et al: A prospective study of disease progression in patients with atherosclerotic renal artery stenosis. Am J Hypertens 1996; 9(11):1055–1061.
17. Strandness DE Jr: Natural history of renal artery stenosis. Am J Kidney Dis 1994; 24(4):630–635.
18. Svetkey LP, Helms MJ, Dunnick NR, et al: Clinical characteristics useful in screening for renovascular disease. Renovasc Dis 1990; 83(7):743–747.
19. McKay DW, Campbell NRC, Parab LS, et al: Clinical assessment of blood pressure. J Hum Hypertens 1990; 4(6):639–645.
20. Baker RH, Ender J: Confounders of auscultatory blood pressure measurement. J Gen Intern Med 1995; 10(4):223–231.
21. Anonymous: Recommendations for human blood pressure determination by sphygmomanometer. Report of a special task force appointed by the Steering Committee, American Heart Association. Circulation 1988; 77(2):501A–514A.
22. Cavallini MC, Roman MJ, Blank SG, et al: Association of the auscultatory gap with vascular disease in hypertensive patients. Ann Intern Med 1996; 124(10):877–883.
23. Anonymous: Recommendations for routine blood pressure measurement by indirect cuff sphygmomanometry. American Society of Hypertension. Am J Hypertens 1992; 5(4 part 1):207–209.

24. Cushman WC, Cooper KM, Horne RA, et al: Effect of back support and stethoscope head on seated blood pressure determinations. Am J Hypertens 1990; 3(3):240–241.
25. Martin LG, Cork RD, Wells JO: Renal vein renin analysis: Limitations of its use in predicting benefit from percutaneous angioplasty. Cardiovasc Intervent Radiol 1993; 16(2):76–80.
26. Mahnensmith RL: Renovascular hypertension: From suspicion to therapy. Emerg Med 1995; 27(3):48–50.
27. Mitty HA, Shapiro RS, Parsons RB, et al: Renovascular hypertension. Radiol Clin North Am 1996; 34(5):1017–1036.
28. Gottlieb RH, Lieberman JL, Pabico RC, et al: Diagnosis of renal artery stenosis in transplanted kidneys: Value of Doppler waveform analysis of the intrarenal arteries. AJR 1995; 165(6):1441–1446.
29. Borrello JA, Li D, Vesely TM, et al: Renal arteries: Clinical comparison of three-dimensional time-of-flight MR angiographic sequences and radiographic angiography. Radiol 1995; 197(3):793–799.
30. Tegtmeyer CJ, Selby JB, Hartwell GD, et al: Results and complications of angioplasty in fibromuscular disease. Circulation 1991; 83(suppl I):I155–I161.
31. Rees CR, Palmaz JC, Becker GJ, et al: Palmaz stent in atherosclerotic stenosis involving the ostia of the renal arteries: Preliminary report of a multicenter study. Radiology 1991; 181(2):507–514.
32. Dean RH, Hansen KJ: Renovascular hypertension. In Moore WS (ed): Vascular Surgery: A comprehensive review, 5th ed. Philadelphia, WB Saunders, 1998, pp 521–541.
33. Dorros G, Jaff M, Jain A, et al: Follow up of primary Palmaz-Schatz stent placement for atherosclerotic renal artery stenosis. Am J Cardiol 1995; 75(15):1051–1055.
34. Acher CW, Belzer FO, Grist TM, et al: Late renal function in patients undergoing renal revascularization for control of hypertension and/or renal preservation. Cardiovasc Surg 1996; 4(5):602–606.
35. Blum U, Krumme B, Flugel P, et al: Treatment of ostial renal-artery stenosis with vascular endoprostheses after successful balloon angioplasty. N Engl J Med 1997; 336(7):459–465.

16

Mesenteric Ischemia

Shahab Abdessalam, MD, and B. Timothy Baxter, MD

∽ · ∽

Mesenteric ischemia remains one of the most difficult diagnostic challenges in contemporary vascular surgery. Although the condition was recognized as early as the fifteenth century, successful revascularization of ischemic bowel without resection did not occur until the 1950s.[1] Basic scientific investigation has led to dramatic progress in understanding the mediators of injury following experimental gut ischemia and reperfusion, including important effects on distant organs. Unfortunately, this progress has not yet had a meaningful impact on patient outcome, inasmuch as the mortality of mesenteric ischemia with infarction remains in excess of 60 percent.[2] While comorbid disease contributes to this high mortality rate, timely diagnosis relative to the onset of ischemia is the most crucial factor in patient outcome. The delay is often caused by failure to consider mesenteric ischemia in the differential diagnosis or a reluctance to order mesenteric arteriography once the diagnosis is considered. Recognizing and establishing the diagnosis of intestinal ischemia requires the input of an entire health care team, a team that is well versed in the clinical features of this rare but deadly problem.

ANATOMY AND PATHOPHYSIOLOGY

Localized ischemia and infarction play an important role in the pathophysiology of a wide array of surgical problems, including appendicitis, strangulation associated with herniation, and segmental ischemic colitis. Rather than discuss these focal processes, this chapter will address four specific entities that affect blood flow in the major arteries or veins of the intestine (Table 16–1). Atherosclerotic stenosis as well as arterial and venous thrombosis and embolization can cause mesenteric ischemia. Understanding the arterial anatomy of the gut provides the basis for understanding differences in the clinical presentation of acute, subacute, and chronic intestinal ischemia.

TABLE 16–1. **Causes of Mesenteric Ischemia**

TYPE OF ISCHEMIA	CAUSE
Chronic mesenteric ischemia	Atherosclerosis and thrombosis
Acute mesenteric ischemia	Embolus
Nonocclusive mesenteric ischemia	Low cardiac output
Mesenteric vein thrombosis	Hypercoagulability

The embryologic foregut, midgut, and hindgut derive their arterial supply from the celiac artery, superior mesenteric artery (SMA), and the inferior mesenteric artery (IMA), respectively.[3] These three major arteries arise from the abdominal aorta (Fig. 16–1). Additionally, branches of the internal iliac artery supply the distal colon. The celiac artery is the first major branch of the abdominal aorta arising from the anterior surface at the level of the twelfth thoracic or first lumbar vertebra. It supplies the stomach, duodenum, liver, pancreas, and spleen. Approximately 1.5 cm below the celiac axis, the SMA originates. It supplies the remainder of the small bowel from the ligament of Treitz, the pancreas, and the ascending and transverse colon. The IMA, which begins midway between the renal arteries and the aortic bifurcation, is the blood supply to the descending and sigmoid colon. The hypogastric arteries (internal iliac arteries) supply the rectum as well as the remainder of the pelvis. All of these vessels divide and anastomose with each other to form a rich vascular network. The major collateral between the celiac artery and the SMA is the anterior pancreaticoduodenal arcade. The meandering mesenteric artery is the important central collateral between the SMA and IMA. The middle and superior hemorrhoidal arteries form an anastomosis between the IMA and hypogastric arteries.

The importance of these collaterals cannot be overestimated inasmuch as gradual occlusion of all three of the vessels has been reported without infarction.[4] Conversely, acute occlusion of a single artery, as might occur from cardiac embolization, can result in rapid segmental infarction.[2, 5] Because of the remarkable ability of the gut to develop compensatory collateral blood flow, ischemia from chronic occlusive disease represents the end stage of progressive occlusion of all major arteries to the gut.[4] Decreased gut perfusion from low cardiac output can cause intestinal infarction.[6–8] Venous outflow occlusion from mesenteric vein thrombosis causes venous hypertension followed by compromised arterial inflow and, finally, infarction.[9, 10]

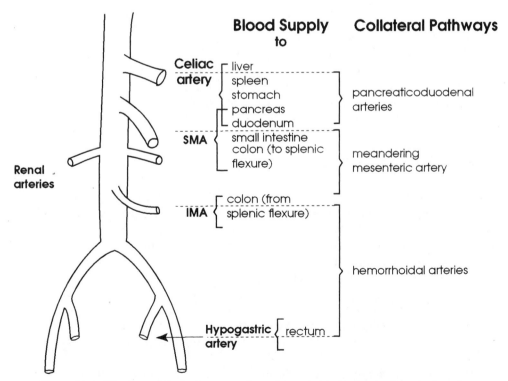

Figure 16–1. The intra-abdominal aorta perfuses the gastrointestinal tract through the celiac artery, the superior mesenteric artery (SMA), the inferior mesenteric artery (IMA), and the hypogastric arteries. The organs perfused by each artery are shown as are the collateral pathways between major arteries.

The basic insult of compromised gut blood flow occurs when the crucial continuous demand for oxygen for cellular viability is not met. The cells of the mucosa are highly active metabolically and are, therefore, exquisitely sensitive to ischemia. The mucosal cells at the tip of the villi are the first to be lost. These early changes affecting the villi may be seen microscopically within 10 minutes of total ischemia.[11] The acute ischemic insult is usually associated with intense peristalsis, which is manifest, clinically, as vomiting, diarrhea, or both. Inflammatory cells, necrotic debris, fibrin, and bacteria accumulate at the surface. With progression, ulcers begin to form on the luminal surface. Fortunately, some degree of collateral blood flow is usually present to attenuate the injury and slow the progression. If flow is not restored, the lamina propria breaks down.[11] Loss of this barrier is a crucial event, allowing egress of fluid and ingress of bacteria. These fluid shifts may lead to significant intravascular volume depletion. The signs of sepsis, including leukocytosis, fever, hypotension, and altered mental status, may appear at this point. Typically, pain is severe but poorly localized within the abdomen until transmural injury causes inflammation of the parietal peritoneum.

There are other local and systemic physiologic responses that arise and contribute to the clinical picture.[3, 12] Autonomic, humoral, and local factors all affect the eventual outcome of the intestine. Autonomic factors including alpha- and beta-adrenergic stimuli cause an initial brief period of vasodilatation followed by sustained vasoconstriction. The humoral factors, angiotensin II and vasopressin, exacerbate local vasoconstriction. The ischemic process causes both local and systemic activation of the immune system. Activated neutrophils may initiate remote organ injury in the lungs or liver.[13] These destructive processes may be greatly amplified following reperfusion of the ischemic bowel.[14] Ongoing experimental work will help to identify pharmacologic approaches that, in the future, may attenuate the inflammatory cascade and reduce morbidity—and mortality—associated ischemia and revascularization.

CLINICAL MANIFESTATIONS

The key to prevention of transmural infarction is early diagnosis. This can only be accomplished if a high index of suspicion is maintained in a patient who fits the "clinical criteria" outlined below. Although these signs and symptoms may be quite nonspecific, when taken together, they are often highly suggestive of the correct diagnosis.

Acute Intestinal Ischemia

Acute ischemia may occur in association with acute embolic occlusion of a mesenteric vessel, as the final thrombotic event in patients with chronic mesenteric ischemia, or from hypovolemic or cardiogenic shock. Of these three, acute embolic occlusion is most readily recognized because of the sudden and dramatic onset of symptoms.[2, 5] It begins with severe, acute abdominal pain and may be followed by prompt emptying of the gastrointestinal tract either by vomiting, a bowel movement, or both. The intense pain is caused by vigorous intestinal contractions, and bowel sounds are usually increased at this stage. Because the patient will often be writhing in pain, it is surprising to find the abdomen soft and minimally tender on physical examination. Abdominal distention is not a consistent feature. The diagnosis is further supported by a history of previous emboli or cardiac dysrhythmias.

Thrombosis of the last patent mesenteric artery in a patient with atherosclerotic occlusive disease will be more insidious than acute embolic occlusion.[2, 5] The more subtle presentation may result because patients are debilitated from malnutrition or because they have long suffered from vague abdominal pain. Although both the weight loss and chronic abdominal pain should help in establishing the correct diagnosis, the crucial diagnostic study, mesenteric angiography, is often delayed by a misdiagnosis such as small bowel obstruction.

The clinical presentation of nonocclusive mesenteric ischemia is more difficult to recognize because of the underlying medical condition of the patient.[7, 8] The signs and symptoms of bowel ischemia usually arise during the course of treatment for some other life-threatening condition. A careful review of the records will identify a period of hypotension, often requiring pharmacologic support, during the previous 72 hours. These patients are often obtunded, and there is a significant delay in recognizing the intestinal ischemia until signs of more advanced ischemic changes or infarction (leukocytosis, abdominal distention, and acidosis) are present.

Chronic Intestinal Ischemia

Although the initial clinical features of chronic mesenteric ischemia are vague, with time, the astute health care provider will identify an emerging pattern of signs and symptoms.[4] Weight loss is invariable and must be present to consider the diagnosis. This is associated with "food fear," avoidance of food because of the associated pain. Abdominal pain occurs within minutes of eating and is initially only associated with large meals. As the atherosclerosis progresses, the patient makes adjustments by eating smaller amounts more often. Eventually these smaller meals also become associated with pain, and caloric intake is no longer adequate; weight loss begins. Diarrhea is often present during this time, presumably related to malabsorption. Other complications of atherosclerosis such as cerebral, coronary, or lower-extremity ischemia and vascular reconstruction usually precede the development of mesenteric ischemia.

Mesenteric Vein Thrombosis

Mesenteric vein thrombosis is a distinct entity that can also cause intestinal infarction.[9, 15] Any extensive infectious process within the mesenteric venous drainage such as appendicitis or diverticulitis can cause thrombosis. It is also seen as a manifestation of hypercoagulable states. This may occur in patients with a history of venous thrombosis and defined abnormalities such as polycythemia vera or a deficiency in antithrombin III, protein C, or protein S. Hypercoagulable states associated with cancer can also cause mesenteric vein thrombosis.

Mesenteric vein thrombosis results in increased venous pressures. This will interfere with capillary flow and result in tissue damage. When this is associated with infarction and peritonitis, the mortality rate is high. Mesenteric vein thrombosis can have a relatively benign course with mild abdominal pain and flu-like symptoms in some patients.[15]

DIAGNOSIS

With suspected acute ischemia, urgent and aggressive diagnostic measures should be undertaken. Unfortunately, laboratory and noninvasive radiologic procedures may not be diagnostic in the early, reversible phase of the process. Development of a rapid and reliable clinical marker has been elusive despite active investigation. Again, however, a pattern of diagnostic findings may help to exclude other more common problems and lead to definitive angiographic assessment.

Laboratory Tests

A serum marker specific for intestinal ischemia has long been sought. This search has proven to be difficult because the liver acts as a filter between the mesenteric venous drainage and systemic venous drainage. Leukocytosis is present in most patients but is, obviously, nonspecific. Metabolic acidosis is a late sign associated with infarction. The BB isoform of creatine kinase is abundant in smooth muscle cells. There are conflicting reports of its sensitivity in gut ischemia.[16] Smooth muscle cells are also rich in phosphate, and elevated serum levels may occur with mesenteric infarction. It is not clear, however, that this is a sensitive marker of ischemia.[16] Peritoneal lavage can be performed in patients with suspected ischemia, and animal studies suggest elevation in peritoneal leukocytes and phosphate in lavage fluid with gut ischemia. This has not been evaluated in clinical trials. D-Lactate is a product of bacterial fermentation not produced in mammalian tissues.[17] Although animal studies suggested it might be a good marker for early ischemia, it was also disappointing in identifying ischemic bowel in clinical trials.

Noninvasive Radiologic Tests

In the past decade, duplex ultrasonography has emerged as a valuable tool in the diagnosis of chronic mesenteric ischemia.[18–20] In the hands of a skilled technician, it can accurately detect stenosis and occlusion in both the celiac artery and SMA. Gaseous distention and pain limit the utility of duplex ultrasonography in the setting of acute ischemia. Keene and colleagues have suggested that these limitations might be overcome using endoscopic transgastric ultrasonography.[21]

Technological advances in computed tomography (CT) have led to a resurgence of interest in this modality.[22, 23] It is invaluable as a tool to exclude other more common causes of abdominal pain. More rapid spiral scanning with timed contrast infusion may allow assessment of bowel perfusion. Bowel wall thickening, intestinal pneumatosis, and portal vein gas are late findings associated with advanced ischemia or infarction. Contrast CT is the definitive diagnostic study for mesenteric vein thrombosis.

Arteriography

Despite the technologic advances in noninvasive diagnosis of other disease processes, angiography remains the single best diagnostic study for bowel ischemia.[5] Because mesenteric ischemia caused by thrombotic occlusion, embolus, and nonocclusive mesenteric ischemia has distinct angiographic features, the underlying process can also be identified (Fig. 16–2). Chronic occlusive disease is ostial and is best seen on lateral view of the aorta. Emboli usually lodge more distally in the superior mesenteric artery. Nonocclusive mesenteric ischemia is associated with narrowing and spasm in the peripheral arcades of the bowel with little filling of mesenteric branches. Besides its diagnostic value in nonocclusive mesenteric ischemia, catheters can be left in place for selective infusion of vasodilators to help reverse local spasm.[7] Furthermore, mesenteric angioplasty (discussed below) can also be performed at the same setting. Because it is the definitive diagnostic study, clinicians should obtain mesenteric angiography when the diagnosis is even remotely considered.

TREATMENT

The goal of treatment of mesenteric ischemia is to restore normal bowel function. The patient's age and overall medical condition and the extent of bowel infarction must be

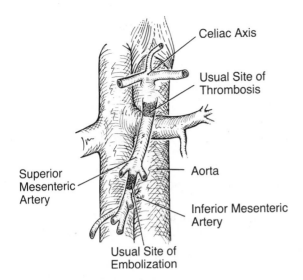

Celiac Axis

Usual Site of
Thrombosis

Superior
Mesenteric
Artery

Aorta

Inferior Mesenteric
Artery

Usual Site of
Embolization

Figure 16–2. The usual site of superior mesenteric artery (SMA) thrombosis is at the origin of the vessel. Embolic occlusion of the SMA typically occurs distal to the ostia. (From Bergan JJ: Operative procedures in acute mesenteric infarction. In Bergan JJ, Yao JST [eds]: Operative Techniques in Vascular Surgery. New York, Grune & Stratton, 1980, p 106.)

considered in choosing the best treatment. Options include local infusion of vasodilators, revascularization by angioplasty or open surgical procedure, and in some unusual cases in which infarction is extensive, observation and supportive therapy alone (Table 16–2).

Whether surgery is anticipated or not, the initial treatment for patients with suspected bowel ischemia is the same: (1) correct intravascular volume loss; (2) optimize cardiac function and mesenteric flow; (3) limit the existing thrombotic or embolic process; and (4) correct electrolyte and acid/base abnormalities. These measures will limit bowel infarction and address the adverse systemic effects of the ischemic process.

Medical Management and Resuscitation

Fluid shifts with bowel ischemia can be dramatic. For this reason, all patients should have a bladder catheter and central venous line to help continuously assess volume status. If blood pressure is labile, an arterial line should be placed. When there are questions about cardiac function, a pulmonary artery catheter can be very helpful. Because of coexistent cardiac disease, hypotension should not always be equated with hypovolemia. Knowing the central venous pressure or pulmonary artery pressure is essential in making the important distinction between cardiogenic and hypovolemic shock.

Saline solutions or plasma may be used to correct the fluid loss. Dextran may also be used and may be of further benefit because of its antiplatelet properties. Regardless of the solution used, a central venous or pulmonary artery catheter is necessary to carefully monitor volume replacement.

During resuscitation, other measures should be directed at improving mesenteric arterial flow. This is best achieved by optimizing cardiac function. Dobutamine may be

TABLE 16–2. **Treatment of Mesenteric Ischemia**

TYPE OF ISCHEMIA	TREATMENT
Chronic occlusive mesenteric ischemia	Bypass, endarterectomy, or angioplasty
Acute embolus to superior mesenteric artery	Embolectomy
Nonocclusive mesenteric ischemia	Circulatory support, local vasodilators
Mesenteric vein thrombosis	Anticoagulation

particularly useful in improving function and selectively improving mesenteric blood flow. Catheters are left in the SMA after arteriography when nonocclusive mesenteric ischemia is diagnosed.[7] Intra-arterial papaverine hydrochloride provides a local vasodilating effect. The infusion continues for one or more 24-hour periods, often with repeat arteriography at the end of each 24-hour period. During this time, the patient must be continually assessed for bowel infarction and peritonitis.

Patients who present after embolization from a cardiac source are at significant risk of recurrent embolization. This risk is dramatically reduced by intravenous heparin infusion. In thrombotic occlusive disease, heparin prevents propagation of newly formed thrombus. Thus, anticoagulant therapy is initiated with heparin sodium while the patient is carefully monitored for any increase in intestinal bleeding owing to bowel infarction and mucosal slough. Long-term warfarin therapy is usually indicated.

When bowel infarction is suspected on clinical grounds, an antibiotic that covers gram-negative and anaerobic organisms should be given. Arterial blood gas values will indicate the need for sodium bicarbonate therapy to correct the acidosis found with bowel infarction.

Nonoperative treatment has a place in the management of nonorganic intestinal ischemia, and angioplasty has been used to treat chronic mesenteric occlusive disease. Surgery, however, remains the most definitive and successful technique for arterial emboli or occlusive disease. When there are obvious physical and radiographic signs of extensive infarction in a severely debilitated and elderly patient, it is not unreasonable in consultation with the family to provide only supportive treatment.

Angioplasty

In those suffering from chronic mesenteric ischemia, newer nonoperative approaches have also been introduced in the last 10 to 15 years. Angioplasty has been used successfully in the coronary and peripheral circulation, so its use in the mesenteric circulation is no surprise. The objective of angioplasty is to dilate significant stenosis (greater than 50 percent) in the celiac artery or SMA.[24] Most authors are reporting initial success rates of greater than 80 percent. As may be seen with angioplasty in other arteries, restenosis is a problem occurring at a rate of 33 percent within 10 months.[24] Whether primary stenting will improve short-term restenosis is unclear.

Surgical Treatment

Surgery continues to have a central role in the management of mesenteric ischemia for two reasons. The first is that surgical revascularization provides the best initial and long-term outlook for the patient.[25] Second, laparotomy may be required to determine the extent of the ischemic process and resect nonviable intestine. In acute embolic occlusion, embolectomy of the superior mesenteric artery by balloon catheter can usually restore normal flow (Fig. 16–3). During surgery, the bowel is carefully examined to determine the need for resection. If the majority of bowel appears ischemic but is not infarcted, a second operation (second look) is performed to observe the condition of the bowel 24 hours after revascularization in the hope that some bowel will recover and resection can be limited.[5]

Acute thrombotic occlusion or chronic mesenteric artery occlusion can be treated with bypass or endarterectomy. The former is more common and can be done with either saphenous vein or prosthetic material (Fig. 16–4). Because all of the arteries will be involved to some degree, bypass to both the celiac artery and SMA provides some

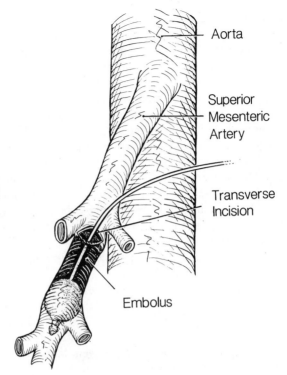

Figure 16–3. Embolectomy of the superior mesenteric artery by means of a Fogarty catheter. (From Bergan JJ: Operative procedures in acute mesenteric infarction. In Bergan JJ, Yao JST [eds]: Operative Techniques in Vascular Surgery. New York. Grune & Stratton, 1980, p 106.)

insurance if one of the grafts eventually fails. Success rates as high as 90 percent have been reported for surgical revascularization.[25]

Postoperative Care

The postoperative phase requires vigilant observation and skilled nursing care. The major areas of focus in the postoperative period should include: (1) observation for signs of

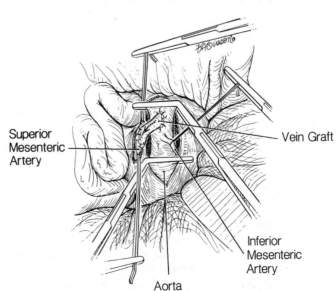

Figure 16–4. Saphenous vein bypass from the aorta to the superior mesenteric artery. (From Bergan JJ: Operative procedures in acute mesenteric infarction. In Bergan JJ, Yao JST [eds]: Operative Techniques in Vascular Surgery. New York, Grune & Stratton, 1980, p 105.)

recurrent ischemia, (2) correction of fluid and electrolyte losses, (3) correction of metabolic acidosis, and (4) monitoring of gastrointestinal function.

The patient must be constantly assessed for signs of intestinal ischemia secondary to recurrent mesenteric embolization or thrombosis of the graft or endarterectomy site. A key symptom would be complaints of new abdominal pain similar to the preoperative pain and not related to the incision site.

Fluid and electrolyte management may be challenging. Hypotension may occur, as the preoperative fluid losses are aggravated by additional fluid loss during surgery and third-space fluid loss postoperatively. Blood pressure measurements, filling pressures, urine output, and vital signs must be carefully monitored.

The patient's cardiac status is a factor to consider during this fluid replacement therapy. If there is compromised cardiac function, frequent central venous or pulmonary artery pressure readings help in attaining a balance between hypovolemia and cardiac overload. Some medications used to improve cardiac function (including digitoxin) may cause vasoconstriction; these drugs may have to be limited or discontinued during this time. Exact intake and output records are important in the fluid management as well as in assessment of renal function.

Many patients with vascular disease are cigarette smokers with some degree of chronic obstructive pulmonary disease. Pulmonary complications such as pneumonia can be prevented with aggressive measures. Vigorous pulmonary care should be started on admission to the intensive care unit. Arterial blood gas analysis provides helpful information regarding oxygen exchange (PO_2) and ventilation (PCO_2). Metabolic acidosis may result from ischemia and/or reperfusion.

A working nasogastric tube is important for gastric decompression. Time for bowel recovery may be prolonged and comparable to that in patients having aortic surgery. When normal bowel sounds have returned and the patient begins passing gas, a liquid diet can be resumed. A period of malabsorption for several weeks postoperatively until the mucosa fully recovers has been reported.

To prevent the complications associated with bed rest, activity should be encouraged as soon as tolerated. Pneumatic compression stockings and subcutaneous heparin should be used for deep venous thrombosis (DVT) prophylaxis. With improvement, the patient is transferred to the floor and discharged after oral intake is adequate.

Patient Education

When the patient has been stabilized and is recovering comfortably, patient education should start. Mesenteric occlusion is usually due to atherosclerosis, so patient education should focus on the following: (1) identification of risk factors such as smoking, high cholesterol levels, hypertension, diabetes, and lack of exercise; and (2) methods to control these risk factors through diet instruction, smoking cessation classes, exercise therapy, and control of blood pressure. After hospital discharge, nursing referral can be made for teaching to be reinforced by the physician's office nurse, a visiting nurse, or through a vascular rehabilitation program.

CONCLUSION

Few challenges in vascular nursing are greater than that of caring for the patient with mesenteric ischemia. Any member of the health care team who recognizes the constellation of signs and symptoms associated with mesenteric ischemia should suggest it be included in the differential diagnosis. Simply considering the diagnosis may help to expedite the evaluation and confirm a diagnosis of mesenteric ischemia. Perioperatively, patients with mesenteric ischemia are extremely challenging because of a combination of sepsis, activation of the inflammatory cascade, and underlying cardiovascular disease. Providing optimal patient care requires knowledge of each of these processes.

Often the immediate need for prompt lifesaving interventions allows time for only a brief nursing assessment focused on the patient's physical status. However, emotional and educational support are also important for both patient and family dealing with a life-threatening illness. Continuous psychological support, combined with skillful assessment and technical expertise, will help reduce stress and put the patient and family at ease.

References

1. Boley SJ, Brandt LJ, Sammartano RJ: History of mesenteric ischemia. Surg Clin North Am 1997; 77(2):275–278.
2. Stoney RJ, Cunningham CG: Acute mesenteric ischemia. Surgery 1993; 114(3):489–490.
3. Rosenblum JD, Boyle CM, Schwartz LB: The mesenteric circulation. Anatomy and physiology. Surg Clin North Am 1997; 77(2):289–306.
4. Baxter BT, Pearce WH; Diagnosis and surgical management of chronic mesenteric ischemia. In Strandness E, Van Berda A (eds): Vascular Diseases: Surgical and Interventional Therapy. New York, Churchill Livingstone, 1996, pp 795–802.
5. McKinsey JF, Gewertz BL: Acute mesenteric ischemia. Surg Clin North Am 1997; 77(2):307–318.
6. Howard TJ, Plaskon LA, Wiebke EA, Wilcox MG: Nonocclusive mesenteric ischemia remains a diagnostic dilemma. Am J Surg 1996; 171(4):405–408.
7. Bassiouny HS: Nonocclusive mesenteric ischemia. Surg Clin North Am 1997; 77(2):319–326.
8. Lock G, Scholmerich J: Non-occlusive mesenteric ischemia. Hepatogastroenterology 1995; 42(3):234–239.
9. Rhee RY, Gloviczki P: Mesenteric venous thrombosis. Surg Clin North Am 1997; 77(2):327–38.
10. Crespo I, Murphy J, Wong RK: Superior mesenteric venous thrombosis masquerading as Crohn's disease. Am J Gastroenterol 1994; 89(1):116–118.
11. Pearce WH, Bergan JJ: Acute intestinal ischemia. In Rutherford RB (ed): Vascular Surgery, 3rd ed. Philadelphia, WB Saunders, 1989, pp 1086–1096.
12. Patel A, Kaleya RN, Sammartano RJ: Pathophysiology of mesenteric ischemia. Surg Clin North Am 1992; 72(1):31–41.
13. Kim FJ, Moore EE, Moore FA, et al: Reperfused gut elaborates PAF that chemoattracts and primes neutrophils. J Surg Res 1995; 58(6):636–640.
14. Koike K, Moore EE, Moore FA, et al: Gut phospholipase A2 mediates neutrophil priming and lung injury after mesenteric ischemia-reperfusion. Am J Physiol 1995; 268(3 pt 1):397–403.
15. Abdu RA, Zakhour BJ, Dallis DJ: Mesenteric venous thrombosis—1911–1984. Surgery 1987; 101:383–388.
16. Kurland B, Brandt LJ, Delany HM: Diagnostic tests for intestinal ischemia. Surg Clin North Am 1992; 72(1):85–105.
17. Murray MJ, Gonze MD, Nowak LR, Cobb CF: Serum D(-)-lactate levels as an aid to diagnosing acute intestinal ischemia. Am J Surg 1994; 167(6):575–578.
18. Bowersox JC, Zwolak RM, Walsh DB, et al: Duplex ultrasonography in the diagnosis of celiac and mesenteric artery occlusive disease. J Vasc Surg 1991; 14:780–786.
19. Jager K, Bollinger A, Valli C, et al: Measurement of mesenteric blood flow by duplex scanning. J Vasc Surg 1986; 3:462–469.
20. Roobottom CA, Dubbins PA: Significant disease of the celiac and superior mesenteric arteries in asymptomatic patients: Predictive value of doppler sonography. AJR 1993; 161(5):985–988.
21. Keen RR, Yao JS, Astleford P, et al: Feasibility of transgastric ultrasonography of the abdominal aorta. J Vasc Surg 1996; 24(5):834–842.
22. Taourel PG, Deneuville M, Pradel JA, et al: Acute mesenteric ischemia: Diagnosis with contrast-enhanced CT. Radiology 1996; 199(3):632–636.
23. Klein HM, Lensing R, Klosterhalfen B, et al: Diagnostic imaging of mesenteric infarction. Radiology 1995; 197(1):79–82.
24. Hackworth CA, Leef JA: Percutaneous transluminal mesenteric angioplasty. Surg Clin North Am 1997; 77(2):371–380.
25. Shanley CJ, Ozaki CK, Zelenock GB: Bypass grafting for chronic mesenteric ischemia. Surg Clin North Am 1997; 77(2):381–395.

PART FOUR

VENOUS DISEASES

17

Venous Thrombosis and Pulmonary Embolism

M. Eileen Walsh, RN, MSN, CVN,
and Karen L. Rice, RN, MSN, CCRN

Venous thrombosis and its life-threatening sequela of pulmonary embolism are major health problems in the United States. Although the exact incidence of venous thrombosis is not known, estimates are derived from its diagnosis and the incidence of pulmonary embolism. More than 600,000–700,000 Americans survive pulmonary embolism each year, whereas 50,000–200,000 die.[1-3] Venous thrombosis is diagnosed in more than 300,000 hospitalized patients annually.[2, 4] Although these statistics support an increase in the incidence of venous thrombosis and a decrease in pulmonary embolism when compared with those of several years ago, it is reasonable to speculate that this is the result of heightened awareness, increased prevention strategies, and improved methods of diagnosis.[5]

A wide variety of medical conditions and surgical procedures make patients potential candidates for deep venous thrombosis (DVT) and pulmonary embolism (PE). Although DVT and PE are most common in the chronically ill, in patients with spinal cord disorders, and in surgical patients, they can occur even in the healthy person with no apparent cause.[6] Because of this, venous thromboembolism affects all fields of nursing.[7]

This chapter focuses on the etiology, clinical manifestations, diagnostic evaluation, treatment, prevention, and nursing management of venous thrombosis and pulmonary embolism. Specific sections include superficial thrombophlebitis, deep vein thrombosis, pulmonary embolism, and venous thromboembolism prophylaxis. Refer to Chapter 2 for a review of anatomy and physiology of the venous system.

VENOUS THROMBOSIS

The topic of venous thrombosis is divided into superficial thrombophlebitis and deep venous thrombosis. Venous thrombosis is an obstruction of a vein in which the thrombus is composed mainly of erythrocytes in a fibrin mesh with few platelets and therefore known as a red thrombus (Fig. 17–1). In 1846, Virchow identified three factors as the

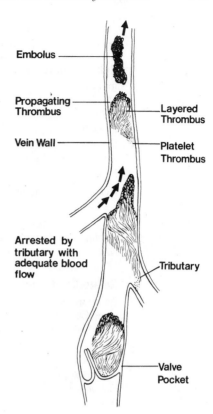

Embolus

Propagating
Thrombus

Layered
Thrombus

Vein Wall

Platelet
Thrombus

Arrested by
tributary with
adequate blood
flow

Tributary

Valve
Pocket

Figure 17–1. Development of deep vein thrombosis and pulmonary embolism. (Reprinted from Critical Care Nursing Quarterly, Vol. 8, No. 2, p. 82 with permission of Aspen Publishers © 1985.)

most important initiators of venous thrombosis: stasis of venous blood flow, damage to the endothelial lining of the vein wall, and changes in the coagulation mechanisms of the blood.[8, 9] These factors are still believed to be of primary importance in thrombus formation, and they contribute to the major risk factors of venous thromboembolism (Table 17–1).[4]

Venous stasis is a state in which blood remains in contact with the venous wall for a prolonged time. It is probably the most important predisposing factor. Because forward movement depends on the action of the voluntary muscles and adequacy of the venous valves, venous stasis can occur when muscles are inactive or when the valves are incompetent.[6, 10] In an immobilized limb, forward venous flow is completely abolished unless the limb is elevated above the level of the heart.

The normal venous endothelium is an intact, smooth, single layer of nonthrombogenic cells containing various substances to prevent platelet adhesion and clot formation.[6, 11] Local venous trauma, however, can result in alteration of this epithelial lining, reducing the intrinsic capacity of the vessel to inhibit thrombus formation. Local platelet aggregation and fibrin entrapment of red blood cells, white blood cells, and additional platelets occur, resulting in thrombus formation.[2]

Changes in the coagulation mechanism of the blood can result from hematologic disorders included in Table 17–1.[10–13] For example, antithrombin III, a circulating anticoagulant, inactivates thrombin and other clotting factors. Therefore an antithrombin III deficiency allows thrombin and other clotting factors to proliferate, increasing the risk of thrombus formation. Malignant conditions result in the production of coagulant materials or reduced fibrinolytic therapy. Surgery can shorten coagulation time and increase the platelet count, as well as cause venodilation in veins distal to the operative site, which correlates with venous endothelial damage.

TABLE 17–1. **Risk Factors for Venous Thrombosis**

Related to Venous Stasis
Immobility
Hip fracture
Length of surgery—more than 30 minutes
Obesity
Stroke
Age (40 and older)
Pregnancy

Related to Vein Wall Damage
Trauma
Fractures, burns
Central venous catheters
Medications
IV drug abuse

Related to Hypercoagulation
Acute myocardial infarction
Congestive heart failure
Antithrombin III deficiency
Protein C deficiency
Protein S deficiency
Activated protein C resistance
Factor V Leiden
Abnormal factor V cofactor activity
Dysfibrinogenemia
Disorders of plasminogen and plasminogen activators
Hyperhomocystinemia
Malignancy
Myeloproliferative disorders
Heparin-induced thrombocytopenia
Nephrotic syndrome
Disseminated intravascular coagulation
Estrogen therapy
Lupus anticoagulant/anticardiolipin antibody
Pregnancy/postpartum state
Surgery
Paroxysmal nocturnal hemoglobinuria
Anticancer drugs
Inflammatory bowel disease
Thromboangiitis obliterans (Buerger's disease)
Behçet's syndrome

Superficial Thrombophlebitis

Superficial thrombophlebitis, estimated to affect 125,000 individuals within the United States, results from both thrombosis and inflammation within a superficial vein.[14, 15] In the lower extremity, the greater or lesser saphenous veins are most often involved. Superficial thrombophlebitis is more commonly seen in women during pregnancy.[12] There is also an increased incidence within the postoperative period and in patients with varicose veins. In the upper extremity, superficial thrombophlebitis is seen in the arm and subclavian veins. Superficial thrombophlebitis is typically associated with a precipitating factor such as trauma, infection, venous stasis, vasculitis, cancer, and/or hypercoagulable state. The specific types of superficial thrombophlebitis are discussed below.

Traumatic superficial thrombophlebitis is the most common type. Trauma to the vein results from a direct injury or an iatrogenic event, such as intraluminal cannulation of a vessel and the administration of intravenous therapy including chemotherapeutic agents, hypertonic solutions (e.g., potassium chloride), specific pharmacologic agents (e.g., benzodiazepines, barbiturates), and radiographic contrast.[14]

Infectious/suppurative thrombophlebitis is a relatively rare but potentially fatal disorder. An infectious process usually develops at the site of a cannulated vein. *Staphylococcus epidermis*, *Staphylococcus aureus*, and many types of Candida are common pathogens. As these microorganisms proliferate, pus accumulates and an abscess forms.[14] This can progress to microorganism seeding in the blood, leading to septicemia and sometimes endocarditis, particularly in those patients with prosthetic heart valves or valvular heart disease.

Superficial thrombophlebitis associated with varicose veins is more likely to develop secondary to trauma and adjacent to venous stasis ulcers. Typically, the greater or lesser saphenous veins are painful, erythematous, and swollen. This type of superficial thrombophlebitis is more common in older patients with longstanding venous insufficiency.

Migratory thrombophlebitis refers to the presence of multiple superficial venous thromboses. Migratory thrombophlebitis frequently occurs in patients with an underlying carcinoma, particularly those with pancreatic cancer. This type of thrombophlebitis also develops in patients with a hypercoagulable problem or an underlying pathology, such as vasculitis.[14]

Clinical Manifestations

Superficial thrombophlebitis is easily recognized on physical examination. The area is erythematous, swollen, and painful along the course of the affected superficial vein. The area is warm and often has a red linear streak. A firm, subcutaneous tender cord may be palpable (see Fig. 4–13). With recent trauma or intravenous cannulation, ecchymosis may be present.

Infectious/suppurative thrombophlebitis, however, is not as easily recognized on physical examination. Most often there are no local signs of thrombophlebitis. The presence of a high-grade fever may indicate suppurative thrombophlebitis. In some cases, septic pulmonary emboli are the first indication of its presence.

Diagnostic Evaluation

Superficial thrombophlebitis is typically diagnosed on the basis of the physical exam alone. An elevated white blood cell count and/or positive blood cultures are typically present. In the lower extremity, a venous duplex ultrasound may be indicated to identify the extent of the thrombus into the sapheno-femoral junction or the deep femoral system.[15]

Treatment

Treatment of superficial thrombophlebitis is based on the type and extent of the disease process. Superficial thrombophlebitis can last for a few days or a few weeks. With traumatic superficial thrombophlebitis, any indwelling catheter should be immediately removed.[16] The affected extremity should be elevated to promote venous return and reduce swelling. The application of local moist heat for 20 to 30 minutes several times a day alleviates pain and reduces inflammation. Compression stockings or an elastic bandage may provide comfort in lower-extremity thrombophlebitis once inflammation begins to resolve.

Nonsteroidal anti-inflammatory drugs (such as ibuprofen) may be administered to relieve symptoms.[17] Aspirin may be given to provide an antithrombotic effect. Other pharmacologic agents, such as antibiotics and corticosteroids, are usually not indicated in noncomplicated situations. Suppurative thrombophlebitis requires surgical excision of the affected vein and its tributaries. In addition, specific antibiotic therapy is administered on the basis of the culture results.

If the thrombus extends into the proximal greater saphenous vein or to the sapheno-femoral junction, more aggressive management is indicated to prevent propagation of the clot into the deep venous system. In this instance, either systemic anticoagulation or surgical ligation proximal to the thrombosis is indicated.[18] The choice of treatment is generally dictated by the overall health status of the patient. Patients at risk of hemorrhagic complications or pregnant women are best treated without anticoagulation using surgical ligation of the affected vein under local anesthesia with conscious sedation if necessary.

Prevention and Nursing Management

The nurse plays an important role in the prevention of superficial thrombophlebitis. Prevention strategies are listed in Table 17–2.

Deep Venous Thrombosis

DVT is an acute, potentially life-threatening condition that necessitates hospitalization. DVT more commonly develops in the veins of the lower extremity. However, the increased use of central venous catheters appears to have increased the incidence of upper-extremity venous thrombosis.

Clinical Manifestations

Patients with DVT may be asymptomatic or symptomatic. Signs and symptoms of DVT vary, depending on the size of the thrombus, location, if the lumen is partially or totally

TABLE 17–2. **Nursing Management: Superficial Thrombophlebitis Prophylaxis**

- Use strict aseptic technique during venous cannulation, intravenous dressing changes, and intravenous therapy.
- Assess intravenous sites every 4–8 hours for signs of thrombophlebitis.
- Check temperature every 4–8 hours.
- Change intravenous tubing every 24–48 hours.
- Change intravenous catheter sites every 72–96 hours.
- Adhere to dilution requirements of intravenous medications.
- Use large veins only for potentially irritating solutions.
- Secure indwelling catheters.
- Pad bed rails of disoriented patients.
- Use arm/leg restraints with extreme caution.
- Avoid using the lower extremity for venous access.
- Use PICC line for long-term access.
- Use a central venous line for select cases.

PICC = peripherally inserted central catheter.

obstructed, and adequacy of collateral circulation. Hence, physical findings may be absent in cases of partial obstruction or when collateral channels reconstitute flow around a complete obstruction.[19] Classic symptoms of DVT include pain, tenderness, and sudden onset of unilateral swelling of the extremity (Fig. 17–2); however, these symptoms can also be related to disorders such as superficial thrombophlebitis, cellulitis, ruptured muscle or tendon, muscle strain, internal derangement of the knee, ruptured popliteal cyst, cutaneous vasculitis, or lymphedema.[1, 6, 10, 11] The presence of calf pain on dorsiflexion of the foot, Homans' sign, is not consistently found in patients with DVT.[6]

With DVT, the collateral venous channels develop in an effort to reconstitute venous flow around the obstruction.[2] This process may cause the superficial veins to visibly dilate. In addition, the inflammatory response of the superficial venous system may be significant enough to exhibit increased local warmth and erythema of the involved extremity.

Obstruction of the large veins, such as iliofemoral veins, commonly manifests some clinical signs and symptoms. Advanced forms of iliofemoral venous thrombosis include phlegmasia alba dolens and phlegmasia cerulea dolens. Phlegmasia alba dolens is commonly seen in postpartum women. The affected limb is swollen, pale, and cool, with nonpalpable pulses. This is caused by a severe perivenous inflammatory reaction extending to the periarterial sympathetic nerve fibers, producing arterial spasm or compression.[11] Phlegmasia cerulea dolens is commonly seen in advanced stages of some cancers. There is almost total occlusion of venous outflow, with increased pressure contributing to arterial inflow obstruction. This can lead to gangrene if untreated. Patients typically have sudden onset of deep pain, massive edema, and cyanosis of the extremity. Hypotension and hemoconcentration may further compound the thrombotic cycle.

Diagnostic Evaluation

Clinical manifestations are not reliable in establishing a diagnosis of DVT, particularly in the early stages. Therefore, objective diagnostic testing is used to confirm the clinical suspicion of venous thrombosis. These tests include venous duplex/color duplex ultrasound, air plethysmography (APG), impedance plethysmography (IPG), radioactive fibrinogen (RF) testing, and ascending venography. In the event of a negative diagnostic finding in the presence of clinical findings, the sensitivity and specificity of the diagnostic

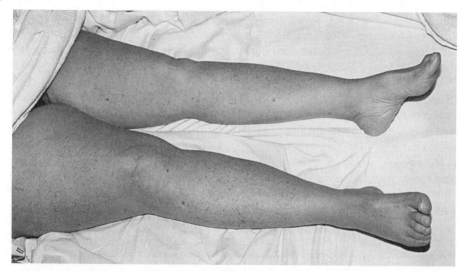

Figure 17–2. Classic symptom of deep vein thrombosis (DVT). Note the unilateral right leg swelling, especially at thigh and calf.

test are evaluated.[4] If the diagnostic test meets the criteria for reliability and accuracy, the same test is repeated in 5 to 7 days. However, if the repeated diagnostic study remains negative for DVT, a differential diagnosis should be explored.

Venous duplex/color duplex ultrasound, now considered the "gold standard," is the most commonly performed and reliable diagnostic modality to identify DVT (see Chapter 5). Venous duplex/color duplex ultrasound allows rapid and clear visualization of thrombi, including identification of unstable or floating thrombi, which may cause emboli.[4, 20, 21] Although duplex ultrasound is reliable and precise in the detection of lower-extremity venous problems, imaging of upper-extremity veins may be more difficult and less precise. APG and IPG measure variations in electrical resistance as a result of changes in blood volume through the use of skin electrodes and pneumatic cuff.[10] Plethysmographic diagnostic methods, although low in cost, are less frequently used because they indicate both intrinsic and extrinsic obstruction of the venous system rather than intraluminal obstruction alone.[11] An example of extrinsic compression frequently identified includes partial obstruction of an iliac vein without DVT due to pressure from a pelvic tumor. However, plethysmographic techniques may be negative in cases of proximal thrombosis associated with good collateral venous channels.[4] These noninvasive techniques are generally used when access to sophisticated ultrasound equipment and technical expertise are unavailable.[11]

RF testing involves the identification of fibrinogen that is attached to thrombi. The radioactive isotope, fibrinogen I^{125}, is administered intravenously with subsequent nuclear scanning at 12 to 24 hours following injection. This diagnostic modality is both highly sensitive and specific for DVT, revealing even small soleal, tibial, and peroneal thromboses.[11] However, there are major limitations due to the cost and the time delay between injection and scanning.[4] In addition, RF is unable to detect thrombi that are free of fibrinogen.

Prior to the development of sophisticated ultrasonography available today, venography was considered the gold standard for the diagnosis of DVT. Ascending venography is performed by the injection of a radio-contrast agent into a superficial vein on the dorsum of the foot. The contrast material mixes with the blood and flows proximally. Radiographic images of the leg and pelvis show the calf, popliteal, and femoral veins, which drain into the external iliac vein. A thrombus is diagnosed by the presence of an intraluminal filling defect, flow diversion, abrupt termination of contrast visibility, and failure to opacify segments or the entire deep venous system. Venography accurately identifies 90 percent of thrombi.[11] In addition, a negative venogram excludes the presence of lower-extremity thrombosis. The small veins and sinuses of the calf, however, may be difficult to visualize, and deep femoral vein opacification in the presence of DVT is only identified in 50 percent of patients.[11] Other limitations of venography include increased cost and increased risk of lower-extremity thrombophlebitis associated with an invasive procedure (see Chapter 6).

Other components of the diagnostic evaluation include blood testing to detect intravascular coagulation. A coagulation profile should be completed including measurement of activated partial thromboplastin time (APTT), prothrombin time (PT) with international normalized ratio (INR), circulating fibrin, monomer complexes, fibrinopeptide A, serum fibrin degradation products, protein C and S, and antithrombin III levels. Chapter 9 discusses these coagulation measurements in more detail.

In the effort to improve clinical outcomes, other diagnostic modalities may need to be included as appropriate. Up to 40 percent of patients with proximal DVT have asymptomatic pulmonary emboli.[4, 11] Approximately 25 percent of those with asymptomatic pulmonary emboli subsequently experience acute signs or symptoms of pulmonary embolism while receiving anticoagulation.[3] Therefore, routine evaluation of patients with DVT involving the iliac or femoral veins should include ventilation/perfusion lung scanning, which is described in the section of this chapter covering pulmonary embolism.

Treatment and Nursing Management

Treatment interventions are based on the location of the thrombus. The goals of treatment are to prevent propagation of the clot, prevent the development of new thrombi, prevent pulmonary emboli, and limit venous valvular damage. The nursing management of the patient closely reflects the implementation of the treatment interventions, which include bed rest, leg elevation, compression stockings, and administration of pharmacologic measures.[22]

If thrombosis is suspected, the patient should be kept on bed rest until examined by the physician. The calf and thigh should be measured at specific points, such as 10 cm above the upper edge of the patella, 10 cm below the tibial crest, and 20 cm below the tibial crest. Any changes from the baseline measurements should be promptly reported to the physician.

Bed Rest. Bed rest is usually recommended for approximately 5 days until the thrombus is stable and has adhered to the intraluminal wall. Progressive ambulation can be started after this period. This length of time varies with physician preference; some patients are currently being treated as outpatients.

Leg Elevation. The affected extremity should be elevated at least 10–20 degrees above the level of the heart to enhance venous return and reduce swelling.[23] Elevation of the foot of the bed is permitted if the head of the bed remains flat, because this will prevent inguinal congestion.[10] Pillows may be used to elevate the affected extremity; they should support the entire length of the leg to prevent compression of the popliteal space. If the thrombosis is located in the upper extremity, the arm can be elevated with a stockinette attached to an intravenous pole. Once ambulation has begun, the patient should be encouraged to avoid prolonged standing and avoid prolonged sitting without leg elevation.[10] If the patient has significant edema, ambulation should be restricted.

Compression Stockings. A compression garment, such as stockings or an elastic bandage, should be worn at all times (Fig. 17–3). Compression promotes venous return and decreases leg swelling.[10] Initially, 4-inch elastic bandages are applied snugly, with consistent tension from the toes to just below the knee with edges overlapped. If an iliofemoral venous thrombosis is present, a 6-inch elastic bandage may be applied above the knee. Once the edema has subsided, the patient should be measured for graded compression stockings (or an upper-extremity sleeve). To fit the stocking correctly, the nurse should measure the largest calf and ankle circumference and the leg length from bottom of heel to bend of knee. Pressure at the ankle should be at least 30–40 mmHg to counteract the high venous pressure; pressure should decrease proximally.

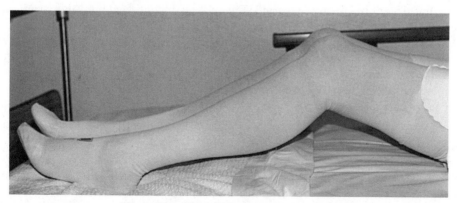

Figure 17–3. Thigh-high compression stockings.

Compression stockings are available in a variety of colors, lengths, and ranges of compression. Knee-high stockings are more effective in the treatment of DVT; they are less expensive and easier to apply, which increases patient compliance. In addition, some physicians believe that compression across the knee joint applies pressure to the popliteal vein, producing venous stasis. Thigh-high stockings are more effective in the treatment of proximal vein DVT.

Pharmacologic Measures. In general, pharmacologic measures consist of anticoagulation with heparin, followed by long-term oral anticoagulation with warfarin. Anticoagulation is essentially prophylaxis because these medications do not actively dissolve thrombus.[24, 25]

Heparin. Heparin, an acidic glycoaminoglycan derived from animal lung or gut mucosa, is the most common treatment of venous thrombosis. Heparin is bound by platelets, vascular endothelium, and antithrombin III, catalyzing the effect of antithrombin III, which inactivates thrombin.[25, 26] Heparin has no thrombolytic activity.

Heparin therapy is initiated after baseline laboratory determinants of APPT, PT with INR, and platelet count are drawn. If a DVT is suspected based on the clinical history and examination, an initial 5000-U intravenous bolus is administered.[23] Once DVT is confirmed, a 5000–10,000-U bolus is given to achieve an immediate therapeutic level. It is then followed by a heparin drip to maintain the APTT ratio between 1.5 and 2.5 times the control. The majority of patients initially require 1000–2000 U per hour to achieve adequate anticoagulation. Laboratory values, including an APTT, are obtained every 6–12 hours and 1–2 hours after any dosage change.[27, 31]

Heparin should be continued for 5–7 days—the usual time the body needs to dissolve the clot completely.[6] Oral anticoagulation should be overlapped with heparin. For iliofemoral thrombosis, a longer period of heparin therapy may be considered.[30–32] Some clinical trials have demonstrated the effectiveness of subcutaneous heparin and low-molecular-weight heparin (LMWH) as treatment for DVT.[28]

Heparin-induced thrombocytopenia is a well-recognized complication of heparin occurring in up to 10 percent patients.[10, 27] Heparin-induced antiplatelet antibodies cause platelet aggregation, leading to thrombocytopenia. The nurse should carefully monitor the platelet count and notify the physician if it is less than 100,000 or 40 percent below pretreatment level.[10] This platelet aggregation may activate the clotting mechanism and result in arterial thromboembolism and extension or recurrence of existing venous thromboembolism, as well as skin slough and wound hematoma[32, 33] (see Chapter 8).

Warfarin. Warfarin (Coumadin) is an oral anticoagulant that inhibits vitamin K–dependent clotting factor synthesis (factors II, VII, IX, and X).[33, 34] Oral anticoagulation with warfarin should begin simultaneously with initiation of intravenous heparin anticoagulation. Warfarin peaks within 36–72 hours and has a duration of 2–5 days. Because warfarin has a very short half-life, there is a period of hypercoagulability that occurs during the first few days of treatment. Heparin should not be discontinued until therapeutic INR values of 2.0–3.0 are maintained.[35, 36]

Oral anticoagulation is generally continued for 3–6 months to prevent recurrent thrombosis in patients with proximal vein thrombosis and symptomatic calf vein thrombosis.[31] Oral anticoagulation is maintained indefinitely in patients with recurrent venous thrombosis, antithrombin III deficiency, protein C deficiency, protein S deficiency, and malignant neoplasm.[17] An anticoagulation flow sheet is a useful tool to document laboratory results and to calculate heparin and warfarin dosages. The nurse should monitor the patient for signs of Coumadin necrosis (see Chapter 8).

Thrombolytic Therapy. Thrombolytic agents, such as streptokinase, urokinase, and recombinant tissue plasminogen activator (rt-PA), are only effective in dissolving existing thrombi during the first 24 hours of the thrombotic event. These agents impair coagulation by increasing fibrinolytic activity through the conversion of circulating plasminogen to plasmin. The only agent approved for intravenous use in both DVT and massive pulmonary embolus is urokinase.[17, 37]

While the patient is anticoagulated or receiving thrombolytic therapy, the nurse should watch for any signs of bleeding[38] (see Chapter 8). If the patient is receiving thrombolytic therapy, the nurse should alert the physician to a fibrinogen level that is less than 100 mg/dl.[17]

Calf Vein Thrombosis

The treatment of calf vein thrombosis remains controversial. Isolated calf vein thrombosis usually does not cause major sequelae and does not place the patient at high risk for pulmonary embolism. However, calf vein thrombi can embolize and propagate proximally to the large deep veins of the thigh. Current studies support the need to treat calf vein thrombosis, which includes the popliteal fossa, with 3 months of anticoagulant therapy.[25] If untreated with anticoagulants, the patient should be monitored with venous duplex/color duplex ultrasound until the high-risk period has passed and the patient returns to full ambulation.

Femoral-Popliteal Venous Thrombosis

Venous thrombosis of the superficial femoral and popliteal veins is the most common type of thrombosis requiring treatment. Anticoagulation is the standard form of therapy. Thrombolysis with an intravenous fibrinolytic agent, such as urokinase, may be useful in appropriate candidates. Treatment continues for about 24 hours until the lysis is complete. Once clot lysis is achieved, the patient should be converted to intravenous heparin followed by long-term anticoagulation (see Chapter 6).

Iliofemoral Venous Thrombosis

Iliofemoral venous thrombosis may not be common, but the devastating sequelae pose more than an increased risk of PE.[25] Advanced states such as phlegmasia cerulea dolens and phlegmasia alba dolens place the patient at risk of limb and life, as discussed earlier in this chapter.

Surgical Management

The primary objective of acute surgical intervention is to eliminate the obstructing thrombus and reconstitute venous outflow, prevent pulmonary emboli, and prevent venous valvular damage. Acute surgical management includes catheter-directed thrombolysis with a fibrinolytic agent, venous thrombectomy with arterial thrombectomy when indicated, and other adjunctive procedures if necessary.[39] Venous thrombectomy with a temporary adjunctive arteriovenous fistula may be recommended as treatment for an occluded iliofemoral vein in a patient with phlegmasia cerulea dolens.[25]

PULMONARY EMBOLISM

PE is the third leading cause of death from cardiovascular disease, exceeded only by atherosclerotic heart disease and stroke.[9] Despite improvements in medical diagnosis and treatment, the actual number of clinically diagnosed cases is significantly less than the true incidence.[4, 40] PE may be the most common preventable cause of death throughout the world.[9]

PE occurs in any clinical setting; it is rarely seen in young healthy patients, whereas the elderly, immobilized, or trauma patients have the highest incidence.[6] An increased risk has also been identified during pregnancy and in the puerperium.[7] Other factors that increase the risk of pulmonary embolism include all types of heart disease, low cardiac output, surgical procedures, the use of oral contraceptives, and having blood group A.[40]

PE is a direct consequence of DVT. More than 90 percent are due to thrombus formation in the deep veins of the legs.[4, 11] However, the incidence of PE increases with more proximal DVT.[41, 42] In addition, the iliac and femoral veins, because of their large size, are the source of most emboli. The upper extremity and the pelvic veins are less common sites. Superficial leg veins generally do not cause pulmonary embolus unless the thrombosis propagates into the larger veins of the deep system. Tumor embolization of the lungs and cardiac tumors involving the right atrium and ventricle may also cause PE, but the incidence is rare.

Clinical Manifestations

The clinical manifestations of PE are directly related to the magnitude of the pulmonary circulatory obstruction caused by migration of a blood clot.[9] Many times symptoms are nonspecific and similar to those of other cardiopulmonary diseases. Symptoms of dyspnea and chest pain have been identified as the most common symptoms of patients with documented PE.[4] However, any abrupt or unexplained episode of hypotension, chest pain, or respiratory distress should be considered suspicious of pulmonary embolism (Table 17–3). Research studies support that PE, as a sudden cause of death identified at autopsy, is suspected in only about 30 percent of this population.[4]

Auscultation of the heart may reveal an accentuated pulmonic second sound (tricuspid

---

TABLE 17–3.
Clinical Manifestations
of Pulmonary Embolism

Most Frequent Signs and Symptoms

Dyspnea
Pleuritic chest pain
Cough
Peripheral edema
Localized rales or wheezes

Associated Signs

Tachypnea
Hypotension
Distended neck veins
Cyanosis
Tricuspid murmur
Acute cor pulmonale

Associated Symptoms

Anxiety
Fever
Orthopnea
Lower-extremity thrombophlebitis

regurgitation murmur). Findings may differ between patients; however, their severity may vary from transient dyspnea to acute right heart failure and cardiopulmonary arrest. Acute cor pulmonale with abrupt onset of cardiovascular collapse, syncope, and sudden death is generally associated with massive pulmonary embolism. Small PE in the pulmonary parenchyma of a relatively healthy patient may be asymptomatic. Yet the same size PE may cause distressing symptoms in a patient with severe cardiopulmonary disease.[9, 41]

Diagnostic Evaluation

Arterial blood gases are normal in approximately 10 percent of patients with PE; however, hypoxemia and primary respiratory alkalosis are common.[4] Routine arterial blood gases are usually not helpful. Although most electrocardiograms are normal, changes may include nonspecific ST-T changes.[9] The electrocardiogram may exhibit changes consistent with right heart strain, but ruling out acute myocardial infarction is also important in ruling out differential diagnoses.

Because PE affects the cardiopulmonary system, a baseline chest x-ray should be obtained. The initial chest x-ray should not demonstrate abnormal findings on the basis of PE, but rather changes in radiodensity associated with other pulmonary disease processes.[9] Congestion is not usually present on x-ray during the early phase of PE. Later, wedge-shaped peripheral infiltrates may be identified. A pleural effusion may also develop if the lung is infarcted and the pleura become inflamed.

A more focused diagnostic modality, a ventilation/perfusion (V/Q) scan, assesses air flow patterns and circulation of the lungs. The perfusion scan demonstrates the distribution of pulmonary artery blood flow and underperfused areas in the lung.[9] The perfusion component of the scan involves intravenous injection of albumin labeled with technetium (^{99m}Tc) or iodine (^{133}I) and should exhibit a radiolucent area of underperfusion.[11] However, pre-existing lung disease, such as pneumonitis, atelectasis, emphysematous bullae, or neoplasm, also demonstrates a defect that produces a false-positive result.[11] Hence, the perfusion scan must be interpreted in conjunction with a recent chest x-ray and the patient's clinical picture. A negative perfusion scan essentially excludes PE, but a positive test may be due to several other causes as described above.[4]

^{133}Xenon ventilation, the ventilation component of a V/Q scan, increases the utility of establishing a diagnosis of PE. It increases the sensitivity of identifying underperfused and underventilated areas by collecting information regarding the distribution of inhaled gas.[9] PE typically causes perfusion defects in an area of normal ventilation. However, ventilation defects are often found in the presence of perfusion defects. Therefore, a positive study produces a mismatch between the ventilation and perfusion components of the scan whereas an inconclusive scan generally warrants further workup to establish a diagnosis.[43, 44]

The V/Q scan may also be repeated 1 to 3 days after the initial scan if PE remains suspected. Many times noninvasive modalities, such as venous duplex/color duplex ultrasound or plethysmography, may be used to rule out PE early to pursue differential diagnoses.[43] These differential diagnoses include pneumonia, acute myocardial infarction, dissecting aortic aneurysm, pneumothorax, and pericarditis.[45, 46]

Pulmonary angiography remains the ultimate standard for establishing a diagnosis of PE.[4] A positive angiogram, via right heart catheterization, demonstrates an internal filling defect in the pulmonary arteries (Fig. 17–4). Although angiography can clearly demonstrate PE, several factors limit its clinical use. Because it is an invasive procedure that requires injection of contrast material, it is associated with some risk.[11] This is particularly true in patients with severe pulmonary hypertension, right-sided heart failure, or respiratory failure.[45] However, sophisticated radiologic equipment and technical expertise are not available in all hospitals. Even those facilities with adequate resources may not provide

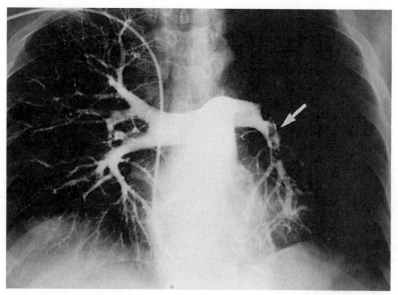

Figure 17–4. Pulmonary angiogram with arrow pointing to filling defect in pulmonary artery. Sudden cut-off of left pulmonary artery branches is demonstrated. (Reprinted from Critical Care Nursing Quarterly, Vol. 8, No. 2, p. 84, with permission of Aspen Publishers, Inc., © 1985.)

testing on nights or weekends. Because of these limitations and the high cost, pulmonary angiography is inappropriate for screening and routine use in establishing the diagnosis of PE.

Echocardiography, including transesophageal echocardiography, provides valuable data to evaluate cardiac function in patients with PE. Although echocardiography cannot visualize most of the pulmonary arterial circulation, it is very useful in evaluating the presence of acute cor pulmonale. More than 50 percent of pulmonary arterial obstructions, pulmonary arterial hypertension, and distention of the right ventricle are due to PE.[9] Thus, echocardiography serves as a useful tool to quantitate the degree of right ventricular distention due to high pressures, which occur with PE. Because the size of ventricular distention can be measured accurately with echocardiography, the effectiveness of fibrinolytic agents can be evaluated during or following thrombolytic therapy.

Treatment

Successful management of PE requires prompt, accurate diagnosis and proper treatment. When PE is suspected, initial therapy is directed toward stabilizing the patient with supportive therapy and initiating antithrombotic therapy.

Supportive Therapy

Supportive measures that improve clinical symptoms should be implemented as soon as possible. The head of the bed should be elevated higher than 30 degrees to minimize dyspnea. Oxygen should be administered by nasal cannula, face mask, or both. In patients with respiratory distress, endotracheal intubation and mechanical ventilation may be required.[11] However, these supportive measures may not be effective alone because the major cause of hypoxia is lack of perfusion of the pulmonary parenchyma.

Small doses of intravenous opiates (i.e., 1–2 mg of morphine) may help the patient's discomfort and apprehension, along with reduction of systemic afterload. However, larger doses may cause respiratory depression. Intravenous access should also be established as soon as possible for rapid delivery of appropriate medications. In addition, intravenous fluid intake should be monitored very closely because of the risk of exacerbation of right ventricular dysfunction.

Heparin

The cornerstone of treatment for PE is intravenous heparin.[31] Maintenance of therapeutic anticoagulation values usually results in improved outcomes. In treating acute PE, APTT values must be closely monitored, particularly after the first 48 hours, to avoid over-anticoagulation. As previously described for DVT, a continuous heparin infusion should be titrated to maintain the APTT at 1.5–2.5 times the patient's baseline.[9] Of equal importance is assuring the patient's level of anticoagulation does not fall into a low range, placing him or her at an increased risk of recurrent and sometimes fatal PE. Initially, the patient may require high doses of heparin, especially with major PE; however, the dose can usually be decreased after the first 24–48 hours. The most common mistake that occurs is to give too little heparin initially when the heparin requirement is high, and too much heparin later, when the heparin requirement is generally low.[9]

Warfarin

Oral anticoagulation with warfarin is generally initiated during heparin administration. However, heparin should not be discontinued until therapeutic anticoagulation with warfarin has been obtained.[9] Heparin is frequently continued for about 5 days in those with a diagnosis of PE. Therefore, administration of a continuous heparin infusion concomitantly with warfarin for 2 to 3 days is not uncommon.[1, 32]

The starting dose of warfarin is usually 5–10 mg daily for the first 2 days. Thereafter the daily maintenance dose is adjusted to yield an INR of 2.0 to 3.0. Oral anticoagulation should be continued for at least 3 months, and sometimes indefinitely.[9]

Thrombolytic Therapy

Three thrombolytic agents, streptokinase, urokinase, and rt-PA, are approved by the Food and Drug Administration (FDA) for treatment of massive pulmonary embolus.[47-52] Indications for thrombolytic therapy include the presence of a large clot, profound refractory hypoxemia, or significant hemodynamic compromise.[47-53] Although the risks associated with thrombolytic therapy may result in a negative outcome, failure to lyse the clot generally leads to pulmonary hypertension and end-stage heart disease. Therefore, early lysis of the thrombus may be lifesaving in situations in which the patient may not survive long enough for spontaneous dissolution to occur.[9]

Thrombolytic therapy is induced into the main pulmonary artery through the catheter used for the pulmonary arteriogram. This technique enables pulmonary arteriography to be repeated at specific intervals to assess the arteriographic effect of the infusion.

Streptokinase. Streptokinase was the first thrombolytic agent employed for treatment of pulmonary embolism and is relatively inexpensive. However, streptokinase does not lyse as rapidly as urokinase and rt-PA and it is more likely to be associated with hypersensitivity.[54] Because of the efficacy of urokinase and rt-PA, and the risk of anaphylaxis, streptokinase is rarely used today.

Urokinase. Urokinase has been used effectively for lysis of pulmonary embolism. Its ability to lyse clots rapidly is superior in comparison to streptokinase but not as rapid as rt-PA in reconstituting venous flow.[56] The treatment guidelines for administration of urokinase are 4400 IU/kg/hour infused over 12–24 hours.

Recombinant Tissue Plasminogen Activator. Research comparing the efficacy of rt-PA to urokinase in massive PE reports that rt-PA (alteplase) is more efficacious. rt-PA dissolves the obstructive embolus more rapidly and completely than urokinase.[9, 48] In addition, administration can be completed in a shorter time frame than other agents. The treatment guidelines for administration of alteplase are 100 mg as a continuous intravenous infusion over 2 hours.[45]

More recently, other thrombolytic agents have become available using recombinant DNA technology, but because of differences in molecular structure, dosing and administration differ between agents.

Precautions. The most serious bleeding complication associated with thrombolytic agents is intracranial bleeding.[47, 57] A retroperitoneal hemorrhage can also be life-threatening. None of these thrombolytic regimens use concomitant heparin therapy in the early stage of PE because of the increased risk of bleeding. If heparin therapy has already been initiated, thrombolytic therapy should not be started until the APTT is 1.5 times the control. Following lytic therapy, it is important to wait until the APTT is under 80 seconds before resuming the heparin infusion.[54]

Vena Caval Interruption

Most patients with DVT—with or without PE—can be successfully treated with heparin. In specific situations, however, heparin cannot be used, and interruption of the vena cava is necessary to prevent recurrent PE and potentially fatal PE. Other indications for filter use are included in Table 17–4. Filters function by intercepting emboli traveling to the pulmonary vasculature. There are several vena caval filters available, including the stainless steel Greenfield filter, nitinol filter, "bird's nest" filter, Venatech filter, and titanium Greenfield filter (Fig. 17–5).[58–63] In recent years, vena caval filters have become smaller in size and may be introduced percutaneously.[58] Filters are inserted through the femoral vein and placed in the vena cava inferior to the renal veins to avoid obstruction of blood flow from the kidneys. Complications after filter placement include recurrent pulmonary

TABLE 17–4. **Indications for Insertion of a Vena Cava Filter**

- Recurrent thromboembolism despite adequate anticoagulation
- Thromboembolism in patient with contraindications or a need to discontinue anticoagulation/thrombolytic therapy
  - Major trauma
  - Recent hemorrhage
  - Recent stroke
- Immediately following pulmonary embolectomy
- Chronic pulmonary embolism with associated pulmonary hypertension and cor pulmonale
- Prophylaxis in high-risk patients
  - More than 50% pulmonary vascular occlusion
  - Large iliofemoral thrombus
  - Septic embolism

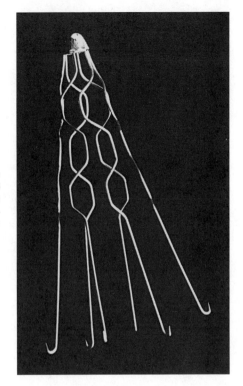

Figure 17–5. A stainless steel Greenfield vena cava filter. (From McCarthy WJ, Fahey VA, Bergan JJ, et al: The veins and venous disease. In James EC, Corry RJ, Perry JF [eds]: Principles of Basic Surgical Practice. Philadelphia, Hanley & Belfus, 1987, p 461.)

emboli, venous insufficiency, air embolism, and improper placement or migration of the device.[22]

Pulmonary Embolectomy

Pulmonary embolectomy is rarely indicated since thrombolytic therapy and vena caval filters have become available.[9] However, when a patient with an acute PE presents with a terminal comorbidity or is not a candidate for lytic agents, emergency pulmonary embolectomy should be considered.[65] Yet most patients with massive PE either die before they can be transported to the surgical suite, or they become hemodynamically stable to the point that the embolectomy is no longer indicated.

Nursing Management

Initial evaluation of the patient with suspected PE should include assessment of the respiratory and cardiovascular systems and vital signs. Initial stabilization of the patient should include oxygen therapy, arterial blood gas, cardiac monitoring, and intravenous access. The head of the bed should be raised to facilitate breathing and promote comfort. Medications should be administered to relieve pain, manage blood pressure changes, treat cardiac dysrhythmia, and reduce fluid overload.[45]

VENOUS THROMBOEMBOLISM PROPHYLAXIS AND NURSING MANAGEMENT

Prophylactic measures to prevent venous thromboembolism are as important as the actual treatment (Table 17–5). These measures can significantly reduce the incidence of DVT

TABLE 17–5. **Nursing Management: Venous Thrombosis Prophylaxis**

- Determine high-risk patients.
- Assess all extremities on a regular basis.
  - Unilateral edema
  - Pain/tenderness
  - Venous distention
  - Cyanosis
- Monitor for low-grade fever to detect thrombophlebitis.
- Use intermittent external pneumatic compression as ordered.
- Apply compression stockings or elastic bandage as ordered.
- Maintain fluid balance to avoid dehydration and/or hypercoagulability.
- Use stool softener to avoid straining, which increases venous pressure.
- Encourage deep breathing during postoperative period.
- Promote activity in the early postoperative period.
  - Ambulation
  - Passive and active range of motion exercises
- Avoid using foot gatch.
- Provide patient education:
  Activity
  - Regularly: walk daily using calf muscle; jog, cycle or swim.
  - Avoid prolonged sitting or exercise, standing in one position.
  - Elevate legs with prolonged sitting.
  - Avoid crossing legs at the knee.
  Clotting
  - Avoid constrictive garments: garters, girdles, tight-fitting stocking.
  - Avoid constrictive shoes or boots.
  Risk Factor Modification
  - Maintain desired weight for height.
  - Avoid cigarette smoking.
  - Discuss estrogen therapy risk with your physician.
  Report to Physician
  - Sudden onset of unilateral leg swelling.
  - Pain or tenderness in an extremity.
  - Sudden dilation of superficial veins.

and PE as well as avoid the complications of the postphlebitic syndrome.[5] Prophylaxis consists of pharmacologic and nonpharmacologic measures. Application of effective prophylaxis depends on the knowledge of the risk factors predisposing to the development of DVT (see Table 17–1).

Venous thromboembolism following surgery is a significant health care problem. Patients may be categorized into low, moderate, high, or very high risk for postoperative venous thromboembolism based on age, type of surgery, and presence of other concomitant risk factors. Other factors that may affect risk include type and duration of anesthesia, intraoperative blood loss with associated hypotension, and the degree and duration of postoperative immobilization.[68–70]

Pharmacologic Measures

Pharmacologic measures include low-dose heparin, LMWH, warfarin, and dextran.

Low-Dose Heparin

Low-dose heparin is safe and effective for moderate-risk general surgery patients; it is less effective in the high-risk group of surgical patients.[22] The usual dose is 5000 U of heparin given subcutaneously beginning 2 hours preoperatively and continued every 8–12 hours until hospital discharge.[41] Low-dose heparin, however, is poorly absorbed after subcutaneous injection; it binds to endothelial cells and many other non-anticoagulant proteins, causing a nonlinear plasma clearance.[68] Therefore, low-dose heparin causes an unpredictable anticoagulant response following administration.[70] It is also associated with an increased incidence of postoperative wound hematoma and a small risk of heparin-associated thrombocytopenia and thrombosis. Hence, patients receiving low-dose heparin should have regular monitoring of the platelet count.

Low-Molecular-Weight Heparin

LMWH is a relatively new classification of heparin used for DVT prophylaxis in general surgical, orthopedic, and spinal cord injury patients.[71–74] LMWH is derived from heparin by either chemical or enzymatic depolymerization.[69] LMWH inhibits factors Xa and IIa activity and results in less bleeding compared with other types of heparin.[68] It is administered subcutaneously and exhibits less variability in anticoagulant response to a fixed dose, thus producing a sustained stable anticoagulant effect. Although laboratory monitoring is not necessary, some physicians continue to follow this practice.[70] The dosage is dependent on the specific drug. It is usually started in the postoperative period.[75–78]

Warfarin

Oral anticoagulants, such as warfarin, inhibit vitamin K–dependent clotting factors II, VII, IX, X, and proteins C and S.[34] When low-intensity warfarin (5–10 mg) is administered the night prior to surgery, therapeutic anticoagulation is usually achieved on the third postoperative day.[69] Other methods, including the two-step and mini-dose regimens, provide lower daily dosages of warfarin (1–2.5 mg and 1 mg, respectively) 1 to 2 weeks prior to surgery.[68–72] These methods were instituted to prevent delays in warfarin and anticoagulant effect, yet avoid the excess bleeding associated with fully therapeutic warfarin during surgery.

Dextran

Dextran is a branched polysaccharide found to be effective in reducing the prevalence of postoperative venous thromboembolism, although less effective than low-dose heparin. The usual dosage is 500–1000 ml intraoperatively, then 500 ml daily for 3 days, then 500 ml every 3 days.[68, 72] Since dextran can contribute to volume overload, it should be avoided in patients with congestive heart failure and renal insufficiency.[11]

Nonpharmacologic Measures

Nonpharmacologic measures include intermittent external pneumatic compression, use of compression stockings, leg elevation, and early mobilization. These measures are beneficial as either primary prophylaxis or as an adjunct combined with pharmacologic measures. Successful prophylaxis with these methods relies on the consistency and accuracy in appropriate use.

External Pneumatic Compression

External pneumatic compression (EPC) reduces the incidence of DVT by augmenting the calf muscle pumps in evacuating the sinuses of blood and reduces venous stasis by stimulating fibrinolytic activity.[5, 11, 67] A synthetic sleeve or boot encircles the extremity and provides alternating periods of compression to the calf alone or the calf and thigh.[75] EPC devices are available in single-chamber and multichamber forms, providing intermittent or sequential pressure (Fig. 17–6).[70] The single-chamber device produces uniform compression of the calves at predetermined time periods, whereas the more frequently used multichamber device produces graded sequential or intermittent compression of the ankles, calves, and thighs.[50]

Proper placement of the single-chamber EPC cuff with the bladder over the calf is important in providing adequate compression. Complications, although rare, may include skin blisters and sensations of warmth/heat. Compression may be initiated at the time of surgery and continued until the patient is ambulatory. EPC is especially effective in patients who cannot tolerate the slightest degree of bleeding (e.g., neurosurgical patients, eye surgery).[68]

Compression Stockings

Compression stockings are useful adjuncts in the prevention of DVT and PE by promoting venous return from the lower extremities.[5, 68] These stockings are made of various materials, such as natural rubber and synthetics, including latex. They are available in a variety of colors, lengths, and ranges of compression with the greatest pressure at the ankle. Most are available as ready-made products. Normal resting venous pressures are 18 mmHg at the ankle to 8 mmHg at the upper thigh (see Fig. 17–3). Patients with preexisting venous disease may have higher resting pressures that would require additional compression for appropriate prophylaxis. Despite the availability of different lengths, knee-high stockings are more effective in the prevention of DVT; they are less expensive and easier to apply. Patients should be taught the proper use and care of compression stockings (Table 17–6).

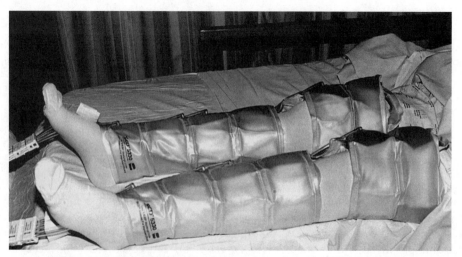

Figure 17–6. Intermittent pneumatic compression device for DVT prophylaxis.

TABLE 17–6. **Teaching Patient About Compression Stockings**

- Wear correct length.
  - Knee high for calf vein thrombosis
  - Thigh high for femoral-popliteal thrombosis
- Wear appropriate pressure gradient.
  - 20–30 mm for venous thrombosis prophylaxis
  - 30–40 mm for venous thrombosis
- Apply stocking by turning all but foot inside out; slide foot into stocking and pull stocking over leg.
- Use rubber gloves to facilitate application.
- Remove stockings at bed time.
- Keep second pair of stockings on hand.
- Replace stocking every 6 months or prn.

Leg Elevation and Early Mobilization

Leg elevation is an important adjunct in DVT prophylaxis. However, its effectiveness is dependent on the angle of elevation.[68] To reduce leg edema, the angle of elevation should be 10–20 degrees above the level of the heart in the nonambulatory patient. All patients should be ambulating as soon as their condition permits.[45] Once ambulation has begun, the patient should be encouraged to avoid prolonged standing and avoid prolonged sitting without leg elevation. Walking and other types of physical activity using the calf muscles should be encouraged on a regular basis.

In summary, nurses play a key role in the detection, treatment, and prevention of venous thromboemblism. An awareness of the signs and symptoms of superficial thrombophlebitis, deep venous thrombosis, and pulmonary embolus, as well as knowledge of patients who are at high risk, is vital in providing optimal nursing care. Nurses are responsible for prevention of deep vein thrombosis by proper assessment, education, and prevention measures. Nurses' adherence to these measures will help reduce the incidence and potentially life-threatening complications of venous thromboembolism.

References

1. Hirsh J, Hoak J: Management of deep vein thrombosis and pulmonary embolism: A statement for healthcare professionals. Circulation 1996; 93:2212–2245.
2. Wakefield TW, Strietert RM, Prince MR, et al: Pathogenesis of venous thrombosis: A new insight. Cardiovasc Surg 1997; 5:6–15.
3. Gray BH, Graor RA: Deep venous thrombosis and pulmonary embolism: The importance of heightened awareness. Postgrad Med 1992; 91:207–220.
4. Colucciello S: Recognizing and treating thromboembolic disease. Emerg Med 1993; 25(11):59–74.
5. Clagett GP, Anderson FA, Heit J, et al: Prevention of venous thromboembolism. Chest 1995; 108(4):312S–334S.
6. Nunnelee J: Minimize the risk of DVT. RN 1995; 58:28–32.
7. Falter HJ: Deep vein thrombosis in pregnancy and the puerperium: A comprehensive review. J Vasc Nurs 1997; 15(2):58–62.
8. Virchow R: Gesammelte abhandlungen zur Wissenschaftlichen mecicin. Frankfurt, AM Von Meidinger Sohn & Co, 1856.
9. Wheeler HB, Anderson FA: Pulmonary embolism. In Gloviczki P, Yao JST (eds): Handbook of Venous Disorders: Guidelines of the American Venous Forum. London, Chapman & Hall Medical, 1996, pp 274–291.
10. Hickey A: Catching deep vein thrombosis in time. Nursing94 1994; 24(10):34–41.
11. Ecklund MM: Optimizing the flow of care for prevention and treatment of deep vein thrombosis and pulmonary embolism. AACN Clinical Issues 1995; 6(4):588–601.

12. Witry SW: Pulmonary embolus in pregnancy. J Perinat Neonatal Nurs 1992; 6:1–11.
13. Lees AJ: Thromboembolic complication in children and adolescents: Who is at risk? J Pediatr Health Care 1995; 9:222–224.
14. Ligush J, Johnson G: Superficial thrombophlebitis. In Gloviczki P, Yao JST (eds): Handbook of Venous Disorders: Guidelines of the American Venous Forum. London, Chapman & Hall Medical, 1996, pp 235–242.
15. Lutter KS, Kerr TM, Roedersheimer R, et al: Superficial thrombophlebitis diagnosed by duplex scanning. Surgery 1991; 110:42–46.
16. Thomas-Masoorli S, Peterson R: Intravenous therapy handbook. Nursing96 1996; 26(10):48–51.
17. Hyers TM, Hul RD, Weg JG: Antithrombotic therapy for venous thromboembolic disease. Chest 1995; 108:335S–351S.
18. Lohr JM, McDevitt DT, Lutter KS, et al: Operative management of greater saphenous thrombophlebitis involving the saphenofemoral junction. Am J Surg 1992; 164:269–275.
19. Greenfield LJ: Venous thromboembolic disease. In Moore WS (ed): Vascular Surgery: A Comprehensive Review. Philadelphia, WB Saunders, 1998, pp 787–799.
20. Mattos MA, Londrey GL, Leutz DW, et al: Color flow duplex scanning for the surveillance and diagnosis of acute deep venous thrombosis? J Vasc Surg 1992; 15:366–376.
21. Comerota AJ, Katz ML, Greenwald LL, et al: Venous duplex imaging: Should it replace hemodynamic tests for deep venous thrombosis? J Vasc Surg 1990; 11:53–61.
22. Fowler SB: Deep vein thrombosis and pulmonary emboli in neuroscience patients. American Association of Neuroscience Nurses 1995; 27(4):224–228.
23. Lilley LL, Guanci R: A cautious look at heparin. AJN 1995; 9:14–15.
24. Berkman SA: Current concepts in anticoagulation. Hosp Pract 1992; 27(2):187–200.
25. Comerota AJ: Acute deep venous thrombosis. In Gloviczki P, Yao JST (eds): Handbook of Venous Disorders: Guidelines of the American Venous Forum. London, Chapman & Hall Medical, 1996, pp 243–259.
26. Hull RD, Raskob GE, Rosenbloom D, et al: Optimal therapeutic level of heparin in patients with venous thrombosis. Arch Intern Med 1992; 152:1589–1595.
27. Warkentin TE, Kelton JG: Heparin-induced thrombocytopenia. Prog Hemost Thromb 1991; 10:1–34.
28. Hull RD, Raskob GE, Pinio GF, et al: Subcutaneous low-molecular-weight heparin compared with continuous intravenous heparin in the initial treatment of proximal-vein thrombosis. N Engl J Med 1992; 326:975–982.
29. Hirsh J: Deep vein thrombosis: Recovery or recurrence? Hosp Pract 1995; 30(3):71–79.
30. Markel, Manzo RA, Bergelin RO, et al: Pattern and distribution of thrombosis in acute venous thrombosis. Arch Surg 1992; 127:305–309.
31. Agnelli G: Anticoagulation in the prevention and treatment of pulmonary embolism. Chest 1995; 107(1):39S–44S.
32. Cosico JN, Rothlauf EB: Indication, management, and patient education: Anticoagulation therapy. MCN 1992; 17:130–135.
33. Hirsh J, Dalen JE, Deykin D, et al: Oral anticoagulants: Mechanism of action, clinical effectiveness, and optimal therapeutic range. Chest 1995; 108(4):231S–245S.
34. Sun J, Chang MW: Initialization of warfarin dosages using computer modeling. Arch Phys Med Rehabil 1995; 76:453–456.
35. Gibbar-Clements T, Shirrell D, Free C: PT and APTT-Seeing beyond the numbers. Nursing97 1997; 7:49–51.
36. Bussey HI, Force RW, Branco TM, et al: Reliance on prothrombin time ratios causes significant errors in anticoagulation therapy. Arch Intern Med 1992; 152:278–282.
37. Turpie AGG: Thrombolytic therapy in acute venous thrombosis. In Yao JST, Pearce WH (eds): Technologies in Vascular Surgery. Philadelphia, WB Saunders, 1992, pp 504–511.
38. Raimer F, Thomas M: Clot stoppers—Using anticoagulants safely and effectively. Nursing95 1995; 25(3):34–43.
39. Lord RSA, Chen FC, Devine TJ, et al: Surgical treatment of acute deep venous thrombosis. World J Surg 1990; 4:694–702.
40. Gulba DC, Schmid C, Borst HG, et al: Medical compared with surgical treatment for massive pulmonary embolism. Lancet 1994; 343:576–577.
41. Goldhaber SZ: Diagnosis, treatment and prevention of pulmonary emboli: Report of the World Health Organization/International Society and Federation of Cardiology Task Force. JAMA 1992; 268:1727–1733.
42. Goldhaber SZ: Pulmonary embolism thrombolysis: A clarion call for international collaboration. J Am Coll Cardiol 1992; 19:246–247.
43. Tapson VF, Davidson CJ, Kisslo KB, et al: Rapid visualization of massive pulmonary emboli utilizing intravascular ultrasound. Chest 1994; 105:888–890.
44. Hull R, Raskob GE, Coates G, et al: Clinical validity of a normal perfusion lung scan in patients with suspected pulmonary embolism. Chest 1990; 97:23–26.
45. Majoros K, Moccia J: Pulmonary embolism—targeting an elusive enemy. Nursing96 1996 26(4):26–31.

46. Hirsh J: Management Guidelines in Venous Thromboembolism: Diagnosis of Pulmonary Embolism. Hamilton, Ontario, Rhone-Poulenc Rorer Canada Inc, 1994.
47. Burns D: Review of thrombolytic use in acute myocardial infarction, pulmonary embolism, and cerebral thrombosis. Crit Care Nurs Q 1993; 15(4):1–12.
48. Sors H, Pacouret G, Azarian R, et al: Hemodynamic effects of bolus vs 2-h infusion of alteplase in acute massive pulmonary embolism: A randomized controlled multicenter trial. Chest 1994; 106:712–717.
49. Goldhaber S: Contemporary pulmonary embolism thrombolysis. Chest 1995; 107:45S–51S.
50. Goldhaber SZ: Pulmonary embolism. Hospital Medicine 1993; 8:24–38.
51. Stein PD, Henry JW, Relyea B: Untreated patients with pulmonary embolism. Chest 1995; 107:931–935.
52. Gisselbrecht M, Diehl JL, Meyer G, et al: Clinical presentation and results of thrombolytic therapy in older patients with massive pulmonary embolism: A comparison with non-elderly patients. J Am Geriatr Soc 1996; 44:189–193.
53. Apple S: New trends in thrombolytic therapy. RN 1996; 59:30–35.
54. Graor RA: Thrombolytic therapy for deep vein thromboses and pulmonary emboli. In Bergan JJ, Yao JST (eds): Venous Disorders. Philadelphia, WB Saunders, 1991, pp 170–181.
55. Hirsch J, Turpie AGG: Use of plasminogen activators in venous thrombosis. World J Surg 1990; 14:688–693.
56. Gonzalez-Juanatey JR, Valdes L, Amaro A, et al: Treatment of massive pulmonary thromboembolism with low intrapulmonary dosages of urokinase: Short-term angiographic and hemodynamic evolution. Chest 1992; 102:341–346.
57. Levine MN, Goldhaber SZ, Califf RM, et al: Hemorrhagic complications of thrombolytic therapy in the treatment of myocardial infarction and venous thromboembolism. Chest 1992; 102(4):364S–373S.
58. Dorfman GS: Percutaneous inferior vena caval filters. Radiology 1990; 174:987–992.
59. Greenfield L, Proctor M: Indications and techniques of inferior vena cava interruption. In Gloviczki P, Yao JST (eds): Handbook of Venous Disorders: Guidelines of the American Venous Forum. London, Chapman & Hall Medical, 1996, pp 306–320.
60. Greenfield LJ: Evolution of venous interruption for pulmonary thromboembolism. Arch Surg 1992; 127:622–626.
61. Nunnelee J, Kurgan A: Interruption of the inerior vena cava for venous thromboembolic disease. J Vasc Nurs 1993; 11(3):80–82.
62. Murphy JP, Dorfman GS, Yedlick JW, et al: LGM vena cava filter: Objective evaluation of early results. J Vasc Intern Radiol 1991; 2:107–115.
63. Greenfield LJ, Cho KJ, Proctor M, et al: Results of a multicenter study of the modified hook-titanium Greenfield filter. J Vasc Surg 1991; 14:253–257.
64. Meyer G, Tamisier D, Sors H, et al: Pulmonary embolectomy a 20 year experience at one center. Ann Thorac Surg 1991; 51:232–236.
65. Meyer JA: Friedrich Trendelenburg and the surgical approach to massive pulmonary embolism. Arch Surg 1990; 125:1202–1205.
66. Comerota AJ, Katz ML, White JV: Why does prophylaxis with external pneumatic compression for deep vein thrombosis fail? Am J Surg 1992: 164:265–268.
67. Ramos R, Salem BI, DePawlikowki MP, et al: The efficacy of pneumatic compression stockings in the prevention of pulmonary embolism after cardiac surgery. Chest 1996; 109(1):83–85.
68. Heit JA: Current recommendations for prevention of deep venous thrombosis. In Gloviczki P, Yao JST (eds): Handbook of Venous Disorders: Guidelines of the American Venous Forum. London, Chapman & Hall Medical, 1996, pp 292–305.
69. Hirsh J: Management Guidelines in Venous Thromboembolism—Prophylaxis of Venous Thromboembolism. Hamilton, Ontario, Rhone-Poulenc Rorer Canada Inc, 1994.
70. Morris BA: Nursing care for the prevention of deep vein thrombosis: Low molecular weight heparins augment conventional interventions. Today's OR Nurse 1995; 17(5):4–29.
71. Fitzgerald RH: Post-discharge prevention of deep vein thrombosis following total joint repalcement. Orthopedics 1996; 19(8)suppl:15–18.
72. Carroll P: Deep venous thrombosis: Implications for orthopaedic nursing. Orthopaedic Nursing 1993; 12(3):33–43.
73. Montgomery KD, Geerts WH, Hollis GP, et al: Thromboembolic complications in patients with pelvic trauma. Clin Orthop Rel Res 1996; 329:68–87.
74. Green D, Twardowski P, Wei R, et al: Fatal pulmonary embolism in spinal cord injury. Chest 1994; 105J:853–855.
75. Green D: Prophylaxis of thromboembolism in spinal cord-injured patients. Chest 1992; 102(6):649S–651S.
76. Nunnelee JD: Low-molecular-weight heparin. J Vasc Nurs 1997; 15(3):94–96.
77. Hirsh J: Low Molecular Weight Heparins. Hamilton, Ontario, Rhone-Poulenc Rorer Canada Inc, 1994.
78. Green D, Chen D, Chmiel JS, et al: Prevention of thromboembolism in spinal cord injury: Role of low molecular weight heparin. Arch Phys Med Rehabil 1994; 75:290–292.

18

Chronic Venous Disease

Tara L. Hahn, MD, and Michael C. Dalsing, MD

ⵥ · ⵥ

Chronic venous disease is a common malady that affects all age groups. Symptoms range from small spider telangiectasias and varicose veins to disabling venous claudication and nonhealing or recurrent venous ulcers. The mainstays of therapy remain nonsurgical, but a renewed interest in this disease has shown some promise for advanced surgical therapy. This chapter discusses the pathophysiology, diagnosis, and treatment of chronic venous disease.

NORMAL ANATOMY AND PHYSIOLOGY

To understand venous disease, a working knowledge of the lower-extremity venous system is imperative. There are three basic components: deep veins, communicating (or perforating) veins, and superficial veins (Fig. 18–1). The deep system is composed of the iliac veins, and the superficial, profunda, and common femoral veins in addition to the popliteal and tibial veins. The greater and lesser saphenous veins compose the superficial system, and the communicating veins create the various connections between the superficial and deep systems. The superficial veins lie within the subcutaneous tissues, whereas the deep veins are located below the fascia and are surrounded by muscle. The perforating veins pierce the fascia to connect the deep and superficial systems.

Key to understanding the etiology of venous disease is the concept of the calf muscles as a pump, the "peripheral heart" (Fig. 18–2 A and B). The lower extremity and infracardiac central veins themselves act as the plumbing system or conduits to direct blood back to the cardiac chambers, while the venous valves act as one-way stopcocks to prevent the reflux of blood into the leg after peripheral pump contraction or when a person assumes an upright position. In this analogy, the deep veins within the gastrocnemius and soleus muscles correspond to the left ventricle. As the calf muscles contract with exercise, the deep venous system is compressed, and blood is propelled or pumped toward the heart. Deep within the muscle pump, pressures can rise to 300 mmHg.[1] As pressure rises in the deep system, the valves in the communicating veins close, preventing not only backflow of blood into the superficial venous system but also the transmission of these high pressures from the deep venous system to the superficial system. Blood is also moved toward the heart in the superficial veins because of compression of the fascia against the skin, even though these pressures may peak at only 100–150 mmHg. Valves in the

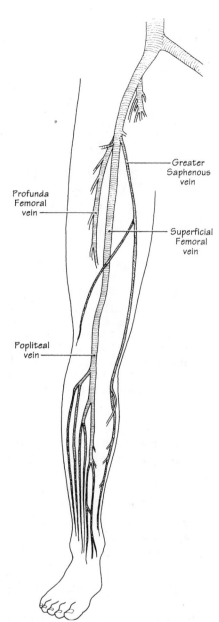

Greater
Saphenous
vein

Profunda
Femoral
vein

Superficial
Femoral
vein

Popliteal
vein

Figure 18–1. An artist's rendition of the veins of the lower extremity. (Reprinted with permission from Dalsing M: Venous valvular insufficiency: Pathophysiology and treatment options. Society of Cardiovascular and Interventional Radiology from Venous Interventions, syllabus V: Venous Interventions, p. 225, © 1995.)

superficial and deep veins open in response to the calf pump to allow blood to move toward the heart. As the pumping action ceases, blood is prevented from refluxing into the leg by the closure of the valves within the deep and superficial veins. Arterial flow begins to fill the venous system during rest. As the venous system fills, the valves in the foot, distal leg, and perforating system will open to allow blood to enter the deep veins within the calf muscle pump.[2]

Normal pressures in a patient's leg can be measured by inserting an intravenous catheter into a vein of the foot. The catheter is connected to a pressure transducer and chart recorder. With the patient lying down, normal venous pressure is approximately 15 mmHg. When the patient stands, gravity exerts its influence in the form of hydrostatic pressure and adds to the baseline pressure. Because the arteries and veins run in parallel, this pressure is exerted equally in both systems. When relaxed, the veins are flat and nondistended. However, as they begin to fill with blood, they become elliptical before

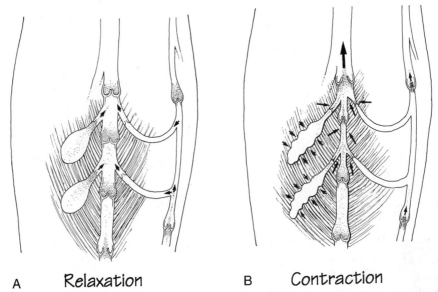

A   Relaxation   B   Contraction

Figure 18–2. A, Veins within the calf muscle pump during relaxation. Note the filling of the deep veins from the perforating veins and lower leg with proper deep venous valve closure in the standing patient. **B,** Veins within the calf muscle pump during muscle contraction with ejection of blood toward the heart. Note the proper closure of the valves of the communicating veins in a nondiseased venous system. (Reprinted with permission from Dalsing M: Venous valvular insufficiency: Pathophysiology and treatment options. Society of Cardiovascular and Interventional Radiology from Venous Interventions, syllabus V: Venous Interventions, p. 225, © 1995.)

proceeding to the circular shape of a fully distended vein. Once the veins become filled to capacity and have assumed a cylindrical shape, any increase in volume will dramatically increase pressure.[1] Ambulatory venous pressure measurements are a physiologic study designed to assess venous function in an active patient. A baseline erect pressure is obtained. This baseline pressure is the pressure exerted on the lower leg as reflected by the venous catheter measurement of a column of blood from the heart to the lower-extremity venous system. This pressure is generally 90 mmHg or higher and is influenced by the height of the patient in addition to other factors. The time it takes to achieve a steady-state pressure after rising from a supine position is called the venous filling time (VFT). The patient then is instructed to perform 10 tiptoe maneuvers at a rate of 1 per second, and the resultant drop in recorded pressure is labeled the ambulatory venous pressure (AVP). After this exercise, the patient remains still until the pressure returns to baseline. The time it takes to return to the baseline erect pressure from the AVP is called the venous refilling time (VRT). Normal AVP values are less than 45 mmHg. If the pressure is greater than 45 mmHg, the sequelae of venous disease are likely because exercise is not effective in decreasing lower leg venous pressures while standing.[3] The VRT reflects the closure of venous valves to prevent blood from refluxing down the leg following exercise. If the VRT is greater than 20 seconds, the venous valvular system is intact and adequately prevents retrograde flow of blood in the veins. If the VRT is less than 20 seconds, valvular reflux is present.

PATHOPHYSIOLOGY AND ETIOLOGY

Chronic venous disease occurs when there is failure of one or more of the components of a normal venous system. Three pathophysiologic states have been defined: venous obstruction, venous valvular insufficiency, and calf muscle pump malfunction.[4]

Primary venous outflow obstruction can occur as a result of either intrinsic or extrinsic factors. Elevated pressures within the venous system result from increased resistance to flow. If the deep system is primarily involved, the increased pressure is eventually transmitted to the communicating system, which then gradually causes communicating vein valve dysfunction. With failure of the communicating vein valves, increased volume and venous hypertension are communicated to the superficial venous system (resulting in the possible appearance of varicose veins), and to the skin and subcutaneous tissues. The superficial system alone can be affected, resulting in a similar visible consequence. Primary causes of obstruction are very uncommon, whereas secondary venous outflow obstruction is often the result of venous thrombosis. Thrombophlebitis is by far the most common cause of venous obstruction.

Extrinsic causes of venous obstruction in the lower limb include compression of iliac and pelvic veins by tumor, retroperitoneal fibrosis, or infection. Left common iliac vein compression by the right common iliac artery as well as external iliac vein compression from the internal iliac artery on either side have been described.[5, 6] The femoral vein can be compressed by a herniation of fat through a femoral hernia defect and by soft tissue tumors limited to the thigh. Aneurysms of the common femoral artery, superficial femoral artery, or the deep femoral artery can compress the thin elastic wall of the femoral vein. Popliteal masses (a popliteal artery aneurysm or Baker's cyst) can compress the popliteal vein and cause obstruction at this distal level.[1]

Internal sources of outflow obstruction other than deep venous thrombus are even less common. Vein wall abnormalities such as absence of the vein (aplasia) or tumors of the vein wall (leiomyomata) have been described.[1] A somewhat less obscure source of obstruction results from intraluminal webs. Such webs have been reported to occur in 20 percent of the population precisely where the left common iliac vein is compressed by the right iliac artery.[7]

Valvular insufficiency may involve one or more of the three venous systems in the lower leg. This incompetence, congenital or acquired, allows for the transmission of high venous pressures to the lower leg on standing, which is not adequately relieved by exercise. Primary valvular insufficiency encompasses a variety of processes. The obvious is congenital absence of valves, a rare cause.[8] Venous valve prolapse, observed as floppy valve cusps, is also seen. These floppy valves can be seen in the very common hereditary varicose veins of the superficial venous system, but they are also observed in the deep and perforating systems. Alternatively, the problem may actually be in the vein itself such that the valve ring dilates, resulting in valve cusps which cannot approximate.[9, 10] Approximately 50–60 percent of deep valvular dysfunction is a result of deep venous thrombosis (DVT), whereas the other 40–50 percent appears to be of a primary etiology.[11] Incomplete or nonexistent recanalization of the vein following DVT can damage the delicate bicuspid leaflets of the venous valves.[12] Even with complete thrombus resorption, scarring can result in damage of these delicate structures.[4] Prolonged exposure to high venous pressures will eventually cause the vein to dilate, preventing the valve cusps from meeting appropriately.[1] Such high pressures can result from an abnormal artery to venous connection (arteriovenous fistula), or from prior proximal valve damage as a result of trauma, DVT, or other cause with resultant pressure on and subsequent failure of even more distal valves. Lower leg venous hypertension is the ultimate effect of venous valvular insufficiency.

Varicose veins are one of the most common sequelae of chronic venous disease. When taken as a whole, 15–20 percent of the adult population is afflicted with superficial varicosities.[13] There are two types of varicose veins—primary and secondary.[14] Primary, or simple, varicose veins (Fig. 18–3) result from superficial vein incompetence. They are often familial in origin and have no underlying etiology. Secondary varicose veins are the result of previous vein pathology. Thrombophlebitis in the deep or superficial system can result in the appearance of varicose veins over time. Also, individuals who are employed in jobs that require prolonged periods of standing (as opposed to intermittent or constant

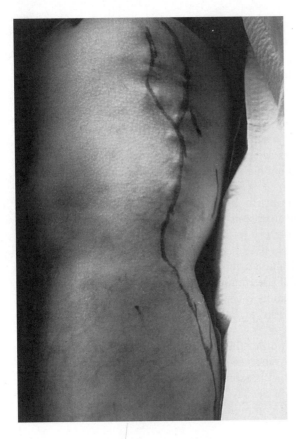

Figure 18–3. Varicose veins on the thigh associated with greater saphenous vein insufficiency. These veins have been marked with permanent ink in preparation for surgery. (Reprinted with permission from Dalsing M: Venous valvular insufficiency: Pathophysiology and treatment options. Society of Cardiovascular and Interventional Radiology from Venous Interventions, syllabus V: Venous Interventions, p. 225, © 1995.)

periods of walking) are at risk. Estrogen has been cited as a factor in varicose vein formation because of its effect on smooth muscle dilation. This may be the reason pregnant women develop varicose veins even within the first trimester of pregnancy, rather than from extrinsic pressure due to an enlarged fundus compressing the iliac veins, as was once believed.[14]

Finally, there can be failure of the calf muscle pump either isolated or in combination with one or the other previously described venous disease states. Returning to the cardiac analogy, calf muscle pump failure is similar to congestive heart failure. The pump eventually is unable to generate the force necessary to eject a satisfactory volume of blood from the leg. The reasons for this are varied. Elderly patients with physiologic muscle wasting may not have the physical muscle strength sufficient to pump the blood out of the leg. This is also true for patients with muscle wasting diseases such as paraplegia, those with trauma injury, or bedridden patients (disuse).[1] Similarly, pathologic conditions that result in muscle fibrosis (e.g., muscular dystrophy, multiple sclerosis) will destroy the calf muscle pump. Thrombus in the deep veins within the gastrocnemius and soleus muscles can prevent blood from entering the pump itself, resulting in a deficient ejection volume. If outflow is obstructed for any reason, the excessive afterload causes dilation of the pump chambers (the veins within the calf muscle). Eventually the perforating vein valves are made incompetent from the excessive pressure placed on them with each pump contraction. The pressures generated by the calf muscle pump are then transmitted to the superficial venous system and surrounding tissue. The overall effect is venous stasis and venous hypertension within the lower extremity.

The final effect of venous stasis and hypertension is the skin changes associated with chronic venous disease. There are theories proposed to explain these changes, but they have yet to be definitively proven. Originally, venous stasis was thought to cause hypoxia as a result of the low oxygen levels associated with excessive venous blood puddling in the lower extremity. This was later brought into question by direct physiologic measurements. Several years later, the fibrin cuff theory became popular. This theory suggests that, as a result of venous hypertension, increased plasma proteins and cells were lost through the capillary wall into the surrounding tissues. Fibrinogen was a major component of these extravasated proteins. The fibrinogen was converted to fibrin by local enzymes, and fibrin buildup was believed to hamper oxygen diffusion through the tissues, resulting in tissue hypoxia.[15, 16] However, fibrin has not been proven to be a deterrent to the diffusing capacity of oxygen. Most recently, white blood cell trapping and then activation have been postulated as a cause for observed skin changes. Patients with chronic venous disease were found to have "trapped" white blood cells within the tissues affected by venous hypertension.[17] The activation of these white blood cells could cause an inflammatory reaction, the normal function of white blood cells. This inflammatory reaction could then be responsible for the skin changes observed.[17] While this appears to be a plausible explanation, definitive experiments are currently under way to verify this theory.

CLINICAL SIGNS AND SYMPTOMS

Venous disease can present in a variety of ways (Table 18–1). Spider veins, also known as telangiectasias, often accompany varicose veins. Patients commonly report feeling a stinging sensation just prior to the development of the spider vein. These appear as fine blue-red branchings just under the surface of the skin. The greatest complaint is their unsightly appearance. However, each spider vein is often accompanied by a larger pathologically dilated vein located deeper in the subcutaneous tissue.[14]

Varicose veins of a hereditary nature will usually appear during the second decade of life. If there is an inciting event, such as thrombosis or trauma, the varicosities generally appear within several years as a natural progression of the disease. These veins appear as blue, dilated, tortuous, and palpable protrusions beneath the skin. They may be isolated or bunched into clusters in the general distribution of the greater or lesser saphenous veins and their branches. Symptoms can range from a dull ache and itching to edema, cramping, and eventually skin damage. Tiredness, heaviness, and pain are commonly reported. The presence of varicose veins and related symptoms can be due to a variety of disease processes, and careful evaluation is required to determine the exact cause. If the pain from varicosities is sufficiently severe to warrant the use of narcotic medications, another source for the pain should be sought.[14]

Even without obvious varicosities, venous disease can result in pain, edema, cutaneous hyperpigmentation (Fig. 18–4A), stasis dermatitis or eczema (Fig. 18–4A), and finally venous ulcers (Fig. 18–4B and C).[18, 19] These changes usually occur just above the medial

TABLE 18–1. **Signs and Symptoms of Chronic Venous Disease**

SIGNS	SYMPTOMS
Telangiectases (spider veins)	Complaints of swelling
Varicose veins	Heaviness
Edema	Pain with standing
Hyperpigmentation	Nocturnal calf muscle cramps
Lipodermatosclerosis	Aching
Venous ulcers	Leg tiredness
	Itching
	Venous claudication

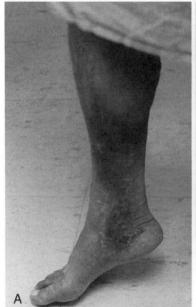

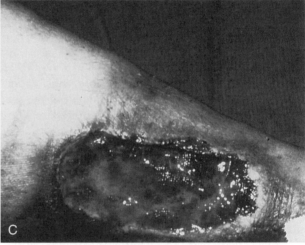

Figure 18–4. A, Lipodermatosclerosis (eczema) and hyperpigmentation in the gaiter area of a patient with chronic venous disease. **B** and **C,** Venous ulcers of the lower extremity in patients with chronic venous disease demonstrating the wide variance in size and depth of such ulcers. (**B** from McCarthy WJ, Fahey VA, Bergan JJ, et al: The veins and venous disease. In James EC, Corry RJ, Perry JF [eds]: Principles of Basic Surgical Practice. Philadelphia, Hanley & Belfus, 1987, p 463.)

malleolus, known as the "gaiter" area. The largest number of perforating veins per area exists in the medial calf. If their associated valves become incompetent or proximal obstruction exists, the high pressures generated by the calf muscle pump can be transmitted to the surface veins and the respective cutaneous capillary beds, resulting in tremendously high venous pressures and skin changes.[1] Similarly, if venous insufficiency is the underlying pathologic process, the high intravenous pressures generated while standing cannot be relieved by exercise. These high pressures generated while standing are most severe in the most dependent areas, the so-called gaiter area.

One of the most severe pain syndromes associated with venous disease is termed venous claudication. Fortunately, this is a rare condition. The characteristics of this condition were described by Cockett and Thomas and consist of leg pain with exercise, iliac vein obstruction, venous hypertension at rest, and increased venous pressures with exercise.[5] Further investigation by Killewich and associates prompted the addition of cyanosis, sensations of increased swelling, and increased prominence of superficial veins to this symptom complex. These investigators also differentiated the pain of venous claudication from the pain of arterial insufficiency by noting a relief of symptoms with 15–20 minutes of rest in combination with elevation of the extremities in the former as opposed to pain relief with cessation of activity and the dangling of the legs in the latter.[20] Nonetheless, there is a wide range of presentations. Some patients are able to function in their everyday routine while others are so debilitated that amputation has been requested.[5] The patients plagued with the most severe disease often have associated deep system incompetence in addition to an obstructive component. This also may be accompanied by superficial and/ or communicating vein incompetence.[19] The signs and symptoms of obstruction are related to both the level of the obstruction and the number and size of collaterals. This was best demonstrated by Labropoulus and associates in their study of venous obstruction.[21] More proximal obstruction is associated with worse symptoms due to the decreased potential for adequate collateral formation. Patients with iliac obstructive disease appear most symptomatic. Patients with femoropopliteal obstruction can rely on collaterals from the long saphenous vein, any duplication of the femoral veins, deep femoral veins, and deep muscular tributaries of the thigh. Those with isolated popliteal occlusion have an even wider network of potential collaterals. However, even a well-developed collateral system does not function as well as a normal caliber vein because these vessels have a higher resistance to flow.[20, 21] Therefore, the calf muscle pump is subjected to elevated outflow resistance, which can eventually cause failure of the pump. The ultimate effect may be a multifaceted venous system malfunction.

DIAGNOSTIC EVALUATION

The diagnosis of potential vein pathology begins with a thorough history and physical examination. A family history of venous disease (varicose veins), past episodes of venous thromboses, and a discussion of symptoms as related to dependency and/or exercise is very important. If leg swelling and pain are noted with standing and relieved by elevation, venous disease becomes a prime diagnostic possibility. The presence of varicose veins confirms venous pathology as one component of the patient's disease complex. The two most common signs and symptoms of chronic venous disease are edema and pain with standing.[16] Chronic venous disease stigmata such as hyperpigmentation or venous ulcers are also significant signs of the disease.

Ambulatory venous pressure measurements, previously described, are a direct measurement of venous hemodynamics and aid in the diagnosis of venous insufficiency. In the diseased state, the veins not only fill from arterial inflow but also from the reflux of blood down the veins. Blood pressure cuffs placed above and below the knee as well as at the ankle can be inflated to compress the greater saphenous vein, the lesser saphenous vein, and essentially all superficial and perforator veins affecting the ankle area. Then VRT measurements can be repeated. If the VRT is still less than 20 seconds, the deep system may be a major component of the reflux seen. With the various cuffs inflated, if the VRT is converted to normal, the problem resides within one or the other superficial or perforating venous systems. The arm-foot pressure differential as developed by Raju is a quantitative measurement for venous obstruction.[22] Venous pressure cannulas are placed in both the hand and the foot. Simultaneously, pressures are measured in the hand and in the foot while the patient is lying down and again after a 3-minute thigh cuff occlusion that induces vasodilation upon cuff deflation. A normal reading after this reactive hyperemia is an arm-foot differential of less than 4 mmHg. With venous obstruction, the pressure difference can range from 6 to 20 mmHg.[22] Direct venous pressure measurements were historically the gold standard for evaluating venous disease but generally have been replaced by noninvasive tests as the techniques were improved and tested against the standard. Duplex scanning and air plethysmographic techniques are the anatomic and functional tests of choice in current medical practice, although, in some cases, invasive testing is still required.[23]

Plethysmography is an indirect method of assessing the venous system and to diagnose obstruction, valve incompetence, or calf muscle pump dysfunction. There are several plethysmographic methods, and all detect changes in blood volume. Obstruction can be determined by evaluating venous capacitance and the rate of venous outflow using impedance plethysmography. With impedance plethysmography, changes in volume are detected as changes in electrical resistance. Patients lie on a table and bilateral thigh cuffs are placed to provide for venous occlusion while electrodes placed on the lower leg measure changes in volume (resistance). A baseline reading is obtained prior to cuff inflation, and then the cuffs are inflated to approximately 50 mmHg to result in occlusion of venous outflow. Once the volume measurement stablizes, a reading is taken and the cuffs are rapidly deflated. The time it takes to return to baseline is noted. Venous capacitance is then determined by subtracting the baseline from the volume plateau. Results are compared to a standard set of normal values.[24] If values lie outside the normal reading, venous obstruction is one component of the patient's venous disease.

Light reflex rheography, similar to photoplethysmography, can quantitate the venous refilling time (VRT) in patients with venous valvular incompetence. A small photoelectrode is placed on the patient's foot. The time for venous refill is measured after 10 plantarflexion/dorsiflexion maneuvers. Normal refill is greater than 20 seconds, whereas reflux is considered to be present if the VRT is less than 20 seconds.[24] Changes in blood volume are detected as changes in light absorption and reflection.[25] With the use of tourniquets, a rough estimation of the localization of reflux (superficial, perforator, deep) is possible much like the intravenous pressure measurement. It does function as an effective screening test for venous insufficiency.

Calf muscle pump function, as well as venous insufficiency, can be evaluated by air plethysmography. A plastic cylinder filled with air is fitted over the calf. This cylinder is connected to a chart recorder and changes in leg volume are detected by increases in pressure within the cylinder. After a baseline reading is taken, patients exercise by ankle dorsiflexion or heel raises to stimulate the calf muscle pump to empty the calf veins. The ejection fraction, the amount of blood propelled cephalad with a single muscle contraction, is determined. After a series of ankle flexions, the volume remaining in the leg is measured and is referred to as the residual volume. The residual volume is considered to be equivalent to the lowest ambulatory venous pressure obtained during exercise. These values can be compared with normal studies to determine the presence and the type of the patient's venous disease.[24] Abnormal resting and residual volumes suggest an abnormal muscle pump. The venous volume refilling time after exercise can be used to characterize venous reflux problems. Because plethysmography cannot give an anatomic depiction of the venous system, many institutions will combine these studies with ultrasonographic techniques to provide a complete venous evaluation.

Ultrasonographic techniques are a direct but noninvasive evaluation of the venous vascular system. A continuous-wave (CW) Doppler uses sound waves generated by a crystal in the Doppler head that are directed into the body to evaluate the underlying veins. By determining the shift in sound frequency as the sound wave hits flowing blood, one can determine blood flow velocity and other flow parameters. Using various maneuvers, one can differentiate between venous obstruction and valvular incompetence. A great deal of skill is required to interpret this examination. If there is a weak signal, one must differentiate between flow in a collateral vessel and flow within a partially recanalized vein. As a general rule, if no signal is obtained over a specific vein location, this area is obstructed. Valve incompetency is demonstrated by noting reflux in a vein segment either by having the patient perform a Valsalva maneuver (forcefully holding a breath to compress the inferior vena cava and propel blood toward the feet) or by compressing a segment of the vein above the probe to force blood distally. However, one competent valve along the path can result in a falsely negative study even though other valves may well be incompetent. The most accurate assessment of insufficiency occurs with the patient standing with weight off the leg being evaluated. A probe is placed over the vein being examined, and the distal leg is compressed. When the compression is released, competent valves will close and prevent backflow. If the valves are incompetent, a retrograde surge of blood will be detected. The drawback to a CW Doppler examination is the inability to be sure which vein is being evaluated because of the possible presence of duplicated veins or large collateral veins. Also, the existence of reflux but not its severity can be determined.

Duplex scanning, currently the most popular and versatile noninvasive venous evaluation, uses B-mode imaging to overcome the limitations of a CW Doppler study (Fig. 18–5). This procedure is able to identify specific venous structures and thereby eliminate the confusion involved with continuous-wave scanning. B-mode imaging uses sound waves to create a picture of the structure being examined. Long segments of vein can be analyzed with this method for easier evaluation of obstruction. In combination with color flow analysis, this method of ultrasonography gives anatomic detail that can be useful for planning surgical procedures. Venous obstruction appears as a segment of vein where there is loss of flow signal. Chronic obstruction can be differentiated from acute thrombosis. Acute thrombosis causes inflammation of the vein resulting in venous distention. Chronic occlusion causes fibrosis of the vein so that it is smaller than normal caliber. Calcifications may be present in a chronic thrombus.[26] One can see recanalization of veins in chronic venous disease as well.

All these findings can be seen in any of the venous structures imaged. With the use of venous compression maneuvers, incompetence of the venous valves can be observed with the maneuvers used and discussed with CW Doppler studies. A reflux time of more than 1.0 seconds is considered abnormal with routine compression maneuvers.[26] As a result of the very precise visualization capable with duplex scanning, evaluation of the perforating veins can even be performed. Of note, incompetent communicating veins can be seen on duplex scanning in approximately two-thirds of patients with lipodermatosclerosis or venous ulcers.[26] When duplex imaging is used in combination with plethysmographic methods, a quantitative and qualitative assessment of the venous system can be achieved with surprising anatomic detail.

Ascending venography has the same purpose in the venous system as arteriography has for arterial disease. It allows for precise anatomic visualization of the entire venous system providing a road map for anticipated surgical procedures. It is performed by placing an

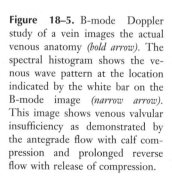

Figure 18–5. B-mode Doppler study of a vein images the actual venous anatomy *(bold arrow)*. The spectral histogram shows the venous wave pattern at the location indicated by the white bar on the B-mode image *(narrow arrow)*. This image shows venous valvular insufficiency as demonstrated by the antegrade flow with calf compression and prolonged reverse flow with release of compression.

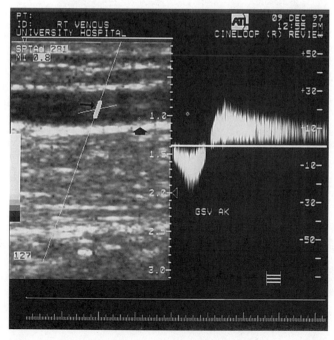

intravenous catheter into a foot vein and injecting contrast dye to fill the venous system. Occasionally during evaluation, the deep system does not fill with contrast dye. This may indicate DVT (Fig. 18–6). However, the placement of tourniquets at the ankle and thigh may help force the contrast agent into the deep system rather than passing only through the superficial veins. The deep veins may be damaged from previous disease rather than from acute thrombosis and the contrast had simply preferentially flowed into the superficial veins prior to the use of tourniquets.

Descending venography is used to detect valvular incompetence and is generally only obtained when surgical intervention is planned. This study is performed by entering another vein in the body (i.e., brachial or contralateral femoral vein) and advancing a catheter to the common femoral vein. This study is then performed in two stages.[27] The initial stage injects contrast material when the patient is at rest and in a semi-erect position with the weight of the patient on the opposite leg. The contrast material is heavier than blood and gently refluxes down the leg, outlining any valves that may be present (Fig. 18–7A).

The second part of the procedure is performed by injection of contrast dye while the patient performs a Valsalva maneuver. Competent valves will prevent reflux of blood down the leg (Fig. 18–7B), whereas incompetence allows reflux down the leg. Reflux is considered pathologic if blood reaches the calf veins in the second stage of the study. The presence or absence of valves has surgical implications. The risks of venography include skin necrosis with extravasation of contrast dye, renal failure from the contrast dye, thrombophlebitis, pulmonary embolus, and allergic reaction to the contrast agent, to mention some of the more common or life-threatening problems.[3]

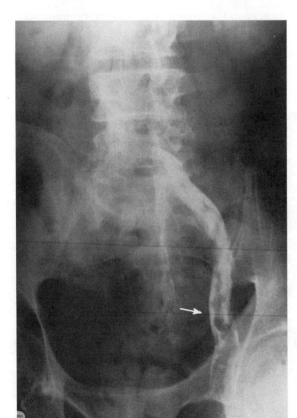

Figure 18–6. A venogram demonstrating deep venous thrombosis of the left common iliac vein. The lumen of the vein is only partially occluded and the thrombus is apparent as areas of the vein not filled with white contrast material (*arrow*).

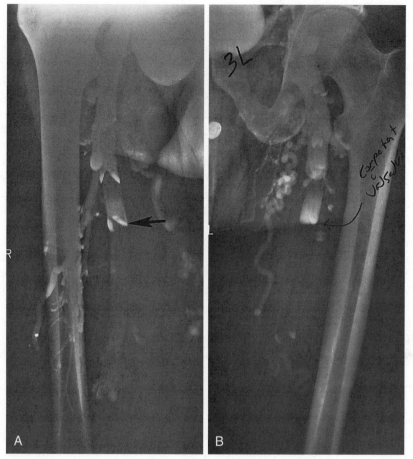

Figure 18–7. Descending venogram with and without Valsalva maneuver. **A,** A picture of the presence of valves in the superficial femoral vein on quiet standing (see *arrow* showing one such valve). **B,** One of the proximal venous valves is competent as the patient performs a Valsalva maneuver.

TREATMENT OPTIONS AND RESULTS

Conservative Medical Therapy

Despite all the advances in modern medicine and in surgical technique, the primary therapy for chronic venous disease has remained unchanged over several decades. The main goals are to treat symptoms and restore as much normal physiologic function to the diseased limb as possible. For conservative therapy to be successful, the full cooperation of the patient is required.[28] Often these measures are uncomfortable or difficult to perform during the normal activities of living. These measures include wearing good-quality compressive stockings (graded 30–40 mmHg at the ankle),[29] elevating the legs whenever possible during the day, avoiding prolonged periods of standing, elevating the foot of the bed 4–6 inches, and applying medicated bandages to ulcerations.[12] Patients must have adequate counseling to perform these tasks well. Elevating the feet does not mean propping them up on the coffee table while sitting to watch TV. The legs must be elevated above the level of the heart for this measure to be effective.

Sclerotherapy

In the event that these conservative measures are unsuccessful or if conservative surgical therapy is potentially curative, it should be considered. Sclerotherapy (needle injection of caustic solutions directly into the vein) has been advocated for the treatment of small varicosities that remain after saphenous vein stripping, small individual varicosities, and telangiectases in the thigh and around the knee. In general, it appears appropriate for patients not afflicted with major superficial, perforator, or deep venous disease. Sclerosing agents such as sodium tetradecyl sulfate or hypertonic saline can be caustic when injected but do eliminate the venous lesions as a result of scar formation. Patients may complain of burning, stinging, or itching upon injection. If there is extravasation of the agent, fat or skin necrosis, ulcerations, and/or hyperpigmentation of the surrounding skin may result. The posttreatment veins are often a brown color as opposed to the blue-red pretreatment color.

Potential complications of sclerotherapy (Table 18–2) include allergic reactions to the sclerosing agent, and toxicity can occur if too many veins are treated (too much sclerosing agent injected) at one setting.[13] Although the immediate postsurgical results are very satisfactory to most patients, the procedure often must be repeated if the larger diseased veins underlying each telangiectasia or small varicosity are not eliminated. Major venous insufficiency, if present, must be surgically managed to prevent recurrence following sclerotherapy.[30, 31]

Venous Bypass

If less invasive measures fail, more aggressive surgical procedures are available for obstructive venous disease. The procedures of cross-femoral venous bypass, saphenofemoral bypass, iliac vein decompression, and inferior vena cava reconstruction have been used to bypass particular obstructed segments of the venous system. Recently, endovascular stenting of certain veins has improved the symptoms of venous occlusive disease.[32] To ensure success after venous reconstruction, it is imperative that the proper patient be selected. Direct venous measurements are thus required to determine which patients are appropriate candidates for surgery and which are not.[18]

These surgical procedures use either native saphenous vein or a piece of polytetrafluoroethylene (PTFE) graft material as the conduit to bypass a nondiseased distal vein to a

TABLE 18–2. **Complications of Sclerotherapy**

ALLERGIC REACTION	TOXICITY
Minor itching	Thirst
Swelling of the lips and tongue	Shivering
Bronchospasm	Headache
Skin blotching	Chest pain
Cardiovascular collapse	Epigastric pain

TREATMENT FOR THESE COMPLICATIONS
Antihistamines
Hydration
Epinephrine
Oxygen
Limit volume of agent injected

disease-free proximal vein. Vena caval reconstructions have been performed and use PTFE grafts as the material of choice because of the lack of comparably sized native vein. Again, venous pressure studies must be obtained to document venous hypertension that would be amenable to vena caval bypass.[18] Iliac vein decompression is utilized in the instance of extrinsic compression by the overlying right iliac artery. If the iliac vein is severely stenosed or occluded, cross-femoral bypass can be performed, but the procedure of choice is direct repair of the involved segment of iliac vein.

The indications for cross-femoral venous bypass include persistent unilateral iliac or common femoral venous occlusion in young patients, patients with subacute onset of progressive leg swelling due to extrinsic compression not amenable to direct surgical cure, and patients with threatened limb loss due to phlegmasia cerulea dolens where thrombectomy or thrombolysis has failed. If compression is due to a neoplastic growth, patient survival should be considered prior to aggressive surgical intervention. The cross-femoral venous bypass operation for proximal iliac or common femoral vein obstruction is performed by gently passing the graft material through a suprapubic subcutaneous tunnel. The saphenous vein or prosthetic graft is then connected to each undiseased femoral vein by an end-to-side technique. The key to the success of this surgery is graft diameter. If the native vein is less than 5–6 mm in diameter, better success will be achieved with an 8-mm diameter PTFE graft.[18] An arteriovenous fistula can be created to increase flow and to improve graft patency in the immediate postoperative period. This fistula can be ligated in 1–3 months if desired.

Indications for a saphenopopliteal bypass are isolated femoral and/or popliteal vein occlusion. In addition, the common femoral and iliocaval system must be patent, a nonvaricosed saphenous vein must exist, and femoral phlebitis must be inactive for 1 year. Finally, conservative therapy to relieve chronic venous disease symptoms must have failed, and abnormal venous pressures of the diseased leg must be present. The procedure uses autogenous vein as the conduit and bypasses extend from distal to proximal nondiseased segments.

Vein Stripping

In the face of superficial venous insufficiency, stripping of superficial varicosities can be employed. This operation should not be performed if deep venous obstruction is a significant component of the patient's problems because the superficial veins may be the only outflow for venous blood. However, it should be considered in cases of combined deep and superficial insufficiency.[33] Vein stripping includes ligation of the greater saphenous vein at the saphenofemoral junction in addition to vein avulsion. Preoperatively, with the patient standing to fully dilate the veins, the varicosities are marked with a permanent marker (see Fig. 18–3) to allow for intraoperative identification of the collapsed veins when the patient is supine. Two incisions are made to define the proximal (groin incision) and distal (ankle incision) extent of the greater saphenous vein in the leg. The saphenofemoral junction is dissected in the groin and all the branches are ligated. A thin, flexible wire (the vein stripper) is placed up the lumen of the saphenous vein from the ankle (Fig. 18–8A) to the groin and secured proximally at the saphenofemoral junction, which is flush ligated with the common femoral vein (Fig. 18–8B). A third incision approximately 6 cm below the knee is made, and the stripper is advanced to this third incision. A second stripper is placed from the ankle and secured at the below-knee incision. The vein stripping device is then briskly removed in a caudad direction, from groin to knee, thereby pulling the vein out of the leg. The distal end of the saphenous vein is removed in a similar fashion through the ankle incision. Small incisions are then made over the previously marked varicosities (Fig. 18–9). The veins are grasped and removed in long segments with a hemostat or other small instrument. Compressive

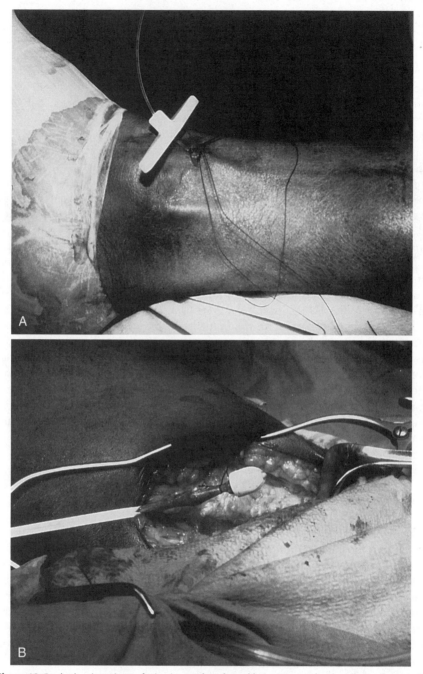

Figure 18–8. A, A vein stripper device inserted at the ankle incision with a handle in place to aid in extracting the vein. **B,** A vein stripper device protruding from the greater saphenous vein at the saphenofemoral junction with cap placed prior to vein removal.

stockings or an elastic bandage are applied in the immediate postoperative period to prevent hematoma formation. Patients are able to resume any activities as tolerated but should avoid prolonged periods of standing or heavy lifting for several weeks.

There are both temporary and definite contraindications to performing a vein stripping procedure (Table 18–3). Complications of vein stripping are rare but include wound infection, DVT, nerve damage, and hematoma formation, to mention the most prominent. Saphenous nerve injury can result in an area of numbness on the lateral foot.[13] Among

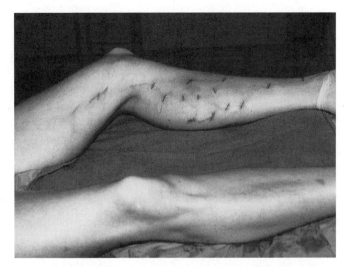

Figure 18–9. The lower leg after completion of a vein stripping procedure with incisions closed. Note the multiple small incisions along previously marked varicosities that were required to remove branches of the greater saphenous vein not extracted by the stripping device.

properly selected patients, recurrent saphenous varicosities will be noted in less than 15 percent of cases.[34] The lesser saphenous vein can be stripped if needed with similar results. Damage to the sural nerve must be prevented during this procedure.

Perforator Vein Ligation

Ligation of perforating veins can be effective treatment for patients with perforating vein incompetence. This can be performed in conjunction with saphenous vein removal. Perforating vein ligation can be performed by an open procedure with direct visualization of the offending veins or with endoscopic instruments. The Linton procedure utilizes an incision along the medial or posterior aspect of the leg and the creation of subfascial flaps. The perforating veins are directly ligated. If a skin ulcer is present, this can be removed simultaneously. If a large amount of soft tissue is affected, including the fascial layers, a skin graft can be placed to speed healing after the diseased tissues are removed.[35]

An angioscopic technique is used[36]; the knee is slightly flexed, and two small (15-mm) incisions are made on the medial aspect of the lower leg near the knee and proximal to areas of induration and inflammation. Subfascial dissection is performed using blunt, balloon, and/or sharp dissection. Some surgeons place a tourniquet on the upper leg to be inflated just prior to subfascial insufflation of carbon dioxide used to improve visualization. The tourniquet is used to prevent air embolus. Under direct enhanced vision with a

TABLE 18–3. **Contraindications to Vein Stripping**

TEMPORARY	DEFINITE
Recent deep thrombophlebitis	Significant arterial disease
Weeping ulcers	Chronic lymphedema
Active cellulitis	Noncorrectable systemic disease
Uncontrolled metabolic disease (i.e., diabetes)	Advanced age
Pregnancy	Bedridden patient
Anemia	
Poor health	

video camera, the perforating veins are clipped with silver clips and then divided. Some physicians have utilized mediastinoscopes through which a long clip applier can be advanced, obviating the need for a second incision. Once all of the vessels have been ligated, the instruments are removed and the incisions closed. Elastic bandages are placed, and the patients are allowed to ambulate the same day.[37] Many surgeons mark the perforating veins preoperatively during duplex evaluation to assure that all offending veins are identified at the time of surgery.

Venous Ulcer Management

Regarding the treatment of venous ulcers, the goals of therapy are twofold: to heal the ulcer and to prevent ulcer recurrence. As with all chronic venous disease, elevation and compression to control edema are paramount to therapy. Conservative therapy with Unna boot application, wet-to-dry dressings, and medicated creams can be attempted. The Unna boot (Fig. 18–10) is a dressing composed of a gauze moistened with zinc oxide and calamine lotion containing glycerin. The boot is applied circumferentially and when dry provides even compression to the damaged skin. Care must be taken not to compromise the circulation by applying the boot too tightly. A compressive bandage (i.e., Ace wrap) is placed over the boot to provide even more compressive support. The boot will need to be changed from twice a week to once every 2 weeks, depending upon the amount of ulcer drainage. Its use must be discontinued if signs of infection develop such as erythema, purulent drainage, warmth, or pain.

Ulcers that have more copious amounts of drainage require more frequent dressing changes or the use of a hydrocolloid dressing.[11] Such hydrocolloid and hydrogel dressings (i.e., Alginate, Sorbsan) are able to absorb many times their weight in discharge fluid. Therefore, these dressings can stay in place longer while maintaining a drier environment for the ulcer and surrounding tissues. With the proper patient selection, successful ulcer healing is generally achieved.[13]

For the recalcitrant or recurrent venous ulcers, skin grafting is an option. These lesions

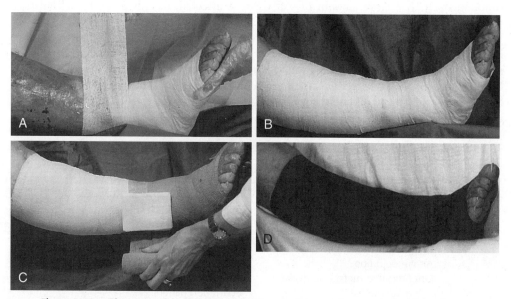

Figure 18–10. Placement of an Unna boot. **A,** Venous ulcers are first wrapped with gauze or a medicated dressing. **B,** Lower leg completely wrapped with gauze. **C,** An extra dressing is placed over the site of the venous ulcer. **D,** An elastic bandage is placed around the entire lower extemity for uniform circumferential compression.

can be extensive, and skin grafting allows for coverage of raw surfaces, thereby speeding the healing process. Once the ulcer has a base of granulation tissue, a split-thickness skin graft can be applied. Skin grafting should be performed only if healing of the ulcer has not occurred with diligent conservative management.

Venous Valve Repair or Replacement

Valve repair and reconstruction can be performed for primary venous valvular incompetence (Fig. 18–11). Valve operations are performed only for end-stage disease symptoms because of the perceived high risk of venous operations. These operations attempt to restore the original anatomic position of the valve cusps so that normal function is possible. A variety of open techniques have been described. The vein is opened so that the valve cusps are visible and using fine Prolene sutures, the cusps are tightened such that they may oppose properly.

Angioscopy can be used to direct the valvuloplasty repair while avoiding the need to open the vein itself. The scope is placed through a side branch and is advanced until the incompetent valve is in view. Again, one or more fine Prolene sutures are used to shore the valve cusps. There may be advantages to the angioscopic technique when compared with the open procedure, which may include decreased operative time, direct visualization of competency of the valves at the time of surgery, and less venous trauma.[35]

These procedures are not without risks, however, which include wound hematoma, wound infection, lymphatic leaks, thrombosis of repaired vein, and recurrent reflux.[38] Long-term results have demonstrated that 70 percent of patients can achieve clinical success with confirmed valve competence following valve repair procedures.[39]

Finally, the use of a transposition procedure or venous valve transplantation has been attempted in patients with complete damage of the venous valves in their lower limb. No valve cusps are present in the lower leg to repair, and therefore more inventive approaches are required. The transposition procedure requires the presence of a competent valve in

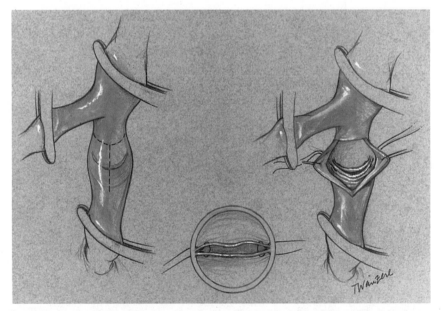

Figure 18–11. An artist's depiction of a venous valve repair in a patient with primary venous valvular incompetency. The vein has been opened and sutures are placed to tighten the valve for proper functioning.

some part of the lower extremity venous system that can be used to provide reflux protection for the incompetent system. The incompetent venous system (often the superficial femoral vein) is ligated proximally and the distal vein is sewn in a position below the available competent valve. This may be applicable in only 2–3 percent of potential patient candidates.[40]

Venous valve transplantation requires finding a competent valve in the upper extremity (or one that can be made competent) and then transplanting it into the lower leg venous system (Fig. 18–12). The valve must be transplanted below all pathologic reflux to be effective. The upper extremity valve is usually obtained from the axillary venous system. The major obstacle to this technique has been the absence of a functional upper extremity valve (40 percent of cases)[40] or incompetence of the transplanted valve over time.[41, 42] Clinically, however, approximately 60 percent of patients severely disabled prior to surgery have been clinically helped for more than 5 years with this approach.[43] There are currently investigations into a valve substitute that might provide an option for patients lacking an appropriate upper extremity venous valve for transplantation.[44]

SUMMARY

Although chronic venous disease symptoms have been documented for centuries, management has not changed dramatically for many years. The mainstays of therapy include elevation and compression to reduce tissue edema. When one or more of the complications of venous disease does occur such as varicose veins, ulcerations, or venous claudication, the most conservative yet effective measures should be attempted first. If these are to no avail, there are several operative therapies available that have been shown to be effective in properly selected patients.

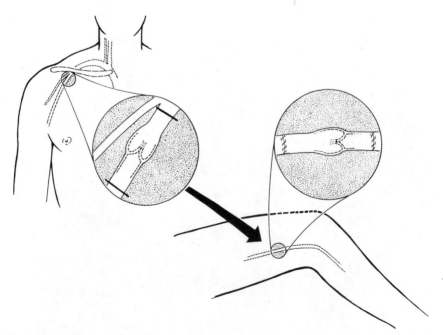

Figure 18–12. The transplantation of a venous valve from the upper arm to the lower leg provides for reflux protection to the lower leg in a patient who otherwise will have no competent valves in the lower leg.

NURSING IMPLICATIONS

Varicose Veins

Patient education should include an explanation of the function of the veins and valves. The patient should be taught the cause of varicose veins as well as preventive measures and should be further informed about recommended treatment as discussed below.

Injection Therapy

A complete health history, including a list of current medications, drug allergies, and hypersensitivities, is obtained from the patient. The patient is advised to avoid platelet-inhibiting drugs for 1 week before treatment. Patients with known cardiac valvular disease should be treated with oral antibiotics.

The procedure and possible adverse effects should be fully explained to the patient. The patient should be told that multiple leg injection bruises will appear 2 to 3 days after treatment and that the legs will look worse before they look better. The patient should be warned of the potential adverse effects, including hyperpigmentation, multiple superficial thrombi, ulceration, nodular fibroses, and blush-mat effects. A consent form should be obtained. Posttreatment instructions should be provided to the patient on discharge as follows:

Activity. Limit vigorous activities such as aerobics, racquet sports, biking, or running for 72 hours. Walking briskly for 30 minutes after treatment is recommended and is thought to enhance the effect of sclerosant agents injected into the veins. It may also decrease the risk of deep venous thrombosis.

Elastic Stockings. Ankle-to-thigh compression dressings should be worn for 72 hours to 3 weeks, depending on the physician's discretion. Prescription compression stockings or elastic wrap bandages may be used. If elastic wrap bandages are used, care must be taken to rewrap as necessary to maintain firm compression. The patient should be taught to wrap the elastic bandage, beginning at the foot and ending at the thigh.

Bathing. The initial compression dressing may be removed so that the patient can bathe only at a designated time to be determined by the physician. This time may vary from 24 hours to 3 days after injection. It must be reapplied promptly after bathing for best results.

Skin Care. Bruising near areas of injection is expected and is usually resolved within 2 weeks. Small, firm, tender, greenish blue nodular areas may also result after sclerotherapy. These are areas of superficial thrombosis and are easily evacuated when the skin is pierced with a large-bore needle and the thrombus is expressed. If untreated, the thrombus will eventually be reabsorbed but will often leave a brownish discoloration of the skin, which may persist for up to 1 year or longer. If the skin is damaged sufficiently, a superficial ulcer may develop that is treated with antibiotic ointments, bandages, and time. The skin will essentially heal but a scar may remain.

Vein Stripping or Perforator Ligation Operation

Preoperative teaching should include an explanation of the function of the veins and valves, information regarding causes of varicose veins, preoperative and postoperative routines, and potential discoloration, bruising, leg swelling, and discomfort after surgery.

The patient should be made aware of possible nerve injury. Operating room nurses should discuss with the surgeon any special equipment that may be needed.

Postoperative Care. Vital signs should be checked regularly. The nurse should monitor the patient for potential hemorrhage by checking leg dressings for excessive drainage. If bleeding is excessive, direct pressure should be applied over the wound, the leg should be elevated, and the surgeon should be notified. If bleeding is minimal, proper elastic support will control it. It is important to ascertain that the bandage is not applied so tightly as to compromise the circulation.

Elastic bandages are applied to the affected leg to decrease hematoma formation and prevent postoperative edema secondary to disruption of perivenous lymphatic vessels that accompany the venous trunks in the lower extremity. When one considers that nearly all lymphatic trunks from the lower extremities are grouped around the long saphenous vein, it is surprising that edema is a rare complication.

Pedal pulses and sensory and motor function of the affected extremity should be checked every 2 hours for the first 8 hours. When the leg is in a dependent position, the patient should wear elastic support below the knee for 1–2 weeks. Leg swelling reduction can also be accomplished by raising the foot of the bed or by using a foam rubber block. Ambulation should be encouraged as soon as possible after surgery.

Venous Reconstruction or Venous Valvular Transplant Operations

An explanation of the procedure should be provided to the patient. As with all surgical procedures, a consent form should be obtained. Patients should be instructed that they will need to be up walking with support hose on the next day. They may have some swelling in the legs as well and will be required to elevate the legs as much as possible (i.e., at night and several times during the day).

Patients must be monitored carefully in the postoperative period for the development of surgical complications. These complications include hematoma formation, incisional bleeding, and swelling of the leg more than anticipated. Adequate compression that does not compromise the circulation will solve these problems, but if this measure is unsuccessful, the physician must be notified. Also, if an arteriovenous fistula was performed for patients undergoing venous bypass procedures, distal pulse checks must be performed to ensure adequate distal circulation. Again, any change in the pulses necessitates physician notification. Because these are major surgical procedures, routine postoperative monitoring, including respiratory, cardiac, and vital signs, must be carefully documented, and results not within standard parameters conveyed to the physician.

Venous Ulceration

Success in healing a venous ulcer can be achieved only if the patient is a ready and willing participant in the plan of care.[28] The patient needs to be educated about venous disease in order to make necessary adjustments in life-style to minimize the effects of the disease. Because the underlying problem in patients with venous ulceration is venous hypertension, nursing care is directed at reducing this high pressure. Efforts to accomplish this involve emphasizing the importance of bed rest, leg elevation, and external elastic support.

A complete assessment of the lower extremities should be performed at each visit, and any abnormalities or changes from baseline should be noted. Pedal pulses and motor/sensory function should be assessed. Thorough documentation of ulcer characteristics should be made at each dressing change to evaluate effectiveness of treatment. Ulcer

TABLE 18–4. **Guidelines for Patients with Venous Disease (With/Without Ulcers)**

HYGIENE

Check skin daily—keep in healthy condition.
- Watch for:
  - Cracking.
  - Breakdown.
  - Change in color/temperature.

If skin is dry use moisturizing lotion.
- Not for use on open wounds.

Wash daily
- Use mild soap.
- Lukewarm water (body temperature).
- Avoid soaking legs in tub.

Wear clean stockings daily.

Use antifungal powder in shoes if feet are moist.

Consult physician for any problems/ concerns.

With venous ulcers:
- Cover Unna boot prior to bathing.
- Sponge bathe to prevent dampening boot.

Prevent injury:
- Avoid bumping, cutting, bruising legs.
- Do not go barefoot.
- Avoid shaving legs with razors.
- Avoid using pillows under knees.
- Avoid:
  - Excess heat/cold.
  - Harsh chemicals.
  - Hair remover creams.
- Test bath water with hands not toes.

ACTIVITY

Exercise regularly
- Even in bed with foot flexing.
- Swimming is good exercise.
  - Not with Unna boot on.
- Walking.
- Cycling.

Avoid excess activity that makes legs swell.

No long periods of standing/sitting.
- If must, leg movement helps.

Automobile trips.
- Stop every 2 hrs to exercise legs.

Leg elevation.
- Decreases swelling.
- Several times a day for 10–15 min.
- Always at night by 6 inches.
  - Blocks under foot of bed.

Elastic support
- Always wear stocking while awake.
- Apply first thing in the morning.
- Wash with mild soap and reuse.
- Discard when elasticity is lost.
- If using elastic bandages:
  - Wrap from toe to below knee.
  - Overlap edges.
  - Wrap snugly.

GENERAL

No smoking.

Nutrition
- Well-balanced diet.
- Reduce sodium.
  - ↓ fluid retention.
- Avoid overeating
  - ↓ weight on legs.
- High-fiber diet.
  - ↓ straining with bowel movement.
  - ↓ pressure on veins.
  - Main sources:
    - Raw fruits.
    - Vegetables.
      - Corn.
      - Celery.
      - Beans.
    - Whole grains.

Clothing
- No constricting garments.
- Wear well-fitting shoes.
- Always wear socks with shoes.
  - Prevents blisters.
- Slowly break in new shoes.
- If feet are swollen:
  - Wear slipper or wide shoe.
- Regular shoe and sock should fit over Unna boot.

TABLE 18–5. **Medical Follow-Up:**
What The Physician
Needs to Know

Sudden weight gain or swelling of the feet, ankles, or legs.
Increase or decrease in temperature of the leg.
Unusual color, amount, or odor of drainage from the wound.
Increase in inflammation, redness, tenderness, or pain in the leg.
Inability to move the legs without pain.
The color of the foot becomes pale.
Skin breakdown occurs.
Fever > 100° F.

characteristics to note include size, condition of granulation tissue, color, odor, consistency and amount of drainage, and condition of the limb (i.e., swelling, redness, warmth, and amount and character of pain). Signs of infection at any time or unsatisfactory progress in ulcer healing within 2 to 3 weeks of treatment necessitate re-evaluation of the patient's treatment regimen. Concurrent medical problems (such as congestive heart failure, lymphedema, malnutrition, and diabetes) must be controlled to afford optimal healing. Providing patients with the guidelines listed in Table 18–4 for proper care may help ensure compliance with prescribed therapy.

Periodic medical check-ups are necessary; all scheduled appointments should be kept. The doctor should be notified if any of the problems listed in Table 18–5 occur. Furthermore, the patients should be encouraged to call the physician with any questions.

References

1. Browse NL, Burnand KG, Thomas ML: Diseases of the Veins: Pathology, Diagnosis, and Treatment. London, Edward Arnold, 1988.
2. Nehler MR, Moneta GL: The lower extremity venous system. Part I: Anatomy and normal physiology. Perspect Vasc Surg 1991; 4:104–116.
3. LaBerge JM, Callen PW: Tutorial 17: Diagnosis of deep venous thrombosis. In Tretotola SO, Savaders SJ, Durham JD (eds): Venous Interventions. Fairfax, The Society of Cardiovascular and Interventional Radiologists, 1995, pp 190–201.
4. Gourdin FW, Smith JG Jr: Etiology of venous ulceration. S Med J 1993; 86:1142–1146.
5. Cockett FB, Thomas ML: The iliac compression syndrome. Br J Surg 1965; 52:816–821.
6. Cockett FB, Thomas ML, Negus D: Iliac Vein Compression—Its relation to iliofemoral thrombosis and the post-thrombotic syndrome. BMJ 1967; 2:14–19.
7. McMurrich JP: The occurrence of congenital adhesions in the common iliac veins, and their relation to thrombosis of the femoral and iliac veins. Am J Med Sci 1908; 135:342–346.
8. Plate G, Brodin L, Eklof B, et al: Physiologic and therapeutic aspects in congenital vein valve aplasia of the lower limb. Ann Surg 1983; 198:229–233.
9. Rose SS, Ahmed A: Some thoughts on the aetiology of varicose veins. J Cardiovasc Surg 1986; 27:534–543.
10. Clarke H, Smith SR, Vasdekis SN, et al: Role of venous elasticity in the development of varicose veins. Br J Surg 1989; 76:577–580.
11. O'Donnell JF Jr: Chronic venous insufficiency: An overview of epidemiology, classification, and anatomic considerations. Semin Vasc Surg 1988; 1:60–65.
12. Nicolaides AN, Hussein MK, Szendro G, et al: The relation of venous ulceration with ambulatory venous pressure measurements. J Vasc Surg 1993; 17:414–419.
13. Dale WA, Cranley JJ, DeWeese JA, et al: Symposium: Management of varicose veins. Contemp Surg 1975; 6:86–124.
14. Lalka, SG: Management of chronic obstructive venous disease of the lower extremity. In Rutherford RB (ed): Vascular Surgery, 4th ed, Vol II. Philadelphia, WB Saunders, 1995, pp 1862–1882.
15. Browse, NL, Burnand, KG: The Cause of Venous Ulceration. Lancet 1982; 2:243–245.
16. Falanga V, Eaglstein, WH: The "trap" hypothesis of venous ulceration. Lancet 1993; 341:1006–1008.

17. Smith PDC, Scurr JH: Current views on the pathogenesis of venous ulceration. In Bergan JJ, Yao JST (eds): Venous Disorders. Philadelphia, WB Saunders, 1991, pp 36–51.
18. Lalka SG, Malone JM: Surgical management of chronic obstructive venous disease of the lower extremity. Semin Vasc Surg 1988; 1:113–123.
19. Dalsing MC: Tutorial 20: Venous valvular insufficiency: Pathophysiology and treatment options. In Tretotola SO, Savaders SJ, Durham JD (eds): Venous Interventions. Fairfax, The Society of Cardiovascular and Interventional Radiologists, 1995, pp 225–238.
20. Killewich LA, Martin R, Cramer M, et al: Pathophysiology of Venous Claudication. J Vasc Surg 1984; 1:507–511.
21. Labropoulos N, Volteas M, Leon M, et al: The role of venous outflow obstruction in patients with chronic venous dysfunction. Arch Surg 1997; 132:46–51.
22. Raju S: New approaches to the diagnosis and treatment of venous obstruction. J Vasc Surg 1986; 4:42.
23. Bays RA, Healy DA, Atnip RG, et al: Validation of air plethysmography, photoplethysmography, and duplex ultrasonography in the evaluation of severe venous stasis. J Vasc Surg 1994; 20:721–727.
24. Araki CT, Back TL, Meyers MG, Hobson RW II: Indirect noninvasive tests (plethysmography). In Gloviczki P, Yao JST (eds): Handbook of Venous Disorders. London, Chapman & Hall Medical, 1996, pp 97–111.
25. Belcaro G, Nicolaides AN, Veller M: Venous Disorders: A Manual of Diagnosis and Treatment. London, WB Saunders Co. Ltd, 1995.
26. Summer D: Direct noninvasive tests for the evaluation of chronic venous obstruction and valvular incompetence. In Gloviczki P, Yao, JST (eds): Handbook of Venous Disorders. London, Chapman & Hall Medical, 1996, pp 130–151.
27. Kistner RL, Feuier EB, Randhawn F, Kawida C: A method of performing descending venography. J Vasc Surg 1986; 4:464–468.
28. Erickson CA, Lanza DJ, Karp DL, et al: Healing of venous ulcers in an ambulatory care program: The roles of chronic venous insufficiency and patient compliance. J Vasc Surg 1995; 22:629–636.
29. Lentner, A, Wienert, V: Influence of medical compression stockings on venolymphatic drainage in phlebologically healthy test persons and patients with chronic venous insufficiency. Int J Microcirc Clin Exp 1996; 16:320–324.
30. Einarsson, E: Compression sclerotherapy of varicose veins. In Eklof B, Gjores JE, Thulesius O, Bergquist D. (eds): Controversies in the Management of Venous Disorders. London, Butterworths, 1989, pp 203–211.
31. Neglen P, Einarsson E, Eklof B: The functional long-term value of different types of treatment for saphenous vein incompetence. J Cardiovasc Surg 1993; 34:295–301.
32. Semba, CP: Tutorial 18: Percutaneous management of deep vein thrombosis. In Tretotola SO, Savaders SJ, Durham JD (eds): Venous Interventions. Fairfax, The Society of Cardiovascular and Interventional Radiologists, 1995, pp 202–213.
33. Padberg FT Jr, Pappas PJ, Araki CT, et al: Hemodynamic and clinical improvement after superficial vein ablation in primary combined venous insufficiency with ulceration. J Vasc Surg 1997; 26:169–171.
34. Larson RA, Toftgren EP, Myers TT, et al: Long-term results after vein surgery: Study of 1000 cases after 10 years. Mayo Clin Proc 1974; 49:114.
35. Rodriguez AA, O'Donnell TF Jr. Reconstructions for valvular incompetence of the deep veins. In Gloviczki P, Yao, JST (eds): Handbook of Venous Disorders. London, Chapman & Hall Medical, 1996, pp 434–445.
36. Gloviczki P, Bergan JJ, Menawat SS, et al: Safety, feasibility, and early efficacy of subfascial endoscopic perforator surgery: A preliminary report from the North American registry. J Vasc Surg 1997; 25:94–105.
37. Sullivan TR Jr, O'Donnell TF Jr: Endoscopic division of incompetent perforating veins. In Gloviczki P, Yao JST (eds): Handbook of Venous Disorders. London, Chapman & Hall Medical, 1996, pp 482–493.
38. Kistner RL, Eklof B, Masuda EM: Deep venous valve reconstruction. Cardiovasc Surg 1995; 3:129–140.
39. Masuda EM, Kistner RL: Long-term results of venous valve reconstruction: A four- and twenty-one-year follow-up. J Vasc Surg 1994; 19:391–403.
40. Raju S: Venous insufficiency of the lower limb and stasis ulceration. Changing concepts and management. Ann Surg 1983; 197:688–697.
41. Raju S, Fredericks R: Valve reconstruction procedures for non-obstructive venous insuficiency: Rationale, techniques, and results in 107 procedures with two-to-eight year follow up. J Vasc Surg 1988; 7:301–310.
42. Bry JDL, Muto PA, O'Donnell TF, Isaacson LA: The clinical and hemodynamic results after axillary-to-popliteal vein valve transplantation. J Vasc Surg 1995; 21:110–119.
43. Raju S, Fredericks RK, Neglen PN, Bass JD: Durability of venous valve reconstruction techniques for "primary" and postthrombotic reflux. J Vasc Surg 1996; 23:357–367.
44. Burkhart HM, Fath SW, Dalsing MC, et al: Experimental repair of venous valvular insufficiency using a cryopreserved venous valve allograft aided by a distal arteriovenous fistula. J Vasc Surg 1997; 26:817–822.

PART FIVE

SPECIFIC PROBLEMS

19

Vascular Access Surgery

Joan Jacobsen, RN, MSN, CVN

⧸⧹ · ⧸⧹

Nurses have a unique role in the management of vascular access, including prevention of complications, patient education, and maintenance of access. Nurses collaborate with members of other disciplines involved in the care of individuals requiring vascular access. These individuals often include vascular surgeons, interventional radiologists, pharmacists, nephrologists, and oncologists.

This chapter discusses two major areas: access for dialysis and vascular access devices. Dialysis access focuses on hemodialysis treatment for the patient experiencing renal failure. Vascular access devices that have their tips in the central vena cava are discussed. The chapter excludes discussion of peripheral intravenous access intended for short-term duration. This chapter emphasizes the adult patient population with special consideration of children addressed as appropriate. Nursing management of both dialysis access and venous access devices is also discussed.

ACCESS FOR DIALYSIS

Treatment of Renal Failure

Hemodialysis is the most commonly employed modality of therapy for patients with end-stage renal disease (ESRD).[1] Elders are the fastest growing age group within the ESRD population. The incidence rate for those 65 years of age and older exceeded 800 cases per million compared with 300 cases per million in those younger than age 65.[2] ESRD is generally characterized by an insidious deterioration in renal function, allowing for advanced planning to obtain long-term vascular access for the provision of hemodialysis. However, the presence of certain physiologic abnormalities may necessitate emergency dialysis. Trauma patients may be treated with continuous arteriovenous hemofiltration. Continuous arteriovenous hemofiltration is performed via large-bore arterial and venous catheters, usually in the femoral vessels.[3] This bedside modality is used to treat patients with refractory fluid overload, complicated acute renal failure, and acid-base and electrolyte derangements, and for those in whom conventional hemodialysis is contraindicated.[4]

Planning for Dialysis Access

Vascular access surgery is often performed well in advance of its anticipated need, allowing 6–12 weeks for adequate dilation and thickening of the vein wall before the fistula is cannulated. Preoperative assessment involves careful evaluation of upper extremity pulses and venous anatomy (Table 19–1). Efforts should be made to preserve the access vessels primarily by avoiding venipuncture in the nondominant arm beginning in the earliest stages of renal failure. Iatrogenic destruction of suitable peripheral veins in a hospital environment reduces the possibility of a successful placement of an autogenous arteriovenous (AV) fistula at the wrist, which is the procedure of choice. Approximately one-half of patients referred for primary access procedures should be suitable for direct fistula at the wrist if these vessels have been preserved.[5]

In devising a strategy for long-term hemodialysis access, one must consider not only the complexity and patency of the procedure but also its potential impact on a future access procedure.[6] Lack of vascular access is a major contributing factor in up to 25 percent of all ESRD patients who die annually in the United States.[1] As a general principle, distal sites are selected first, providing a long vein segment for cannulation and preserving proximal sites for future access procedures. The chosen site should allow for ease of access for cannulation and should be positioned so as to assure patient comfort during hemodialysis.[5]

Maintenance of adequate vascular access requires the prospective identification of anatomic lesions that result in access thrombosis, the most common cause of failure with access fistula.[7] Before creating a radiocephalic fistula, the radial and ulnar pulses are palpated. Doppler systolic pressures at the wrist are obtained if the surgeon remains uncertain as to their adequacy. In addition, the Allen test is performed to ascertain the ability of the ulnar artery to perfuse the hand if the radial artery should thrombose or be ligated subsequent to fistula creation. Careful preoperative evaluation of the potential collateral circulation of the limb is done to predict and prevent ischemia; such evaluation is especially crucial with the diabetic and peripheral vascular disease (PVD) population.[8]

Primary Arteriovenous Fistulae

A primary AV fistula directly connects, via an anastomosis, an artery and a vein.[9] The autogenous AV fistula remains the standard method of achieving long-term vascular access for hemodialysis purposes. Best results are achieved by anastomosing the radial artery to the cephalic vein at the wrist (known as the Brescia-Cimino fistula). Preferences for the radiocephalic fistula are based on factors such as superior long-term patency rates, lower incidence and ease of managing infectious complications, and a decreased incidence of other complications such as aneurysm formation.[10]

Lack of a suitable native vessel limits the creation of a primary AV fistula. As the proportion of elderly and diabetic patients entering hemodialysis centers increases, the proportion of patients with arterial and venous anatomy suitable for endogenous fistula consruction has decreased.[7] Constructing a Brescia-Cimino wrist fistula may be precluded by the presence of atherosclerotic changes in the radial artery, thrombosis of the cephalic vein, or a cephalic vein that is small, fragile, or too thin walled to adequately mature and

TABLE 19–1. **Planning for Hemodialysis Access**

Preservation of primary access vessels	Allen test
Impact on future access procedures	Collateral circulation evaluation
Radial and ulnar pulse assessment	

sustain multiple needle punctures. In the geriatric population, superficial veins become more tortuous and the incidence of atherosclerosis increases, making vascular access more difficult to achieve and maintain once hemodialysis is initiated and the access is cannulated.[2]

Other anatomic possibilities for direct fistulae include connecting the ulnar artery to basilic vein and brachial artery to basilic or cephalic vein (Table 19–2). The latter provides a long segment of vein for cannulation and is a reasonable site for primary access if the forearm vessels are unsuitable. The brachial artery to the basilic or cephalic vein also offers an ideal option after late failure of a forearm fistula. Patency rates of these veins compare with or are superior to those used for radiocephalic fistulae.

Rivers and colleagues described a technique for transposing the basilic vein, which usually lies deep in the upper arm, and anastomosing it to the brachial artery via an anterolateral tunnel for easy and safe cannulation.[6] The reported cumulative 49 percent patency rate at 30 months is comparable to the primary patency of wrist fistulae and secondary patency of polytetrafluoroethylene (PTFE) grafts. For patients lacking any suitable superficial veins, the dialysis access choice is generally between a transposed autologous vein and the placement of a prosthetic graft. Rivers and colleagues stated that basilic vein transposition has been an underused autologous alternative to prosthetic dialysis angioaccess.[6]

If no upper-extremity vessels are suitable for access, use of a lower-extremity fistula is possible. However, because of a significantly higher complication rate (most notably infection), lower-extremity fistulae are of little value except for young children or for patients in whom repeated infections preclude use of the upper extremities.

Surgical Procedure

Venous anatomy is assessed by observation and manual palpation or by engorging veins using a tourniquet or blood pressure cuff inflated below systolic pressure. Once the veins are adequately visualized, they are marked with an indelible pen to facilitate their location in the operating room. Local anesthesia is often sufficient for creating a fistula at the wrist or antecubital fossa. If a more proximal procedure is anticipated, brachial or axillary nerve block or general anesthesia is used.

In the operating room, the entire arm is prepared, allowing for use of a more proximal artery and vein if the distal vessels are inadequate. The skin is incised and the artery and vein are localized. Various anastomotic connections between vessels are possible (Fig. 19–1); in each, the artery and vein are surgically connected. Each type of anastomosis has inherent advantages and disadvantages that are outlined in Table 19–3.

After the artery and vein are sutured and before the incision is closed, a thrill should be easily palpable over the anastomosis and within the proximal vein segment. The presence of a strong arterial pulse without a thrill suggests outflow obstruction in the vein that requires surgical correction to prevent fistula thrombosis. The proximal vein is

---

TABLE 19–2. **Primary Arteriovenous Fistula Sites**

Most Preferred Site
Radial artery to cephalic vein at wrist (Brescia-Cimino fistula)

Alternate Choices
Ulnar artery to basilic vein
Brachial artery to basilic or cephalic vein
Transposition of basilic vein to brachial artery

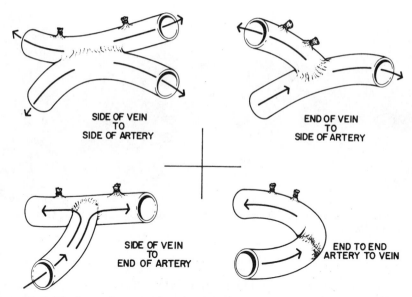

Figure 19–1. The four major types of arteriovenous anastomoses commonly constructed between the radial artery and the cephalic vein at the wrist. (Adapted from Fernanco ON: Arteriovenous fistulas by direct anastomosis. In Wilson SE, Owen ML [eds]: Vascular Access Surgery. Chicago, Year Book, 1980.)

inspected and may be probed with a Fogarty embolectomy catheter or carefully dilated. If attempts at correction do not produce a thrill, creation of another fistula is considered.

After surgical formation of a fistula, arterial pressure is transmitted directly into the adjoining vein, which dilates and develops a hypertrophied muscular wall amenable to repeated needle puncture (Fig. 19–2). This process, referred to as arterialization or maturation, typically occurs over 2 to 6 months.[7] Ideally, the fistula should not be used before 4 weeks of maturation because premature cannulation is often associated with hematoma formation and early thrombosis.[5]

Bridge Fistula

An AV shunt or bridge fistula communicates between an artery and vein resulting from a conduit anastomosed separately to each vessel.[9] A bridge fistula is considered when an autogenous fistula cannot be constructed or fails. Successful primary AV fistula in the

TABLE 19–3. **Types of Arteriovenous Anastomoses**

TYPE	ADVANTAGES	DISADVANTAGES
Side of artery to side of vein	Technically easiest to construct; highest flow rate	
End of artery to side of vein (ligation of distal artery)	Limited flow turbulence; less likelihood of arterial "steal"	Lower flow rate than side to side
Side of artery to end of vein (ligation of distal artery and vein)	Highest proximal venous flow; minimal distal venous tension	Technically more difficult to construct than other types of fistula
End of artery to end of vein (ligation of distal artery and vein)	Least likelihood of arterial "steal" and venous hypertension	Lowest flow rate of 4 types

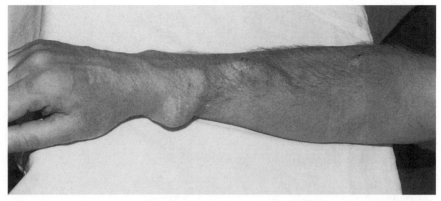

Figure 19–2. Photograph depicting mature, arterialized fistula. (Courtesy of James O. Mensoian, MD, Boston, MA.)

dominant arm is preferred over a synthetic graft bridge fistula in the nondominant arm. The patient population for bridge fistula is usually elderly and anemic (hematocrit of 20–25%), and up to 50 percent are diabetic.[1]

A bridge fistula can be formed between most superficial arteries and veins of acceptable size (Fig. 19–3). Arm placement of synthetic graft fistula is preferred, usually between the radial artery and the cephalic or basilic vein in the antecubital fossa. Placement is either done through a straight (distal radial artery to basilic vein) or loop (brachial artery to basilic vein) configuration. After insertion, bridge fistulae are easily palpated and punctured. However, use of a bridge fistula should be avoided for several weeks to allow the graft material to incorporate into surrounding tissues and to minimize the risk of extravasation from the graft when the needles are removed. A synthetic graft fistula may be used in 2 weeks. With new modifications in prosthetic PTFE manufacturing, cannulation can be done safely within the first 24 hours.[5] PTFE is the most commonly used material in construction of bridge fistulae. PTFE grafts are more prone to infection and thrombosis than endogenous AV fistulae.[7, 11] Patency rates of PTFE grafts at 1 year generally exceed 70 percent.[12]

Physiology of Arteriovenous Fistulae

The local, systemic, and hemodynamic effects of surgically created AV fistulae vary, depending on the nature of the fistula (i.e., acute versus chronic), the anatomic configuration, and location on the vascular tree (i.e., proximal versus distal vessels). With all fistulae, the direction of blood flow in the artery and vein proximal to the fistulous connection is normal. Most fistulae created for therapeutic use have a diameter greater than 75 percent of the proximal arterial lumen, resulting in backflow of the blood in the distal artery toward the fistula and retrograde flow in the distal vein away from the fistula. Venous hypertension may develop in the limb distal to the fistula because of this reversal in flow. In addition, as the fistula matures over the ensuing 4 to 6 weeks, the vein thickens and dilates, leading to valvular incompetence, further increasing distal venous pressure.

When a fistulous opening is created, there is a fall in peripheral vascular resistance (PVR) because arterial flow is shunted directly into a vein, bypassing the usual arteriole-capillary-venule circuit. This fall in PVR is compensated for by an increase in cardiac output that increases flow through the fistula. Although proximal venous outflow is also increased, significant central venous pressure elevation normally does not occur because of the large capacity of venous vessels. Flow rates in fistulae created between small-caliber

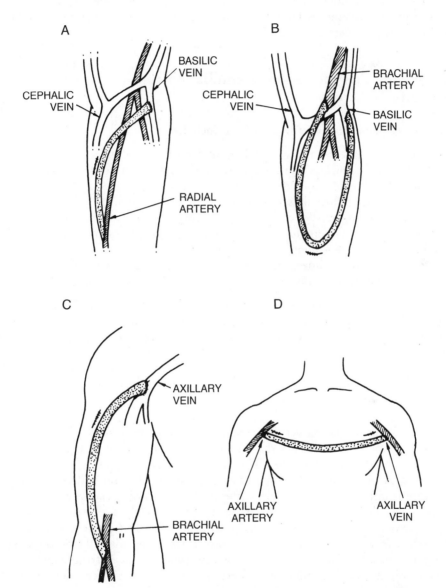

A

BASILIC
VEIN

CEPHALIC
VEIN

RADIAL
ARTERY

B

BRACHIAL
ARTERY

CEPHALIC
VEIN

BASILIC
VEIN

C

AXILLARY
VEIN

BRACHIAL
ARTERY

D

AXILLARY
ARTERY

AXILLARY
VEIN

Figure 19–3. Bridge fistulae of the upper extremity. **A,** Straight graft between radial artery and basilic vein. **B,** Loop graft between brachial artery and basilic vein. **C,** Straight graft between brachial artery and axillary vein. **D,** Straight graft between axillary artery and contralateral axillary vein. (From Bennion RS, Wilson SE: Hemodialysis and vascular access. In Moore WS [ed]: Vascular Surgery: A Comprehensive Review. Philadelphia, WB Saunders, 1991.)

arteries (i.e., radial, tibial) and adjacent veins vary from 150–600 ml/minute, whereas larger-caliber fistulae (i.e., axillary, femoral) have flow rates of 800–1600 ml/minute.[9]

In addition to these hemodynamic alterations, several histologic changes develop as a result of creating a fistula. The smooth muscle of the proximal artery hypertrophies, dilates, and elongates. With time, the muscle layer atrophies and the artery becomes aneurysmal. In the venous limb, smooth muscle and fibrous tissue increase. Eventually, the vein may develop atherosclerosis. The vein also elongates and continues to dilate for up to 8 months postoperatively.

Percutaneous Central Venous Cannulation for Hemodialysis Access

Indications for percutaneous catheter dialysis include:

1. acute renal failure requiring a limited number of treatments;
2. chronic renal failure in the immediate postoperative period after surgical creation of an internal fistula (to allow for "maturation" of fistula);
3. fistulae that have thrombosed in patients with renal transplant;
4. urgent need for transfer from peritoneal dialysis because of complications (i.e., severe peritonitis, abdominal complications, or catheter dysfunction);
5. acute exogenous poisoning; and
6. physiologic abnormalities, including hyperkalemia, pulmonary edema in the presence of oliguria, metabolic acidosis, severe neurologic symptoms, or pericarditis.

During hemodialysis, blood is removed from the cannulated vein, circulated through the dialyzer, and returned to the patient either via a peripheral vein or through the second lumen of a double-lumen catheter. The two most common dialysis access routes are the subclavian and femoral veins.

Subclavian Access

To catheterize the subclavian vein percutaneously, the patient is placed supine in Trendelenburg's position (which dilates the vein and minimizes risk of an embolism) with the head rotated to the opposite side. The skin is disinfected and a local anesthetic is administered. A 16-gauge needle and a subclavian catheter are inserted into the vein, and a guidewire is introduced through the catheter. The subclavian catheter is removed and exchanged for a dialysis catheter that can be used immediately. A chest roentgenogram is done to rule out pneumothorax or hemothorax before dialysis treatment is initiated.

Subclavian vein catheters can be used for several weeks, avoiding the need for repeated needle punctures of the skin. The catheter is kept patent between treatments by filling it with heparinized saline solution and clamping it or by intermittent flushing with the above solution.

Major complications of subclavian vein catheterization (Table 19–4) include pneumothorax, hemothorax, and subcutaneous hematoma. Other less common or frequent compli-

TABLE 19–4. **Subclavian Vein Catheter Complications**

Major Complications	Less Common Complications
Pneumothorax	Air embolism
Hemothorax	Subclavian vein thrombosis
Subcutaneous hematoma	Infection

cations include air embolism, subclavian vein thrombosis, and infection. Stenosis and thrombosis occur more frequently in catheters left in place longer than 4 weeks.

Femoral Access

During femoral vein catheter insertion, the patient lies supine with the leg externally rotated and the knee slightly flexed. Elevating the buttocks on a pillow allows fuller extension of the groin crease. The skin around the femoral vein site is shaved, disinfected with povidone-iodine, and draped. Local anesthesia is achieved with lidocaine. After palpating the femoral artery, the physician inserts a 16-gauge cannula at a 45-degree angle into the femoral vein located approximately 1–2 cm medial to the femoral artery. If the femoral vein is entered, blood should drip freely from the outer tip of the catheter. A guidewire is inserted through the cannula and threaded into the common iliac vein and inferior vena cava (IVC). With the guidewire in place, the cannula is removed and a dialyzing catheter is threaded over the guidewire into the IVC. If blood returns freely, the catheter is connected to the arterial end of the dialyzer and dialysis is begun.

If the femoral vein catheter is left in place, meticulous care of the insertion site with sterile technique is essential. As with subclavian vein catheters, interim patency is maintained either by instillation of heparinized saline solution and capping or by intermittent irrigation with heparin flush solution.

The most frequent complication with femoral vein cannulation is bleeding from the vein puncture site. Other less frequent complications include femoral vein thrombosis predisposing the patient to the risk of pulmonary embolism; infection; traumatic formation of AV fistulae between the femoral artery and vein, usually resulting from inadvertent puncture of the artery; and femoral nerve damage.

Complications of Hemodialysis Access

The morbidity and mortality associated with chronic long-term hemodialysis patients are in large part determined by the ability of nephrologists, dialysis staff, and vascular surgeons to establish and maintain adequate vascular access.[7] Patients undergoing chronic hemodialysis are most frequently hospitalized to manage complications of dialysis access (Table 19–5). Among those hemodialysis patients older than 65 years of age, there are more vascular access–related hospital admissions than any other age group, accounting for 24 percent of all hospital admissions compared with less than 19 percent of those younger than 65 years.[2] A discussion of the most common complications of chronic hemodialysis access follows.

Thrombosis

Thrombosis is the most common complication of an arteriovenous fistula. The incidence of thrombosis depends on the type of fistula, the diameter and quality of the artery and

TABLE 19–5. **Complications of Hemodialysis**

Thrombosis	Congestive heart failure
Infection	Distal ischemia
Aneurysm formation	Neuropathy
Distal venous hypertension	

vein, the site of the AV anastomosis, and the materials used. Thrombosis occurring within 1 month of vascular access placement is often due to technical errors in fistula construction or premature use.[7] The autogenous radiocephalic AV fistula is associated with a fairly high early failure rate of 10–15 percent.[12]

Maintaining vascular access patency is an ongoing challenge. Late thrombosis of autogenous fistulae is often due to venous fibrosis and stenosis secondary to repeated venipuncture. This fibrotic process may be detected early if increasing pressure is noted in the venous return line during dialysis, suggesting outflow obstruction. Other routine measurements used to identify venous stenosis prospectively include urea recirculation determination caused by sluggish flow and color Doppler evaluation.[7] Increased venous pressure warrants an angiogram that may define the area of obstruction, allowing surgical revision before total occlusion occurs. Chronic fibrosis is usually limited to the venous anastomosis and can often be corrected surgically by local endarterectomy or patch angioplasty.

Late thrombosis of a prosthetic graft is usually due to obstruction at the site of venous outflow. As with autogenous fistulae, angiography is indicated if function is inadequate. This study may detect a number of surgically correctable problems, including technical anastomotic errors, thrombus within the graft, or extrinsic graft compression within the subcutaneous tunnel. Forty percent of thrombosed bridge fistulae can be salvaged with surgical thrombectomy and/or revision. The remaining 60 percent require construction of a new fistula.[12] Implantation of a new graft or fistula has a greater likelihood of achieving long-term patency than does a declotting procedure.

About 20 percent of dialysis access thromboses occur in the absence of an identifiable anatomic lesion.[7] Hypotension, intravascular volume depletion, and prolonged compression of the fistula during sleep may lead to markedly decreased fistula flow and subsequent thrombosis. Specifically, considering the elderly patient's propensity for lower diastolic pressure, careful blood pressure monitoring of elders to prevent hypotensive episodes during and immediately after the dialysis treatment becomes more important. The frail elderly person must perfuse the access in order for it to remain patent and prevent system problems. Accordingly, volume replacement may be indicated for some hypotensive geriatric patients.[2]

Thrombolytic therapy offers an alternative to surgical thrombectomy for acute thrombosis of an established dialysis access site. Urokinase is the lytic agent of choice, offering a short half-life and nonantigenicity. These qualities allow repeated administration for recurrent thrombosis. Contraindications to thrombolytic therapy of a clotted access graft include suspected graft infection, as well as contraindication to anticoagulant/fibrinolytic therapy or severe allergy to angiographic contrast material, because repeat angiograms are necessary to determine the efficacy of treatment.

Percutaneous transluminal angioplasty (PTA) also provides a nonsurgical alternative for access grafts that are failing because of arterial anastomotic and venous outflow stenosis. However, restenosis is unavoidable; recurrence rate of 25 percent within 1 year has been reported.[13] Most restenosis can be successfully treated by repeat angioplasty.[7] Mizumoto and associates reported the development of directional atherectomy (DA) as a new therapeutic modality for vascular access stenosis.[14] An atherectomy device may be used to remove stenotic tissue, which may prolong the period before restenosis. Therapeutic alternatives such as PTA or DA are methods available as outpatient procedures and do not preclude surgical revision at a later date.[14]

Consequences of long-term patency following multiple angioplasty procedures may be equivalent to that of surgically revised fistulae. However, comparison of long-term patency rates after revascularization is difficult due to trends in surgical reporting.[15] The benefit of successful angioplasty and repeated angioplasty procedures is prolonging the usable life of the original fistula without extending it farther up the arm with a surgical procedure.

Infection

Infection is the most common complication of vascular access surgery after thrombosis and is a frequent cause of hospitalization in hemodialysis patients.[16] Infection may prematurely end the function of autogenous or prosthetic fistulae. The routine use of perioperative antibiotics has helped to decrease the incidence of infections.

Local signs and symptoms of infection include cellulitis over the graft, purulent drainage from a puncture site, and the presence of an inflammatory pseudoaneurysm near the prosthetic graft anastomosis. Systemic manifestations include leukocytosis, fever, malaise, and positive blood cultures. In bacteremic patients, appropriate intravenous antibiotic therapy is used to combat the specific organism(s) isolated.

An infection of a bridge fistula usually requires removal of the prosthetic material, ligation of the artery and vein, and drainage of any local abscess. If possible, creation of another vascular access site should be delayed until all signs of infection have resolved, so as to minimize the risk of seeding and infecting a new area. Preferably, a different extremity should also be used for the new access.

Ena and associates described the epidemiology of *Staphylococcus aureus* infections in hemodialysis patients.[17] The findings of their study supported the hypothesis that *S. aureus* isolates causing infections in hemodialysis patients are of endogenous origin, specifically in the nares. These data provide a rationale for using antimicrobial therapy to eradicate *S. aureus* nasal carriage among hemodialysis patients. However, additional studies are needed to identify those at highest risk of infection who would benefit from prophylaxis.

Aneurysm Formation

Dilation or true aneurysm formation of the central venous limb of an autogenous fistula often requires no treatment and actually may increase the ease of cannulation. Surgical intervention should be considered, however, if the overlying skin is thin and rupture threatens or if a thrombus within the aneurysmal segment impairs blood flow or makes needle insertion difficult. True aneurysms of prosthetic bridge fistulae usually occur as a result of repeated cannulation in the same area. Dilation of the entire graft may also occur secondary to degeneration of the prosthetic material. This occurs far less frequently with PTFE than with bovine heterografts.

False aneurysms or pseudoaneurysms rarely occur with autogenous fistulae. The incidence increases with prosthetic bridge fistulae. Pseudoaneurysm formation occurs in focal regions subjected to repeated needle punctures in certain PTFE cannulation sites, as well as following use of oversized needles and use of improper techniques of graft puncture at hemodialysis.[18] Pseudoaneurysms are repaired by excising the damaged graft segment and replacing it by interposing segments of PTFE.

Distal Venous Hypertension

Increased venous pressure may occur in tissues distal to the fistula, resulting in chronic edema and the development of varicosities. In extreme situations, discoloration, pigmentation changes, and even ulceration may develop. This problem may worsen as the fistula matures and valvular incompetence develops. Treatment involves ligating the vein just distal to the fistula. Some surgeons routinely ligate the distal vein at the time of fistula creation to avoid distal venous hypertension whereas others, citing its infrequent occurrence, advocate ligation only after symptoms develop.

Congestive Heart Failure

Right heart strain or congestive heart failure (CHF) secondary to therapeutic fistulae is exceedingly rare, even with rapid flow rates. Congestive failure may occur when fistula flow increases cardiac output as little as 20 percent.[9] However, venous return to the heart increases considerably when a large proximal artery is connected directly to an adjacent vein. The heart compensates by increasing heart rate, stroke volume, and cardiac output as necessary to maintain fisutla flow.

Surgical revision of the fistula may be necessary if CHF develops subsequent to fistula maturation and does not respond to conventional medical therapy. The fistula may be banded with a circumferential extrinsic Teflon cuff to decrease flow through the graft. Unfortunately, decreased flow may result in thrombosis, requiring creation of a new fistula.

Distal Ischemia

Distal vascular insufficiency may develop as a consequence of excessive flow through a fistula, resulting in reversed flow in the distal artery toward the fistula. Reversed flow is sometimes seen with side-to-side fistulae at the wrist. This alteration in the direction of flow has been labeled "steal." When it is of sufficient magnitude and cannot be compensated by collateral flow, it results in ischemic manifestations.[8]

This "steal" syndrome rarely produces clinically significant symptoms. About 10 percent of hemodialysis patients may complain of coolness, some numbness, and pain during dialysis.[8] The problem is self-correcting and symptoms reverse completely within about 1 month. The majority of patients affected with distal ischemia are diabetics and have severe obstructive disease of the arteries distal to the brachial artery. The "steal" may be corrected by ligation of the artery (usually the radial) just distal to the fistula.

Neuropathy

A small number of patients with radiocephalic fistulae report carpal tunnel symptoms (i.e., numbness in the distribution of the median nerve).[12] Nerve conduction studies can confirm or discount the the diagnosis. It is theorized that tissue edema and median nerve compression may result from venous hypertension. It is also thought that nerve ischemia may result from arterial "steal" syndrome. Some patients with intolerable symptoms have been managed by the conventional surgical division of the carpal ligament to relieve median nerve compression.

Nursing Management of Patients With Hemodialysis Access

Preoperative Considerations

Chronic renal failure is generally an insidious process allowing time for planning and preparation. This includes planning to address both psychosocial and physiologic needs. Consideration of hemodialysis as a treatment modality involves a major adjustment in the daily activities of an individual with ESRD. The individual needs information and education about the hemodialysis process (i.e., equipment, fistula formation, etc.), the commitment of time for dialysis, the arrangements for travel to a dialysis center, consideration of other options available for dialysis, and the impact of renal failure related to the patient's perception of health and well-being.

Primary access vessels (Table 19–6) should not be used for venipuncture, intravenous cannulation, or invasive monitoring lines in patients with acute or progressive renal disease. All involved hospital personnel must be informed of the need to preserve the selected vessels beginning with the earliest indication of renal failure.[5] Posting a sign over the patient's bed can inform other providers of the need to preserve vessels. Adequate hydration, weight control, hypertension treatment, avoidance of smoking, and control of local dermatitis or cellutitis are all measures that may help increase the chance of being able to perform and maintain an autogenous AV fistula at the wrist.[5]

Perioperative Considerations

Dialysis patients have certain particular needs when they come to the operating room. The perioperative nurse should first note the cause of the patient's renal failure.[19] A patient with newly diagnosed renal failure will have different needs than a patient with chronic renal failure who has had multiple access operations. To provide optimal nursing care, it is essential that the nurse be sensitive to the patient's level of acceptance of his or her disease and its processes.[19] Other areas that need to be assessed include: (1) the ability of the patient to lie still during the vascular access procedure under local anesthesia; (2) the ability of the patient to follow directions and cooperate during the procedure; and (3) the impact of positioning requirements on the patient's skin integrity.

Postoperative Considerations

Postoperative nursing management after creation of an AV fistula includes elevating the patient's operative arm on a pillow or with a sling for 24 hours to minimize the development of upper-extremity edema. Some swelling nearly always occurs but resolves in several weeks.

The dressing is checked frequently for excessive bleeding. The initial dressing is left intact overnight unless excessive bleeding occurs. Once the initial dressing is removed, the surgical incision is inspected for evidence of infection, including erythema, warmth, excessive tenderness, and drainage. Any suspicion of infection should be reported to the surgeon.

Assessment of adequate fistula function includes palpation for a thrill that is generated as high-pressure arterial blood flows into a contiguous vein. Also, a bruit should be audible on auscultation over the venous limb with a stethoscope. The absence of these findings suggests thrombosis and should be reported to the surgeon. Constricting dressings and blood pressure cuffs on the operative arm are avoided because they restrict venous flow.

Before discharge, the patient is taught to:

1. Avoid wearing tight clothing, hanging things over the arm, or carrying heavy objects, so that blood can flow freely through the fistula.
2. Check blood flow through the fistula several times daily by feeling for a thrill or

TABLE 19–6. **Primary Access Vessels**

Arteries	Veins
Radial	Cephalic
Brachial	Cubital fossa veins (basilic, antecubital, and cephalic)

listening for a bruit. Report loss of thrill or bruit to the physician or nurse immediately.

3. After the sutures are removed, keep the area over the fistula clean and dry. Apply lotion to keep skin moisturized.

4. Exercise the operative arm by squeezing a rubber ball or lifting a 1-pound weight (soup can) for 10–15 minutes several times daily to promote enlargement of the vein.

5. Report any redness, swelling, excessive tenderness, or drainage to the physician or nurse immediately.

6. Bathing, swimming, and other similar activities can be safely resumed several weeks after surgery.

Continuing Care

Highly functional hemodialysis vascular accesses and access devices are the patient's avenue to adequate and optimal dialytic therapy.[20] To achieve long-term success with vascular access, a team approach is needed. This team includes the patient, family/support system, nursing staff, nephrologist, radiologist, and the vascular access surgeon. Once the vascular surgeon successfully creates a primary or bridge fistula, the dialysis staff must correctly care for it.[21] Technique and the method of needle placement in the fistula are major factors in achieving the optimal flow rate, maintaining the fistula site for future use and avoiding gross disfigurement of the fistula limb.[22]

In a typical work-week, a dialysis nurse performs 64 needle cannulations, and 1248 cannulations in 1 year. Needle cannulation experience increases quickly as a dialysis nurse is prepared and completes 1 year of work, but experience does not equal expertise.[21] Bacterial contamination of the vascular access and subsequent infection may occur because of poor needle cannulation technique.[23] Some nurses are taught to insert the arterial needle in the direction of blood flow, pointing toward the venous anastomosis (antegrade cannulation) as indicated in Figure 19–4. Others are taught to direct the arterial cannulation toward the arterial anastomosis of the access (retrograde cannulation). There is little convincing evidence that either technique is preferable and both have their benefits.[20]

It is important to rotate needle cannulation sites to prevent compromise of both skin and vascular access integrity.[23] For each year on dialysis, the patient undergoes 312 needle cannulations. Dialysis staff need to educate patients concerning rotation of needle sites.[21] Patient resistance to needle rotation is only natural. Patient-preferred sites generally have been used repetitively, form scar tissue, and offer little discomfort.[20]

Finally, assessment of the patient for presence or absence of vascular access infection should be done before every dialysis treatment. The use of strict aseptic technique by the nursing staff providing vascular access care is essential; adherence to this standard decreases the risk of bacterial contamination of the access during the dialysis procedure.[23]

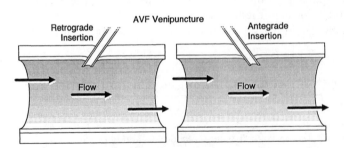

Figure 19–4. Retrograde and antegrade puncture of an arterialized vein.

TABLE 19–7. **Benefits of Vascular Access Devices**

Conducive to self-care
Decrease in nosocomial infections
Elimination of multi-venipunctures
Use in non–acute care settings, i.e., patient homes
Outpatient procedure for placement
Potential placement in home environment by skilled providers

VASCULAR ACCESS DEVICES

Use of Vascular Access Devices

The vascular access devices (VADs) discussed in this chapter include those that have the distal tip in the superior vena cava. Accordingly, peripheral intravenous (IV) sites and midline and midclavicular peripherally inserted catheters will not be addressed. All the VADs presented can be used for blood withdrawal or sampling, blood product administration, and long-term IV therapy.

The availability of dependable long-term vascular access is an important consideration in the provision of chemotherapy, total parenteral nutrition (TPN), or long-term antibiotics. VADs are commonly used to provide initial therapy for such patients. In addition, persons with acquired immunodeficiency syndrome (AIDS), sickle cell disease, burns, Crohn's disease, and osteomyelitis frequently may require such access. In the United States, an estimated 2.75 million central venous catheters are placed per year. Of these, approximately 386,000 are tunneled catheters and an additional 135,000 are totally implanted venous access port devices.[24]

The increased use of VADs is consistent with "patient-focused" care trends. These devices offer many benefits to patients (Table 19–7). They are conducive to self-care and promote a decrease in nosocomial infections, especially with their increased use in home settings. Nosocomial blood stream infections, such as intravascular device–related sepsis, cost approximately $6000 per patient.[25] However, these infections are largely preventable. There is also a convenience factor with the potential for placement of nontunneled, peripherally inserted central catheters (PICCs) within home settings. The major overall advantage of using VADs is to eliminate multiple venipunctures in the management of long-term therapies for patients with chronic conditions.[26]

The selection of the appropriate VAD is best made as an interdisciplinary decision. Several factors require consideration (Table 19–8). Safety considerations of the device design include its necessary length and diameter of the catheter; the number of lumens; and Dacron cuff to prevent infection and secure the catheter.[27, 28] Patient characteristics

TABLE 19–8. **Factors to Consider for Appropriate Vascular Access Device Selection**

Safety Considerations	Patient Characteristics
Length and diameter of catheter	Competency level
Number of lumens	Manual dexterity
Use of Dacron cuff	Visual acuity
Type of therapy	Home environment
	Caregiver support
	Elderly or pediatric patient
	Cosmetic appearance concerns
	Anxiety with needle stick into a port

requiring consideration include competency level, manual dexterity, visual acuity, the home environment, caregiver support, and whether the patient is elderly or pediatric. The type of therapy determines the type of line needed. A central line is required for hyperalimination and is highly recommended for irritating, sclerosing, or vesicant agents.[29] Support systems available for use of the VAD in a home setting need careful assessment. Support systems include the availability of home nursing and proximity of follow-up care.

Cost is a factor in the choice of appropriate VAD. The expense of initial insertion of a nontunneled device may be less than an implanted port; however, if the device is used longer than 6 months, the port may be more economical when considering maintenance costs. Therefore, length of treatment and cost of VAD maintenance need to be considered when choosing the appropriate device.

The patient provides input into the selection of an appropriate device. Issues for the patient to consider include cosmetic appearance, concerns with activity or work limitations, anxiety with a needle stick into a port, site care, and catheter flushing requirements.[29]

Currently, polyurethanes, silicone elastomer (Silastic), and elastomeric hydrogel are the most frequently used materials in the manufacture of VADs.[27] Rather than acting as passive conduits, the biomaterials used in VADs elicit active responses from both the host and the endogenous microflora of the host. These interactive responses are involved in the most common complications of venous access: infection, inflammation (phlebitis), and thrombosis.[30] Research continues in the development of new biomaterials and antimicrobial agents with improved activity within the microenvironment of the biofilm.[31]

Long-term catheters need to be radiopaque to allow for visualization of the catheter tip on initial insertion or any time that displacement is suspected. The confirmation of catheter tip by chest radiograph is recommended by Standards of Practice of Intravenous Nurses Society, Access Device Guidelines from the Oncology Nursing Society, and Central Venous Catheter Working Group of the Food and Drug Administration (FDA).[27]

General Management Principles of Vascular Access Devices

Flushing

Flushing requirements vary with each device. Flushing these catheters cleanses their internal diameters of fibrin buildup and debris.[28] Macklin suggested using a pulsating motion to create enough turbulence to allow the solution to "scrub" the catheter wall.[32] However, regardless of which VAD is being flushed, a low pressure should be used. Excessive pressure especially when using syringes of 3 ml or less can cause catheter fracture. The need to maintain positive pressure, which prevents the reflux of blood into the cannula and possible clot development, is of critical importance. To achieve positive pressure when flushing, close the clamp on the catheter or withdraw the syringe while injecting the last 0.2 to 0.5 ml of flush solution.[29] The Intravenous Nurses Society recommends a flushing volume of heparinized saline solution equal to two times the internal volume of the catheter and of a concentration of heparin that will not alter the patient's clotting factors.[29]

A study reported by Mayo and associates identified that Groshong catheter valves frequently allow blood to enter the catheter lumen.[33] When the lumens were flushed weekly with saline, the refluxed blood clotted and adhered to the intraluminal catheter surface, causing obstruction. When heparinized saline flushes were used, blood still occasionally refluxed into the catheters, but the incidence of adherent clots was significantly less. The authors also cited financial advantages for using heparinized saline flush solution versus urokinase treatment for occlusions.

Dressings/Care of Exit Site

Dressing type, frequency of care, and frequency of insertion site assessments remain controversial issues.[25, 28, 29, 34] Using ointments after cleansing the exit site remains controversial also. Evidence supporting the value of using an antimicrobial ointment to prevent infection is lacking.[25, 28] Dressings may consist of sterile gauze and tape covering, a transparent, semipermeable membrane, or a highly permeable transparent membrane.[34] Gauze dressings should be changed every 48–72 hours, depending on agency policy and whenever the dressing is soiled or loose. Transparent dressings may be changed every 2–7 days.

Blood Withdrawals

Several techniques can be used to obtain blood samples, including discarding, reinfusing, mixing; or a Vacutainer or syringe can be used. The most commonly reported procedure in the adult population is the discard method.[28] The amount discarded varies from 3 to 10 ml. Blood is withdrawn and discarded, the sample is collected, and the VAD is flushed with normal saline.

Blood samples used for coagulation studies should be drawn peripherally because heparin adheres to the internal catheter lumen. A study reported by Mayo and colleagues confirmed the difficulty in obtaining reliable coagulation tests with blood samples drawn through tunneled central catheters that have been flushed with heparin.[35] Even after 25 ml of blood discard, the differences between the activated partial thromboplastin time (APTT) of catheter blood and peripheral blood were statistically significant, reflecting trace amounts of heparin. It is important to differentiate between statistical and clinical significance. Test results from catheter blood that falls into the higher end of normal could be considered clinically reliable even if they are slightly higher than results from peripheral blood. When the objective is to confirm that a patient has normal coagulation tests before an invasive procedure, this would be acceptable. However, if the results are used to monitor anticoagulant therapy or to evaluate a coagulopathy, then peripheral blood should be used for sampling.

Clamping

Tunneled and nontunneled catheters have open tips except for the Groshong catheter. Therefore these external catheter lumens need to be clamped when not being used to prevent blood from backing up into the catheter. The Groshong catheter has a solid blunt tip with a three-position valve on the side (Fig. 19–5). Providing positive pressure into a Groshong catheter opens the valve to allow fluid infusion; significant negative pressure opens its valve inward, allowing blood aspiration. When pressures are equalized, the valve is closed. As a result, the Groshong catheter does not need to be clamped.[29]

Tunneled Catheters

Tunneled catheters are recommended for patients requiring prolonged administration of chemotherapeutic agents, antibiotics, or TPN. Tunneled catheters have many benefits, including: (1) insertion can be done as an outpatient procedure; (2) catheters can remain in place indefinitely; (3) only a clean dressing is needed for care; and (4) they do not

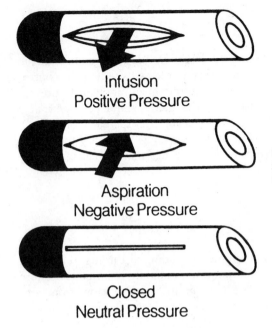

Infusion
Positive Pressure

Aspiration
Negative Pressure

Figure 19–5. Tip of the Groshong catheter illustrating the unique valve. (Courtesy of Bard Access Systems, Inc., Salt Lake City, UT.)

Closed
Neutral Pressure

require a needle stick.[25] Tunneled catheters are beneficial for patients in whom port placement would be impractical, such as obese or chronically thrombocytopenic patients.[26]

These one- to three-lumen catheters have external parts; therefore, body image needs to be considered when discussing tunneled catheters as an option for long-term vascular access. Catheter care and maintenance also need to be considered, including procedures for site care, flushing, and cap changes.

Tunneled catheters are inserted in the operating room and are tunneled subcutaneously to an exit site on the chest wall some distance from the entry into the subclavian or external jugular vein (Fig. 19–6).[25] The catheter is advanced into the superior vena cava or right atrium. Certain conditions such as superior vena cava syndrome, neck or mediasti-

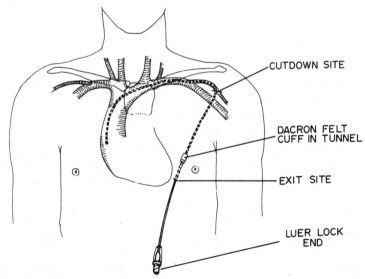

CUTDOWN SITE

DACRON FELT
CUFF IN TUNNEL

EXIT SITE

LUER LOCK
END

Figure 19–6. Diagrammatic representation of Broviac catheter in proper position, with tip in right atrium. (From Bennion RS, Wilson SE: Hemodialysis and vascular access. In Moore WS [ed]: Vascular Surgery: A Comprehensive Review. Philadelphia, WB Saunders, 1991.)

nal tumor, bilateral radical neck resection, an infected median sternotomy, torso burns, or trauma may preclude cannulation of the neck or chest.[36] In such cases, the femoral vein provides an alternate insertion site, and the catheter is advanced into the inferior vena cava. A primary concern with long-term femoral vein catheterization is the presumed increase in the risk of bacteremia compared with lines at other sites because of the proximity to the perineum. Goldstein and associates cite a catheter-related sepsis rate of only 4.9 percent for femoral vein access in pediatric patients with burns, which compares favorably with results ranging from 2 percent to 13 percent obtained with catheters at other sites.[37]

Both Broviac and Hickman catheters have a Dacron felt cuff 30 cm from the Luer-Lok end, allowing fibrous tissue ingrowth of the cuff to provide a barrier to the migration of bacteria from the skin into the venous system. Intraoperative roentgenograms are used to confirm proper positioning of the catheter tip. These catheters are heparinized and capped with Luer-Lok caps or may be used immediately. An occlusive gauze or transparent dressing is used over the exit site until the wound has healed.

Goldfarth and Coldwall suggested consideration of bedside placement of Groshong catheters.[38] The physician has the option to place chronic venous catheters in the operating room or at the bedside using the Groshong catheter insertion tray including trocar for passing the catheter. According to Goldfarth and Coldwall, infection rates for bedside placements are comparable to those for lines placed in operating rooms.[38] The authors also cite cost savings of approximately $2450 per catheter for a bedside procedure versus operating room placement.

Peripherally Inserted Central Catheters

The Intravenous Nurses Society (INS) defined a peripherally inserted central catheter (PICC) as one inserted via a peripheral vein with the tip residing in the vena cava.[39] The advantages of a PICC include ease of insertion, lack of sutures, a reduced potential of infection, and reduced risk of pneumothorax, hemothorax, or air embolism as compared with conventional tunneled catheters (Table 19–9).[25] Insertion of a PICC is done in a nonsurgical setting by a variety of providers, including specially credentialed registered nurses, without the use of local or general anesthetics.[40]

The catheter lumens are external, nontunneled, and may not be sutured. Maintenance care is similar to that of the tunneled central catheters. Therefore, body image issues and self-care abilities require assessment prior to the placement of a PICC. For patients who participate in frequent exercise or strenuous manual work or who have active children, a PICC may not be the best device because of the increased risk of dislodgement or limitation of the upper extremity.[28]

PICCs are a good selection for patients who have or have had chest injury, radical neck dissection, radiation fibrosis within the chest, fungating chest tumor, or neck veins that cannot be cannulated, or are malnourished or are physically unable to undergo a surgical procedure.[28] PICCs can be used for patients who have limited peripheral access.[39] Hagle

TABLE 19–9. **Advantages of Peripherally Inserted Central Catheters**

Ease of insertion without local or general anesthetic
Decreased potential of infection
Decreased risk of pneumothorax
Placement in nonsurgical setting
Placement by nonphysician providers, including registered nurses

suggested that a PICC should not be considered a "last resort" but rather a "first choice" for patients with poor peripheral veins.[29] PICCs should be used for patients who need several weeks or months of treatment. For example, adults with osteomyelitis require a minimum of 14–19 catheter changes during a standard 6- to 8-week antibiotic course using peripheral intravenous therapy.[29] These individuals are candidates for a PICC. Currently it is not known if there are limits for the length of time a single PICC may be used. The INS position paper for peripherally inserted central catheters indicates that consideration may be given to leaving a PICC in place for up to 1 year.[39]

PICCs are not effective for rapid, large-volume infusions.[28] Also, small-gauge PICCs are not recommended for blood sampling because of the propensity for catheter collapse.[28] Blood sampling needs an 18-gauge or larger catheter.[29] However, if the catheter is too large, blood flow around the catheter may be inadequate to dilute the medication being infused, resulting in increased chemical irritation to the vein.[27]

PICCs are inserted from the antecubital area into the central venous system with the tip residing in the superior vena cava. A variety of techniques may be used for PICC insertion, including a through-the-introducer technique, short-term peripheral catheter used as a stylet, or over-wire Seldinger method similar to the technique used to insert subclavian catheters.[27] Donaldson and associates advocated using an ultrasound-guided venipuncture for peripheral insertion of central venous catheters in the pediatric population.[41]

After insertion, a chest radiograph is recommended to confirm the location of the catheter tip. A measurement of the amount of catheter left externally is recorded. The extruding catheter is measured at subsequent dressing changes to monitor for possible dislodgement.[42] When the external catheter length changes, the tip location also changes and the appropriateness of the infusion medium must be evaluated.[29] The catheter may be trimmed so that the tip lies in the proximal segment of the axillary vein. This placement, called a peripherally inserted catheter (PIC)[29] or a midline catheter,[27] does not require a postprocedure radiograph. PICCs may be removed with gentle pulling by registered nurses.[29] Extreme care must be taken with removal to maintain catheter integrity for the entire length. After removal, the length of the catheter is measured and compared with the documented length.[32]

Subcutaneous Access Ports

With venous access ports, a catheter is attached to a plastic or metal port and both lie completely beneath the skin (Fig. 19–7). The port consists of a dense, resealable silicone

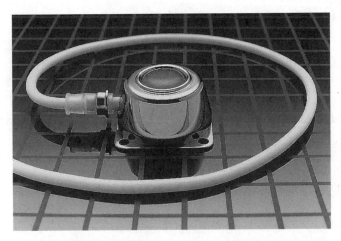

Figure 19–7. Port-A-Cath implantable venous access system. (Copyright Pharmacia Deltec, Inc., St. Paul, MN.)

septum overlying a small reservoir body of plastic, rubber, or metal. The port lies perpendicular to the skin. The advantages of implanted ports include greater freedom of activity, less maintenance, superior cost-effectiveness, and better cosmetic acceptability as compared with external devices.[26] The minimal care requirements and subcutaneous placement make the venous access port an excellent long-term access option for the elderly or pediatric population. Ports are the only VADs that are completely protected from a pediatric patient and cannot be pulled out.[41] However, accessing the port requires a needle stick. Port access should not be used by individuals undergoing treatments that cause prolonged myelosuppression.[28]

Ports for venous access are generally implanted in the infraclavicular fossa. Mid-arm to upper-arm placement of peripheral ports is an alternative when arm veins are still intact or when implantation in the neck or chest is inadvisable.[43] Peripheral arm port devices are much smaller in all dimensions than the conventional chest port (Fig. 19–8). Arm port devices should be placed in the nondominant arm whenever possible.[44] Implanted arterial ports are used for patients requiring access to the arterial system for infusion therapy. Site location depends on the organ targeted for drug delivery. The liver is the most common organ targeted. Therefore, the most common location for an arterial port catheter is the common hepatic artery.[45]

Surgical technique for insertion of access ports is similar to that for tunneled catheters. A catheter cut to the appropriate length is advanced into the superior vena cava. A port is then attached and sutured into the subcutaneous pocket. The port is accessed by percutaneous insertion of specially designed noncoring needles, which allows the septum to reseal when the needle is withdrawn (Fig. 19–9).

An alternative to surgically placed central venous access is placement of chest wall ports and arm ports in radiology suites by interventional radiologists. Advantages of interventional radiologic port placement include timeliness, decreased cost, and use of image-guided techniques that allow a high successful procedure rate and aid in minimizing procedural complications.[44, 46] A greater than 50 percent cost reduction and comparable infection rates of 4–16 percent support nonsurgical port placement.[24] Schuman and Ragsdale described the use of a treatment room in a freestanding cancer center for placement of arm ports; only hospital inpatients are taken to the operating room for arm port placement.[47]

Insertion of a totally implantable subcutaneous port in the upper body may be difficult or contraindicated in some clinical situations. Multiple previous placements of catheters to the great vessels of the upper part of the body may further complicate permanent access to those veins. Difficult or contraindicated subclavian or jugular vein access is a

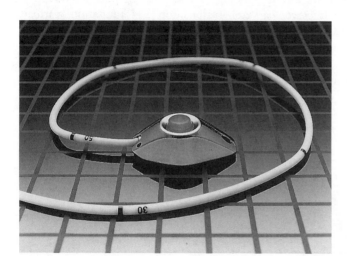

Figure 19–8. P.A.S. Port implantable peripheral venous access system. (Copyright Pharmacia Deltec, Inc., St. Paul, MN.)

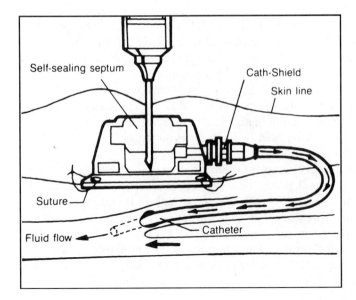

Figure 19–9. Diagrammatic representation of subcutaneous venous access port (Port-A-Cath) showing perpendicular needle insertion. (Copyright Pharmacia Deltec, Inc., St. Paul, MN.)

clinical situation that can occur in approximately 8 percent of overall long-term port placements. Bertoglio and colleagues evaluated the feasibility of femoral percutaneous port access as an alternative to accessing the subclavian or jugular veins.[48] They concluded that the percutaneous femoral route should be considered a safe alternative.

Complications of Vascular Access Devices

Placement and maintenance of central VADs are not without potential complications (Table 19–10). The risk of developing complications is an important issue for several reasons, including obtaining adequate informed consent prior to placement. Patients must be apprised of the possible problems associated with placement and use of the devices.[49]

Early complications of percutaneous catheterization are most often related to technique, with pneumothorax being the most frequently encountered serious complication. Other complications include major venous or arterial injury, lymphatic fistulae, neurologic injury, cardiac dysrhythmia or tamponade, and improper catheter placement.[50]

Infection and occlusion are common late complications of VADs. Less common complications are serious and in some cases life-threatening. These rare complications include catheter pinch-off and catheter fracture, catheter malposition and migration, cardiac perforation, extravasation, breakage, and defective devices.[51]

TABLE 19–10. **Complications of Vascular Access Devices**

Early Complications	**Common Complications**
Pneumothorax	Infection
Venous or arterial injury	Occlusion
Lymphatic fistulae	**Less Common Complications**
Neurologic injury	Catheter pinch-off and fracture
Cardiac dysrhythmia	Catheter malposition and migration
Improper catheter placement	Cardiac perforation
	Extravasation
	Breakage
	Defective devices

Infection

Infection is the most common complication of VADs.[52] The risk of infection is increased the longer a catheter remains in place; this risk is considered cumulative and increases with time.[53] Also additional lumens per catheter increase the risk of infection due to the increased manipulation of the system.[25, 26] Much of the risk of infection of a percutaneous central catheter relates to the manner used to insert the catheter. The risk for significant colonization of the catheter may be related to the cumulative experience of the physician inserting the catheter.[54]

Infections may be local or systemic. Local infections occur at the site where the device exits the body (exit site), along the subcutaneous tunnel of catheters, and in the port pocket of implanted ports. Systemic infection (septicemia) is confirmed when the same organism is isolated from a culture of a catheter segment and peripheral blood with no clinical evidence of any other apparent source.[52] Catheter-related blood stream infections are particularly troublesome because of the dramatic morbidity, a case fatality rate of 14 percent, and their iatrogenic nature.[54] The most common cause of infections is *Staphylococcus epidermidis*.[53]

Prevention of local infection centers on catheter care that in many instances is done by the patient. The nurse must teach the patient handwashing, aseptic technique, thorough site care, and daily assessment. Another method of prevention is the use of antimicrobial-coated catheters which have been shown to decrease the rate of catheter-associated infections.[25]

Treatment of VAD infection depends on several factors, which include: (1) the causative organism; (2) extent of infection; (3) type of device; and (4) physical condition of patient.[52] Many exit site infections of tunneled catheters can be treated successfully with antibiotic therapy and do not require catheter removal.[25] The salvage of an infected subcutaneous port is more difficult, with the majority requiring removal.[55] A major controversy regarding treatment of VAD-related infection is whether to remove the device. Most clinicians agree that the VAD should be removed under the following circumstances: confirmed VAD-related septicemia or tunnel infection; the signs and symptoms of septicemia persist despite antibiotic therapy; or the causative organism is fungi or bacilli.[52]

Occlusion

Occlusion occurs in all catheter types and is the second most common problem associated with VADs.[26, 52] Catheter occlusion results most frequently from a blood clot or drug precipitate. There may be several variables related to venous thrombogenicity, including catheter diameter, catheter tip placement, normal physiologic response to access device insertion, left-sided catheter placement, and hypercoagulability associated with certain malignancies.[26, 52, 56] Occlusions may be classified as either total occlusion or partial occlusion. Resistance when attempting to flush the device, the inability to infuse fluids, and no blood return on aspiration are indicative of a total occlusion.[29] A partial occlusion or persistent withdrawal occlusion is a relatively frequent complication. In this instance there is sluggish or absent blood withdrawal from a VAD even though fluids may be easily infused.[57] There may also be a "positional blood draw"; when a patient changes position or performs Valsalva's maneuver, blood can be aspirated. A fibrin sheath is generally the reason for partial occlusion. Fibrin sheaths have been reported as early as 24 hours after device insertion and will develop in virtually all catheters left in place for more than 1 week.[57] The sheath eventually covers the catheter tip, acting as a one-way valve or flap. The flap allows fluids to be infused but prevents blood from being withdrawn because the tip becomes occluded from the vacuum that is created when negative pressure is applied.

Blood-clotted catheters can usually be cleared via gentle flushing with heparinized saline solution of a thrombolytic agent such as single-dose urokinase (Abbokinase Open-Cath, Abbott Laboratories, North Chicago, IL). Urokinase works on the endogenous fibrinolytic system. It converts plasminogen to the enzyme plasmin. The plasmin then breaks down the fibrin with the thrombus, which leads to resolution of the clot. Urokinase is the preferred thrombolytic agent due to few side effects and decreased expense.[58] Urokinase can be used in pediatrics for catheter-related thrombi.[59] If catheter patency is not restored after the prescribed procedure has been followed, the physician should be notified because another cause of occlusion may exist.

Occlusions caused by lipid materials have been reported with the use of prolonged infusion of TPN. Urokinase has been shown to be ineffective in clearing occlusion of lipid deposits. The use of an ethanol solution has been reported to restore patency without complications.[32, 58] Drug precipitation or mineral deposits can cause abrupt occlusion during or immediately after infusion. Hydrochloric acid has been used to dissolve insoluble mineral precipitates that occur as a result of high concentrations of calcium or phosphorus in TPN or other IV therapies.[32, 58]

Other Complications

Other complications that occur rarely include catheter pinch-off and fracture, catheter malposition and migration, cardiac perforation, extravasation, and device breakage.[51] Catheter pinch-off is the anatomic, mechanical compression of a catheter as it passess between the clavicle and first rib of the costoclavicular space. Catheter fracture is the complete or partial breakage that occurs internally with the migration of a catheter fragment. Catheter migration indicates malposition of a catheter that at one time used to be in the proper location. There is increased risk of catheter migration if the catheter is short, or the tip is in the innominate vein or at the junction of innominate vein and superior vena cava.[60] Cardiac perforation may occur during insertion or as a late complication because of catheter migration into the heart.[51] Extravasation is primarily associated with needle dislodgement from implanted ports, but it may also be caused by backtracking of fluid resulting from a partially or totally occluded catheter.[26] If there is a sheath solidly encasing a VAD from its tip to its venous entry point, fluid exiting the lumen may flow retrograde and backtrack along the outside of the catheter. Incidence of extravasation secondary to fibrin sheath formation ranges from 1.2 to 2.6 percent.[57] The most commonly reported cause of breakage is catheter rupture caused by forceful flushing.[51]

Many of the above problems require removal of the catheter. This presents a serious problem for individuals with limited access choices. Lowell and associates described a technique for the exchange of tunneled polymeric silicone catheters and implantable infusion ports without incurring the risk of a new venipuncture.[61] The catheter exchange procedure using a guidewire is performed in the operating room using local anesthesia.

Nursing Management of Patients With Vascular Access Devices

Preoperative Interventions

Prior to the insertion of a VAD, accurate assessment of the patient and significant other's ability to manage the care and maintenance of the device is critical. Components of this assessment include manual dexterity, visual acuity, cognitive ability, and willingness to participate with the management of the VAD. Methods for improving compliance behavior for patients with access devices include encouraging participation in treatment decisions from the time of diagnosis and selection of an access device; reinforcing education on care of the access device; exploring the patient's perception of disease and treatment; and incorporating support from the family, community, and health care professionals.[62] Patients who need VADs placed frequently have cancer or other debilitating chronic illnesses. The health care team needs to consider the trajectory of illness in the plan of care for managing the device.

Postoperative Interventions

For patients undergoing insertion of external catheters or subcutaneous infusion ports, broad-spectrum antibiotics should be administered prophylactically immediately before and for 24 hours after placement to minimize the risk of infection. With use of aseptic technique, the catheter or port should be aspirated and irrigated with heparinized saline solution to assure adequate patency. If the VAD is to be used for continuous infusions, the use of an electronic infusion device is recommended as the standard of practice.[29]

Patient education for self-care is an important independent function of professional nursing practice. Patients need to be empowered as active partners in their care. They should be provided with the opportunity to develop the ability to take control of the use and care of their access devices. Knowing and using the proper techniques for VAD care reduce the risk of infection of other complications.[26, 49] In the present environment of health care with shortened lengths of stay in hospitals and limited time that nurses have to accomplish essential care, practicing nurses employed in hospitals cannot be held entirely responsible for all patient education. Coordination of efforts needs to extend beyond the hospital into clinics, doctor offices, and community agencies.[62] Nursing staffs in clinics can provide community nurses with information on the care and use of ports via telephone and continuing education classes.[26] A "troubleshooting" guide can be developed for both patients and providers to prevent or reduce access device complications.[62]

The steadily increasing number and greater life expectancy of patients requiring maintenance hemodialysis, and the broadened indications for long-term vascular access to treat other medical problems, continue to challenge the expertise and creativity of the vascular surgeon. Nurses need to keep pace with advancements in vascular access surgery, as nurses provide an essential role in patient preparations, maintenance of functional access sites, and prevention and early detection of complications, which might obviate the need for further access surgery.

References

1. Davidson IJA: Vascular access surgery—general considerations. In Davidson IJA (ed): On Call in Vascular Access. Austin, Landes, 1996, pp 1–10.
2. Culp K, Taylor L, Hulme PA: Geriatric hemodialysis patients: A comparative study of vascular access. Am Neph Nurs Assoc J 1996; 23:583–592.
3. Tominage GT, Ingegno M, Ceralgi C, et al: Vascular complications of continuous arteriovenous hemofiltration in trauma patients. J Trauma 1993; 35:285–289.
4. Johnson CL, Hiatt JR: Vascular access for trauma, emergency surgery, and critical care. In Wilson SE (ed): Vascular Access: Prinicples and Practice. St. Louis, Mosby, 1996, pp 67–78.
5. White GH: Planning and patient assessment for vascular access surgery. In Wilson SE (ed): Vascular Access: Principles and Practice. St. Louis, Mosby, 1996, pp 6–11.
6. Rivers SP, Scher LA, Sheehan E, et al: Basilic vein transposition: An underused alternative to prosthetic dialysis angioaccess. J Vasc Surg 1993; 18:391–397.
7. Berkoben M, Schwab SJ: Maintenance of permanent hemodialysis vascular access patency. Am Neph Nurs Assoc J 1995; 22:17–24.

8. Haimov M, Schanzer H, Skladani M: Pathogenesis and management of upper-extremity ischemia following angioaccess surgery. Blood Purif 1996; 14:350–354.

9. Gordon IL: Physiology of the arteriovenous fistula. In Wilson SE (ed): Vascular Access: Principles and Practice. St. Louis, Mosby, 1996, pp 29–41.

10. Fernando HC, Fernando ON: Arteriovenous fistulas by direct anastomosis for hemodialysis access. In Wilson SE (ed): Vascular Access: Principles and Practice. St. Louis, Mosby, 1996, pp 129–136.

11. Enzler MA, Rajimon T, Lachat M, et al: Long-term function of vascular access for hemodialysis. Clin Transplant 1996; 10:511–515.

12. Wilson SE: Vascular interposition (bridge fistulas) for hemodialysis. In Wilson SE (ed): Vascular Access: Principles and Practice. St. Louis, Mosby, 1996, pp 157–169.

13. Newman G, Davidson C, McCann R, et al: Functional restenosis rate after hemodialysis graft angioplasty. J Am Soc Nephrol 1991; 2:341.

14. Mizumoto D, Watanabe Y, Kumon S, et al: The treatment of chronic hemodialysis vascular access by directional atherectomy. Nephron 1996; 74:45–52.

15. Kumpe DA, Durham JD, Mann DJ: Thrombolysis and percutaneous transluminal angioplasty. In Wilson SE (ed): Vascular Access: Principles and Practice. St. Louis, Mosby, 1996, pp 239–261.

16. Ready AR, Buckels JAC: Management of infection: vascular access surgery in hemodialysis. In Wilson SE (ed): Vascular Access: Principles and Practice. St. Louis, Mosby, 1996, pp 198–211.

17. Ena J, Boelaert JR, Boyken LD, et al: Epidemiology of *Staphylococcus aureus* infections in patients on hemodialysis. Infect Control Hosp Epidemiol 1994; 15:78–81.

18. Back MR, White RA: The biologic response of prosthetic dialysis grafts. In Wilson SE (ed): Vascular Access: Principles and Practice, St. Louis, Mosby, 1996, pp 137–149.

19. Stein P: Perioperative considerations of vascular access for dialysis. Assoc Oper Room Nurs J 1994; 60:947–958.

20. Hartigan MF: Vascular access and nephrology nursing practice: Existing views and rationales for change. Adv Renal Replac Ther 1994; 1:155–162.

21. Brouwer DJ: Hemodialysis: A nursing perspective. In Henry ML, Ferguson RM (eds): Vascular Access for Hemodialysis-IV. Chicago, Gore and Precept Press, 1995, pp 131–151.

22. Stansfield G: Cannulation of arteriovenous fistulae. Nurs Times 1987; 83:38–39.

23. Thomas-Hawkins C: Nursing interventions related to vascular access infections. Adv Renal Replac Ther 1996; 3:218-221.

24. Foley MJ: Radiologic placement of long-term central venous peripheral access system ports (PAS port): Results in 150 patients. J Vasc Interven Rad 1995; 6:255–262.

25. McClane C: Intravascular medication delivery devices and monitoring systems. Crit Care Nurs Clin North Am 1995; 7:675–684.

26. Dearborn P, DeMuth JS, Requarth AB, et al: Nurse and patient satisfaction with three types of venous access devices. Onc Nurs Forum 1997; 24:34S–40S.

27. Hadaway LC: Comparison of vascular access devices. Semin Onc Nurs 1995; 11(3):154–166.

28. Winslow MN, Trammell L, Camp-Sorrell D: Selection of vascular access devices and nursing care. Semin Onc Nurs 1995; 11(3):167–173.

29. Hagle ME, McDonagh JM, Rapp CJ: Patients with long-term vascular access devices: Care and complications. Ortho Nurs 1994; 13(5):41–52.

30. D'Amelio LF, Greco RS: Biologic properties of venous access devices. In Wilson SE (ed): Vascular Access: Principles and Practice, St. Louis, Mosby, 1996, pp 42–53.

31. Khardori N, Yassien M: Biofilms in device-related infections. J Indust Microbiol 1995; 15:141–147.

32. Macklin D: How to manage PICCs. Am J Nurs 1997; 97(9):26–33.

33. Mayo DJ, Horne MK, Summers BL, et al: The effects of heparin flush on patency of the Groshong catheter: a pilot study. Onc Nurs Forum 1996; 23:1401–1405.

34. Treston-Aurand J, Olmsted RN, Allen-Bridson K, et al: Impact of dressing materials on central venous catheter infection rates. J Intraven Nurs 1997; 20:201–205.

35. Mayo DJ, Dimond EP, Kramer W, et al: Discard volumes necessary for clinically useful coagulation studies from heparinized Hickman catheters. Onc Nurs Forum 1996; 23:671–675.

36. Wickham RS: Advances in venous access devices and nursing management strategies. Nurs Clin North Am 1990; 25:345–364.

37. Goldstein AM, Weber JM, Sheridan RL: Femoral venous access is safe in burned children: An analysis of 224 catheters. J Pediatr 1997; 130:442–446.

38. Goldfarth PM, Coldwall D: Chronic venous access: Bedside placement technique and complications. Canc Prac 1994; 2:279–283.

39. Intraven Nurs Soc: Position paper: Peripherally inserted central catheters. J Intraven Nurs 1997; 4:172–174.

40. Donovan MS, Thomas KD, Davis DC, et al: Peripherally inserted central catheters: Placement and use in a family practice hospital. J Am Board Fam Pract 1996; 9:235–240.

41. Donaldson JS, Morello FP, Junewick JJ, et al: Peripherally inserted central venous catheters: US-guided vascular access in pediatric patients. Radiology 1995; 197:542–544.

42. Sansivero GE: Taking care of PICCs. Nurs 1997; 27(5):28.

43. Lilienberg A, Bengtsson M, Starkhammer H: Implantable devices for venous access: Nurses' and patients' evaluation of three different port systems. J Adv Nurs 1994; 19:21–28.

44. Kaufman JA, Salamipour H, Gellar SC, et al: Long-term outcomes of radiologically placed arm ports. Radiology 1996; 201:725–730.

45. Almadrones L, Campana P, Dantis EC: Arterial, peritoneal, and intraventricular access devices. Semin Onc Nurs 1995; 11:194–202.

46. Simpson KR, Hovsepian DM, Picus D: Interventional radiologic placement of chest wall ports: Results and complications in 161 consecutive placements. J Vasc Interven Rad 1997; 8:189–195.

47. Schuman E, Ragsdale J: Peripheral ports are a new option for central venous access. J Am Coll Surg 1995; 180:456–460.

48. Bertoglio S, DiSomma C, Meszaros P, et al: Long-term femoral central venous access in cancer patients. Eur J Surg Onc 1996; 22:162–165.

49. Eastridge BJ, Lefor AT: Complications of indwelling venous access devices in cancer patients. J Clin Onc 1995; 13:233–238.

50. Hye RJ, Stabile BE: Complications of percutaneous vascular access procedures and their management. In Wilson SE (ed): Vascular Access: Principles and Practice, St. Louis, Mosby, 1996, pp 92–103.

51. Ingle RJ: Rare complications of vascular access devices. Semin Onc Nurs 1995; 11:184–193.

52. Rumsey KA, Richardson DK: Management of infection and occlusion associated with vascular access devices. Semin Onc Nurs 1995; 11:174–183.

53. Masoorli S: Managing complications of central venous access devices. Nurs 1997; 27(8):59–63.

54. Farr BM: Understaffing: A risk factor for infection in the era of downsizing? Infect Control Hosp Epidemiol 1996; 17:147–149.

55. Barnes JR, Lucas N, Broadwater JR, et al: When should the "infected" subcutaneous infusion reservoir be removed? Am Surg 1996; 62:203–206.

56. Brown-Smith JK, Stoner MH, Barley ZA: Tunneled catheter thrombosis: Factors related to incidence. Onc Nurs Forum 1990; 17:543–549.

57. Mayo DJ, Pearson DC: Chemotherapy extravasation: A consequence of fibrin sheath formation around venous access devices. Onc Nurs Forum 1995; 22:675–680.

58. Kupensky DT: Use of hydrochloric acid to restore patency in an occluded implantable port: a case report. J Intraven Nurs 1995; 18:198–201.

59. Ruble K, Long C, Connor K: Pharmacologic treatment of catheter-related thrombus in pediatrics. Pediatr Nurs 1994; 20:553–557.

60. Collin GR, Ahmadinejad AS, Misse E: Spontaneous migration of subcutaneous central venous catheters. Am Surg 1997; 63:322–326.

61. Lowell JA, Shikora SA, Bothe A: A technique for the exchange of tunneled polymeric silicone catheters and implantable infusion ports. Am J Surg 1995; 169:631–633.

62. McDermott MK: Patient education and compliance issues associated with access devices. Semin Onc Nurs 1995; 11:221–226.

20

Amputation in the Vascular Patient

Jacqueline Helt, RN, BS, CVN, and Joan Jacobsen, RN, MSN, CVN

ᥰ · ᥰ

The word *amputation*, like *cancer*, is more often considered than spoken. It is frequently the fear of amputation that compels the patient to seek medical attention when "circulation problems" in the legs are suspected. This is not surprising inasmuch as amputation was the only treatment available for advanced arterial occlusive disease in the not-so-distant past. Amputation was frequently above the knee, "the acknowledged safest site for early healing."[1] It often confined the patient to a wheelchair for life and carried a high mortality rate.

With improved vascular surgical techniques, revascularization is considered the primary, optimal method of treating lower-extremity ischemia. Unfortunately not all patients are candidates for this type of intervention, and amputation remains the only alternative. This situation reinforces a negative image of amputation as a failure to save the leg instead of the positive relief of symptoms and restoration of functional ability. For the elderly patient over the age of 70, the initial choice of revascularization or amputation holds special significance. This group of patients is less likely to maintain an independent existence after amputation, thus underscoring the importance of a decision for or against revascularization.[2]

The incidence of amputation sharply increases after the age of 55.[3] In addition, approximately 50–70 percent of all lower-extremity amputations involve persons diagnosed with diabetes mellitus.[4, 5] Despite an increasingly older and more debilitated population, the outlook is promising. The perioperative mortality rate has decreased. Rehabilitation is an integral part of the treatment process, and prosthetic technology is advancing rapidly. Amputation may be the end, the loss of a part, but it may also be the end of pain and a new beginning. Amputation and rehabilitation are synonymous in the minds of the vascular health care team. The challenge is to impart this conviction to vascular patients who regard themselves as too old or too sick to be rehabilitated.

Nurses in many health care settings are in a unique position to help ease a patient's suffering and offer hope. Nursing interactions with the patient and family have a direct impact on recovery and rehabilitation. The purpose of this chapter is to provide the background information necessary to render competent, compassionate nursing care to meet the physical and psychosocial needs of patients undergoing lower-extremity amputation. Approximately 80 percent of amputations involve the lower extremity; therefore the focus of this chapter is on below-knee and above-knee amputations.[6] Upper-extremity amputation as a result of arterial occlusive disease is rare and is not addressed.

TABLE 20–1. **Variables to Evaluate
When Amputation Is Considered**

- Presenting symptoms, i.e., gangrene, rest pain, infection
- Comorbidities, i.e., cardiac, pulmonary, renal, other
- Angiographic evaluation of arterial status
- Risks and benefits of each procedure option
- Potential for prosthetic ambulation

SURGICAL PROCEDURE

Indications for Amputation

There is controversy regarding which patients with lower-extremity arterial occlusive disease can be successfully revascularized. Because vascular reconstruction may not prevent loss of an extremity or prolong life, careful judgment is required with emphasis on the individual's quality of life.[3] The multitude of variables involved in the decision for or against amputation are listed in Table 20–1. The advanced-age populace requires serious consideration of the validity of aggressive revascularization versus primary amputation based on the increased mortality rates of revascularization procedures for older adults.[2] Despite the differences of opinion, it is generally agreed that all patients with arterial insufficiency and limb-threatening symptoms should be thoroughly evaluated for revascularization before amputation is considered. Nontraumatic indications for amputation are indicated in Table 20–2.

Failed Revascularization

Ischemic symptoms vary from mild to severe and limb-threatening. Intermittent claudication is a relatively benign manifestation; a small percentage of patients with claudication eventually require amputation as their disease and symptoms progress. Although claudication is not an indication for amputation, some patients require amputation when revascularization originally performed for relief of claudication has failed. Vascular patients often have multiple procedures, including revascularization surgery, angioplasty, thrombolytic therapy, and surgical revision, before an amputation is the only remaining option. During a 20-year study period, Hallett reported that among the limbs that required minor and major amputations, arterial surgery had been performed on 26–32 percent.[7]

Rest Pain

Ischemic rest pain is characterized by severe burning pain in the toes and forefoot that is intensified by elevation and somewhat relieved by dependency. The pain often wakens the

TABLE 20–2. **Nontraumatic
Indications for Amputation**

- Failed revascularization
- Rest pain
- Ischemic ulceration/gangrene
- Infection
- Massive muscle necrosis
- Phlegmasia cerulea dolens

patient from a sound sleep and becomes progressively more constant and severe. High doses of narcotics in addition to elevating the head of the bed on blocks or sleeping in a sitting position fail to bring relief. This unremitting pain results in a cycle of sleeplessness, exhaustion, lack of appetite, and general debilitation. Rest pain is an indication for amputation when revascularization is not possible and pain cannot be controlled by any other means. Patients who fit this description and do not have gangrene should be treated conservatively until a level of demarcation has emerged.[8] Ischemic rest pain can also occur in a residual limb, necessitating revision of a below-knee amputation to an above-knee amputation.

Ischemic Ulceration/Gangrene

The majority of scenarios leading to amputation begin when patients with absent peipheral sensation sustain a pivotal event initiating the causal chain to an amputation. This event is frequently footwear-related, followed by ulceration and faulty wound healing.[9] Ischemic ulceration (failure of a wound to heal because of inadequate blood flow) often precedes gangrene (tissue death). Both of these conditions are extremely painful, debilitating, and limb-threatening. This is due to the progression of necrosis and/or the superimposed infection that finds little resistance from ischemic tissues. Most foot lesions resulting in amputation are located around the digits.[10] Humphrey and associates found that the primary indication for amputation in the majority (77 percent) of non–insulin-dependent diabetes cases was gangrene.[11]

Vascular patients with foot ulcers, especially those with diabetes, run a high risk of developing new foot ulcerations. In a prospective study by Apelqvist and colleagues, 50 percent of the patients developed a new ulcer within 2 years of observation.[12] All subsequent amputations in this study were precipitated by a foot ulcer; this stresses the need for lifelong observation of the vascular and diabetic foot at risk.

Infection

The diabetic foot is especially vulnerable to infection of all types: local, diffuse (cellulitis), and necrotizing. Uncontrolled sepsis, as in "gas" gangrene (*Clostridium* infection), is an indication for immediate amputation to preserve life. Intravenous antibiotic therapy combined with early debridement of all dead or infected tissue is essential to preserve as much viable tissue as possible. For the patient with diabetes, glycemic control is critical. Poor glycemic control is an important predictor for amputation even after adjustment for other risk factors, including cardiovascular disease, peripheral arterial disease, and peripheral neuropathy.[13] Improved understanding of the pathophysiology of diabetic foot ulceration, infection, and the pattern of ischemia characteristic of diabetic patients can lead to a decrease in the number of amputations.[14] At present, the amputation rate in the diabetic population is documented at 8.1 per 1000 patients.[15]

Massive Muscle Necrosis

Massive muscle necrosis is generally a sequela of an acute embolic or thrombotic event. Because collateral vessels have not yet developed, severe ischemia ensues within hours. There is rapid progression of symptoms (pain, pallor, pulselessness, paresthesias, paralysis, and poikilothermia), edema of the muscles within the fascial sheath (compartment syndrome) secondary to ischemia or reperfusion, and the development of systemic toxicity with renal failure. A high-level amputation is usually necessary.

Venous Disease

Venous ulcers, when uncomplicated by arterial insufficiency, can be treated adequately with conservative measures no matter how extensive, painful, or infected. Despite the patient's fears to the contrary, amputation of the leg is rarely indicated for venous ulcers. On rare occasions, extensive deep venous thrombosis (phlegmasia cerulea dolens) may lead to venous gangrene and amputation.

In summation, major lower-limb amputation is indicated in limb- or life-threatening situations after careful consideration of the risks and benefits of all available alternatives.

Selection of Amputation Level

The objective of preoperative evaluation is to determine the most distal level at which healing will occur and function be restored after removal of all dead or infected tissue. This concept of preservation of tissue and restoration of function is dictated by the knowledge that a higher amputation results in increased morbidity and mortality and decreased rehabilitation potential, primarily as a result of increased demand on the myocardium. Ambulating with a transtibial prosthesis increases energy requirements by 30 percent.[16] The metabolic cost of walking with an above-knee amputation is increased up to 100 percent, which often limits endurance and functional ambulation for the amputee with coexisting cardiopulmonary disease.[17, 18]

The various amputation levels are clearly elucidated in Figure 20–1. The most common are toe, transmetatarsal, below-knee (BK), and above-knee (AK) amputations. Most AK amputations (AKA) will heal without difficulty as a result of the rich collateral circulation

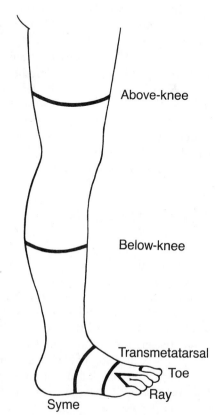

Figure 20–1. Potential levels of amputation in the lower extremity.

in the thigh. Prediction of healing below this level requires careful evaluation of all factors that affect wound healing, including surgical technique, postoperative care, and nutritional status, as well as arterial circulation, particularly tissue perfusion.

The earliest attempts to judge the appropriate level of amputation focused on the presence of palpable pulses, angiographic findings, skin color and temperature, character and location of pain, and, most notably, the presence of incisional skin bleeding at the time of surgery. An armamentarium of objective, diagnostic methods exists to help determine the level at which healing will occur. In addition to Doppler pressure measurements and pulse volume recordings, diagnostic tools include photoplethysmographic pressures, laser Doppler blood flow studies, xenon 133 skin blood flow studies, and transcutaneous oxygen determinations. In a pilot study by Yablon and associates, no patient with a transcutaneous partial pressure of oxygen measurement of less than or equal to 15 mmHg healed his or her incisional wound during the rehabilitation stay.[19] The extent to which these technologies are used will depend on the availability of equipment, the accuracy of each laboratory, and the costs involved. However, these tests have not been consistently more reliable than clinical judgment in predicting wound healing at a given level.[20, 21] Most surgeons use a combination of objective data and assessment of the appearance of the tissues at the time of surgery, particularly bleeding, to decide on the site of amputation.

It is generally thought that most patients requiring a lower-extremity amputation will heal at the below-knee level. If the intention is to fit a prosthesis, BK amputation (BKA) is preferred to all other levels.[22] The qualitative evaluation by Hagberg showed that the higher the level of amputation, the lower the usefulness of the prosthesis.[23] Therefore, it is routine to attempt a BKA rather than an AKA when a major amputation is indicated. However, the results of an outcome study by McWhinnie and coworkers question this practice of maximizing the ratio of BKA to AKA in patients with end-stage arterial disease.[24] Their study concluded that increasing the proportion of BKA from one-third to two-thirds of lower-limb amutations did not improve rehabilitation rates as determined by the number of patients able to walk at 2 years after amputation (26 percent of study participants).[24]

Some clinical situations contraindicate a primary BKA approach. The presence of ulcers, gangrene, or infection extending to the midcalf precludes healing at a standard BK level. Revision to a higher BK level where healing would occur results in a limb that is too short for a functional prosthesis. A severely contracted knee has great potential for nonhealing because of the difficulty with positioning the stump to promote healing. A stroke on the affected side may result in a nonfunctional limb. Dependent rubor at the chosen level is generally considered a contraindication because healing is unlikely. Each case must be determined individually because of the importance of preserving the knee.

Techniques of Amputation

Amputation is among the oldest of operative procedures; information about amputation was recorded in the Vedas of ancient India (3500–1800 BC).[25] Although not technically difficult and a relatively short procedure, amputation requires the meticulous technique of an experienced surgeon who can maximize skin viability through delicate handling of tissues. General principles include amputation after demarcation if possible, debridement of gross infection, and the use of antibiotics. Technical details include gentle handling of tissue, preservation of the blood supply, careful hemostasis to avoid hematoma formation, careful approximation of skin edges, and limitation of tension on the sutures.

Amputations are classified according to the level and type of operative procedure. The following surgical techniques are only a representative sample of currently acceptable surgical approaches.

Open Amputation

Open amputation involves creating soft tissue flaps at the chosen level. The skin edges are not closed. The wound is packed and traction is applied to the flaps to prevent retraction of skin and muscle. Skin and muscle retraction causes an exposed bone end that does not heal. This procedure is generally indicated for trauma or infection, allowing for both drainage and regular observation of tissue viability until closure at a later date.

Guillotine amputation is an open procedure in which all the tissues are cut at the same level through a circular incision. Given this name in sixteenth-century France, this was the standard method of amputation until modern times. Today guillotine amputation is reserved for extremely ill patients who require quick control of rapidly spreading infection such as gas gangrene. Because there are no tissue flaps, future bone revision and/or skin grafting is necessary to obtain wound closure.

Closed Amputation

Closed amputation is the most commonly used technique when amputations are necessitated by vascular disease. The incision is made through presumably healthy tissues, and skin flaps are shaped for primary (sutured) closure.

Above-Knee Amputation

Generally, a fish-mouth incision is used with an AKA. Equal anterior and posterior, or slightly longer anterior, flaps are made at approximately midthigh level (Fig. 20–2). The

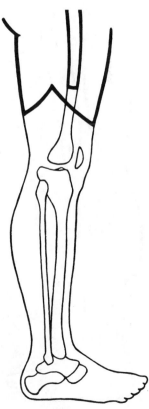

Figure 20–2. Above-knee amputation with a slightly longer anterior flap to cushion the femur, which was divided at midthigh level.

soft tissues are elevated from the femur and retracted, allowing the bone to be divided (cut) straight across. The nerves are gently pulled distally, sectioned, and allowed to retract. Blood vessels are ligated carefully. The skin and deep fascia are drawn distally and the incision is closed primarily. Sutures are loosely placed to prevent skin necrosis when edema develops. A drain may or may not be used.

Below-Knee Amputation

In the BK procedure, a long posterior myocutaneous flap is fashioned from the calf muscles (Fig. 20–3). This flap serves to pad the bone end and provide a rich blood supply to the incision. The tibia is divided in the upper-third section and the front edge is beveled at a 45–60-degree angle; the sharp edges are filed flat. The fibula is divided approximately 0.5–1 inch shorter than the tibia. The periosteum is carefully cut, rather than stripped. The remaining tissues are handled as in an AKA.

Nonsurgical Amputation

Autoamputation is described in ancient Greek writing of the Hippocratic era (approximately 400 BC), when surgical amputation was generally not practiced.[26] Nature was allowed to take its course; that is, if the gangrenous part did not become secondarily infected, it was allowed to demarcate, mummify, and eventually fall off. An entire limb could be treated this way combined with occasional debridement of dead tissue. Care was taken to protect any viable tissue. The process usually took several months. Today, autoamputation is reserved for small, well-demarcated areas of gangrene, such as individual

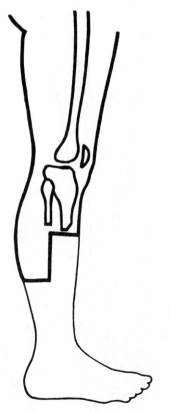

Figure 20–3. Below-knee amputation with a long posterior myocutaneous flap that has a rich blood supply and pads the tibia and fibula when swung forward to the anterior incision. Tibia and fibula are divided at nearly equal lengths.

TABLE 20–3. **Complications of Amputation Surgery**

- Myocardial infarction
- Venous thromboembolism
- Poor wound healing
- Bleeding
- Hematoma formation
- Infection
- Flexion contracture
- Wound dehiscence secondary to trauma
- Phantom sensation
- Phantom pain

digits or parts thereof. The mummified part does not separate until healing has occurred at the line of demarcation.

Complications of Amputation Surgery

Among patients who have undergone lower-extremity amputation as a result of arterial occlusive disease, the frequency of concomitant heart disease has been estimated to be as high as 75 percent, which contributes to increased mortality, with the cause of death most often myocardial infarction.[27] Venous thromboembolism from immobility is also a major cause of mortality. Figures vary, but mortality is generally highest in high thigh amputation or hip disarticulation. BK amputations have traditionally been associated with lower risk.

Survival rates of amputees are dismal. Nagashima studied survival rate at 3 years after primary amputation.[28] The results of this study indicated a higher rate of survival (66.7 percent) for individuals with diabetic gangrene as the cause of their amputation versus those with arterial occlusive disease, who had a 52.3 percent survival rate at 3 years.[28] Five-year survival rates following amputation of a lower extremity are estimated at 35–40 percent.[16] Dawson and associates studied the late outcomes of limb loss after failed infrainguinal bypass and determined that the long-term survival rate was poor (72 percent at 1 year and 53 percent at 3 years)[29] and was not related to the traditional risk factors for atherosclerosis.[29] Because of the systemic nature of vascular disease, continued risk of losing the contralateral leg exists. This risk is approximately 20 percent within the 2 years following amputation.[16]

Common complications of amputation are listed in Table 20–3. Eneroth and coworkers studied risk factors for failed healing in amputation for vascular disease and found that a preoperative hemoglobin greater than 120 g/L gave a higher risk of failure at 35 percent.[8] Smokers had a failure rate of 31 percent at 6 months after amputation.[8] Common complications can be minimized through insightful preoperative assessment, meticulous surgical technique, thorough postoperative medical and nursing care, and early mobilization.

PREOPERATIVE MANAGEMENT

Rehabilitation in the Preoperative Period

Rehabilitation is a dynamic, action-oriented process carried out by an extensive interdisciplinary team consisting of a surgeon, physiatrist, physical therapist, prosthetist, nurses, social worker, nutritionist, the patient, and the patient's significant others. The degree of involvement of each team member will vary according to the needs of the patient.

Rehabilitation is initiated preoperatively when possible. This is actually a preventive phase of care. The focus of rehabilitation at this time includes:

1. maintaining mobility and activity of the other limbs
2. establishing cardiac and pulmonary reserves
3. preventive care for the uninvolved limb, i.e., foot care
4. general conditioning exercises
5. psychosocial evaluation
6. vascular assessment to determine amputation level
7. patient education about the rehabilitation experience[18]

Realistic advice on prostheses before surgery is very important for the vascular patient. The presence of arthritis, gait abnormality, or neurologic deficit may contribute to nonreferral for limb fitting.[22] Memory, attention and concentration, and organizational abilities are cognitive skills necessary for the effective use and maintenance of a prosthetic limb.[30] These are some components of preoperative assessment for prosthetic consideration.

For optimal patient, family, and staff satisfaction, the rehabilitation team, including participation by members of an amputee support group, should be available during the preoperative period. During this time a relationship can be established; an assessment of the patient's physical and emotional status, home situation, and lifestyle can be made; myths can be dispelled; and realistic goals can be defined. Both the patient's and the significant others' fears, frustrations, and depression can be decreased through proper emotional and physcial preparation preoperatively. The patient and family may be overwhelmed by the sheer number of members on the health care team. It is helpful to provide the patient with a list of names of health team members.

Amputee Clinical Pathways

Coordination of patient care among health care professionals is essential for all patients. The interdisciplinary treatment programs needed to provide rehabilitation, including those for amputees, are naturally conducive to coordination and collaboration among team members. The concept of the clinical path tool is to develop and improve guidelines for care collaboration, based upon an optimal sequence of activities and outcomes, i.e., mobility without a prosthesis, independent functioning, and so on.[31] A clinical pathway identifies and describes the requirements for care that occur in a predictable way.[32]

Duration of in-hospital stay is the most important cost-generating factor for amputation surgery.[33] An amputation clinical path is used to manage these costs and lower the average length of stay while maintaining or increasing patient care quality.[34] Clinical paths are the tools of a case manager or care coordinator and are integral to a managed care system of services. However, it must be emphasized that clinical paths are guidelines and that as patient conditions or circumstances warrant, there will be clinical judgments made by physicians and other providers to deviate from these guidelines.

Separate, unique clinical paths for amputees may be designed for the acute care inpatient stay and rehabilitation episode of care, which includes prosthetic training. Clinical paths are generally organized by category. For the acute care clinical path, these categories may include treatments, tests, medications, consults, activities, teaching, and discharge planning (Table 20–4). Rehabilitation categories typically include functional activities of daily living, therapies designed to increase mobility with and without a prosthesis, residual limb care, body image, self-care education, and use of needed equipment (Table 20–5). The acute care clinical path time sequencing would be by days,

TABLE 20–4. **Acute Care Amputee Clinical Pathway**

	PREOP	**OR DAY**	**PO DAY 1**	**POD 2**	**POD 3–5**	**POD 5–6**
Treatments	NPO p MN IV fluids	NPO preop Clear liq.—postop VS q 2 hr Foley cath	VS q 4 hr Adv diet D/C Foley Dressings, elastic wrap Foot care	VS q 8 hr	VS q 8 hr	Soft stump dressing or RRD Desensitize stump
Meds		IV ABX Pain meds Inj./PCA DVT prophylaxis	Stool softener	PO pain meds		
Consults	Rehab/PT SW Amputee support group		PT		Home health services	
Activity	PT to increase strength Active as tolerated	BR with stump elevated	D/C stump elevation Avoid flexion Wheelchair transfers PT begins	Ambulate without prosthesis Balance activities		Safe in transfers, ADLs
Teaching	Pre-op teaching		PT exercise plan Safety measures	Care of residual limb	Equipment informa- tion	Stump care Intro to prosthesis DME Medication F/U care
Discharge Planning	Identify discharge needs; home vs. rehab. vs NH			Preliminary discharge plans Wheelchair prescription	Support group meeting informa- tion	DME take home or delivered Home care arranged

OR = operating room; POD = postoperative day; NPO = nothing by mouth; p MN = after midnight; IV = intravenous; VS = vital signs; I/O = intake & output; D/C = discontinue; RRD = rigid removable dressing; ABX = antibiotics; PCA = patient-controlled analgesia; DVT = deep venous thrombosis; PO = by mouth (oral); PT = physical therapy; SW = social worker; BR = bed rest; ADLs = activities of daily living; DME = durable medical equipment; F/U = follow-up; NH = nursing home.

whereas the rehabilitation path would be described by weeks. These sample paths are not intended to be inclusive of all activities of care for individuals undergoing an amputation. Instead they are provided as a sample of a clinical path format using a simple, tabular listing of activities to be accomplished within a time frame, i.e., day or week.

Nursing Assessment and Intervention

Preoperatively, the nursing focus should be on supporting the patient and the family through their pain, suffering, and decision making. In addition, nurses assist in preparing

TABLE 20–5. **Rehabilitation Amputee Clinical Pathway**

	WEEK 1	WEEK 2	WEEK 3
Functional ADLs	Moderate assist with LE	Minimal assist with LE	Independent functioning of ADL's
Mobility	Maximum—moderate assist with w/c, transfers, ambulation	Minimal assist transfers, ambulation with assistive device, w/c independent	Independent transfers and ambulation (may use assistive device)
Residual Limb Care	Understands limb care (inspection, hygiene, shaping)	Shaping with supervision	Independent inspection, hygiene, elastic wrap or shrinker
Body Image	States impact of amputation	Aware of support services	Participates with support group
Self-Care Education	Aware of needs	Participates in training and cares	Understands meds, diet, risk factors
Equipment	Identify equipment needs	Uses adaptive equipment/ assistive device with supervision	Independent with adaptive equipment and assistive devices

ADLs = activities of daily living; LE = leg exercise; w/c = wheelchair.

the patient physically for surgery and rehabilitation (Table 20–6). Four general areas that are assessed include: (1) physical functioning, such as ambulation and self-care; (2) social factors, such as financial, living, or structural arrangements; (3) psychologic needs; and (4) vocational needs.[35]

Physiologic Focus of Nursing Care

As with any major surgery, the risk of postoperative complications is markedly reduced if the patient is in optimal medical condition, particularly in terms of control of cardiac condition, diabetes, and sepsis. To maximize the patient's potential, nursing care goals encompass the concerns as identified in Table 20–7.

Infection Control. Infection control is directed not only at stabilization of existing infections but also at the prevention of new infection. Strict adherence to infection control principles and routine monitoring of parameters is essential. Amputation level is frequently dictated by the degree of infection control that can be achieved preoperatively. Because

TABLE 20–6. **Preoperative Nursing Assessment and Interventions**

- Assess patient and family needs and responses to clinical situation.
- Prepare patient physically for surgery and rehabilitation.
- Function as coordinator of health care team.
- Provide support and information.

TABLE 20–7. **Physiologic Focus of Preoperative Nursing Care**

- Infection control
- Avoidance of trauma
- Pain management
- Preservation of mobility
- Prevention of venous thrombosis
- Promotion of adequate nutrition

of the direct relationship between inadequate diabetes control and infection, diabetes is monitored carefully and all efforts are made to control blood sugar levels. Utilization of an endocrinologist or a diabetes clinical nurse specialist is an excellent practice.

Avoidance of Trauma. For the patient with arterial occlusive disease, further skin breakdown may necessitate a higher level of amputation or may introduce infection to a noninfected leg before surgery. If arterial disease is present, a skin break on the opposite leg could lead to pain and ulceration, delayed rehabilitation, or, in the worst scenario, a bilateral amputation and a loss of opportunity for prosthetic ambulation.

Pain Control. Providing comfort is essential to enabling the patient to participate in preoperative conditioning exercises and rehabilitation. The patient is reassured that postoperatively incisional pain usually decreases significantly within a week and can be managed successfully with positioning and analgesia. An assessment about prior pain experiences is done; patients usually know whether their tolerance is high or low.

Phantom sensation and phantom pain are addressed. Phantom sensation is the feeling that all or part of the amputated limb is still present. Frequently only the most distal part is affected with tingling, numbness, or a pressure sensation. Traditionally thought to be permanent and problematic in only 5–10 percent of patients, it appears that the incidence may be 85 percent or higher.[36] Phantom pain may be continuous or intermittent. It may disappear as the rehabilitation progresses, or it may last throughout life. When the pain persists for more than 6 months, the prognosis for spontaneous improvement is poor and it can be extremely difficult to treat successfully.[18]

The cause of phantom pain is not well defined. The usual explanation for phantom limb sensation and pain is that the remaining nerves in the affected limb continue to generate impulses that flow through the spinal cord and the thalamus to the somatosensory areas of the cerebral cortex.[18] Appropriate management of phantom limb symptoms include preventing long periods of pain before the amputation.

Preservation of Mobility. Maintaining full range of motion and strengthening muscles is a joint responsibility of nursing and physical therapy. The nurse reinforces the rationale for regular exercise, particularly "push-up" exercises from the chair or bed that strengthen arms for the use of a walker. The nurse's role includes supervision or assistance in performing the scheduled exercises as recommended by the physical therapist. The patient needs to remain active, particularly if several weeks of antibiotic therapy and multiple debridements are necessary preoperatively.

Prevention of Venous Thrombosis. Patients who are immobilized, obese, aged, hypercoagulable, or who have a previous history of venous thrombosis are at increased risk of deep venous thrombosis and pulmonary embolism. Instruction regarding prevention of this potentially fatal complication is given. Because venous stasis is the primary mechanism, a program of regular exercise of the lower extremities is recommended. Subcutaneous low-dose heparin or intermittent compression devices are also effective and are indicated when the patient cannot exercise independently.

Promotion of Nutrition. Multiple surgical procedures and repeated or lengthy hospitalizations of the frail elderly or the diabetic patient with sepsis frequently result in anemia, malnutrition, immunosuppression, and debilitation. Poor nutrition, reflected by an albumin level of less than 3.5 g/dl, severely impairs wound healing. Nutritionists are essential for evaluating the patient's nutritional status, setting goals, determining food preferences, and suggesting supplements. The nurse supervises adequate intake of the recommended diet and oral supplements when ordered. Appetite may be stimulated by scheduling exercises or activities before meals. Monitoring the patient's weight on a regular basis is indicated. Serum transferrin levels are also important nutritional markers.

Psychosocial Focus of Nursing Care

> You ought not to attempt to cure eyes
> Without head,
> Or head without body,
> So you should not treat body
> Without soul.
>
> *Socrates*[26]

This ancient principle of treating the whole person is essential to understanding the implications of amputation and formulating a comprehensive care plan for the amputee patient. The impact of amputation is profound. Amputation results in disfigurement, leading to a negative body image and potential loss of social acceptance. In addition, there is a loss of body function (mobility) that affects one's independence and/or livelihood. Grief associated with these losses is expected.

The grieving process may begin long before the patient reaches the hospital, while the patient is at home comtemplating an amputation. Nurses are adept at recognizing the stages of grief: denial, anger, regression, depression, and acceptance. The stages may occur in any order, can repeat or be absent or exaggerated. Statements of guilt or blaming and frequent requests for second opinions regarding the necessity for amputation are common behaviors exhibited by a potential amputee.

The nursing focus at this point is best directed toward establishing a trusting relationship with the patient and significant other. If the patient had established a relationship with nursing staff on a certain ward during a prior admission, re-establishing that link may be helpful. Active listening is critical. Discussion about the patient's life, work, family, and values may provide the background information to explain the patient's feelings. Seeking out the patient's strengths in prior situations and focusing on them is therapeutic.

The patient's specific fears are identified so that appropriate information may be provided. The most common fears are experiencing pain, dying, and losing independence. Another fear is the reaction of others to the change in body image. Reassurance is given that these fears are normal. Patients and their families tend to overestimate the functional impairment associated with lower-extremity amputation. Therefore, it is beneficial to arrange a meeting with a person who has experienced the kind of amputation that is anticipated. Contact with an amputee support group is helpful at this time.

The nurse should reassure the patient that the surgical procedure itself is short and, unless there are complications, does not require transfer to an intensive care unit postoperatively. Most patients are out of bed within 24–48 hours and discharged to a rehabilitation facility within 3–7 days or home with help within 1–3 weeks. A small percentage of patients are discharged to nursing homes permanently; some elderly debilitated amputees may go to a nursing home for short-term rehabilitation.

POSTOPERATIVE MANAGEMENT

Promoting Functional Independence

Functional Screening and Rehabilitation Outcomes

The major goal of rehabilitation is to improve functional ability, and it is important to be able to measure this.[37] With the present need to reduce medical expenditures, an effective method of screening patients prior to rehabilitation hospitalization was sought. Muecke and colleagues did a retrospective evaluation of postamputation rehabilitation patients who had received a Functional Independence Measure (FIM) assessment on admission and discharge as part of routine inpatient evaluation.[38] The FIM was developed in 1983 by a national task force as an instrument for measuring the progress in regaining function in patients with multiple disabilities. This study provided preliminary evidence that the least functional patients as a group benefited the most from hospitalization and stayed fewer days; however, individual outcomes were highly variable and not predicted well by the FIM on admission.[38] Similarly, in a study by Leung and coworkers, the results indicated that neither the admission FIM nor the change in FIM score helped to differentiate between those who achieved a rehabilitation end-point of ambulation with a prosthesis and those who did not.[37]

Any attempt to use a screening instrument that measures current level of functioning to predict outcome of rehabilitation is subject to significant limitations.[38] Individuals with a high level of functioning on admission to a rehabilitation center will do best on discharge while those with the lowest level of functioning have the greatest capacity to improve. Therefore, FIM scores or any other screening tool should not be used as the only criterion for admission to a rehabilitation program.

Successful rehabilitation can be defined as independence in carrying out daily activities with or without a prosthesis, or even while confined to a wheelchair.[3] Amputee follow-up varies from setting to setting, and measurement of idealized outcomes has not been uniformly applied. Esquenazi and associates identified functional outcome lists for lower-limb amputations with prosthetic restoration.[18] For example, some of the components in the transtibial level outcome list include: (1) ambulation with prosthesis on level surfaces, ramps, and curbs; (2) independence in dressing; (3) independence in donning and doffing prosthesis; (4) standing for up to 2 continuous hours; (5) comfort with falling techniques; and (6) climbing stairs step over step. The authors warn that functional outcome lists are idealized goals and patients may not achieve these levels of function because of comorbidities.[18]

Identifying functional outcomes benefits both the amputee and the rehabilitation team by clarifying goals of the individual rehabilitation program that is designed to meet unique patient needs. The essence of rehabilitation is the individual's achievement of functional goals that correspond to his or her maximal level of independence, lifestyle, and quality of life. In the future, these additional components need to become integral parts of the evaluation of the rehabilitation of amputees.

Physical Therapy Program

The physical therapy (PT) program goals are identified in Table 20–8. Success of a PT program is enhanced by prompt initiation of therapy, open communication with other team members, and clear, concise instruction to the patient.

Active range-of-motion, strengthening, and conditioning exercises are done slowly three or four times each day. While supine, adduction and abduction is done at the hip;

TABLE 20–8. **Physical
Therapy Goals**

- Maintain or regain physical strength.
- Maintain range of motion.
- Prevent contractures.
- Prevent residual limb edema.
- Promote mobility.
- Promote self-care.
- Assist with adjustment to limb loss.
- Evaluate and prepare for prosthesis fitting.

the knee is flexed and extended; and thighs and buttocks are lifted off the bed. For upper extremities, the trapeze bar is used to strengthen biceps and push-ups from the bed or chair strengthen triceps. When resting in bed, flexion of the knee and external rotation of the hip is avoided. The residual limb is elevated for only the first 24 postoperative hours. The limb is not dangled from the bed or the wheelchair due to the potential of edema. Lying prone promotes hip extension.

Ambulation training begins on the first or second day after surgery with the aid of walker, crutches, parallel bars, or temporary prosthesis such as the immediate postoperative prosthesis or an air splint. Early ambulation with the elderly amputee reduces complications such as pneumonia, thromboembolism, residual limb edema, infection, and loss of balance.[16] Weight-bearing on the residual limb is carefully monitored if a temporary prosthesis is used. Body alignment has changed; therefore, new patterns of balance and mobility must be learned. Transfers to the wheelchair, commode, and shower-tub seat are taught. Transfers help strengthen the opposite leg. In addition, they provide a psychologic lift as normal activities are resumed. Until long-distance independent ambulation is achieved, the patient may be mobile with a wheelchair. The therapist recommends the appropriate type of wheelchair and teaches the patient and the significant other how to operate it safely.

Residual Limb Care

A crucial aspect of postoperative management is residual limb care. The objectives of treatment include control of residual limb shrinkage, prevention of edema, prevention of trauma, and reduction of wound pain. This can be achieved by wrapping the residual limb (either AKA or BKA) with an elastic wrap. Wrapping with an elastic bandage is done at surgery, after suture removal, or after complete healing of the incision; the initiation of wrapping depends on the dressing technique and the physician's preference. Initially reapplication occurs every 1–2 hours, extending to every 4–5 hours. Effective wrapping provides the tightest compression distally while avoiding circular turns and is smooth, without wrinkles. Figure-of-eight turns encourage proper limb shape and proximal joint extension. Figure 20–4 demonstrates a generally accepted method of wrapping a BKA limb. Wrapping of an AKA limb is shown in Figure 20–5. The key to successful residual limb care with an elastic bandage is even compression. Unfortunately, due to the number of individuals wrapping and rewrapping the limb, i.e., therapists, nurses, physicians, and patients, consistency is difficult to achieve. Skin breakdown and distal edema can be problems in postoperative residual limb care with elastic bandages.

Patients are taught wrapping techniques. However, elderly patients may not have the balance and coordination necessary to wrap effectively. For this reason, the therapist may adapt a method to meet the individual patient's needs. In some cases, a shrinker is used.

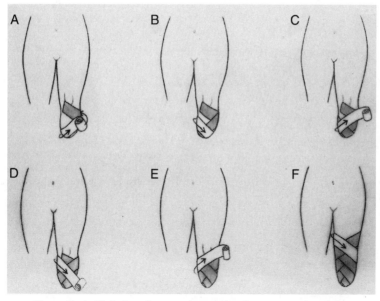

Figure 20–4. Technique for wrapping a below-knee amputation stump.

Shrinkers are graduated-compression elasticized garments that are conical in shape. They are applied like a sock and are held in place by garters or a waist belt attachment as shown in Figure 20–6. Like elastic bandages, shrinkers must be properly positioned, removed regularly for skin care, and washed to avoid irritation. Shrinkers are more expensive than elastic wraps, and smaller shrinkers must be purchased periodically as the limb is shaped and shrinks in size. There is a danger of excessive pressure over bony areas with a shrinker, and there is no protection of the limb with unexpected falling.

For the transtibial amputee, a rigid removable dressing (RRD) provides a safe method to achieve early mobility and rapid prosthetic fitting. Use of an RRD reduces the problems of skin breakdown and distal edema frequently experienced with use of an elastic

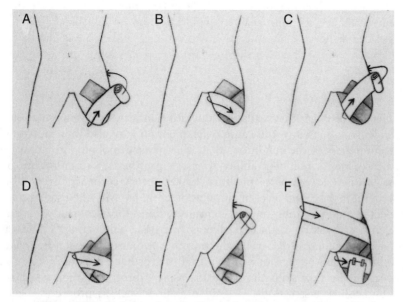

Figure 20–5. Technique for wrapping an above-knee amputation stump.

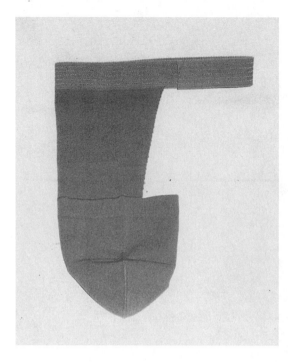

Figure 20–6. Example of a shrinker, an elasticized, socklike garment that may be recommended for a patient who cannot learn to wrap effectively.

bandage.[39] The transtibial plaster cast extends only up to the knee level for easy removal and is suspended by a stockinette to a supracondylar suspension cuff. Underneath the RRD, residual limb socks are added to provide continuous controlled compression. In addition, knee extension exercises and partial weight-bearing exercises while wearing the RRD can be done using a TheraBand (a strip of rubberized material supplied at various tensile strengths). Patients are taught to push the residual limb into a TheraBand held between two hands or stretched between the wheelchair siderails.[16]

Residual limb care includes desensitization and stump hygiene. Desensitization prepares the stump for weight bearing and decreases phantom limb pain. Techniques of desensitization include light tapping and rubbing. In addition, scar massage prevents adherence to underlying tissues, which is a predisposing factor in late stump breakdown. Stump hygiene includes daily washing with mild soap to avoid infection or skin breakdown. Prosthetic socks are replaced daily.

Prosthetics

Often the medical problem that leads to amputation influences postamputation mobility. Medical problems unrelated to the cause of amputation may also influence mobility and ambulation. Awareness of the conditions that affect patient mobility are important in the evaluation of a patient's potential ability to use a prosthesis.[40] Comorbidity of at least one chronic disease, i.e., diabetes mellitus, hypertension, coronary artery disease, and degenerative joint disease, and level of amputation correlate with the use of a prosthesis.[37] In a retrospective study by Johnson and colleagues, the authors concluded that regardless of age, patients with more medical problems had poor ambulation.[40] Thus age alone should not determine prosthetic rehabilitation.[16] Any person previously walking (or a potential walker) should be considered for a trial of prosthetic walking.[42]

Also, incorporating new skills necessary for using a prosthesis requires the ability to understand and follow instructions. Cognitive abilities such as procedural learning and memory, attention and concentration, and problem solving are skills involved in using and maintaining a prosthesis.[30] Intellectual impairment is a prime cause of failure in rehabilitation programs.[42]

Readiness for a temporary prosthesis is evaluated. The residual limb needs to be healed prior to active prosthetic training. Wound healing is age dependent. Although wound healing in the elderly follows the classical phases (inflammatory, proliferative, and remodeling), the phases occur at a delayed rate. Therefore, age is more important than the indication for amputation in predicting the time it takes until gait training with a prosthesis is initiated.[44] The skin of the residual limb should be free of lesions or adherent scar. A conical shape of the distal end of the residual limb is desired. Full range of motion is necessary for ambulation with a prosthesis. Other considerations include patient motivation, strength, previous functional level, and the condition of the opposite leg. The use of a temporary prosthesis such as the one shown in Figure 20–7, particularly for AK amputees, can be especially helpful in the evaluation of the patient's strength, balance, and ability to handle the increased energy demands necessary for prosthetic ambulation.

Selecting the most appropriate components for prosthetic restoration of the residual lower limb is an extremely challenging task in view of the variety and complexity of new prosthetic components, socket fabrication techniques, suspension systems, and available materials.[18] For example, the endoskeletal type of prosthesis (Figs. 20–8 to 20–10) has the weight-bearing mechanical structures covered with a foam plastic material and elastic stocking that not only looks but also feels like a real leg. Total-contact sockets with flexible inserts (Fig. 20–11) provide even pressure distribution. A modular-design prosthesis allows for interchangeability of parts (socket, pylon, foot) resulting in decreased costs because a

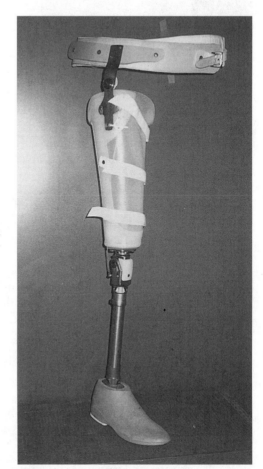

Figure 20–7. Temporary above-knee prosthesis with waist attachment. Note Velcro straps that allow adjustments of socket size to accommodate limb changes.

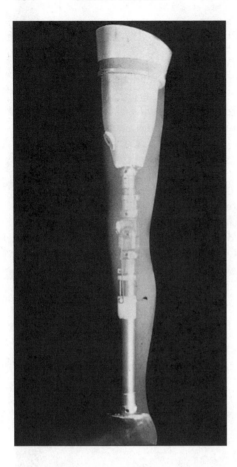

Figure 20–8. Finished Bock endoskeletal prosthesis showing the components within a cosmetic cover. (From Otto Brock Orthopaedic Industry, Minneapolis, MN, with permission.)

broken or ill-fitting part may be exchanged rather than replacing the entire prosthesis. New prosthetic ankle-foot components have been developed in the last several years as a result of a better understanding of the biomechanics of human locomotion and technical advances in materials technology (Fig. 20–12).

The three phases of gait training are listed in Table 20–9. One of the goals in the clinical rehabilitation of the amputee is to maximize the endurance of ambulation with a prosthesis. Data suggest that amputees walk less "efficiently" than normal and have a tendency to fatigue at shorter ambulation distances.[17] Efforts to achieve maximum endurance have focused on trying to reduce the abnormally elevated metabolic cost of walking through several approaches, including the development of lighter weight prosthetic

TABLE 20–9. **Phases of Gait Training With Prosthesis**

Basic stage
  • Donning and doffing prosthesis
  • Parallel bars
  • Weight shifting
  • Initial ambulation
Intermediate stage
  • Ambulation outside of parallel bars with appropriate assistive device
Advanced stage
  • Stairs, ramps, curbs, obstacles, etc.

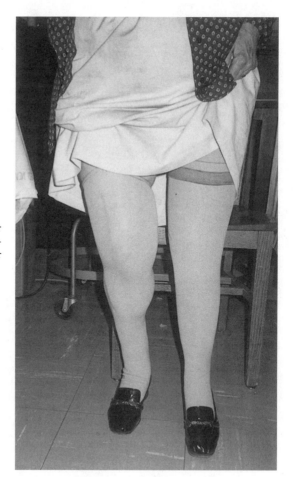

Figure 20–9. Elderly amputee demonstrates her left, above-knee prosthesis. Right leg has undergone multiple surgical procedures and vascular repair.

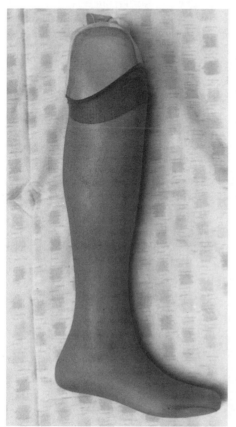

Figure 20–10. Below-knee, endoskeletal prosthesis with flexible socket. It is ultra-lightweight, as the components are made of titanium. (Courtesy of Roger W. Chin, Certified Orthotist-Prosthetist, New York.)

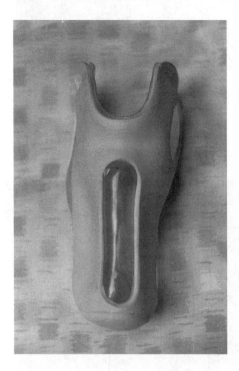

Figure 20–11. Flexible insert for flexible-socket, below-knee prosthesis. (Courtesy of Roger W. Chin, Certified Orthotist-Prosthetist, New York.)

limbs.[45] However, a reduction in prosthetic mass alone does not reduce metabolic energy consumption.[46] Gitter and associates found that amputees are able to conserve effectively the additional mechanical work that is required to propel a heavier limb during a push-off and early swing of ambulation by recovering this energy during the terminal swing deceleration of the limb and transferring it to the trunk.[45] Amputees appear to have the ability to self-optimize their gait during a range of prosthetic masses without any adverse effect on metabolic cost or net mechanical work.

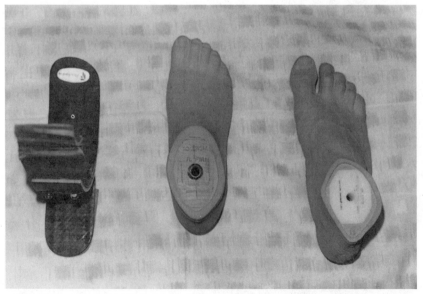

Figure 20–12. Energy-storage feet. From left to right: Flex-Foot; Sten-Foot; Seattle Foot. (Courtesy of Roger W. Chin, Certified Orthotist-Prosthetist, New York.)

Postoperative Nursing Management

Nursing Care of the Residual Limb

Because some vascular amputations are performed through relatively ischemic tissue, it is imperative to provide a clean, comfortable, and nontraumatic environment to enhance wound healing. Two types of wound management, soft dressing technique and rigid dressing (plaster cast) technique, provide good results.

Soft Dressing Technique. A more traditional system of wound management involves the use of a soft, light dressing held in place with a cotton stockinette. The residual limb is generally elevated on one pillow for the first 24 hours to prevent edema. Thereafter, it is maintained flat to prevent hip contractures.

Advantages of this technique include ease of application by the surgeon in the operating room, minimal possibility of pressure injury from elastic, circular bandages or rigid materials, and easy observation of the wound postoperatively. The "sock" dressing is useful until suture removal in 3–4 weeks.

Disadvantages include inadequate edema control and minimal protection from dehiscence secondary to a fall. In addition, this technique will not effectively prevent knee flexion in the face of ischemic pain or spasm. A common variation of the soft-dressing technique attempts to remedy these disadvantages through the application of elastic wrap. A rigid posterior splint placed at the time of surgery or a bulky dressing with an external prefabricated foam padded knee immobilizer may be helpful in this situation.

Rigid-Dressing (Plaster Cast) Technique. In this technique, a drain may be placed and the incision covered with a small fluff dressing and a sterile stockinette. All bony prominences are well padded, and an elasticized plaster cast is applied from distal limb to thigh level. If desired, a pylon (a rigid rod with a detachable foot) is secured to this cast; this is an immediate postoperative prosthesis (IPOP) (Fig. 20–13). A belt attachment provides suspension and prevention of slippage of the pylon. The limb is elevated for 24 hours and then positioned flat. Ambulation may begin as early as the first postoperative day with partial weight bearing for patients with an IPOP. Active participation of the prosthetist in

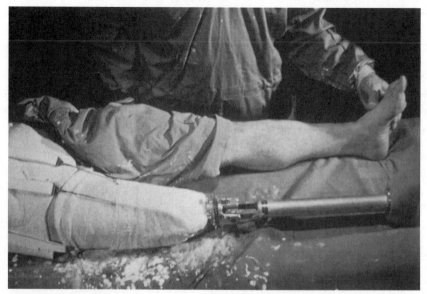

Figure 20–13. Rigid-dressing technique using plaster cast, pylon, and detachable foot. Note suspension apparatus. (Courtesy of Vern Houston, PhD, CPO, New York.)

the operating room and on several scheduled occasions for cast removals and reapplications is essential if a pylon has been attached. Cast removal is indicated for wound inspection if ischemia, pressure injury, or sepsis is suspected.

Advantages of either casting technique include prevention of postoperative edema, reduced pain as a result of incision immobilization, prevention of knee flexion contractures, and protection against trauma. Healing is promoted through control of edema and limited weight bearing with the IPOP. Folsom studied the efficacy of an IPOP program and found that the average interval from amputation to ambulation was 15.2 days for the BK amputees and 9.3 days for the AK amputees.[47] There is psychologic benefit to the patient by replacing the amputated limb immediately with a prosthesis.

However, there are some disadvantages to the rigid-dressing technique. The wound cannot be observed. The cast is heavy and cumbersome for elderly or debilitated patients. There is a potential for pressure injuries on bony prominences. The "beeper foot" (weight-bearing indicator) in the IPOP is ineffective with a hearing-impaired patient. Finally, use of an IPOP requires a very active role by the rehabilitation department and a large, highly skilled interdisciplinary team.

Additional Considerations. Impaired skin integrity is a common nursing diagnosis for amputees.[48] In addition to dressing techniques, care of the residual limb includes other assessments and interventions. Bleeding immediately postoperatively may occur. Drainage areas are marked on dressings, which are reinforced as needed. In the later postoperative period, a hematoma or frank oozing may occur, delaying wound healing. Pallor, poor capillary refill, coldness, petechiae, cyanosis along the incision, or diffuse mottling of the limb is indicative of ischemia. A severely ischemic residual limb may require revision of the limb to a higher level.

The typical signs of infection, including redness, purulent drainage, or elevated temperature, need to be monitored. Infection should be treated promptly according to hospital protocol. Minor redness at suture sites may be normal inflammation. Redness and tenderness at the distal part of a BK limb may be related to constant knee flexion that presses the limb tip into the mattress. The knee should be positioned properly in extension. Splinting the knee to maintain full range and prevent distal pressure may be necessary.

Pain Management. An option for acute postsurgical analgesia is the use of epidural medication. This approach can provide excellent sensory analgesia for several days after surgery.[18] Other pain management strategies include use of patient-controlled analgesia (PCA) or scheduled dosing. Oral analgesics may typically be used for pain relief beginning on postoperative day 3 or 4. A complaint of severe pain may indicate ischemia, pressure areas, or infection.

Phantom limb sensation (the feeling that the leg is still there) occurs in almost every amputee and does not usually require treatment. It is most strongly felt in the immediate postoperative period. Phantom limb pain also begins in the immediate postamputation period, generally subsides, and is seldom a long-term problem.[18] However, for a few amputees, phantom limb pain results in a chronic pain syndrome. Some modalities commonly used to diminish severe phantom limb pain include transcutaneous electrical nerve stimulation (TENS), percussion, vibration, massage, acupuncture, biofeedback, hypnosis, and relaxation techniques. Invasive techniques such as sympathectomy, neuroma excision, and epidural spinal cord stimulation may also be considered.[18]

Psychosocial Adjustment

Most amputees exhibit signs and symptoms of depression during the postoperative period. Crying easily, lack of appetite, difficulty sleeping, withdrawal, and wanting to sleep all the time can be indications of depression. The patient may express feelings of helplessness and hopelessness. Depression must be differentiated from the exhaustive state that frequently follows lengthy periods of pain and sleeplessness. For exhausted patients, sleeping on and off all day for 2 or 3 days is therapeutic. Because depression may be a reaction to the fear of never walking again, early mobilization is a key therapeutic modality. Reassurance is helpful; however, most patients may not believe they will walk again until they actually begin doing it.

In addition, the effects of an amputation impact the entire family system. During the acute phase of rehabilitation, the family of an amputee needs support. With appropriate nursing interventions, the family may be more effective in supporting the patient and in adapting to the long-term consequences of the amputation. Involving family members in a family support group may assist families in resolving the crisis of the acute phase and preparing for a life with a chronic disability.[49]

Discharge Planning

Discharge planning involves input from the entire team and begins on admission. As the discharge date draws nearer, plans are finalized. Some of the variables impacting the length of hospitalization after amputation include status of the incisional wound, presence of postoperative complicatons, and progress in activities of daily living.

The interdisciplinary team has a responsibility to plan and implement the rehabilitation program and to provide patient education and emotional support until the patient is integrated into the family and community.[18] Some areas that need assessment are listed in Table 20–10. Eligibility for support services needs to be considered. The elderly vascular patient is typically on a fixed income with Medicare coverage; however, there may be limitations with Medicare for home care benefits.

One discharge option is for the patient to go directly home with support services. Prior to discharge, an amputee should be able to transfer from the wheelchair, demonstrate the proposed home exercise program, perform essential activities of daily living independently, and, if possible, safely ambulate short distances independently with a walker or crutches.[43] In this situation, patient teaching is reinforced for a home exercise program, wound care, stump wrapping, foot care, and medications. Equipment needs are identified and equipment procurement is arranged. Examples of durable medical equipment (DME) typically needed in a home setting include assistive devices (walker or crutches) for short-distance ambulation; a wheelchair (Fig. 20–14) for longer distances until endurance improves or a prosthesis is fitted; and bathroom equipment, including a shower-tub bench, a hand-held shower, and safety bars for the toilet and tub area (Fig. 20–15). For some patients, a raised toilet seat or commode may be indicated.

For the amputee who returns to a home setting, referral to a home health care agency is routine to ease the transition back to normal activities. The home care nurse and the physical therapist ensure continuity of the rehabilitation plan, monitor the patient's

TABLE 20–10. **Components of Discharge Plan to Home Setting**

- Availability of assistance, i.e., family, friends
- Transportation needs, i.e., wheelchair van arrangements
- Ability to manage nutrition, i.e., grocery shopping, food preparation
- Medication management, i.e., obtaining medications
- Status of home environment, i.e., stairs
- Eligibility for support services, i.e., home nursing care, mobile meals

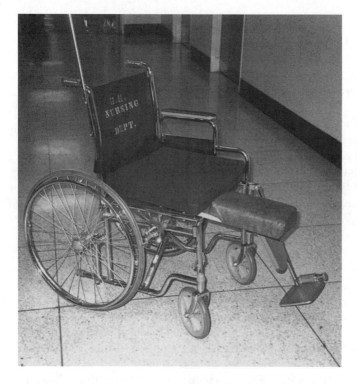

Figure 20–14. Standard amputee wheelchair, with foam seat cushion, seat extender to support limb, self-propelling wheels, removable arms, and detachable foot rests. Notice that wheels are set back 2 inches to prevent tipping backward.

progress, evaluate the home for safety, provide emotional support, and serve as resource personnel. If needed, a home health aide can assist with personal care needs; this provides some relief to the family.

Some patients still drive a car. They are referred to the Motor Vehicle Department for information regarding a handicapped person's parking permit and validation of the driving license. This may require a driving test for some amputees. If necessary, the car is adapted with hand controls. The three major U.S. car manufacturers (GM, Ford, and Chrysler) have programs to support adaptive equipment needed for automobiles and vans.

Fitting of a permanent prosthesis and gait training are accomplished most efficiently through an amputee clinic or rehabilitation center with the assistance and expertise of a multidisciplinary team. This occurs in either inpatient or outpatient settings depending on the assessment by the team to meet the needs of the amputee. For the bilateral amputee, the severely compromised elderly amputee, or the amputee with multiple comorbidities, inpatient therapy is typically recommended. A center or clinic close to home is preferable, reducing travel time and expense for the patient and the family during the 2–4 weeks necessary for an inpatient gait training program.

Another postoperative discharge option for a new amputee is direct transfer to a rehabilitation center or subacute rehabilitation facility. This could be a temporary situation until the residual limb is ready for a prosthesis and would include prosthetic gait training. Direct transfer to a skilled nursing facility with rehabilitation services on a permanent basis may best serve the needs of patients who have long-term care needs and are unable to live independently.

Extending Rehabilitation Into the Community

Ambulation a year after surgery is frequently limited. Several studies identify that amputees may be able to ambulate with a prosthesis within their home environment but have serious

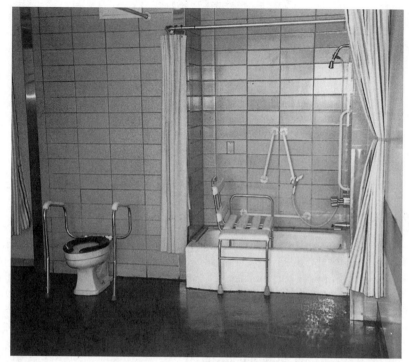

Figure 20–15. Bathroom equipment for an amputee includes a shower-tub bench, hand-held shower, and safety grab bars.

impairment with ambulation in the community.[3, 22, 43, 50] To achieve the highest level of independent living, consideration is given to the various needs arising from the totality of life experiences.[6] Current rehabilitative efforts regarding home mobility are satisfactory; however, attention to community mobility and recreation would improve reintegration to normal living after amputation.[50] One activity that can influence reintegration to normal living is involvement in a support group.

Amputee Support Groups

Support groups play an integral role in holistic care by providing opportunities for peers and interdisciplinary team members to meet the unique needs of amputees. Amputee participation in support groups promotes self-preservation, social acceptance, intimacy, self-expression, and achievement. Acceptance of the amputation is critical to survival; it can influence the level of activity of the lower-extremity amputee.[6]

Amputee support groups provide amputees opportunities to share experiences. New amputees learn about circumstances of other amputees, i.e., same etiology, same concerns and fears, and same initial problems of pain, movement, and body image. Amputee support groups also provide opportunities to obtain resource information such as available community services, possible home adaptations, and the process of rehabilitation. Role models promote independence and share information about organizations that support independent activites such as fishing and golfing. Family participation in the support group activities is also encouraged because an amputation to one person has a major impact on the entire family group.

TABLE 20–11. **Developing an Amputee Support Group**

- Identify need for support group (institution or community)
- Collaborate with other disciplines for support/assistance
- Determine meeting format
- Develop communication system
- Identify group activities
- Solicit funding
- Promote peer visitation

Development of an Amputee Support Group

Nurses have opportunities to assist with the development of amputee support groups (Table 20–11). Initially the need for a support group within the institution or community should be assessed. Support for the development of an amputee support group can be solicited from many disciplines involved within a health care facility. Opportunities for collaboration would typically include physical therapists, occupational therapists, orthotists, prosthetists, chaplains, social workers, psychologists, and patient and family educators.

After the need for an amputee support group is identified, other things to consider include the meeting format, communication system, activities, funding, and peer visitation. The meeting format may be formal with scheduled speakers or consist of an informal sharing of experiences and emotions. Guest speakers present information on various aspects of care, including residual limb care, prosthetic care, and foot care.[36] Group facilitators should be aware that it is impossible to meet the needs of all members, all the time, especially if the group is composed of long-term amputees and new amputees. The group should design its communication system. This system may include a newsletter produced by group members or a sponsoring organization. The group may request, plan, and enjoy social activities such as outings and picnics. Of course, some financial planning needs to be considered. Funding is necessary for the support group's activities, meeting space, newsletter printing and postage, and refreshments.

An important component of an organized amputee support group is peer visitation. Amputees participating in a peer visitation program make hospital visits to individuals preoperatively and provide support to new amputees and their families after the surgery. Training for amputees to function as a peer visitor is beneficial and recommended.

Finally, because nurses support a holistic approach to care, they are most appropriate to facilitate amputee support groups. Facilitating a support group requires many skills. The specific techniques of active listening and questioning are used by successful facilitators during the meeting itself.[51] Support group facilitators need to maintain a balanced perspective and keep some emotional distance.[52] A successful support group develops a sense of "group ownership" with its participants. Group members gradually become less dependent on the facilitator and other professionals who are involved in the support group. Concurrently, successful support group members initiate plans for activities and use of facilitators and other care providers as resources. Such behaviors reflect successful adjustment to amputation experiences.

CONCLUSIONS

In conclusion, the incidence of arterial occlusive disease continues to increase as the numbers of elderly and individuals with diabetes increase. Although amputation is the inevitable result for some individuals, new developments in the field of prosthetics have made ambulation an attainable goal for most vascular amputees. Prompt initiation of therapy is essential for this group; this is especially crucial because of the markedly decreased life expectancy as a result of the generalized nature of the atherosclerotic disease process. Prompt restoration of function to increase the quality of the remaining life is best accomplished through the efforts of an interdisciplinary rehabilitation team that views amputation as the first step in rehabilitation.

References

1. Haimovici H: Amputation of lower extremity. In Haimovici H (ed): Vascular Surgery, 2nd ed. Norwalk, CT, Appleton-Century-Crofts, 1984, pp 1087–1119.
2. Bunt TJ, Malone JM: Amputation or revascularization in the >70 year old. Am Surg 1994; 60:349–352.
3. Weiss GN, Gorton A, Read RC, et al: Outcomes of lower extremity amputations. J Am Geriatr Soc 1990; 38:877–883.
4. VanHoutum MH, Lavery LA: Outcomes associated with diabetes-related amputations in the Netherlands and in the state of California, USA. J Intern Med 1996; 240:227–231.
5. Fylling CP, Knighton DR: Amputation in the diabetic population: Incidence, causes, cost, treatment, and prevention. J Enterostom Ther 1989; 16:247–255.
6. Medhat A, Huber PM, Medhat MA: Factors that influence the level of activity in persons with lower extremity amputation. Rehab Nurs 1990; 15:13–18.
7. Hallett JW, Byrne J, Gayari MM, et al: Impact of arterial surgery and balloon angioplasty on amputation: A population-based study of 1155 procedures between 1973 and 1992. J Vasc Surg 1997; 25:29–37.
8. Eneroth M, Persson BM: Risk factors for failed healing in amputation for vascular disease. Acta Orthop Scand 1993; 64:369–372.
9. Reiber GE: Who is at risk of limb loss and what to do about it? J Rehabil Res Dev 1994; 31:357–362.
10. Isakov E, Budoragin N, Shenhav S, et al: Anatomic sites of foot lesions resulting in amputation among diabetics and non-diabetics. Am J Phys Med Rehabil 1995; 74:130–133.
11. Humphrey LL, Palumbo PJ, Butters MA, et al: The contribution of non-insulin dependent diabetes to lower extremity amputation in the community. Arch Intern Med 1994; 154:885–892.
12. Apelqvist J, Larsson J, Agardh CD: Long-term prognosis for diabetic patients with foot ulcers. J Intern Med 1993; 233:485–491.
13. Lehto S, Pyorala K, Ronnemaa T, et al: Risk factors predicting lower extremity amputations in patients with NIDDM. Diabetes Care 1996; 19:607–612.
14. Gibbons GW, Marcaccie EJ, Burgess AM, et al: Improved quality of diabetic foot care, 1984 vs 1990. Arch Surg 1993; 128:576–581.
15. American Diabetes Association: Clinical practice recommendations 1996. Diabetes Care 1996; 19:Suppl 1.
16. Cutson TM, Bongiorni D, Michael JW, et al: Early management of elderly dysvascular below-knee amputees. J Prosthet Orthotics 1994; 6(3):62–66.
17. Czerniecki JM: Rehabilitation in limb deficiency. 1. Gait and motion analysis. Arch Phys Med Rehabil 1996; 77:S3–S8.
18. Esquenazi A, Meier RH: Rehabilitation in limb deficiency. 4. Limb amputation. Arch Phys Med Rehabil 1996; 77:S18–S28.
19. Yablon SA, Novick ES, Jain SS, et al: Postoperative transcutaneous exygen measurement in the prediction of delayed wound healing and prosthetic fitting among amputees during rehabilitation. A pilot study. Am J Phys Med Rehabil 1995; 74:193–198.
20. Bacharach JM, Rooke TW, Osmundson PJ, et al: Predictive value of transcutaneous oxygen pressure and amputation success by use of supine and elevation measurements. J Vasc Surg 1992; 15:558–563.
21. Dwars BJ, van den Broek TA, Rauwerda JA, et al: Criteria for reliable selection of the lowest level of amputation in peripheral vascular disease. J Vasc Surg 1992; 15:536–542.
22. Houghton AD, Taylor PR, Thurlow S, et al: Success rates for rehabilitation of vascular amputees: Implications for preoperative assessment and amputation level. Br J Surg 1992; 79:753–755.
23. Hagberg E, Berlin OK, Renstrom P: Function after through-knee compared with below-knee and above-knee amputation. Prosthet Orthot Int 1992; 16:168–173.
24. McWhinnie DL, Gordon AC, Collin J, et al: Rehabilitation outcome 5years after 100 lower-limb amputations. Br J Surg 1994; 81:1596–1599.
25. Sanders GT: Lower Limb Amputations: A Guide to Rehabilitation. Philadelphia, FA Davis, 1986.
26. Majino G: The Healing Hand—Man and Wound in the Ancient World. Cambridge, Mass, Harvard University Press, 1975.

27. Roth EJ, Wiesner SL, Green D, et al: Dysvascular amputee rehabilitation, the role of continuous noninvasive cardiovascular monitoring during physical therapy. Am J Phys Med Rehabil 1990; 69:16–22.
28. Nagashima H, Inoue H, Takechi H: Incidence and prognosis of dysvascular amputations in Okayama Prefecture (Japan). Prosthet Orthot Int 1993; 17:9–13.
29. Dawson I, Keller BP, Brand R, et al: Late outcomes of limb loss after failed infrainguinal bypass. J Vasc Surg 1995; 21:613–622.
30. Phillips NA, Mate-Kole C, Kirby RL: Neuropsychological function in peripheral vascular disease amputee patients. Arch Phys Med Rehabil 1993; 74:1309–1304.
31. Coffey RJ, Othman JE, Walters JI: Extending the application of critical path methods. Qual Mgt Health Care 1995; 3(2):14–29.
32. Mikulaninec CE: An amputee clinical path. J Vasc Nurs 1992; 10(2):6–9.
33. Solomon D, Ven Rij A, Barnett R, et al: Amputations in the surgical budget. N Z Med J 1994; 107:78–80.
34. Schaldach DE: Measuring quality and cost of care: Evaluation of an amputation clinical pathway. J Vasc Nurs 1997; 15:13–20.
35. Yetzer EA, Kauffman G, Sopp F, et al: Development of a patient education program for new amputees. Rehabil Nurs 1994; 19:355–358.
36. Bowser MS: Giving up the ghost: A review of phantom limb phenomena. J Rehabil 1991; July/Aug/Sept:55–62.
37. Leung EC, Rush PF, Devlin M: Predicting prosthetic rehabilitation outcome in lower limb amputee patients with the functional independence measure. Arch Phys Med Rehabil 1996; 77:605–608.
38. Muecke L, Shekar S, Dwyer D, et al: Functional screening of lower-limb amputees: A role in predicting rehabilitation outcome? Arch Phys Med Rehabil 1992; 73:851–858.
39. Wu Y, Krick H: Removable rigid dressing for below-knee amputees. Clin Prosthet Orthot 1987; 11:33–44.
40. Johnson VJ, Kondqiela S, Gottschalk F: Pre- and post-amputation mobility of trans-tibial amputees: Correlation to medical problems, age, and mortality. Prosthet Orthot Int 1995; 19:159–164.
41. Cutson TM, Bongiorni DR: Rehabilitation of the lower limb amputee: A brief review. J Am Geriatr Soc 1996; 44:1388–1393.
42. Penington GR: Benefits of rehabilitation in the presence of advanced age or severe disability. Med J Aust 1992; 157:665–666.
43. Andrews KL: Rehabilitation in limb deficiency. 3. The geriatric amputee. Arch Phys Med Rehabil 1996; 77:S14–S17.
44. Scremin AME, Tapia JI, Vichick DA, et al: Effect of age on progression through temporary prostheses after below-knee amputation. Am J Phys Med Rehabil 1993; 72:350–354.
45. Gitter A, Czerniecki J, Meinders M: Effect of prosthetic mass on swing phase work during above-knee ambulation. Am J Phys Med Rehabil 1997; 76:114–121.
46. Czerniecki JM, Gitter AG, Weaver K: Effect of alterations in prosthetic shank mass on the metabolic costs of ambulation in above-knee amputees. Am J Phys Med Rehabil 1994; 73:348–352.
47. Folsom D, King T, Rubin JR: Lower extremity amputation with immediate postoperative prosthetic placement. Am J Surg 1992; 164:320–322.
48. Heafey ML, Golden-Baker SB, Mahoney D: Using nursing diagnosis and interventions in an inpatient amputee program. Rehabil Nurs 1994; 19:163–168.
49. Winterhalter JG: Group support for families during the acute phase of rehabilitation. Holistic Nurs Pract 1992; 6(2):23–31.
50. Nissen SJ, Newman WP: Factors influencing reintegration to normal living after amputation. Arch Phys Med Rehabil 1992; 73:548–551.
51. Overbeck B, Overbeck J: Starting/running support groups. Dallas, TLC Group, 1992, p 13.
52. Galinsky MJ, Schopler JH: Negative experiences in support groups. Soc Work Health Care 1994; 20:77–95.

21

Vascular Trauma

Judith M. Jenkins, RN, MSN, and Jennie P. Daugherty, RN, MSN, CS

Trauma is the leading cause of death in the United States for individuals under the age of 44 years, and the fourth most common cause of death for all age groups.[1] Approximately 150,000 Americans die annually from traumatic injuries and an additional 400,000 people suffer permanent disability. The impact on society can be quantified in lost wages, disability, and subsidized health care, as well as lost productivity for both the patient and family. Trauma is both a preventable disease and a serious public health problem with cumulative costs in excess of 100 billion dollars per year.[2]

Patients often present with multiple injuries, most commonly as a result of motor vehicle crashes, gunshot wounds, stab wounds, or falls. Improved patient survival and functional recovery are related to advancements in prehospital care, regionalization of trauma care, adherence to the Advanced Trauma Life Support (ATLS) guidelines, advances in surgical critical care, and early transition to rehabilitation.

Vascular trauma presents an especially challenging subset of patients. Patients are at risk for both loss of life from the sequelae of hemorrhagic shock and loss of limb from ischemia. Further, vascular trauma is not usually an isolated injury, but one of a constellation of injuries requiring thoughtful consideration of treatment priorities. Diminishing physiologic reserve may not permit definitive reconstruction at the initial operation, but may require a temporizing procedure to bridge the patient until revascularization can be accomplished. This represents a strategic departure from conventional principles used in elective vascular surgery.

This chapter addresses the mechanism and pathophysiology of vascular injuries, examines injuries by anatomic location, and explores the concept and application of damage control principles to vascular surgery. The trauma patient with a vascular injury presents a challenge both physiologically and psychosocially. The chapter concludes with nursing implications pertinent to these issues.

MECHANISM OF INJURY

Mechanism of injury combines the action of forces and its effect on the human body. When a force pushes tissue beyond its limits, injury occurs. Injury can be caused by either penetrating or blunt forces. Knowledge of the mechanism and circumstances of the injury predicts its nature and severity. Urban environments foster penetrating injuries from gunshot or stab wounds, whereas farming and hunting accidents are more common in rural settings. Motor vehicle crashes, falls, and suicide attempts transcend environment.

Penetrating Trauma

Penetrating trauma is produced when a foreign object passes through tissue.[2] The ensuing injury is more predictable than blunt trauma because of the finite wound path. Gunshot and stab wounds are the most common injuries, although vascular penetration can occur as a result of displaced bone fragments or impaled objects.

The degree of damage from a gunshot wound depends on the caliber and velocity of the missile. The greatest damage results from a large-caliber, high-velocity gun. The extent of injury is proportional to the amount of kinetic energy (KE) that is lost by the missile:

$$KE = \frac{\text{mass} \times (V1^2 - V2^2)}{2 \times g}$$

V1 is impact velocity, and V2 is exit or remaining velocity.[2] Kinetic energy is proportional to the mass of the bullet and to the velocity. Therefore, high-velocity injuries, such as those caused by military weapons, produce more tissue destruction than low-velocity handgun injuries.

Conversely, stab wounds are less likely to produce severe vascular injury. Small knives are often used, sparing deep vascular structures, except in the neck where vessels are more superficial. Wounds occur more frequently on the left side of the body because most assailants are right-handed. Stab wounds may also be created by impaled objects, shards of glass, or bone fragments. Damage is usually confined to the wound path.

Penetrating injuries most commonly involve the intestines, liver, spleen, and truncal vascular structures. The resulting impact can be direct, that is, laceration from the missile or its fragments, or indirect, compression and temporary cavitation of the surrounding soft tissue. The vascular injury resulting from the blast effect causes perforation with free bleeding, vessel transection with exsanguination or thrombosis, or arteriovenous fistula formation from contiguous arterial and venous wounds.

Blunt Trauma

Blunt trauma is defined as an injury in which there is no communication with the outside environment. Motor vehicle crashes, falls, and assaults are the usual cause. Multiple injuries are common and, because of the diffuse pattern of injury, are usually more life-threatening than penetrating trauma.

Injury occurs as a result of deceleration, acceleration, shearing, crushing, compression, or a combination of forces. Direct impact causes the most injury. Indirect forces are transported internally, with energy dissipating to internal structures. The extent of injury from an indirect force depends on the transmission of energy from an object to the body. As energy is released, tissues become displaced and injury occurs.

Deceleration or compression produces avulsion and thrombosis of small vessels, whereas acceleration/deceleration and shearing injuries cause intimal flaps and secondary thrombosis. Vascular structures that are tightly attached to musculoskeletal structures, such as the thoracic aorta, are more prone to injury.

PATHOPHYSIOLOGY OF INJURY

Penetrating trauma produces laceration, transection, or perforation of an artery or vein. Complete transection can result in arterial thrombosis, leaving distal perfusion dependent on available collaterals. Conversely, partial disruption of an artery or vein may produce exsanguinating hemorrhage unless the bleeding is controlled or until the circulating volume is sufficiently depleted for the hemorrhage to stop. Successful volume resuscitation can cause hemorrhage to resume unless the injured vessel has been repaired.

Blunt trauma creates stress on the artery wall from lateral displacement or stretching, often without apparent disruption. Visually, the vessel may appear uninjured; however, the lumen may be occluded by an intimal flap, producing ischemia. Arterial spasm is common after small-vessel trauma. It is usually transient, but may be sufficient to jeopardize distal perfusion and tissue viability (Fig. 21–1). Evidence of distal ischemia should always be evaluated and not assumed to be due to arterial spasm.

Arteriovenous (A-V) fistula formation or pseudoaneurysms are infrequent late findings following arterial trauma. An injury that produces an A-V fistula may be surprisingly free of significant blood loss at the time of injury. Penetrating trauma can produce a concomitant laceration of the artery and the adjacent vein. Blood flows directly from the artery into the vein or into the adjacent hematoma and then into the vein. As healing begins, the hematoma retracts, allowing direct blood flow between the artery and the vein. The hemodynamic consequences of an A-V fistula involving a large artery include tachycardia,

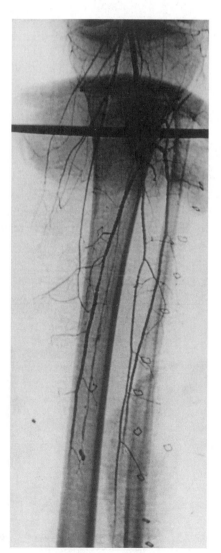

Figure 21–1. Arterial spasm associated with fracture of the tibia and fibula.

increased cardiac output, high-output cardiac failure, and compromised distal perfusion as arterial circulation is diverted from the periphery.

Pseudoaneurysms occur following an incomplete arterial laceration. A pulsating hematoma is created with continued arterial bleeding. Frequently, pseudoaneurysms are asymptomatic, discovered only in the course of evaluating concomitant injuries (Fig. 21–2). Symptoms result from compression of surrounding structures rather than ischemia as distal perfusion usually remains intact. Repair is indicated to prevent expansion, rupture, or thrombosis.

EXTRACRANIAL VASCULAR INJURIES

Relative to its size, the cervical region contains a greater variety and concentration of anatomic structures than any other area of the body. The airway, vessels, thoracic duct, pharynx, esophagus, spinal cord, spinal column, lower cranial nerves, muscle, and soft tissue are all at risk for injury.[3] Neck trauma resulting in vascular injury is most commonly due to penetrating trauma caused by gunshot or stab wounds. Blunt injuries are considered uncommon, though one series found a 0.67 percent incidence of blunt carotid trauma following motor vehicle crashes.[4] The probable mechanism of injury for most internal carotid artery (ICA) injuries is rapid deceleration, resulting in hyperextension and rotation of the neck, which stretches the ICA over the upper cervical vertebrae, producing an intimal tear.[5]

The neck is divided into three anatomic zones. Diagnosis and management is guided by the primary zone of injury and the neurologic status of the patient. Zone I extends from the clavicle to the cricoid cartilage, and includes the proximal carotid arteries, the subclavian vessels, the major vessels of the chest, the upper mediastinum, esophagus, trachea, and thoracic duct. Because of the potential for great-vessel involvement, arteriography is recommended in stable patients to define the injury and to determine the best course for surgical exposure.

Zone II extends cephalad from the cricoid cartilage to the angle of the mandible, and includes the carotid and vertebral arteries, jugular veins, esophagus, and trachea. It is the area most susceptible to injury and accessible to evaluation and repair. Historically, violation of the platysma muscle mandated surgery; however, the selective utilization of observation, arteriography, and endoscopy in asymptomatic patients has been demonstrated to reduce the incidence of negative surgical exploration.[6]

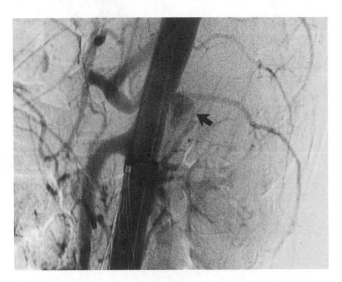

Figure 21–2. Pseudoaneurysm of the abdominal aorta *(arrow)* following a gunshot wound to the abdomen with injury to the stomach, pancreas, and T-12 paraplegia.

Zone III originates at the angle of the mandible and terminates at the base of the skull. Surgical exposure is difficult or impossible in this area. Arteriography is indicated to define surgically manageable carotid or vertebral artery lesions and, therapeutically, to embolize inoperable injuries.[7]

Carotid duplex imaging in the emergency environment is limited by cost, availability, and personnel. Also, the distal ICA may be difficult to visualize when an associated or suspected cervical spine injury precludes flexion, extension, or rotation of the neck.[6]

A thorough clinical examination, augmented by arteriography, endoscopy, and bronchoscopy, dictates the management strategy. As in elective surgery, revascularization of a neurologically compromised patient may convert an ischemic deficit into a hemorrhagic stroke with devastating consequences. Thus, patients with mild to moderate deficits should be considered for revascularization, although heparin therapy, followed by warfarin for 3 to 6 months, has been shown to be efficacious in reducing neurologic morbidity and mortality.[4] Patients with severe deficits are usually managed nonoperatively or with ligation. Unlike patients with chronic vascular disease, a young trauma patient with an intact contralateral vascular bed has an increased chance for recovery with minimal sequelae.

The initial management of extracranial vascular injuries is dictated by the principles of the ATLS—**A**irway, **B**reathing and **C**irculation.[8] The airway is secured, ventilation assisted, if indicated, and hemorrhage controlled. Volume resuscitation with crystalloid and blood must be initiated immediately in response to hemodynamic stability. A brief neurologic examination should be obtained before sedation or paralytics are administered. Finally, any patient with a mechanism of injury suspicious for an associated cervical spine injury requires cervical spine immobilization until such injury is ruled out or until operative exposure dictates mobilization. Table 21–1 summarizes the nursing considerations for patients with extracranial vascular injuries

Penetrating neck wounds should not be probed, cannulated, or locally explored because manipulation may dislodge a clot and produce exsanguinating hemorrhage. Nasogastric tubes should be avoided, if possible, until after anesthesia is induced because gagging and vomiting may also dislodge a tamponading clot.[3]

The operative options for extracranial vascular trauma are much the same as for elective revascularization. The decision process, however, is influenced by the neurologic status of

TABLE 21–1. **Extracranial Injuries: Nursing Considerations**

- ABCs
  - O_2 administration to maintain $SaO_2 > 92\%$
  - Intubation and assisted ventilation, if indicated
  - 2 large-bore IV catheters for volume resuscitation
- Neurologic examination prior to sedation/paralytics
- Assess for hematoma formation
  - Tracheal deviation
  - Airway compromise
- Assess for delayed chest injuries
  - Auscultate for bilateral breath sounds
  - Monitor SaO_2
  - Assess for Beck's triad
    - Hypotension
    - Jugular venous distention
    - Muffled heart tones
- Cervical spine immobilization for suspected cervical spine injuries

SaO_2 = oxygen saturation in arterial blood; IV = intravenous.

the patient.[3] When possible, proximal and distal control of the injured vessel is secured. The internal jugular vein may be repaired or ligated without neurologic consequences. Carotid reconstruction requires debridement to normal intima to achieve a technically satisfying repair and reduce the incidence of thrombosis or distal embolization and stroke. Repair options, thereafter, include primary closure, patch angioplasty with autogenous tissue or polytetrafluoroethylene (PTFE), resection with end-to-end anastomosis, and ligation. Shunts are indicated only when backbleeding is inadequate, although the nature of the injury may make shunt insertion both technically impossible and inordinately time-consuming.

Vertebral artery injuries are rare, due largely to its protected anatomic location along the vertebral column. Frequently patients are asymptomatic. Proximal vertebral artery injuries—those located in Zone I—are more accessible for repair. Options include primary repair, reimplantation to the subclavian artery, anastomosis to the adjacent carotid artery, and ligation. Injuries occurring in Zones II and III are difficult, if not impossible, to expose because of the overlying vertebral column. Arteriography with therapeutic embolization to occlude the injured vertebral artery is recommended. The incidence of neurologic sequelae following ligation or embolization is minimal.

Subclavian artery injuries present a challenge for surgical exposure and control because of the anatomic proximity of the aorta and great vessels. A supraclavicular incision, median sternotomy, or both, may be necessary depending on the location of injury. An anterolateral thoracotomy extending into a supraclavicular incision and a median sternotomy, the so-called "trapdoor" approach, may be indicated to expose the proximal left subclavian artery at its origin from the aorta. Reconstructive options include primary repair, an interposition graft with PTFE, or a subclavian-to-carotid anastomosis for proximal injuries with sufficient length of normal artery.

THORACIC INJURIES

Thoracic vascular injuries occur primarily in the civilian environment. These are injuries of the "urban war zone," and the majority of experience is from inner-city trauma centers.[9] Gunshot or stab wounds account for an overwhelming majority of thoracic vascular trauma, although deceleration injuries to the aorta are not uncommon following motor vehicle crashes. All are catastrophic, present as surgical emergencies, and have variable outcomes.

Presentation includes external or internal hemorrhage (manifested as hemothorax, mediastinal hematoma, or cardiac tamponade), thrombosis with distal ischemia, or intimal disruption with a variable vascular exam. The presence of palpable distal pulses does not preclude proximal injury or rupture because an associated hematoma can be contained by the perivascular tissues, allowing for the transmission of a pulse. A high index of suspicion may save a life. Markers suspicious for thoracic vascular injury include:

- bullet trajectories that cross the midline;
- a first or second rib fracture;
- sternum, clavicle, or scapula fractures;
- flail chest; or
- massive left hemothorax

All are indicative of an enormous energy transfer to the thoracic cavity. The presence of more than 2000 ml of blood in the chest and continued bleeding of greater than 250 ml/hr from the chest tube are relative indications for thoracotomy.[10]

Arteriography is not indicated, nor usually an option, in these patients due to hemodynamic instability. Further, the patient may have concomitant life-threatening injuries that preclude extensive preoperative evaluation. Only those tests that influence the strategic management plan should be obtained in the Emergency Department. Operative management must be directed at the source of hemorrhage, leaving other injuries for subsequent repair. This concept will be explored further in the section on Damage Control.

Table 21–2 outlines the nursing considerations for patients with thoracic and abdominal vascular injuries. Each injury type will be explored separately, although the nursing challenges are the same.

Aortic Arch and Great Vessels

Patients with aortic injuries have a 50–85 percent mortality, infrequently surviving the prehospital environment. Those patients that arrive in the Emergency Department alive have tamponaded the injury, avoiding immediate exsanguination. Aggressive volume resuscitation may cause a sufficient rise in blood pressure to defeat this compensatory mechanism, resulting in exsanguinating hemorrhage unless the injured vessel is expeditiously controlled.

Injury to the aortic arch, innominate artery, right subclavian, and proximal carotid arteries is best managed via a median sternotomy with or without supraclavicular extension. The clavicle is not excised for supraclavicular exposure except in life-threatening injuries because doing so jeopardizes upper-extremity function. Aortic and carotid artery

TABLE 21–2. **Thoracic/Abdominal Vascular Injuries: Nursing Considerations**

- ABCs
  - O_2 administration to maintain $SaO_2 > 92\%$
  - Intubation and assisted ventilation, if indicated
  - 2 large-bore IV catheters for volume resuscitation
- Enhance pulmonary function
  - Endotracheal suctioning
  - Aggressive pulmonary toilet following extubation
  - Pain control
  - Early mobility
- Improve hemodynamics
  - Crystalloid and blood product resuscitation
  - Assess hemodynamic parameters—BP, HR, PA pressures
  - Monitor chest tube output
- Assess neurovascular status
  - Glasgow Coma Scale
  - Moving all extremities
  - Palpate pulses distal to injury
  - Bilateral blood pressures
- Enhance gastrointestinal motility and nutritional status
  - Early enteral feedings
  - Advance to oral feedings after extubation
  - TPN for intolerance to enteral feedings
  - Provide stress ulcer prophylaxis in the absence of enteral feedings
- DVT prophylaxis
  - Enoxaparin
  - Sequential compression devices

SaO_2 = oxygen saturation in arterial blood; IV = intravenous; BP = blood pressure; HR = heart rate; PA = pulmonary artery; TPN = total parenteral nutrition; DVT = deep venous thrombosis.

repair options include primary repair, knit Dacron patch angioplasty, or graft interposition. The innominate artery can be repaired primarily or with a synthetic bypass from the aorta for proximal injuries.

Associated injuries to the trachea or esophagus are common. Esophagoscopy and bronchoscopy are indicated for patients with a high index of suspicion for injuries to these organs. Pulmonary contusions are common and patients may require prolonged ventilatory management, early tracheostomy, and aggressive pain control to enhance chest wall excursion.

Descending Thoracic Aorta

Aortic disruption is the leading cause of immediate death following blunt trauma caused by motor vehicle crashes or falls.[11] On deceleration, tears occur at points of anatomic fixation from a combination of shear stress, bending stress, and tension. The result is intimal and/or medial tears, or complete disruption and immediate death. Aortic tears produce pseudoaneurysms or partial circumferential hematomas tamponaded by the peri-aortic tissue. The most common site for disruption is distal to the origin of the left subclavian artery adjacent to the ligamentum arteriosum (Fig. 21–3).

A high index of suspicion is essential to diagnosis and patient survival. A widened

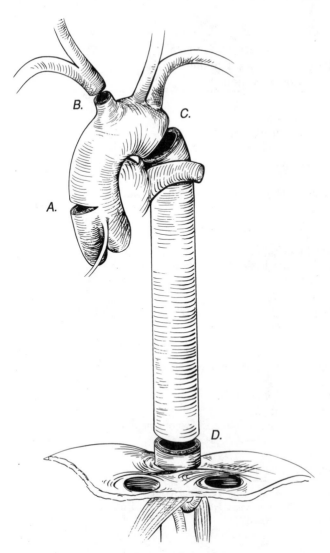

Figure 21–3. Sites of aortic rupture. The most common site is *C*, adjacent to the ligamentum arteriosum, followed by sites *A, D,* and *B.*

mediastinum found on chest x-ray (CXR) indicates the presence of mediastinal blood and should be reassessed with an upright or reverse Trendelenburg CXR.[10] Signs of a wide mediastinum include increased mediastinal width (greater than 8 cm), apical capping, loss of the aortic knob, or deviation of the nasogastric tube. If the repeat CXR is positive, the decision must be made for further assessment with aortography (Fig. 21–4) or computerized tomography (CT).

Surgical exposure is achieved via a posterolateral thoracotomy. The anesthesiologist must avoid hypertension on induction because this may cause fatal rupture of the surrounding hematoma. Repair options include primary suture repair or graft interposition. Once hemorrhage is controlled, the operation is more technically satisfying in the young trauma population because of the absence of associated atherosclerotic disease.

Spinal cord ischemia, resulting in paraplegia, may be reduced by limiting aortic cross-clamp times to less than 30 minutes and by close placement of the proximal and distal clamps to minimize intercostal artery hypoperfusion.[7] Still, the incidence of paraplegia is as high as 10 percent. If a long cross-clamp time is anticipated, a shunt or partial cardiopulmonary bypass should be utilized to preserve distal perfusion.

Cardiac Tamponade

Cardiac tamponade is a life-threatening emergency caused by penetrating or blunt trauma. Because it is both a symptom and an injury, the underlying cause must be addressed simultaneously for definitive resolution.[11]

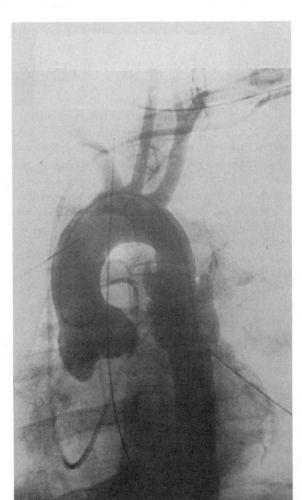

Figure 21–4. Aortic disruption at the ligamentum arteriosum.

The pericardial sac normally contains 25 ml of serous fluid to cushion and protect the heart. The addition of blood or air from traumatic injury causes diminished venous return to the right atrium with subsequent ineffectual myocardial contraction, decreased stroke volume, and decreased cardiac output. Decline in cardiac performance is directly related to the speed with which the pericardial sac must accommodate blood and fluid, as well as the total volume to be accommodated.[11] Thus, slow leaks into the pericardial sac are tolerated for a period of time allowing for diagnosis and treatment.

Diagnosis of cardiac tamponade can be difficult because the symptoms may be obscured by the symptoms of hypovolemic shock and concomitant life-threatening injuries. Beck's triad is the classic constellation of diagnostic signs and includes hypotension, jugular venous distention (JVD), and muffled heart tones. Recognition of JVD may be concealed by the cervical collar, and heart tones are difficult to assess in a noisy trauma resuscitation room. Other symptoms include a narrowed pulse pressure and an increased central venous pressure, quickly assessed by vigorous venous backflow upon central line insertion. A high index of suspicion can be lifesaving.

Management options are twofold: pericardiocentesis (percutaneously aspirating the pericardial sac to provide for adequate cardiac contractility) or resuscitative Emergency Department thoracotomy. Patients with blunt trauma, or without "signs of life," are not candidates for thoracotomy because survival in these circumstances is virtually zero. "Signs of life" include detectable blood pressure, palpable pulse, pupillary activity, and respiratory effort in the absence of sedation. The goal of Emergency Department thoracotomy is to control hemorrhage, enhance myocardial and cerebral perfusion via aortic cross-clamping and/or open cardiac massage, and direct volume resuscitation. Still, the prognosis is poor for patients requiring this heroic intervention.

ABDOMINAL VASCULAR INJURIES

Hemorrhagic shock is the most common cause of death in patients with abdominal vascular injuries. The primary mechanism of injury is penetrating trauma secondary to gunshot or stab wounds, although iatrogenic injuries resulting from diagnostic procedures, operative procedures of the abdomen or spine or after therapeutic procedures, such as the intra-aortic balloon pump (IABP), can also produce vascular injury.[12] Consequences of penetrating injuries include intimal flap formation with secondary thrombosis, vessel wall defects with hemorrhage, or complete transection of the artery or vein. Rapid deceleration following motor vehicle crashes or falls causes avulsion of small branches from their origin or intimal tears with thrombosis, often associated with seat belt injuries (Fig. 21–5).

Clinical presentation depends on whether there is active hemorrhage (associated with profound hypotension, tachycardia, and abdominal distention) or a contained hematoma (characterized by hypotension responsive to volume resuscitation). Peripheral pulses may be diminished or absent, although this is an unreliable sign because distal pulses will not be palpable with a systolic blood pressure less than 80 mmHg or in the presence of hypothermia. Penetrating wounds that cross the midline are markers for vascular injury, as well.

Table 21–2 summarizes the nursing considerations for the patient with an abdominal vascular injury. Interventions for these patients are much the same as for patients with thoracic injuries and, as such, are presented conjointly.

Management of the patient with an abdominal vascular injury begins with the principles of the ATLS. The airway is secured, ventilation assisted, if indicated, and volume resuscitation initiated with crystalloid and blood products. During the initial evaluation, the presence of a life-threatening intra-abdominal hemorrhage must be expeditiously determined and intervention initiated to control the bleeding. Operative goals include identifying and exposing the injured vessel, achieving hemostasis, and restoration of end-organ

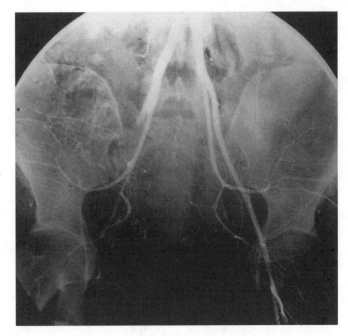

Figure 21–5. Right iliac artery occlusion secondary to seat belt injury.

perfusion.[13] The decision to repair, ligate, or temporize the injury is determined by weighing the benefits of immediate hemostasis against the risk of ischemia. Unlike elective procedures where revascularization is completed prior to closure, the trauma patient *in extremis* cannot physiologically tolerate a complicated or time-consuming definitive procedure. Patients *in extremis* are characterized clinically by hypothermia, coagulopathy, and acidosis (Table 21–3).[10] In such circumstances the decision must be made to temporize the injury for reconstruction at a second operative setting. This concept will be discussed further in the section on Damage Control.

Arteriography is not indicated in penetrating trauma prior to surgery because impending exsanguination mandates immediate management. There is value, however, to therapeutically embolizing deep bleeding vessels that are not amenable to surgical repair. Situations for such an intervention include bleeding associated with complex pelvic fractures, as well as mesenteric and remote hepatic bleeding. There is currently no role for duplex imaging in abdominal vascular trauma, although ultrasound may provide useful information in the hands of trained personnel.

The patient is prepared for surgery from the clavicle to the knees. This allows access to the chest, if thoracotomy is needed, and to the groin, if femoral access is required for line placement or harvesting autogenous tissue. A midline incision extending from the xiphoid process to the symphysis pubis is preferred. Because opening the abdomen can result in loss of tamponade with exsanguination and cardiac arrest, the anesthesiologist must be prepared to volume resuscitate the patient upon opening the abdomen.[10] Aortic

TABLE 21–3. **Definition of**
in Extremis

Hypothermia	Core temperature < 35° C
Coagulopathy	Diffuse oozing from cut surfaces
	Prothrombin time > 15 seconds
	Platelets < 75,000
Acidosis	Base deficit > −15 mmol/L

control to stop hemorrhage can be achieved with the aortic occluder placed at the diaphragmatic hiatus or via thoracotomy for thoracic aortic control. Thoracotomy, however, has the disadvantage of promoting hypothermia by exposing another body cavity and provides more cut surfaces from which to bleed.[10] Bleeding from the vena cava can usually be controlled manually or with sponge stick pressure.

Abdominal Aorta and Iliac Arteries

Hemorrhage from injury to the abdominal aorta and iliac arteries is brisk and rapidly fatal. The etiology is most often penetrating trauma, although blunt injury with intimal disruption of the iliac artery can occur following a seat belt injury (Fig. 21–5). Clinical presentation includes shock, abdominal distention ultimately limiting respiratory excursion, abdominal pain, and, less frequently, acute lower-extremity ischemia. Expeditious surgical intervention is mandatory for survival. Isolated pelvic hematomas associated with pelvic fractures or blunt trauma are not explored unless there is evidence of injury to the aorta.

Proximal control of hemorrhage is achieved using the methods described previously. In some cases, digital compression is sufficient until the source of hemorrhage can be isolated. Repair options include primary repair, synthetic patch angioplasty, graft interposition, or extra-anatomic bypass in the setting of massive fecal contamination, frequently associated with concomitant iliac and colon injuries. The external and common iliac arteries should be repaired, whereas the internal iliac artery can be ligated with impunity. It may be necessary to accept an iatrogenic stenosis or temporize the injury for subsequent reconstruction in the patient *in extremis*. Definitive repair can be accomplished once the patient's physiologic condition permits.

Vena Cava and Iliac Veins

The etiology of vena cava and iliac vein injuries is primarily penetrating, including penetration resulting from displaced bone fragments associated with pelvic fractures. Injuries to the vena cava are frequently retrohepatic and are associated with massive liver injury from blunt trauma. It is best to manage these nonoperatively, if possible, because the technical exigencies of exposure and control of hemorrhage, combined with hypothermia and coagulopathy, make the operative mortality and morbidity higher than the risk of conservative management.

Surgical repair is often hampered by the difficulty in identifying a finite source of venous hemorrhage, loss of proximal control of hemorrhage, or vessel tearing during mobilization and dissection. Further, branches of the vena cava can be easily avulsed from their origins resulting in further hemorrhage. Proximal aortic control may be necessary to reduce massive venous hemorrhage, whereas packing or ligation may be necessary to control pelvic hemorrhage. Options for repair include simple venorrhaphy or, for complete transection, end-to-end anastomosis. Ligation may be indicated for exsanguinating hemorrhage, accepting the risk of chronic lower-extremity edema.

Visceral Injuries

The celiac axis is most commonly injured following penetrating trauma. Clinical presentation includes signs of hemorrhagic shock and hemoperitoneum. Ligation may be necessary to prevent exsanguination. This is usually well tolerated in the absence of pre-existing atherosclerotic disease because of the rich collateral supply from the superior mesenteric artery (SMA). The splenic artery can also be ligated followed by splenectomy, whereas the hepatic artery should be repaired, if possible.

The mechanism of injury for the SMA is primarily penetrating, although a direct blow or lap belt can produce injury as well. As with celiac axis injuries, patients with injury to the SMA present with an acute abdomen and shock. Ischemic bowel may be encountered at operation. Mortality is reportedly 70–90 percent as a result of massive hemorrhage. The exigencies of the situation may dictate SMA ligation and resection of ischemic bowel. If repair is possible, options include primary repair or bypass with autogenous tissue. Reperfusion of ischemic small bowel and colon can result in cardiac arrest; therefore, mannitol and sodium bicarbonate should be administered prophylactically prior to removing the cross-clamp.[10] A planned second-look operation is mandatory should the patient survive the damage control operation.

Injury to the superior mesenteric vein (SMV) should be repaired if possible, although it can be ligated with a low incidence of small bowel ischemia. Of note, patients requiring SMV ligation will have massive fluid requirements related to bowel edema and fluid sequestration.[10]

Renovascular injuries require repair or nephrectomy. Revascularization options include suture repair and bypass. For the patient *in extremis*, nephrectomy may be lifesaving; however, it is advisable to determine the function of the contralateral kidney prior to nephrectomy. Although it may be necessary to render a patient anephric to preserve life, it is preferable to know this beforehand.[10]

Retroperitoneal Hematoma

The presence of a retroperitoneal hematoma is indicative of massive bleeding from either a visceral organ of the retroperitoneum or a major vascular structure. Complex pelvic fractures are notoriously associated with retroperitoneal bleeding and hemodynamic instability. CT scan is the most effective tool for the preoperative diagnosis of retroperitoneal injuries, although they are often discovered at the time of celiotomy. This can be catastrophic because if the retroperitoneum is opened, tamponade of venous bleeding is lost, and the patient may exsanguinate.[10]

Management of a retroperitoneal hematoma is governed by the patient's hemodynamic stability as well as the location and mechanism of injury. The crucial operative decision revolves around whether to open and explore the hematoma. To make this decision, retroperitoneal hematomas are classified according to zones (Fig. 21–6).[10]

Zone I is defined as the central medial zone and includes the duodenum and pancreas, and the major abdominal vasculature. Presentation is often dramatic and associated with a high mortality rate. In general, Zone I hematomas require exploration, regardless of the mechanism of injury.[10]

Zone II is lateral to Zone I and incorporates the kidney and retroperitoneal portion of the colon and its mesentery. These injuries are often associated with hematuria, and are managed nonoperatively. Zone III includes the entire pelvis; pelvic fractures account for the majority of injuries in this area. In blunt trauma, the hematoma is not explored for fear of losing compensatory tamponade. Exploration is indicated, however, following penetrating injury because hemorrhage is commonly the result of iliac vessel damage amenable to repair. In practice, large retroperitoneal hematomas may overlap zones, but the source of the injury is usually apparent.[10]

PERIPHERAL VASCULAR INJURIES

The scope and ultimate outcome of a peripheral vascular injury depends significantly on the mechanism of injury. Peripheral vascular injuries in the urban environment are most

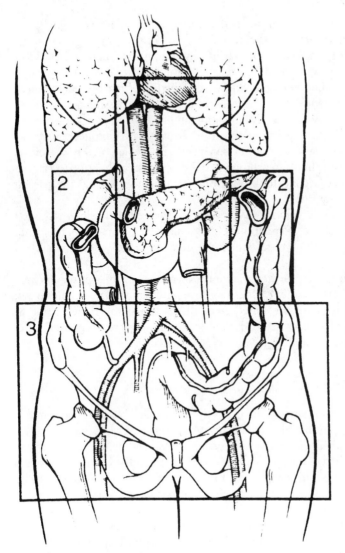

Figure 21–6. Zones of the retroperitoneum. Zone 1 is the central medial zone, containing the pancreas, duodenum, and major vessels. Zone 2 contains the kidneys and the retroperitoneal colon. Zone 3 contains the major vessels of the pelvis and the rectum. (From Morris JA Jr, Eddy VA, Rutherford EJ: The trauma celiotomy: The evolving concepts of damage control. Curr Prob Surg 1996; 33(8):627.)

commonly due to penetrating trauma. Stab wounds to the upper extremity are most common, whereas gunshot wounds are more common in the lower extremity (Fig. 21–7). Motor vehicle crashes and falls are the most frequent causes of blunt injury. Blunt peripheral vascular injuries are more morbid than penetrating trauma owing to associated fractures, dislocations, and crush injuries to muscles and nerve trunks.[14]

Clinical findings are categorized as either "hard" or "soft." "Hard" findings include physical evidence of arterial occlusion (the 6 Ps: pulselessness, pain, pallor, poikilothermia, paresthesia, paralysis), arterial bleeding, rapidly expanding hematoma, and palpable thrill or audible bruit, although this is difficult to assess in a noisy trauma resuscitation room. Hard signs of arterial injury mandate immediate operative intervention or arteriography if the patient is hemodynamically stable.

"Soft" findings include a history of active bleeding at the scene, close proximity of the wound or blunt injury to a major artery, small nonpulsatile hematoma, or a neurologic deficit. As previously discussed, the absence of a palpable distal pulse or definitive ischemic findings does not preclude an injury.

Table 21–4 summarizes the nursing considerations for the patient sustaining a peripheral vascular injury. As with all trauma patients, management begins with the principles

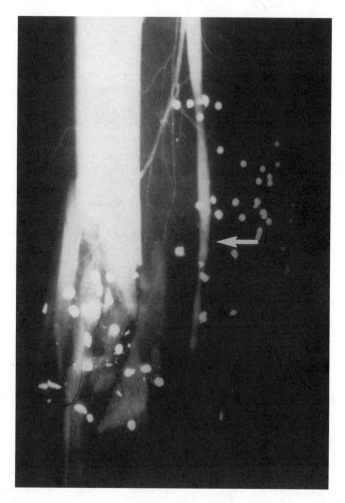

Figure 21–7. Shotgun injury to the femur with intimal disruption *(arrow)* of the superficial femoral artery.

of ATLS. The airway is secured and ventilation assisted, if indicated. Volume resuscitation is initiated via two large-bore intravenous (IV) lines with crystalloid and blood products. Depending on the clinical presentation and mechanism of injury, three management options are available: observation, therapeutic embolization, and surgical intervention.

Selective observation, although controversial, has been advocated in asymptomatic

TABLE 21–4. **Peripheral Vascular Injuries: Nursing Considerations**

- ABCs
  - O_2 administration to maintain $SaO_2 > 92\%$
  - Intubation and assisted ventilation, if indicated
  - 2 large-bore IV catheters for volume resuscitation
- Assess neurovascular status
  - Palpate pulses distal to injury
  - Assess motor and sensory function
  - Bilateral blood pressures
- Provide pain control to enhance mobility and pulmonary toilet
- Early mobility
- Physical therapy/occupational therapy intervention

SaO_2 = oxygen saturation in arterial blood; IV = intravenous.

patients with arteriographic evidence of minimal injury. Patients are observed in the hospital for 24 hours, and must be amenable to close follow-up in the outpatient setting.[15]

Therapeutic embolization is beneficial in the setting of low-flow A-V fistulae, pseudoaneurysms, active bleeding from unnamed arteries, or as an adjunct to surgical intervention for injuries that are difficult to expose or control. This is particularly useful for the distal profunda femoris and tibial artery branches that are inaccessible to operative repair.

Immediate surgical intervention is indicated for most peripheral vascular injuries to preserve limb viability and functional outcome. The entire injured extremity is prepped and draped, along with the contralateral extremity if the need for autogenous tissue is anticipated. Proximal and distal control is secured, and the artery inspected and debrided to normal intima. A Fogarty catheter is passed proximally and distally to remove any intraluminal thrombus inhibiting perfusion. Repair options include patch angioplasty, suture repair, resection with end-to-end anastomosis, graft interposition, and bypass. Autogenous tissue is preferred, although PTFE may be utilized. PTFE has the advantage of being more resistant to infection than other synthetic materials and has an acceptable long-term patency in the above-knee position, especially in nonatherosclerotic trauma patients.

Temporary intraluminal shunts may be necessary when definitive revascularization must be delayed for fracture fixation, complex tissue repair, or other life-threatening injuries. This damage control technique has the advantage of providing limb perfusion while buying time for a more complete assessment of soft tissue, nerve, and bone injuries.[14]

Concomitant orthopedic injuries are common following both blunt and penetrating trauma and contribute to an increased incidence of limb loss. Arterial injuries are usually repaired first to restore perfusion. An exception to this mandate is a situation of massive musculoskeletal trauma with severe instability; surgeon preference is also a factor. A temporary intraluminal shunt followed by external fixation of the fracture may be required to sufficiently stabilize the extremity prior to definitive revascularization. The goal of reconstruction is limb salvage with functional recovery.

Associated nerve injury determines the patient's long-term prognosis and functional recovery. Repair of a mangled extremity, defined as massive orthopedic, nerve, soft tissue, and vascular injuries, may be difficult or impossible. Primary amputation is recommended in such circumstances to expedite functional recovery and reduce the expected incidence of sepsis.[14, 16]

Upper-Extremity Vascular Injuries

Distal subclavian and axillary artery injuries are uncommon. Penetrating trauma is the primary mechanism of injury. Ischemic symptoms may be absent or equivocal because of the rich collateral supply in the shoulder; therefore, a high index of suspicion augmented by arteriography is often necessary for a definitive diagnosis. A median sternotomy may be necessary to achieve proximal arterial control. The presence of a concomitant brachial plexus injury following blunt trauma is the primary determinant of functional recovery (Fig. 21–8).[14]

Brachial, radial, and ulnar artery injuries are usually iatrogenic, resulting from arterial line placement or brachial catheterization for arteriography. Brachial artery injuries should be repaired. Single-vessel forearm injury can be ligated; however, injury to both arteries requires repair of one to preserve perfusion to the hand. The ulnar artery is repaired preferentially because it is the dominant vessel to the palmar arch.[14]

Femoral and Popliteal Injuries

Injuries to the proximal profunda femoris artery should be repaired if possible because this is a rich source of collaterals to the pelvis, buttocks, thigh, and lower extremity.[17]

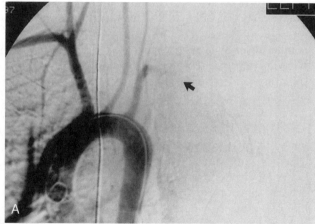

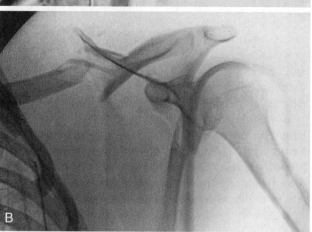

Figure 21–8. Subclavian artery thrombosis *(arrow)* associated with an avulsion of the brachial plexus **(A)** and sternoclavicular dissociation **(B)** following a motor vehicle crash. Surgical management included saphenous vein graft interposition to the axillary artery and a two-compartment forearm fasciotomy.

Ligation or embolization may be necessary, however, in the setting of hemodynamic instability. The superficial femoral artery requires repair unless amputation for a mangled extremity is imminent.

The outcome of penetrating injury to the popliteal artery and vein is dependent on the mechanism of injury. Amputation rates following shotgun blasts are significantly higher than those following gunshot or stab wounds owing to the associated soft tissue destruction and ensuing septic complications. Instability of the knee or frank dislocation are the most common causes of popliteal injury following blunt trauma. Surgical exposure can be achieved from either a medial approach or posteriorly, if the injury is isolated. Repair options include primary repair, graft interposition, or bypass.

Tibial Artery Injuries

An isolated injury to one tibial artery rarely produces limb ischemia in the setting of sufficient collateral perfusion. Single-vessel injuries can be ligated or embolized with impunity, whereas injury to the tibioperoneal trunk or two vessels mandates repair. The surgical exposure to tibial injuries is the same as in elective revascularization—a medial approach for the posterior tibia and peroneal arteries, and an anterolateral approach for the anterior tibial artery. Functional recovery requires satisfactory reconstruction of associated bone, nerve, and soft tissue injuries accompanied by early and diligent rehabilitation.

COMPARTMENT SYNDROME

Compartment syndrome occurs as a result of vasodilatation and interstitial fluid shifts following injury or reperfusion. Swelling ensues, compromising venous return and diminishing arterial perfusion. This ominous series of circumstances yields irreversible muscle ischemia and necrosis in as little as 2–4 hours.

The development of a compartment syndrome should be anticipated if a prolonged period of shock or arterial occlusion has occurred, there is a combined arterial and venous injury, arterial or venous ligation is required, or massive crush injury with swelling is present. Compartment pressures greater than 30 mmHg are abnormal and greater than 45 mmHg mandate fasciotomy.[14]

Early signs of extremity compartment syndrome include pain disproportionate to the injury or surgery, neurosensory changes, and increased compartment pressures. Late findings include the loss of distal pulses and motor deficits, indicative of irreversible ischemic damage to the nerve and muscle (Table 21–5). Many trauma patients will not recognize or be able to communicate an increase in pain or neurosensory changes because of sedation and paralytic agents. Further, extremity swelling is common following injury and/or massive volume resuscitation. The distinction between expected edema and compartment syndrome is difficult but critical to limb salvage. A high index of suspicion in patients at risk may prevent devastating consequences.

Lower-extremity fasciotomies should decompress all four compartments via medial and lateral incisions (Fig. 21–9). Inadequate decompression provides little gain for functional limb recovery. Thigh and upper-extremity fasciotomies are rare. Wound closure options following fasciotomy include primary skin closure if the skin edges can be comfortably reapproximated or skin grafting. Meticulous wound care is necessary prior to closure to reduce the incidence of wound infection and sepsis.

IATROGENIC INJURIES

Iatrogenic injuries are those injuries that occur as a result of a therapeutic or diagnostic procedure. Sequelae can be as benign as thrombophlebitis following peripheral IV insertion or life-threatening, such as hemorrhage or dissection following an arterial catheterization. Cardiac catheterization accounts for the greatest incidence of iatrogenic injuries, followed by peripheral arterial cannulation for an indwelling arterial catheter. The increased use of such therapeutic modalities as percutaneous stent placement, transluminal angioplasty, IABP insertion, and peripheral vascular angiography has increased patient vulnerability to iatrogenic injury.

Morbidity from an iatrogenic injury includes hemorrhage, hematoma formation, thrombosis, A-V fistula formation, pseudoaneurysm formation, dissection, and embolization. Hematoma development is the most common complication of arterial catheteriza-

TABLE 21–5. **Compartment Syndrome**

Early Signs
• Compartment pressures > 30 mmHg
• Pain disproportionate to injury or surgery
• Decreased sensation
Late Signs
• Absent distal pulses
• Inability to move extremity

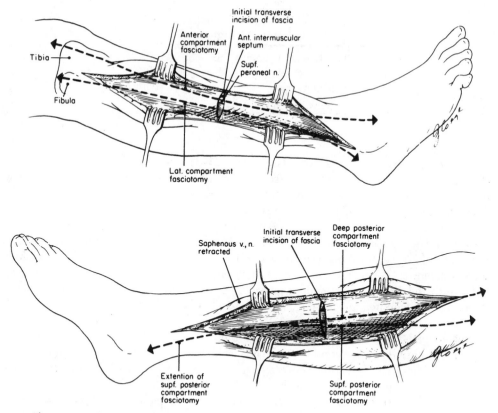

Figure 21–9. Four-compartment fasciotomy via a medial and lateral incision. (From Bongard F, Wilson S, Perry M (eds): Vascular Injuries in Surgical Practice. Norwalk, CT, Appleton & Lange, 1991.)

tions, and does not require surgical intervention unless there is concomitant nerve compression causing motor or sensory deficits. Hemorrhage can usually be managed with direct pressure, though primary suture repair may be indicated for large-bore defects.

The incidence of A-V fistula formation, pseudoaneurysm, and dissection is minimal; however, definitive repair requires suture closure or obliteration and bypass. Embolization from the site of cannulation is most frequently seen in elderly patients with pre-existing atherosclerotic disease. Clinically, the patient may be asymptomatic or have signs of distal ischemia, jeopardizing digits, limbs, or visceral organ perfusion. Such dramatic cases require intervention; options include embolectomy, thrombolysis, and/or anticoagulation.

DAMAGE CONTROL

Vascular injury is often part of a complex constellation of injuries requiring a creative management strategy to preserve tissue perfusion while addressing the exigencies of the patient at risk for exsanguination. The concept of damage control is not new to vascular surgery. Precedent exists in the management of ruptured abdominal aortic aneurysms, where the presence of concomitant ileofemoral occlusive disease is accepted in deference to impending physiologic exhaustion. Vascular trauma is especially challenging in the context of damage control because of the inherent conflict between the need for elaborate and time-consuming reconstruction and the urgent need to abbreviate the procedure before the patient reaches physiologic exhaustion.[18]

The patient *in extremis* is approaching physiologic exhaustion, characterized by hypo-

TABLE 21–6. **Damage
Control Techniques**

- Extraluminal balloon tamponade
- Temporary intraluminal shunt placement
- Ligation
- Primary amputation

thermia, coagulopathy, and acidosis (see Table 21–3). Historically, this condition was referred to as "irreversible shock." These patients have depleted their physiologic reserve and are incapable of tolerating an extensive operative procedure. Recognition of the patient *in extremis* is crucial to patient survival.[10]

Damage control is a minimalist procedure designed to maximize the patient's chances for survival.[19] Ischemia takes a lower priority than hemorrhage but should be addressed early unless doing so threatens systemic viability.[18] Techniques such as extraluminal balloon tamponade, intraluminal shunt placement, ligation, and primary amputation are strategies to diminish the effects of impending physiologic exhaustion (Table 21–6).[20] The role of arteriography is limited to defining and therapeutically embolizing inaccessible sites of hemorrhage.

Extraluminal balloon placement in the wound track may be useful to tamponade hemorrhage until definitive control can be achieved. Conversely, intraluminal shunt placement is a temporizing technique directed at the preservation of distal perfusion while other life-threatening injuries are addressed. The shunt is inserted in the injured artery briefly during orthopedic fixation or left in place until the patient can tolerate definitive revascularization.

Ligation should be considered for any patient approaching physiologic exhaustion. It is especially useful for surgically inaccessible vessels, those requiring complex repair, or when shunt insertion is technically impossible or inordinately time-consuming.[18, 21] Figure 21–10 illustrates that many arteries in the abdomen can be ligated with relative impunity. The ICA can be ligated as a lifesaving measure with a reasonable chance of neurologic recovery in a young trauma patient with an intact contralateral vascular bed. All limb veins can be ligated with impunity, though concomitant fasciotomy may be necessary to reduce the amputation rate following popliteal vein and major lower-extremity artery ligation.[18]

The decision for primary amputation is difficult, but easier in exsanguinating patients whose diminishing physiologic reserve renders them unable to tolerate a prolonged multispecialty reconstruction. A guillotine amputation is the most expeditious and best physiologically tolerated primary procedure. Revision and definitive closure are accomplished when the patient is hemodynamically stable.

Morbidity includes hemorrhage and postoperative ischemia. The patient *in extremis* is at risk for hemorrhage from coagulopathy, multiple cut surfaces, and the inherent risk that a temporary intraluminal shunt, if placed, may become dislodged due to inadequate fixation or changing wound geometry associated with resuscitation. Ischemia is difficult to diagnose in the hypotensive patient with severe hypothermia, limb edema, and peripheral vasoconstriction. Peripheral pulses are often not palpable in these circumstances. Fasciotomy or a minimalist revascularization procedure may be indicated at the bedside if the patient cannot tolerate transport to the operating room.

Damage control is followed by a period of secondary resuscitation in the surgical intensive care unit. The goals of this phase include aggressive rewarming, replacement of blood and clotting factors, correction of acid-base imbalances, and the aggressive use of cardiopulmonary support. When the goals have been achieved (Table 21–7), the patient is ready for reconstruction and consideration of definitive repair.[10]

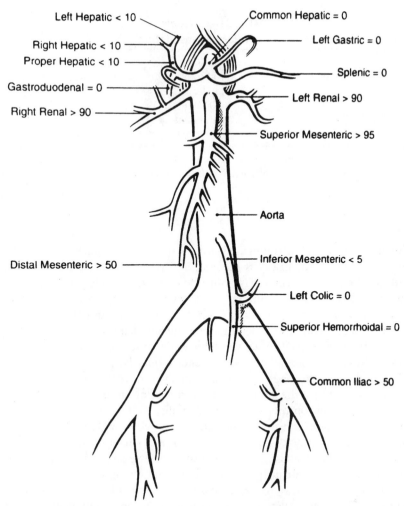

Figure 21–10. Diagram summarizing the risk of ischemia associated with the ligation of named arteries in the abdomen. (From Morris JA Jr, Eddy VA, Rutherford EJ: The trauma celiotomy: The evolving concepts of damage control. Curr Prob Surg 1996; 33(8):665.)

The concept of damage control defies the traditional view of vascular surgery that arterial reconstruction must be immediate, complete, and a high priority. It is no longer acceptable to perform a technically satisfying operation only to have the patient die as a result of physiologic exhaustion.[10] Application of this minimalist approach in the multiply injured patient is prudent and places the value of life over limb.

NURSING IMPLICATIONS

The trauma patient with a vascular injury presents a physiologic challenge. Patients often present with multiple injuries. Some present *in extremis* requiring techniques to temporize the injury until physiologic reserve is restored and definitive reconstruction can be accomplished. The nurse is integral to efforts focused on achieving the patient's best functional outcome. The principles of vascular nursing described in previous chapters apply to trauma patients; however, special considerations dictated by injury will be addressed here (Table 21–8).

TABLE 21–7. **Goals of Secondary Resuscitation**

Temperature	>36° C
Coagulation	Prothrombin time < 15 seconds
	Platelets > 75,000
Cardiovascular	SvO_2 > 65%
	Hematocrit > 35%
Acid-base	Serum lactate < 2.5 mg/dl

Data from Morris JA Jr, Eddy VA, Rutherford EJ: The trauma celiotomy: The evolving concepts of damage control. Curr Probl Surg 1996; 33(8): 612–700.
SvO_2 = venous oxygen saturation.

The initial management of trauma, regardless of injury or mechanism, is dictated by the principles of ABC. The airway is secured, and ventilation assisted, if indicated. The presence of life-threatening hemorrhage must be expeditiously identified and intervention initiated to control bleeding. A minimum of two large-bore IV lines is required for volume resuscitation. Crystalloid and blood replacement is initiated immediately in response to hemodynamic stability. Volume resuscitation may dictate that a high-volume infuser (Level I Technologies Inc.) be utilized to deliver sufficiently large quantities of fluids.

Once the ABCs have been addressed, patients should be assessed for life-threatening injuries, followed by a thorough secondary survey for less serious injuries. Dramatic injuries can quickly capture the attention of the resuscitation team; however, it is imperative that the focus remain on the ABCs over disability.

Multiple injuries require creative management strategies within the limitations of the patient's physiologic tolerance. The initial assessment, including the prehospital exam, dictates the management strategy. A complete vascular assessment includes an appraisal of the patient's neurologic exam prior to the administration of sedation or paralytics; the presence of pulses, sensation, movement, color, and temperature of the extremities and sites distal to the injury; and bilateral blood pressures. Accurate and complete documentation is crucial for future reference.

Only those tests that influence the strategic management plan should be obtained in the Emergency Department. Multiply injured patients must reach definitive care expeditiously to achieve the best clinical outcome. A CXR is mandatory for all trauma patients prior to transport out of the trauma resuscitation bay. This defines the presence of multiple rib fractures, a hemopneumothorax requiring chest tube insertion, and transmediastinal bullet trajectories. An anterior-posterior (AP) pelvic x-ray is indicated to identify complex pelvic fractures at high risk for hemorrhage or the presence of transabdominal bullet trajectories.

TABLE 21–8. **Trauma Nursing Implications**

- ABCs
- Management of patient *in extremis*
- Pain control
- Early mobility
- DVT prophylaxis
- Patient/family intervention and education
- Early initiation of discharge planning

DVT = deep venous thrombosis.

TABLE 21–9. **Management
of Patients *in Extremis***

- Hypothermia
  - Warm room to 85° F
  - Warm infused fluids to 40° C
  - Warming blankets
  - Heat and humidify ventilated air
- Coagulopathy
  - Administer blood/blood products
  - Obtain clotting studies
  - Treat hypothermia
- Cardiopulmonary management
  - Aggressive volume resuscitation
  - Sedation
  - Pulmonary care and support

By definition, patients *in extremis* are hypothermic, coagulopathic, and acidotic. Table 21–9 outlines the nursing strategies for the management of these critically ill patients. Hypothermia causes cardiac dysrhythmias, a left shift in the oxyhemoglobin dissociation curve that inhibits the release of oxygen to the tissues, and inhibition of the clotting cascade.[10] The treatment of hypothermia involves a dual strategy: preventing heat loss and providing heat gain.[10, 22] Preventing heat loss includes warming the room to greater than 85° F, the thermoneutral zone for humans, and warming infused fluids to 40° C using the Level I countercurrent warming system.[10] Providing heat gain can be accomplished with the use of conductive warming devices (Bair Hugger), applying warm blankets to the body and head, heating and humidifying air in the ventilator circuit, and warming infused solutions. Heroic measures to treat hypothermia include continuous arteriovenous or veno-venous rewarming and body cavity lavage via CT or peritoneal lavage catheters. Most patients requiring such aggressive modalities, however, cannot physiologically tolerate these interventions, or are sufficiently physiologically exhausted that the measures are of little benefit.

Coagulopathy is treated with aggressive blood and blood product replacement, including fresh frozen plasma and platelets. Patients often require massive transfusion, defined as administration of greater than 20 units of red blood cells in 24 hours.[23] It is imperative that the nurse keep up with blood losses, obtain clotting studies as indicated, and aggressively treat hypothermia.

Cardiopulmonary management to reverse lactic acidosis is accomplished by maximizing oxygen delivery and minimizing oxygen consumption. Oxygen delivery is enhanced via aggressive crystalloid and blood replacement, whereas oxygen consumption can be minimized by treating fever, shivering, and seizures. The goal is to maintain the mixed venous oxygen saturation (SvO_2) at 65–70 percent.[10] Ventilatory support is necessary, accompanied by positive end-expiratory pressure (PEEP) and pressure support.

Pain control and sedation is fundamental to recovery. Adequate pain management maintains comfort, enhances pulmonary function, reduces oxygen consumption, promotes mobility, and, following damage control techniques, prevents dislodging the temporary intraluminal shunt or evisceration of abdominal contents if the abdomen is open. Conversely, sedation can obscure the signs of impending compartment syndrome. Swelling from musculoskeletal trauma or extravascular fluid shifts further complicates the diagnosis. A high index of suspicion for patients at risk, combined with a low threshold for evaluating compartment pressures, may prevent functional limb loss.

Mobility and early intervention by the rehabilitation team (physical therapy, occupational therapy, and speech therapy for concomitant head injury) maximizes the opportunity for a functional recovery. The presence or absence of spinal fractures should be determined early so that the patient can be out of bed. While mobility may be impaired by associated orthopedic injuries or a closed head injury, even limited activity such as transfer from the bed to the chair promotes pulmonary toilet and minimizes the risk of deep venous thrombosis (DVT).

DVT prophylaxis should be instituted immediately in patients at high risk for pulmonary embolus—spinal cord injuries, pelvic and lower-extremity fractures, multiple severe injuries mandating bed rest or impaired mobility, and patients older than 50 years. Contraindications for anticoagulation or enoxaparin include severe closed head injury, coagulopathy, or a visceral organ injury at risk for hemorrhage. These patients must have a sequential compression device or, if the risk for DVT is expected to exceed 60 days, be considered for insertion of a vena caval filter.

Anticoagulation is recommended following blunt carotid injury[4] or ligation of the iliac, femoral, or popliteal veins. Compliance with warfarin therapy or follow-up prothrombin time assays is low in the trauma population; therefore, patient selection for this treatment regimen must be critically considered.

Once the goals of acute care have been achieved, the patient is ready for discharge from the hospital. Transfer to a rehabilitation setting, once acute care is completed, focuses the patient's goals and resources on functional recovery. Further, the appropriate utilization of trauma beds provides the community at large with acute care resources for future trauma patients.

CONCLUSION

Vascular trauma produces a challenging subset of patients at risk for both loss of life from hemorrhagic shock and loss of limb from ischemia. Often, vessel injury is not an isolated event, but one of a constellation of injuries requiring thoughtful consideration of treatment priorities. Diminishing physiologic reserve dictates a damage control strategy, delaying definitive reconstruction until the patient is hemodynamically stable. At the very least, all patients with a vascular injury are at risk for hemorrhagic shock and require diligent attention to the principles of Advanced Trauma Life Support.

Exemplary nursing care is fundamental to positive patient outcomes. Accurate assessment, aggressive intervention, and a high index of suspicion for potential complications impacts recovery. This chapter describes the therapeutic strategies and associated nursing implications for patients sustaining vascular trauma in hopes that loss of life and limb can be minimized and functional recovery improved.

References

1. Veise-Berry S, Beachley M: Evolution of the trauma cycle. In Cardona VD, Hurn PD, Mason PJB, et al (eds): Trauma Nursing: From Resuscitation through Rehabilitation, 2nd ed. Philadelphia, WB Saunders, 1994, pp 3–16.
2. Weigelt JA, Klein JD: Mechanism of injury. In Cardona VD, Hurn PD, Mason PJB, et al (eds): Trauma Nursing: From Resuscitation through Rehabilitation, 2nd ed. Philadelphia, WB Saunders, 1994, pp 91–113.
3. Thal ER: Injury to the neck. In Feliciano DV, Moore EE, Mattox KL (eds): Trauma, 3rd ed. Stamford, CT, Appleton & Lange, 1996, pp 329–343.
4. Fabian TC, Patton JH, Croce MA, et al: Blunt carotid injury: Importance of early diagnosis and anticoagulant therapy. Ann Surg 1996; 223(5):513–525.
5. Zelenock G, Kazmers A, Whitehouse W, et al: Extracranial internal carotid artery dissections. Arch Surg 1982; 117(4):425–432.
6. Klyachkin ML, Rohmiller M, Charash WE, et al: Penetrating injuries of the neck: Selective management evolving. Am Surg 1997; 63(2):189–194.

7. Yellin AE, Weaver FA: Vascular system. In Donovan AJ (ed): Trauma Surgery: Techniques in Thoracic, Abdominal, and Vascular Surgery. St. Louis, Mosby, 1994, pp 207–262.
8. American College of Surgeons: Advanced Trauma Life Support Course Book. Chicago, ACS, 1993.
9. Wall MJ, Granchi T, Liscum K, et al: Penetrating thoracic vascular injuries. Surg Clin North Am 1996; 76(4):749–760.
10. Morris JA Jr, Eddy VA, Rutherford EJ: The trauma celiotomy: The evolving concepts of damage control. Curr Probl Surg 1996; 33(8):612–700.
11. Hurn PD, Hartsock RL: Thoracic injuries. In Cardona VD, Hurn PD, Mason PJB, et al (eds): Trauma Nursing: From Resuscitation through Rehabilitation, 2nd ed. Philadelphia, WB Saunders, 1994, pp 466–511.
12. Feliciano DV, Burch JM, Graham JM: Abdominal vascular injury. In Feliciano DV, Moore EE, Mattox KL (eds): Trauma, 3rd ed. Stamford, CT, Appleton & Lange, 1996, pp 615–633.
13. Mullins RJ, Huckfeldt R, Trunkey DD: Abdominal vascular injuries. Surg Clin North Am 1996; 76(4):813–832.
14. Weaver FA, Papanicolaou G, Yellin AE: Difficult peripheral vascular injuries. Surg Clin North Am 1996; 76(4):843–859.
15. Frykberg ER, Crump JM, Dennis JW, et al: Nonoperative observation of clinically occult arterial injuries: A prospective evaluation. Surgery 1991; 109(1):85–96.
16. Moniz MP, Ombrellaro MP, Stevens SL, et al: Concomitant orthopedic and vascular injuries as predictors for limb loss in blunt lower extremity trauma. Am Surg 1997; 63(1):24–28.
17. Edwards, WH, Jenkins JM, Mulherin JL, et al: Extended profundoplasty to minimize pelvic and distal tissue loss. Ann Surg 1990; 211(6):694–702.
18. Aucar JA, Hirshberg A: Damage control for vascular injuries. Surg Clin North Am 1997; 77(4):853–862.
19. Rotondo MF, Schwab CW, McGonigal MD, et al: Damage control: An approach for improved survival in exsanguinating penetrating abdominal injury. J Trauma 1993; 35(3):375–383.
20. Porter JM, Ivatury RR, Nassoura ZE: Extending the horizons of "damage control" in unstable trauma patients beyond the abdomen and gastrointestinal tract. J Trauma 1997; 42(3):559–561.
21. Pourmoghadam KK, Fogler RJ, Shaftan GW: Ligation: An alternative for control of exsanguination in major vascular injuries. J Trauma 1997; 43(1):126–130.
22. Eddy VA, Morris JA Jr: Secondary resuscitation: An organ systems approach. Trauma Quarterly 1993; 10(1):71–87.
23. Phillips TF, Soulier G, Wilson RF: Outcome of massive transfusion exceeding two blood volumes in trauma and emergency surgery. J Trauma 1987; 27(8):903–910.

INDEX

Note: Page numbers in *italics* refer to illustrations; page numbers followed by t refer to tables.

Upper extremity(ies) *(Continued)*
  incisions in, 307, *307–308*
  monitoring after, 312–313
  patient education after, 313–314
  traumatic injury and, 308
  wound care after, 313
  sympathectomy in, 310–311, 311t
  thrombolectomy in, 308
bridge fistula of, 394, *395*
deep vein thrombosis in, 30
evaluation of, 88–89
vascular anatomy of, 292–293, *293*
vascular trauma to, 460, *461*
veins of, 26, 27
venous assessment of, 68–69
venous imaging of, 79
Urokinase, 149–150, 169
  for pulmonary embolism, 356
  half-life of, 170
  loading dose for, 170
  occlusion clearing with, 412
  recombinant, for lower extremity arterial ischemia, 253
  used in thrombolysis, 119
Urokinase infusion nursing protocol, 118t

— V —

VAD. See *Vascular access device (VAD).*
Vagus nerve, postoperative injury to, 283t
Valve(s), lymphatic, 34
  venous. See *Venous valve(s).*
Valvulotome, stainless steel, 148–149
  flexible, *149*
  rigid, *148*
Varicose vein(s), 69
  cause of, 31
  compression stockings for, 375
  examination of, 70–71, *71*
  formation of, estrogen in, 368
  hereditary nature of, 369
  in chronic venous disease, 367–368, *368*
  primary, 367
  sclerotherapy for, 376, 376t
    nursing interventions in, 383–384
  secondary, 367
  stripping of, 377–379, *378–379*
    complications of, 378–379
    contraindications to, 379t
    nursing interventions for, 383–384
Vascular access device (VAD), 403–413
  appropriate, selection of, 403t, 403–404
  benefits of, 403t
  blood withdrawal from, 405
  care of exit site of, 405

Vascular access device (VAD) *(Continued)*
  central catheter as, peripherally inserted, 407t, 407–408
  clamping of, 405, *406*
  complication(s) of, 410t, 410–412
    catheter fracture as, 412
    catheter pinch-off as, 412
    infection as, 411
    occlusion as, 411–412
  costs of, 404
  dressings for, 405
  flushing of, 404
  patients with, nursing management of, 412–413
  postoperative interventions for, 413
  preoperative interventions for, 412–413
  principles of, 404–405
  subcutaneous port as, 408–410, *408–410*
  tunneled catheter as, 405–407, *406*
  use of, 403t, 403–404
Vascular endoscopy, 150, *150*
Vascular prosthetic grafts, 146–147
Vascular rehabilitation, 197–208. See also *Rehabilitation, vascular.*
Vascular surgery, 131–158. See also specific surgery, e.g., *Carotid endarterectomy.*
  access for, 390–413
    devices in, 403–413. See also *Vascular access device (VAD).*
  in hemodialysis, 390–402. See also *Hemodialysis access.*
  bypass in. See *Bypass surgery.*
  endoscopy in, 150, *150*
  intraoperative nursing care in, 131–133, *132–133*, 134t–135t, *135*, 135–136
  of aorta. See *Aortic surgery.*
  prosthetic grafts in, 146–147
  thrombolytic agents in, 149–150
Vascular system. See also *Arterial system; Venous system.*
  clinical assessment of, 50–72
  diseases of, percutaneous treatment of, 100–129. See also specific procedure, e.g., *Arteriography.*
  noninvasive testing of, 74–99
    B-mode ultrasonography in, 76
    color duplex ultrasonography in, 76–77
    Doppler ultrasonography in, 74–75, *75–76*
    instrumentation in, 74–77
    plethysmography in, 77
    quality control in, 97, 99
  physical examination of, preparation for, 50–51
  resistance in, 4
Vascular trauma. See *Trauma.*
Vasospasm, in upper extremity ischemia, treatment of, 311–312

Vasospastic phenomenon, 11
Vein(s), 21–31. See also named vein, e.g., *Subclavian vein.*
  anatomy of, 21–26, 364, *365*
    congenital variations in, 24–25
    gross, *23*, 23–26
    macroscopic, *22*, 22–23
    microscopic, 21–22
  arm, in bypass surgery, *243*, 243–244
  compliance of, 27
  function of, 21
  in bypass surgery. See under *Bypass surgery.*
  in calf muscle, pumping of, 364, *366*
  neural and hormonal influences on, 28–29
  normal hemodynamics of, 27–28, *29*
  obstruction of, 29–30
  of lower extremity, 24–25, *24–26*
  of upper extremity, 26, 27
  pathophysiology of, 29–31
  perforating, ligation of, in chronic venous disease, 379–380
  physiology of, 26–29, 364–366
  prosthetic, in bypass surgery, 244
  stripping of, 377–379, *378–379*, 379t
  thrombosis of. See *Deep vein thrombosis (DVT); Thrombophlebitis, superficial.*
  varicose. See *Varicose vein(s).*
Vena cava, injury to, 456
  interruption of, for pulmonary embolism, 356–357, *357*
  indications for, 356t
Vena cava filters, percutaneous replacement of, complications of, 122–123
  indications for, 122
  nursing management for, 123
  technique of, 122, *123*
Venography, 107–109
  complications of, 109
  indications for, 107–108
  nursing management for, 109
  of chronic venous disease, ascending, 373–374, *374*
    descending, 374, *375*
  of deep vein thrombosis, 348
  technique of, *108*, 108–109
Venous access ports, 408–410, *408–410*
Venous bypass surgery, 376–377
Venous claudication, 31
Venous disease, as indication for amputation, 419
  chronic, 364–386
    ambulatory venous pressure measurements in, 371
    ascending venography in, 373–374, *374*
    calf muscle pump function in, 372

ISBN 0-7216-7657-X